SURGICAL RECONSTRUCTION *of the* FACE *and* ANTERIOR SKULL BASE

SURGICAL RECONSTRUCTION *of the* FACE *and* ANTERIOR SKULL BASE

Anthony J. Maniglia, M.D.
The Julius W. McCall Professor and Chairman
Case Western Reserve University
School of Medicine
University Hospitals of Cleveland
Cleveland, Ohio
Clinical Professor
University of Miami School of Medicine
Miami, Florida

Fred J. Stucker, M.D.
Professor and Chairman
Louisiana State University
School of Medicine in Shreveport
Shreveport, Louisiana

David W. Stepnick, M.D.
Associate Professor
Case Western Reserve University
School of Medicine
University Hospitals of Cleveland
Cleveland, Ohio

W.B. SAUNDERS COMPANY
A Division of Harcourt Brace & Company
Philadelphia London Toronto Montreal Sydney Tokyo

W.B. SAUNDERS COMPANY
A Division of Harcourt Brace & Company

The Curtis Center
Independence Square West
Philadelphia, Pennsylvania 19106

Library of Congress Cataloging-in-Publication Data

Surgical reconstruction of the face and anterior skull base / [edited by] Anthony J. Maniglia, Fred J. Stucker, David W. Stepnick.—1st ed.

p. cm.

ISBN 0–7216–6993–X

1. Face—Surgery. 2. Surgery, Plastic. I. Maniglia, Anthony J. II. Stucker, Fred J. III. Stepnick, David W. [DNLM: 1. Face—surgery. 2. Facial Bones—surgery. 3. Reconstructive Surgical Procedures—methods. WE 705 S96135 1999]

RD523.S846 1999 617.5′2059—dc21

DNLM/DLC 98–25699

SURGICAL RECONSTRUCTION OF THE FACE AND ANTERIOR SKULL BASE ISBN 0–7216–6993–X

Printed in the United States of America

Last digit is the print number: 9 8 7 6 5 4 3 2 1

To my mother, Norma, and to my late father, Benedicto. Their dedication, foresight, drive, and inspiration ensured a graduate education for their five children and a work ethic that resulted in successful careers over the years.

To my late beloved wife, Josephine, and to my son, Victor. They provided me with support and endured loneliness and lack of companionship while I was caring for my patients and developing my academic career.

Without my excellent education and degree provided by my alma mater, The School of Medicine of the University of São Paulo, Ribeirão Prêto, Brazil, I could not have accomplished my goals. My numerous teachers provided me with invaluable education and training.

I am also indebted to my patients who allowed me to care for them and provided me with the opportunity to do research and develop new knowledge. My aspirations and dreams have indeed come to fruition.

You can never repay your parents as your teachers
You can only pass on what they have given you . . .
(Talmud)

AJM

To my wife, Debbie, to whom I owe a newfound equanimity. Her wisdom and inspiration are profoundly appreciated.

To my three siblings, Thomas B. Stucker, M.D., J. Paul Stucker, M.D., and Joan E. Tobin, whose overt excellence is a constant and continuous stimulus.

Common sense is the knack of seeing things as they are,
and doing things as they ought to be done.
(C.E. Stowe)

FJS

To my wife, Paula, and to our children, Geoffrey Ryan and Elisabeth Nicole, who are a constant source of joy and inspiration.

To my mother, Mrs. William J. Stepnick, for her love and nurturing.

And in memory of my father, whose support and guidance has shaped me more than he ever had a chance to know.

DWS

CONTRIBUTORS

ROBERT F. AARSTAD, M.D.
Associate Professor and Vice-Chair, Department of Otolaryngology-Head and Neck Surgery, Louisiana State University School of Medicine in Shreveport, Shreveport, Louisiana
Cartilage Grafts in Nasal Reconstruction

GREGORY A. ANTOINE, M.D., F.A.C.S.
Assistant Professor, Case Western Reserve University School of Medicine; Chief, Craniomaxillofacial Surgery, Department of Otolaryngology-Head and Neck Surgery, MetroHealth Medical Center, Cleveland, Ohio
Complex Midface Fractures

JAMES E. ARNOLD, M.D.
Professor, Department of Otolaryngology-Head and Neck Surgery, Case Western Reserve University School of Medicine; Chief, Division of Pediatric Otolaryngology, Department of Otolaryngology-Head and Neck Surgery, Rainbow Babies and Children's Hospital, University Hospitals of Cleveland, Cleveland, Ohio
Midfacial Degloving for Nasal, Sinus, and Skull Base Lesions

TARANEH AZAR, M.D.
Resident, Department of Otolaryngology-Head and Neck Surgery, Case Western Reserve University School of Medicine; Resident, Department of Otolaryngology-Head and Neck Surgery, University Hospitals of Cleveland, Cleveland, Ohio
History of Reconstructive and Cosmetic Septorhinoplasty

NICHOLAS J. CASSISI, D.D.S., M.D.
Professor and Chairman, Department of Otolaryngology, University of Florida College of Medicine; Active Attending, Shands Teaching Hospital and Clinics, Inc., and Veterans Affairs Medical Center, Gainesville, Florida
Maxillofacial Prosthetics

FRANCISCO J. CIVANTOS, M.D.
Assistant Professor, University of Miami School of Medicine; Co-Director, Miami Center for Skull Base Surgery, Jackson Memorial Hospital and University of Miami Hospital and Clinics/Sylvester Comprehensive Cancer Center, Miami, Florida
Skeletal Reconstruction Following Extended Maxillectomy

RICHARD E. DAVIS, M.D.
Assistant Professor, Division of Facial Plastic and Reconstructive Surgery, Department of Otolaryngology, University of Miami School of Medicine; Director, Facial Plastic and Reconstructive Surgery, University of Miami Hospital and Clinics/Sylvester Comprehensive Cancer Center, Miami, Florida
Skeletal Reconstruction Following Extended Maxillectomy

PAUL C. DRAGO, M.D.
Attending Physician, Piedmont Medical Center, Private Practice, Rock Hill, South Carolina
Subtotal Nasal Reconstruction

PAUL E. GOCO, M.D.
Instructor in Surgery, Department of Surgery, Uniformed Services University of the Health Sciences, Bethesda, Maryland; Staff, Facial Plastic and Reconstructive Surgery Department, Madigan Army Medical Center, Tacoma, Washington
Evolution of the Management of Rhinophyma and Related Diseases

JEFFREY A. GOLDSTEIN, M.D., F.A.C.S.
Associate Professor of Surgery (Plastic Surgery) and Pediatrics, Case Western Reserve University School of Medicine; Chief of Plastic and Reconstructive Surgery and Medical Director, Craniofacial Center, University Hospitals of Cleveland and Rainbow Babies and Children's Hospital, Cleveland, Ohio
Treatment of Congenital Craniofacial Anomalies

GÖSTA GRONSTRÖM, M.D., D.D.S., Ph.D.
Senior Lecturer, Department of Otolaryngology, University of Gothenburg; Consultant, Ear, Nose, and Throat Clinic, Sahlgrenska University Hospital, Gothenburg, Sweden
Osseointegrated Percutaneous Titanium Implants

DENIS K. HOASJOE, M.D., F.R.C.S.(c)
Clinical Assistant Professor, Department of Otolaryngology, Louisiana State University School of Medicine in Shreveport, Shreveport, Louisiana; Private Practice, Baytown, Texas
Evolution of the Management of Rhinophyma and Related Diseases

DAVID J. HOWARD, F.R.C.S., F.R.C.S., Ed.
Senior Lecturer in Laryngology, Institute of Laryngology and Otology, University College London; Consultant, Head and Neck Surgeon, Royal National Throat, Nose, and Ear Hospital, London, UK
Management of Carcinoma of the Ethmoids, Craniofacial Resections, and Alternatives for Reconstructions

GENE HOWARD, M.D.
Associate Professor, Department of Otolaryngology, University of South Carolina School of Medicine, Charleston, South Carolina
Concepts in Orbital Reconstruction and Optic Nerve Decompression

T. IIZUKA, M.D., D.D.S., Ph.D.
Associate Professor, Craniomaxillofacial Surgery, Facial Plastic and Reconstructive Surgery, Faculty of Medicine, University of Berne; Senior Maxillofacial Surgeon and Professor, Craniomaxillofacial Surgery, Facial Plastic and Reconstructive Surgery, University Hospital of Berne, Berne, Switzerland
Reconstruction of the Midface and Fronto-orbital Region Following Tumor Resection and Trauma

KURT LÄDRACH, M.D., D.M.D.
Assistant Professor, Department of Craniomaxillofacial Surgery, University Hospital/Inselspital, Berne, Switzerland
Reconstruction of the Midface and Fronto-orbital Region Following Tumor Resection and Trauma

KIMLYN LONG, M.D.
Resident, Department of Plastic Surgery, Cleveland Clinic Foundation, Cleveland, Ohio
Cranial Bone for Midface and Skull Reconstruction

VALERIE J. LUND, M.S., F.R.C.S., F.R.C.S., Ed.
Professor of Rhinology, Institute of Laryngology and Otology, University College London; Consultant, Otorhinolaryngologist, Royal National Throat, Nose, and Ear Hospital and Moorfield's Eye Hospital, London, UK
Management of Carcinoma of the Ethmoids, Craniofacial Resections, and Alternatives for Reconstructions

ANTHONY J. MANIGLIA, M.D.
The Julius W. McCall Professor and Chairman, Department of Otolaryngology-Head and Neck Surgery, Case Western Reserve University School of Medicine; Director, Department of Otolaryngology-Head and Neck Surgery, University Hospitals of Cleveland, Cleveland, Ohio; Clinical Professor, Department of Otolaryngology, University of Miami School of Medicine, Miami, Florida
History of Reconstructive and Cosmetic Septorhinoplasty; Subtotal and Total Nasal Reconstruction—Flaps and Bone Grafts; Midfacial Degloving for Nasal, Sinus, and Skull Base Lesions; Oculoplastic Techniques for Reconstruction of Upper and Lower Eyelids; Reconstructive Surgery of the Midface for Large and Massive Defects: Cancer, Fungal Infections, Gunshot Wounds; Reconstructive Techniques of the Anterior Mandibular Arch; Simultaneous Rhinoplasty and Functional Endoscopic Sinus Surgery

JOÃO JAIRNEY MANIGLIA, M.D.
Professor of Otolaryngology, Federal University School of Medicine; Attending Physician, Hospital de Clinicas, Curitiba, Paraná, Brazil
Midfacial Degloving for Nasal, Sinus, and Skull Base Lesions; Oculoplastic Techniques for Reconstruction of Upper and Lower Eyelids;

JOSÉ VICTOR MANIGLIA, M.D.
Dean, School of Medicine, Professor and Chairman, Department of Otolaryngology-Head and Neck Surgery, State of São Paulo-Rio Prêto School of Medicine; Hospital de Base, Otolaryngology-Head and Neck Surgery, S.J. Rio Prêto, São Paulo, Brazil
Midfacial Degloving for Nasal, Sinus, and Skull Base Lesions; Oculoplastic Techniques for Reconstruction of Upper and Lower Eyelids

RICARDO FABRÍCIO MANIGLIA, M.D.
Ear, Nose, and Throat Resident, University Hospital, Medical Faculty, Federal University of Paraná State, Brazil
Oculoplastic Techniques for Reconstruction of Upper and Lower Eyelids

LAWRENCE J. MARENTETTE, M.D.
Associate Professor, Department of Otolaryngology, University of Michigan School of Medicine, Ann Arbor, Michigan
Reconstructive Surgery of the Midface for Large and Massive Defects: Cancer, Fungal Infections, Gunshot Wounds

JEFFREY S. MASIN, M.D.
Clinical Instructor, Department of Otolaryngology-Head and Neck Surgery, Case Western Reserve University School of Medicine; Attending Physician, Department of Otolaryngology-Head and Neck Surgery, MetroHealth Medical Center, Cleveland, Ohio
History of Reconstructive and Cosmetic Septorhinoplasty

FREDERICK J. MENICK, M.D.
Associate Clinical Professor, Division of Plastic Surgery, University of Arizona College of Medicine; St. Joseph's Hospital, Tucson, Arizona
Aesthetic Subunits of the Nose and Reconstructive Application

LINDSEY MORGAN-LUNDIE, M.I.M.P.T., H.N.C.
Maxillofacial Prosthetics
Maxillofacial Prosthetist, Queen Elizabeth Site, University Hospital Birmingham NHS Trust, Edgbaston, Birmingham, UK
Anaplastology and Its Application to Facial Rehabilitation

CHERIE-ANN NATHAN, M.D.
Assistant Professor, Louisiana State University School of Medicine in Shreveport; Department of Otolaryngology/Head and Neck Surgery, Louisiana State University Medical Center, Shreveport, Louisiana
Alloplasts in Facial Reconstruction

J. DAVID OSGUTHORPE, M.D.
Professor of Otolaryngology, University of South Carolina School of Medicine, Charleston, South Carolina
Concepts in Orbital Reconstruction and Optic Nerve Decompression

FRANK A. PAPAY, M.D.
Assistant Clinical Professor, Ohio State University College of Medicine, Columbus; Head, Section of Craniofacial and Pediatric Plastic Surgery, Staff, Department of Plastic and Reconstructive Surgery, Cleveland Clinic Foundation, Cleveland, Ohio
Cranial Bone for Midface and Skull Reconstruction

WILLIAM PATE, M.D.
Associate Professor in Clinical Otolaryngology, Department of Otolaryngology, Louisiana State University School of Medicine in Shreveport; Chief, Otolaryngology, Overton Brook Veterans Affairs Hospital, Shreveport, Louisiana
Alloplasts in Facial Reconstruction

DAVID A. PHILLIPS, M.D.
Former Resident Physician, Department of Otolaryngology-Head and Neck Surgery, Case Western Reserve University School of Medicine, Cleveland, Ohio; Charleston Eye and Ear Clinic, Charleston, West Virginia
Midfacial Degloving for Nasal, Sinus, and Skull Base Lesions

DAVID W. PROOPS, M.B., B.D.S., F.R.C.S.
Honorary Senior Lecturer in Otolaryngology and Paediatrics, University of Birmingham; Consultant, Otolaryngologist, Queen Elizabeth Site, University Hospital Birmingham NHS Trust, Edgbaston, Birmingham, UK
Osseointegrated Percutaneous Titanium Implants; Anaplastology and Its Application to Facial Rehabilitation

J. RAVEH, M.D., D.M.D.
Professor, Faculty of Medicine, University of Berne, Berne, Switzerland
Reconstruction of the Midface and Fronto-orbital Region Following Tumor Resection and Trauma

ALAIN SABRI, M.D.
Chief Resident, Case Western Reserve University of Medicine, University Hospitals of Cleveland, Cleveland, Ohio
Reconstructive Techniques of the Anterior Mandibular Arch

FRANK J. SCACCIA, M.D., F.A.C.S.
Attending Surgeon, Riverview Medical Center, Red Bank, New Jersey
Simultaneous Rhinoplasty and Functional Endoscopic Sinus Surgery

BARRY SHIPMAN, D.M.D.
Director, Prosthodontic and Maxillofacial Prosthetics, Associate Professor, Division of Oral and Maxillofacial Surgery, Department of Surgery, University of Miami School of Medicine, Miami, Florida
Skeletal Reconstruction Following Extended Maxillectomy

ROBERT C. SPRECHER, M.D.
Assistant Professor, Department of Otolaryngology-Head and Neck Surgery, Case Western Reserve University School of Medicine; Attending Physician, Division of Pediatric Otolaryngology, Department of Otolaryngology-Head and Neck Surgery, Rainbow Babies and Children's Hospital, University Hospitals of Cleveland, Cleveland, Ohio
Midfacial Degloving for Nasal, Sinus, and Skull Base Lesions

DAVID W. STEPNICK, M.D.
Associate Professor, Department of Otolaryngology-Head and Neck Surgery, Case Western Reserve University School of Medicine; Director, Residency Training Program in Otolaryngology-Head and Neck Surgery, University Hospitals of Cleveland, Cleveland, Ohio
History of Reconstructive and Cosmetic Septorhinoplasty; Midfacial Degloving for Nasal, Sinus, and Skull Base Lesions; Free Flap Reconstruction Techniques of the Skull Base; Reconstructive Surgery of the Midface for Large and Massive Defects; Cancer, Fungal Infections, Gunshot Wounds; Reconstructive Techniques of the Anterior Mandibular Arch; Reconstructive Techniques for Defects After Resection of Carcinoma of the Lip; Simultaneous Rhinoplasty and Functional Endoscopic Sinus Surgery

FRED J. STUCKER, M.D.
Professor and Chairman, Department of Otolaryngology-Head and Neck Surgery, Louisiana State University School of Medicine in Shreveport, Shreveport, Louisiana
Cartilage Grafts in Nasal Reconstruction; Subtotal Nasal Reconstruction; Evolution of the Management of Rhinophyma and Related Disease; Facial Soft Tissue Defects and Nasal Deformities in the Pediatric Patient; Alloplasts in Facial Reconstruction

ANDERS TJELLSTRÖM, M.D., Ph.D.
Associate Professor, Department of Otolaryngology, University of Gothenburg; Sahlgrenska University Hospital, Gothenburg, Sweden
Osseointegrated Percutaneous Titanium Implants

GLENN E. TURNER, D.M.D., M.S.D.
Associate Professor, Department of Prosthodontics, University of Florida College of Dentistry; Active Staff, Shands Teaching Hospital and Clinics, Inc., and Veterans Affairs Medical Center, Gainesville, Florida
Maxillofacial Prosthetics

MICHAEL J. WAKE, M.B., C.L.B., B.D.S., F.D.S.R.C.S.
Consultant, Oral and Maxillofacial Surgeon, Queen Elizabeth Site, University Hospital Birmingham NHS Trust, Edgbaston, Birmingham, UK
Anaplastology and Its Application to Facial Rehabilitation

STEVEN WORROLLO, M.I.M.P.T.
Maxillofacial Prosthetist and Laboratory Manager, Queen Elizabeth Site, University Hospital Birmingham NHS Trust, Edgbaston, Birmingham, UK
Anaplastology and Its Application to Facial Rehabilitation

JAMES E. ZINS, M.D.
Chairman, Department of Plastic Surgery, The Cleveland Clinic Foundation, Cleveland, Ohio
Cranial Bone for Midface and Skull Reconstruction

PREFACE

Life is short, art is long, occasion fleeting . . .
(Hippocrates, 460–370, BC.)

The goal of the physician and surgeon is to follow the best pathway that leads to preservation of form and function, restoration of health, and ideally happy outcome. In this pursuit, *Surgical Reconstruction of the Face and Anterior Skull Base* addresses the importance of the anatomic landmarks of the head and neck; pertinent physiologic principles; focused areas of pathology; and issues related to current management of some specific traumatic, infectious, neoplastic, and congenital diseases involving this area. Often, appropriate procedures cause deformities that may be treated by a variety of surgical techniques or by anaplastology or prosthodontic prostheses. One must always act in the best interest of the patient, however, in order to achieve good results. The outcomes and complications should be carefully considered along with alternative modalities of treatment.

About 3000 years ago in ancient India, Shushruta stated, *Only the union of medicine and surgery constitutes the complete doctor. The doctor who lacks knowledge of one of these branches is like a bird with only one wing.* Indeed, this statement has stood the test of time and is very valid even today.

A cadre of illustrious international contributors allowed this textbook to come to fruition. This multidisciplinary group of authors has made significant contributions in the difficult area of head and neck medicine and surgery. The editors are grateful for their time and effort to produce such excellent chapters. We hope that this work will become a valuable resource for physicians, surgeons, and others in the specialties of otolaryngology–head and neck surgery, general plastic surgery, oral–maxillofacial surgery, neurosurgery, ophthalmology, and anaplastology.

There are many ways to achieve similar results in medicine and surgery. Our approach represents our viewpoints and experiences that helped result in the compilation of this work. Medicine and surgery are always in evolution and progress. The history of surgery, especially as it relates to the contribution of our predecessors in the area of reconstructive and plastic procedures of the head and neck, is very rich. *We have seen so far because we have stood on the shoulders of giants,* as Sir Isaac Newton stated.

AJM
FJS
DWS

ACKNOWLEDGMENTS

My deepest appreciation and gratitude go to more than 130 residents, more than 2000 medical students, and more than 50 national and international fellows. They provided me with the inspiration, challenge, and opportunity to transmit knowledge and afford excellent quality of patient care in an academic setting. During my teaching, I have always had the opportunity to learn from them. The nurses, staff, and clerical personnel also contributed a great deal. My faculty co-workers and colleagues provided the necessary contribution for world-class achievements and cross-fertilization of ideas.

AJM

The editors are grateful to Stephanie Smith Donley for her assistance in bringing this textbook to press. We appreciate her continued diligence and expert editorial advice as we worked together with our contributing authors.

AJM
FJS
DWS

CONTENTS

The Color Plates are part of the Frontmatter

COLOR PLATES

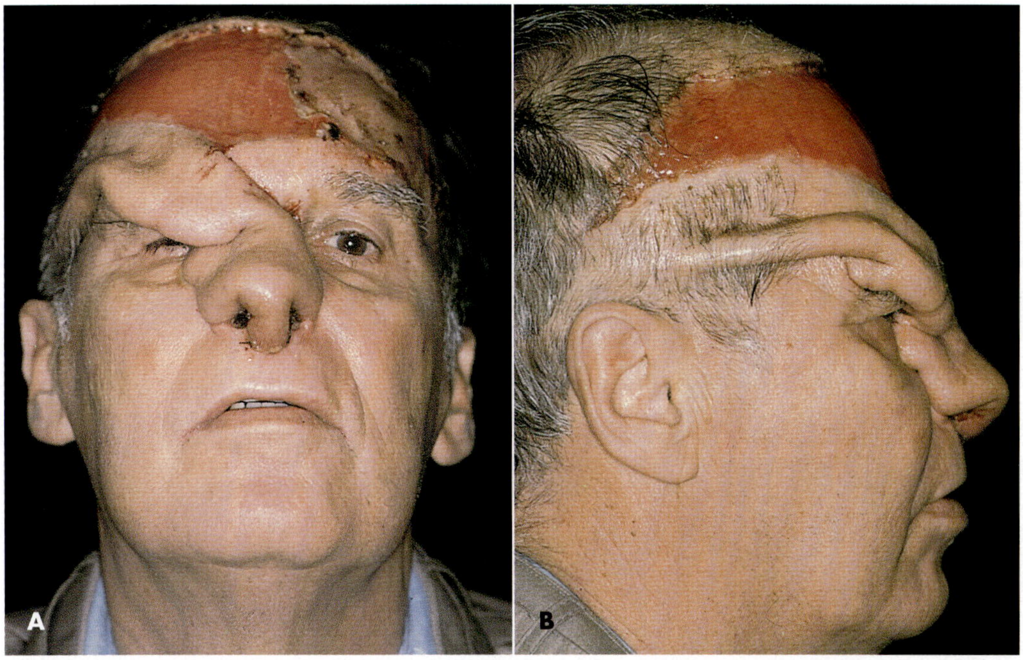

Figure 5–12. *A* and *B*, Front-basal and lateral views of the patient 3 weeks postoperatively. The full-thickness skin graft of the supraclavicular area was a total success.

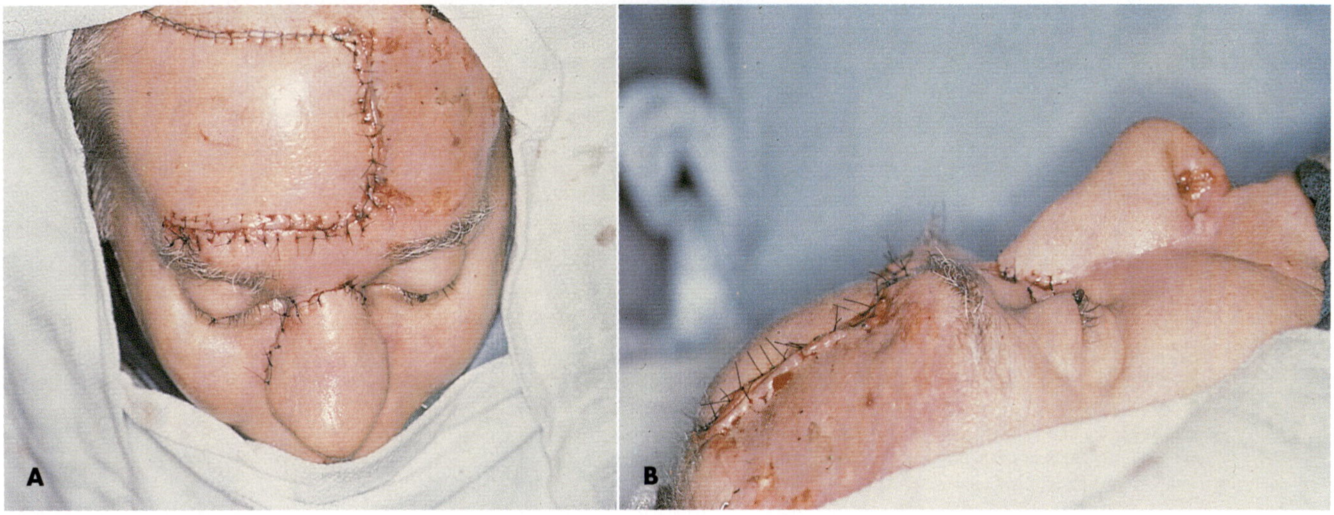

Figure 5–15. *A* and *B*, Front and lateral surgical views taken right after the forehead flap was divided and tailored and the proximal end returned to the donor site.

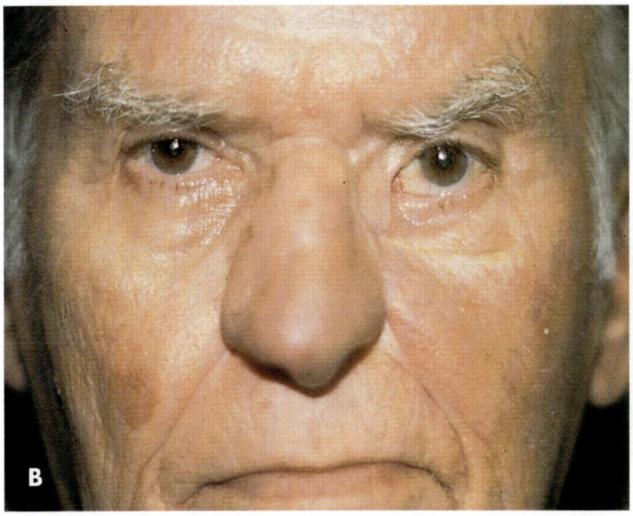

Figure 5–24. *B*, Front view of the patient 10 years after the initial resection. He has no evidence of disease. No additional refinement procedures were performed on this patient because of lack of desire on his part.

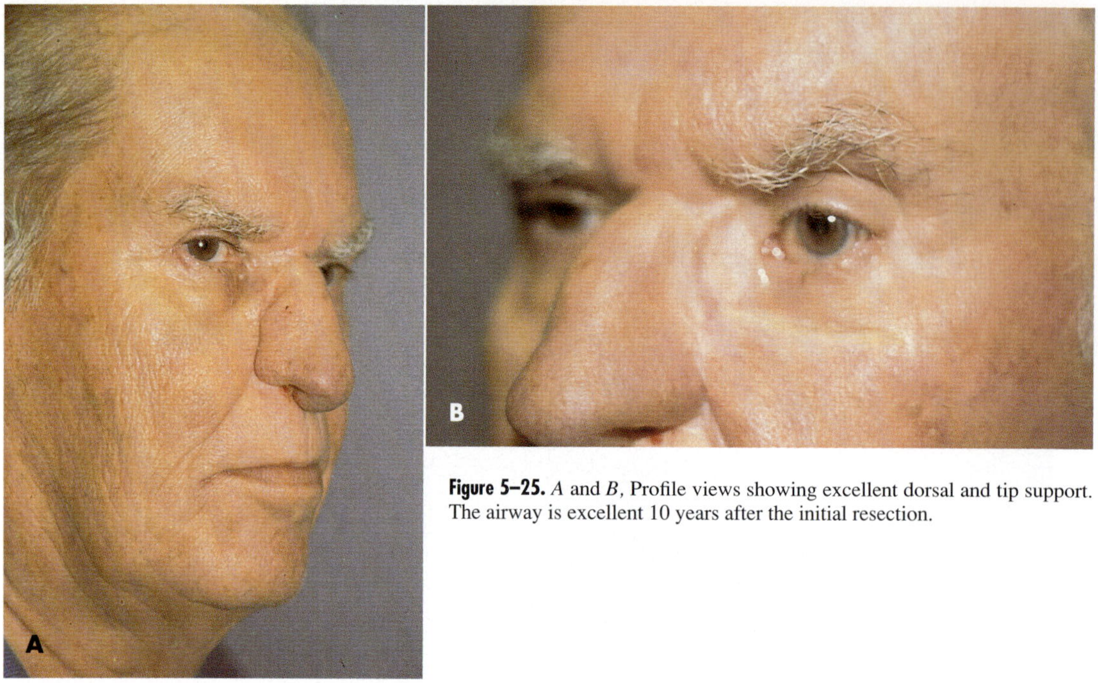

Figure 5–25. *A* and *B*, Profile views showing excellent dorsal and tip support. The airway is excellent 10 years after the initial resection.

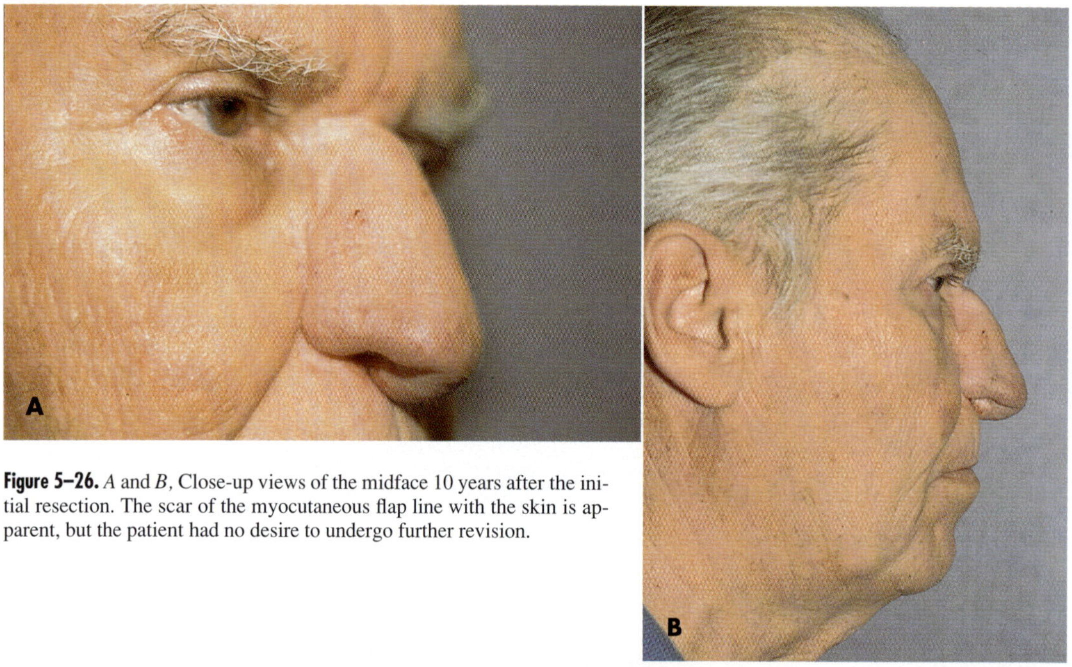

Figure 5–26. *A* and *B*, Close-up views of the midface 10 years after the initial resection. The scar of the myocutaneous flap line with the skin is apparent, but the patient had no desire to undergo further revision.

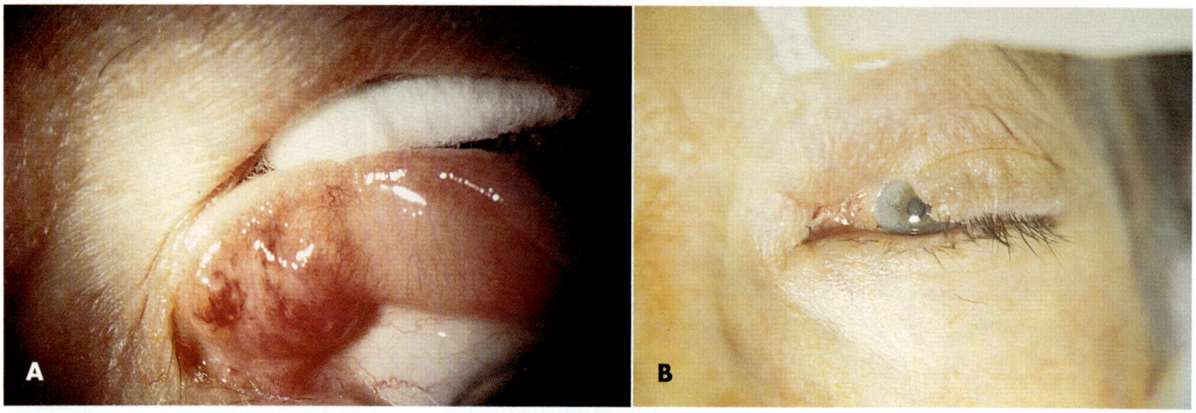

Figure 8–23. *A*, Preoperative view of upper lid tumor. *B*, Tissue defect after tumor-free margins were obtained.

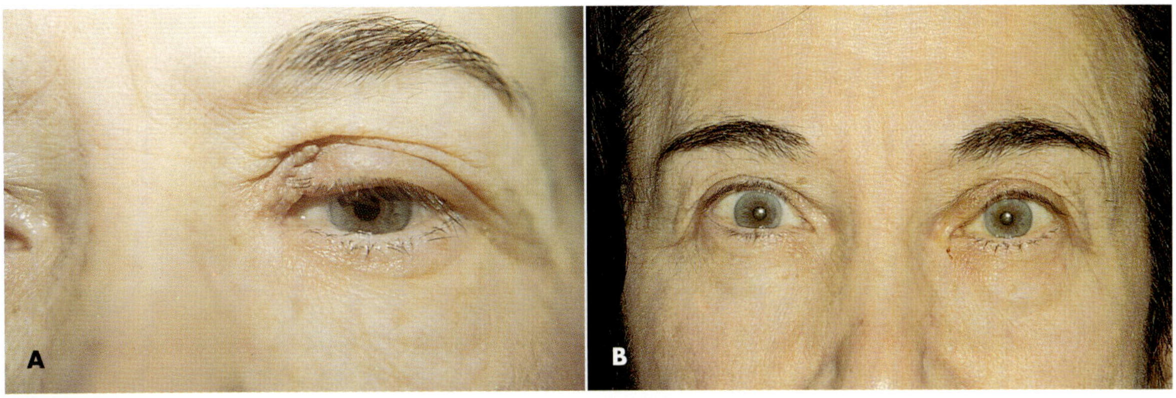

Figure 8–24. *A,* After reconstruction, which consisted of the following: Lid was everted, and tarsus was divided horizontally. Flap of tarsus and conjunctiva was mobilized inferomedially to the defect and sutured to the lid margin and the medial canthus. *B,* Reconstructed eyelid showing symmetrical extent of lashes, excellent function, and good contour.

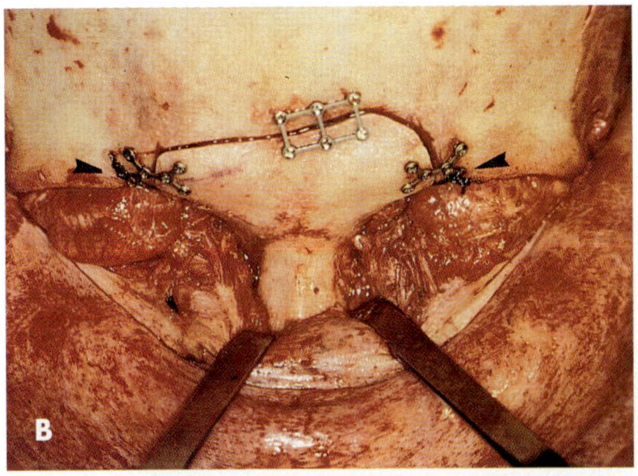

Figure 10–2. Replacement of the osteomized segment and canthal ligament fixation. *B,* Repositioned frontonasal segment fixed with titanium microplates (Leibinger). Arrows show the thread fixed to the contralateral side, which allows not only medial adjustment of the canthal ligaments but also adjustment in an inward posterior direction.

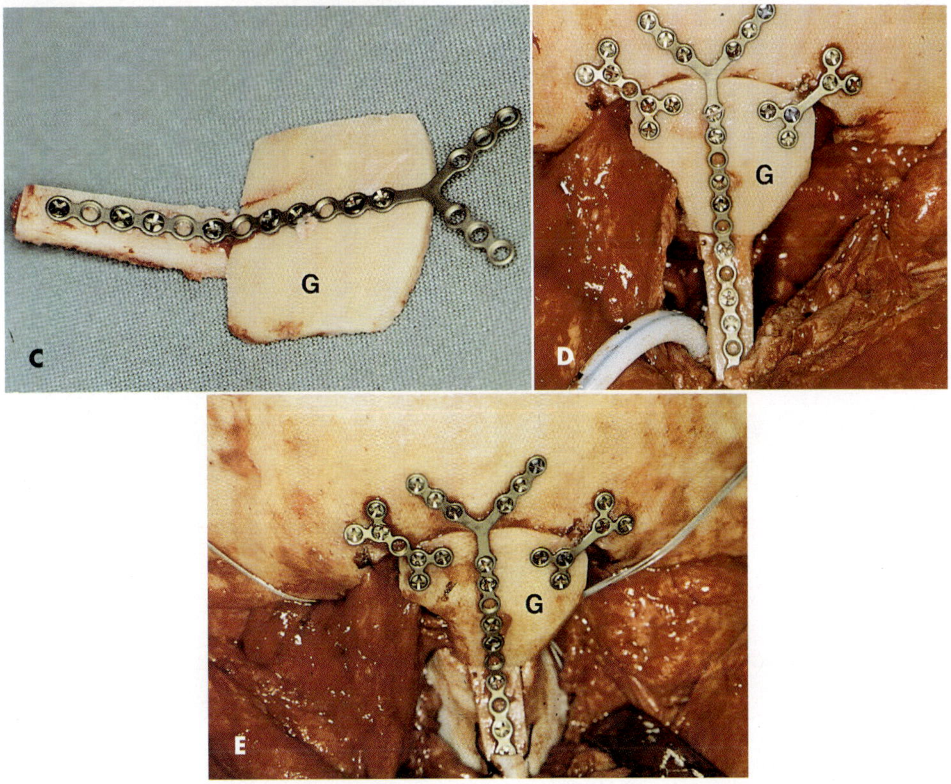

Figure 10–3. Reconstruction following loss of the fronto-orbital segment. *C* and *D,* Calvarial external table grafts (G) fixed to the newly designed miniplate (Leibinger), contoured previous to the resection. *E,* Adjusted frontonasal frame and lateral walls (G). The threads for the canthal ligament fixation are not yet fixed to the frontal bone.

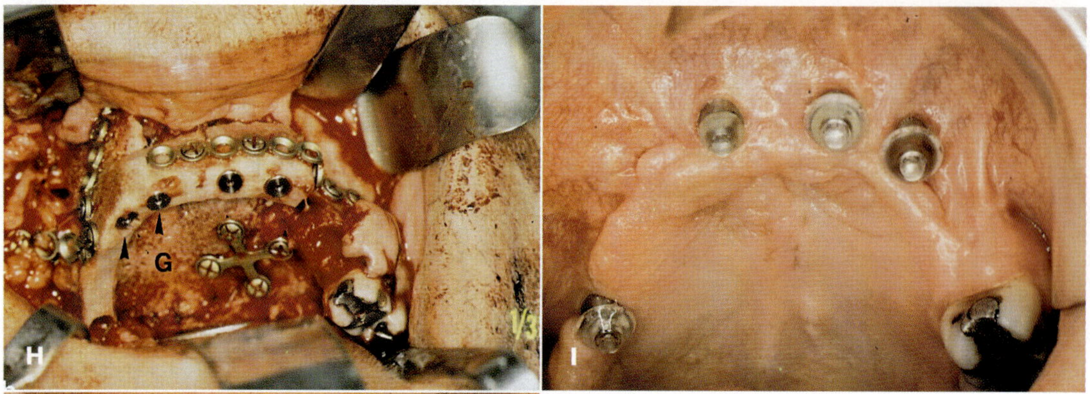

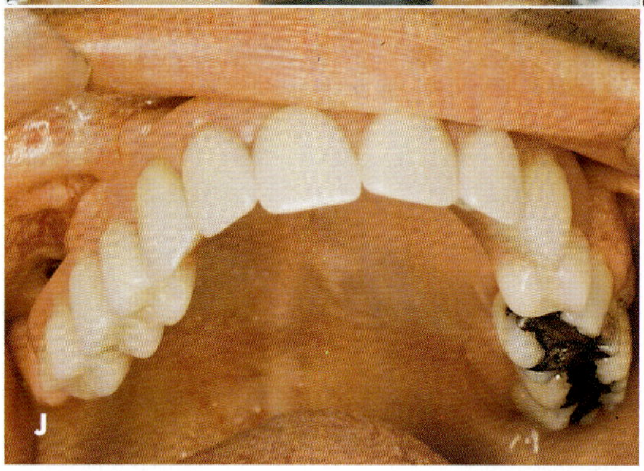

Figure 10–4. *H,* Intraoperative view illustrating fixation of the graft and dental implants *(arrows). I* and *J,* The exposed dental implants—consolidation of the local mucosal flaps and the definitive denture.

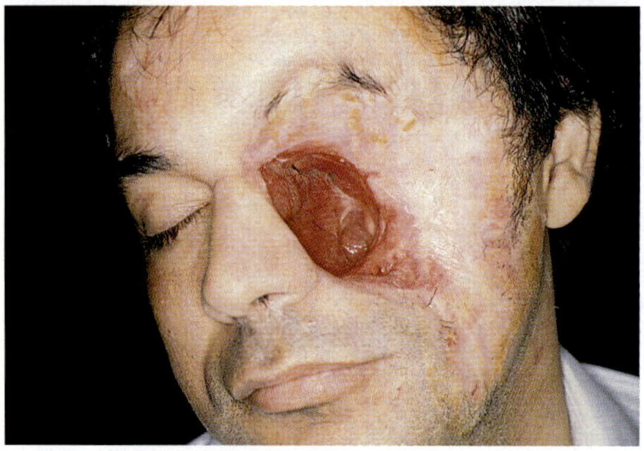

Figure 13–5. Close-up view of healed defect after 1 year. The sphenoid sinus cavity is also visible.

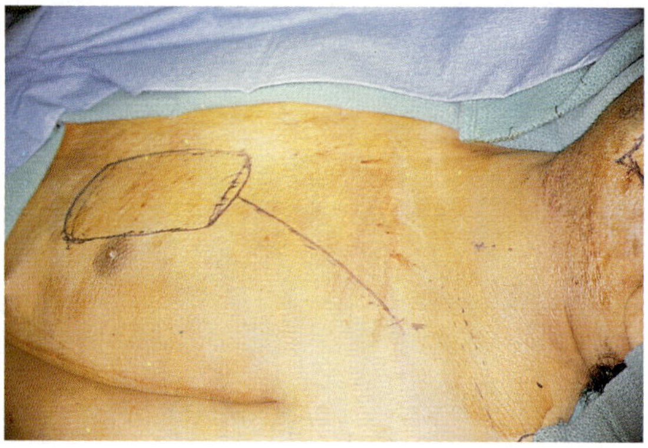

Figure 13–6. Views of the chest wall showing an outline of the pectoralis major flap (PMF).

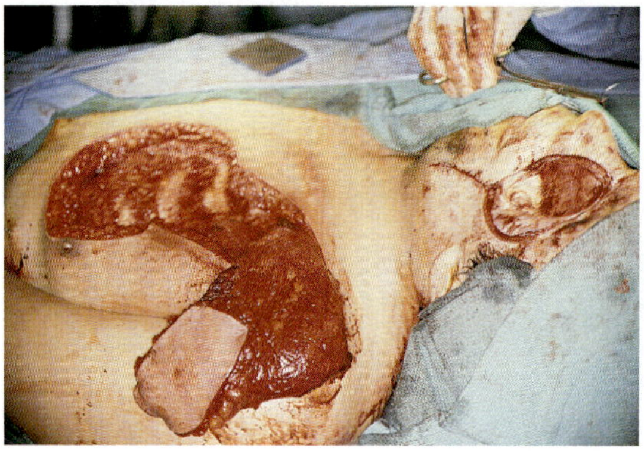

Figure 13–7. The PMF is dissected and elevated, ready for trimming and transfer.

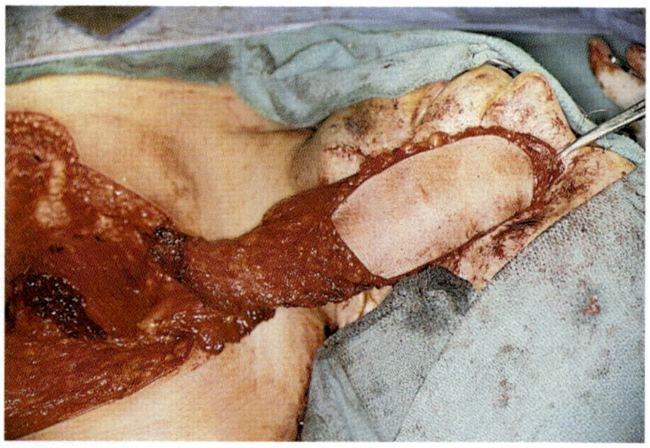

Figure 13–8. The PMF is trimmed and tried for size on the defect.

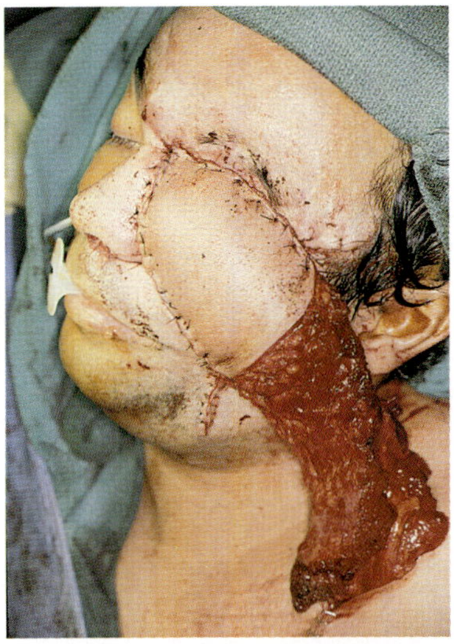

Figure 13–10. The PMF sutured in place to reconstruct the defect. The pedicle is externally placed.

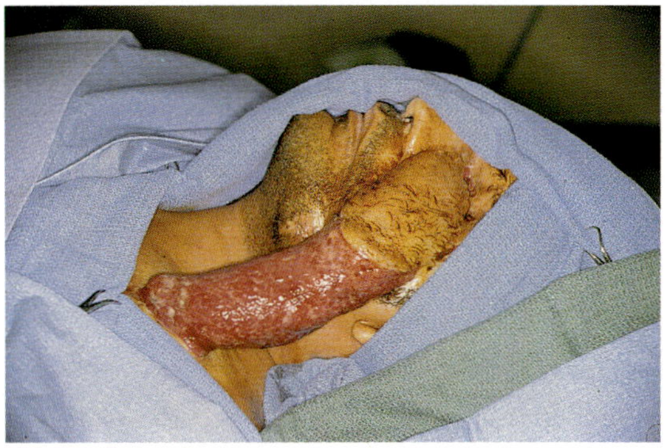

Figure 13–11. Three weeks after transfer of the PMF, the pedicle is constricted with a large Penrose drain. There is a good autonomic blood supply on the face derived from blood vessels from local tissues.

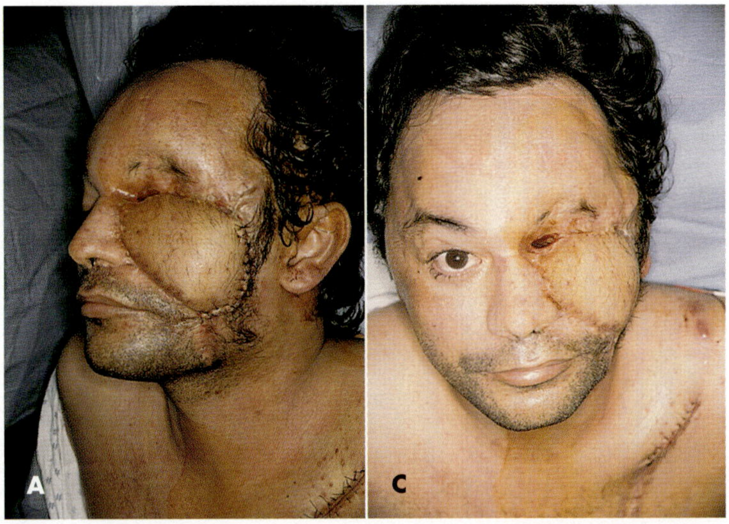

Figure 13–12. *A*, Profile view 3 weeks after the pedicle was severed. A small defect still exists at the junction of the frontal bone and the tip of the PMF. *C*, Frontal view.

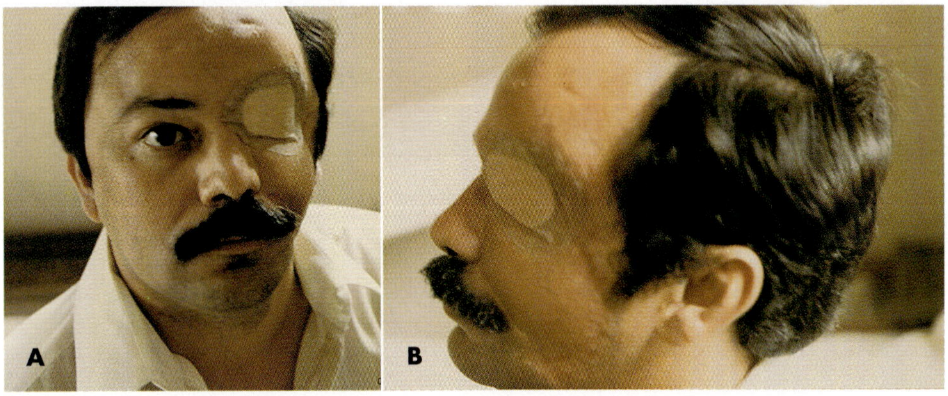

Figure 13–13. *A*, Frontal view 1 year postoperatively showing good bulk and color matching of the flap. *B*, Lateral view.

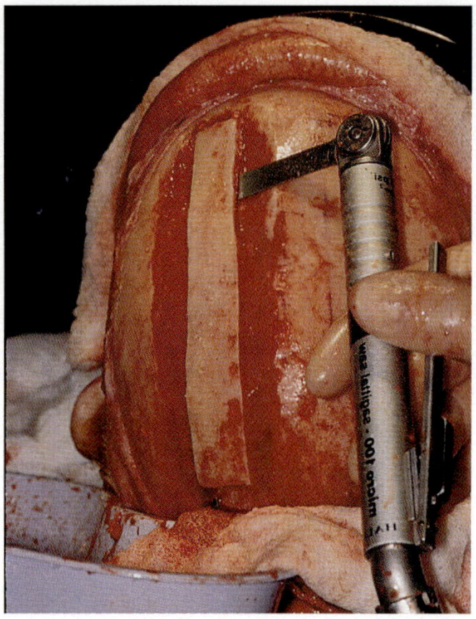

Figure 14–4. Use of the oscillating saw to harvest calvarial bone from the outer table. Note how the peripheral saucerization of the donor site facilitates blade angulation.

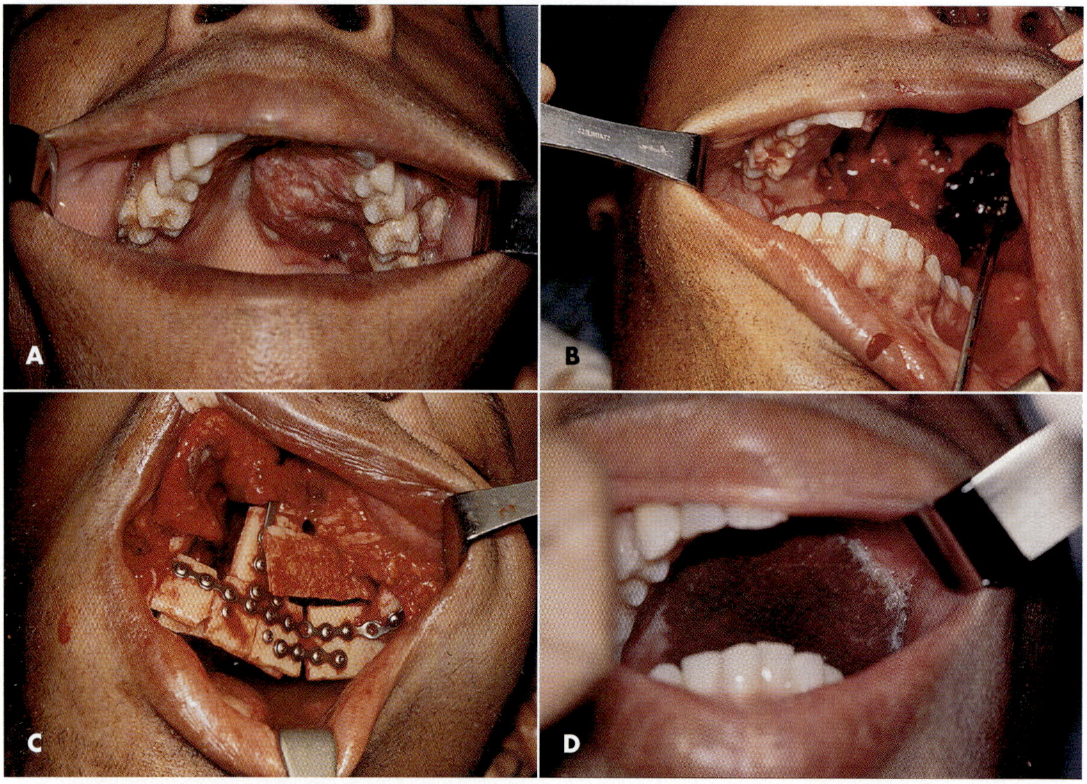

Figure 14–7. *A*, Presenting lesion. *B*, Surgical defect with preservation of the contralateral alveolus. *C*, Surgical defect following reconstruction with autologous calvarial bone grafts. *D*, Palatal contour 4 months following radiotherapy.

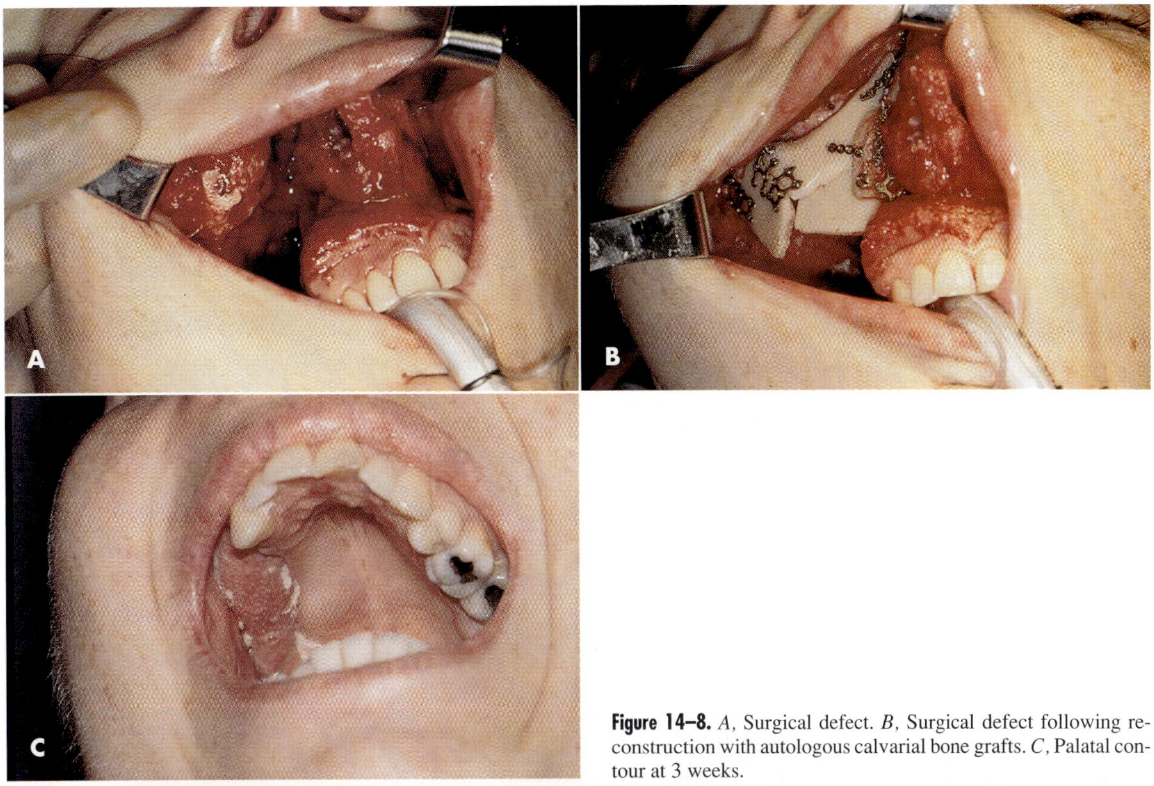

Figure 14–8. *A*, Surgical defect. *B*, Surgical defect following reconstruction with autologous calvarial bone grafts. *C*, Palatal contour at 3 weeks.

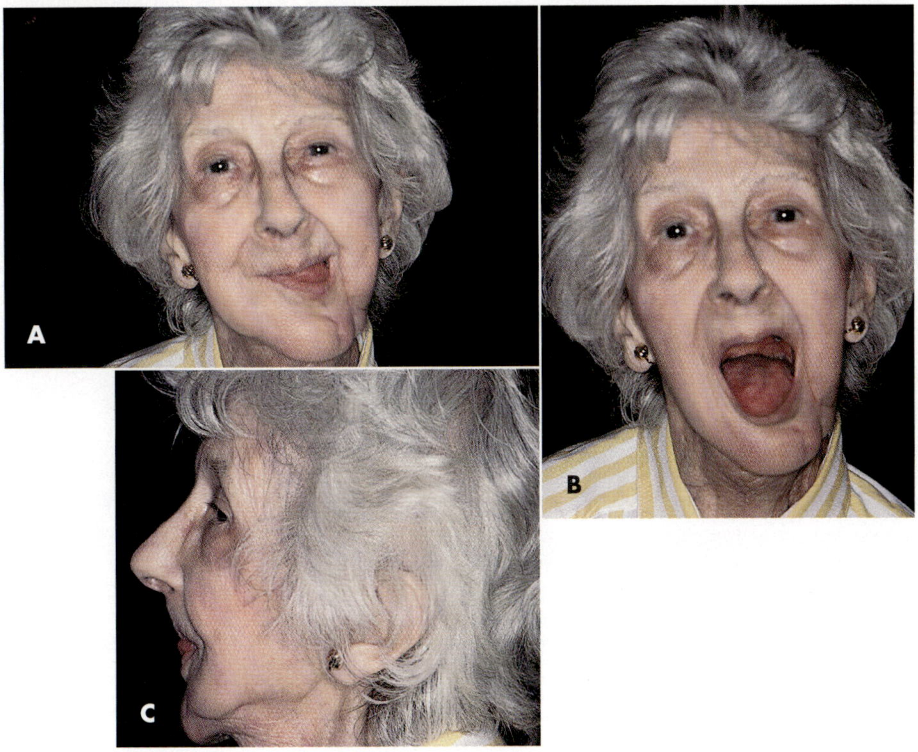

Figure 16–6. This patient underwent anterior mandibulectomy and trapezius-scapular spine mandibular reconstruction in 1987. Although she has a reasonable profile *(A)* and retains the ability to open her mouth and move her tongue *(B)*, the frontal view *(C)* shows the typical appearance of such a patient in whom external fixation was used to secure relatively thin, oddly shaped bone fragments. This technique is primarily of historical interest because better techniques are available today.

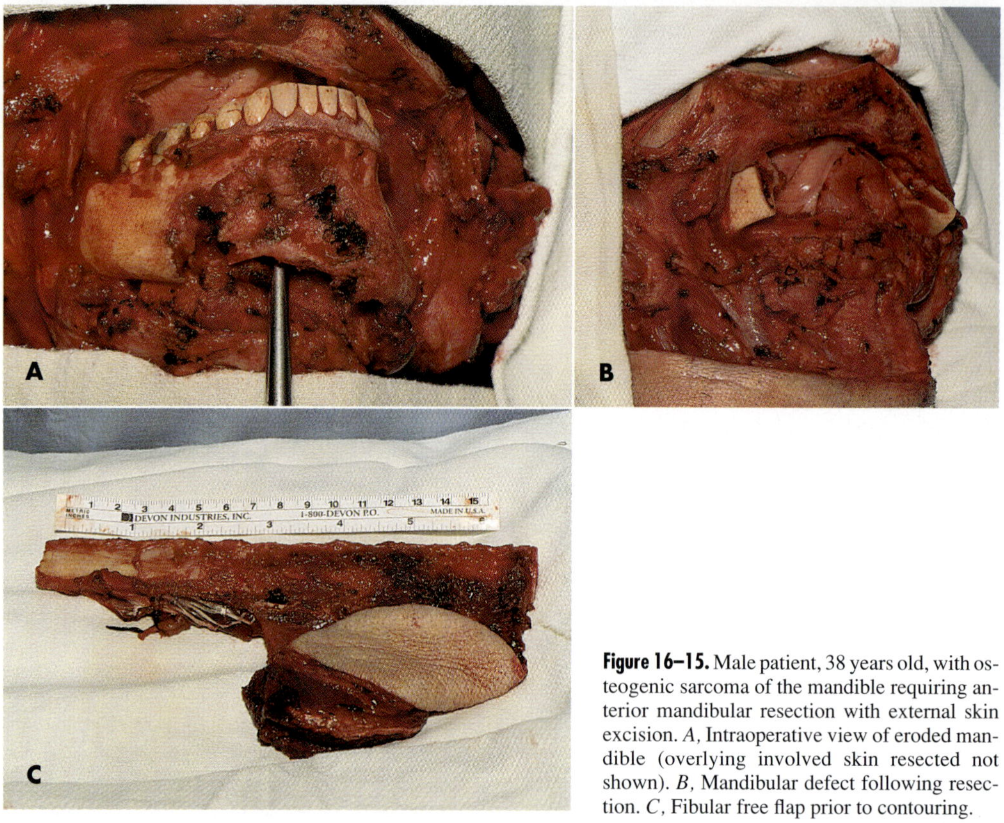

Figure 16–15. Male patient, 38 years old, with osteogenic sarcoma of the mandible requiring anterior mandibular resection with external skin excision. *A*, Intraoperative view of eroded mandible (overlying involved skin resected not shown). *B*, Mandibular defect following resection. *C*, Fibular free flap prior to contouring.

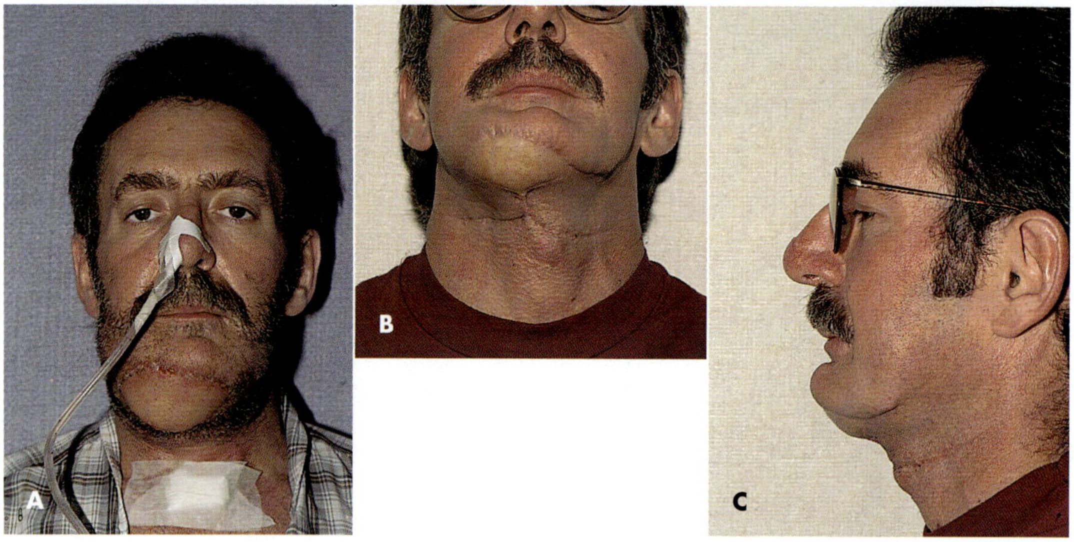

Figure 16–16. *A*, Early postoperative view. *B*, Frontal view, *C*, Lateral view showing excellent cosmetic results coinciding with similarly good functional results.

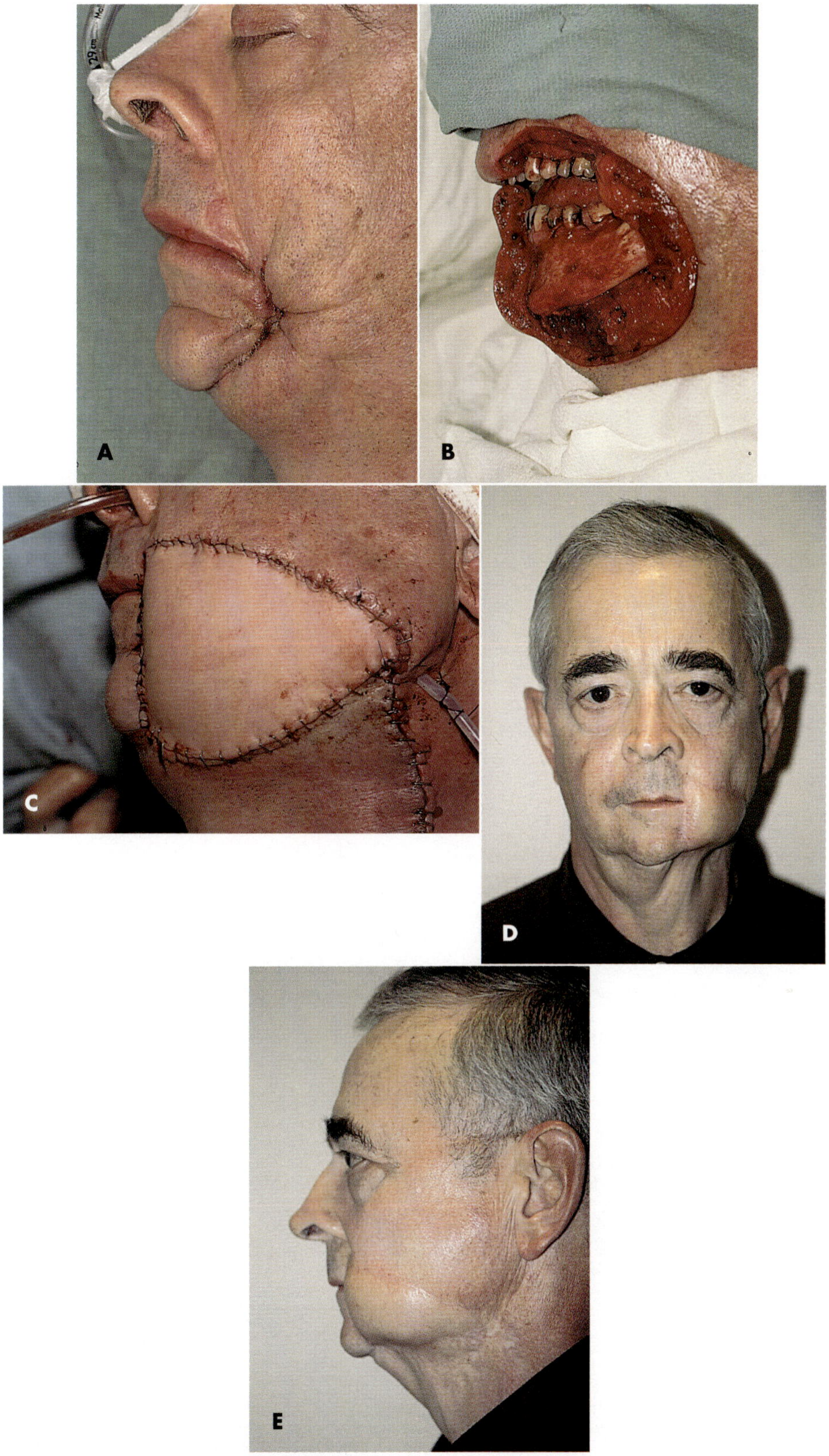

Figure 17–16. *A,* Preoperative view of patient showing retraction and skin changes as a result of carcinoma in the commissure region. *B,* Intraoperative view, following excision after clear margins were obtained. *C,* Intraoperative view of scapular free flap in position. Note that the flap has been turned in on itself to create an epithelial lining inside the mouth as well. The intervening segment, now attached to the remaining lip, has been deepithelialized. *D* and *E,* Postoperative views, following radiation and eventual secondary revision, 36 months later. The patient is now free of disease at 4 years.

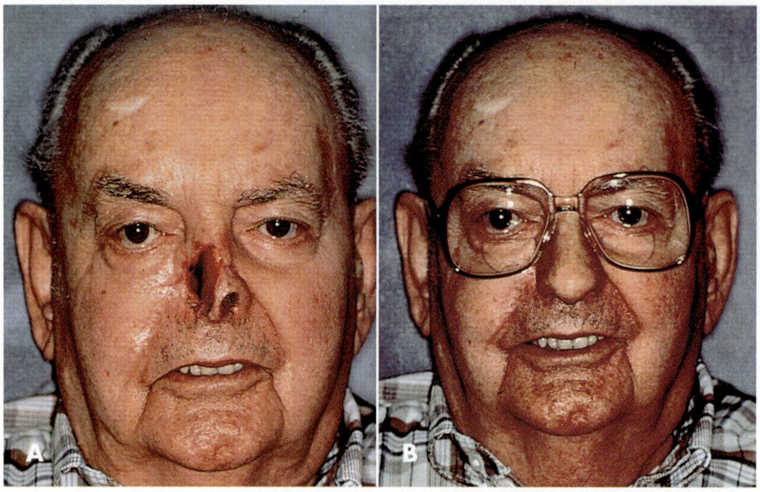

Figure 19–1. Partial rhinectomy. *A,* Nasal defect. *B,* Full face with prosthesis and eyeglasses in place.

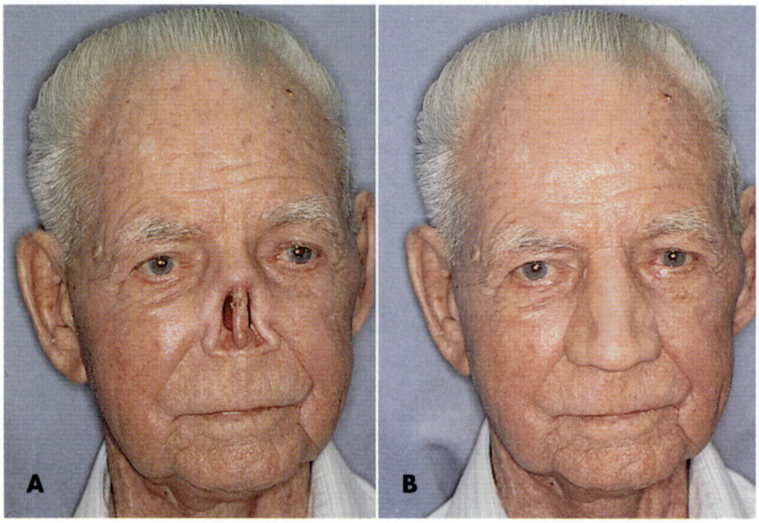

Figure 19–2. Rhinectomy with alae and nasal septum remaining. *A,* Full face showing defect. *B,* Prosthesis is too wide.

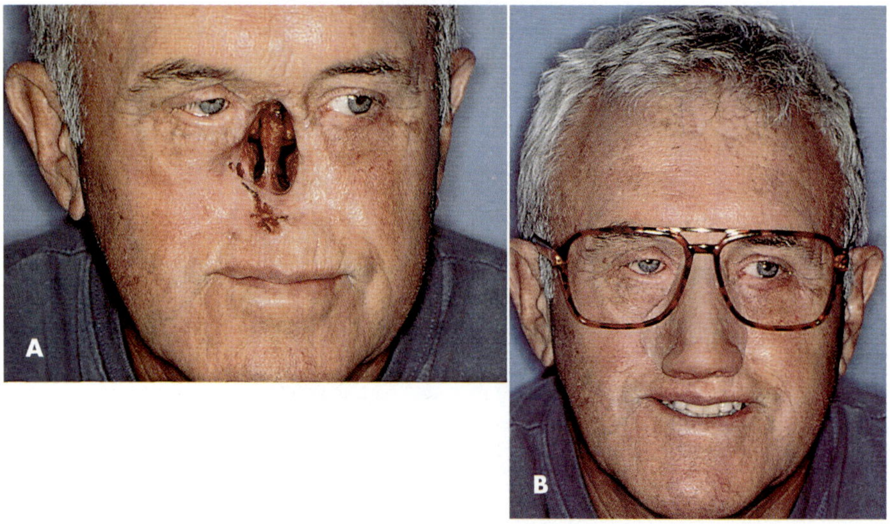

Figure 19–3. Good tissue base. *A,* Full face showing the defect. *B,* Prosthesis in place with eyeglasses.

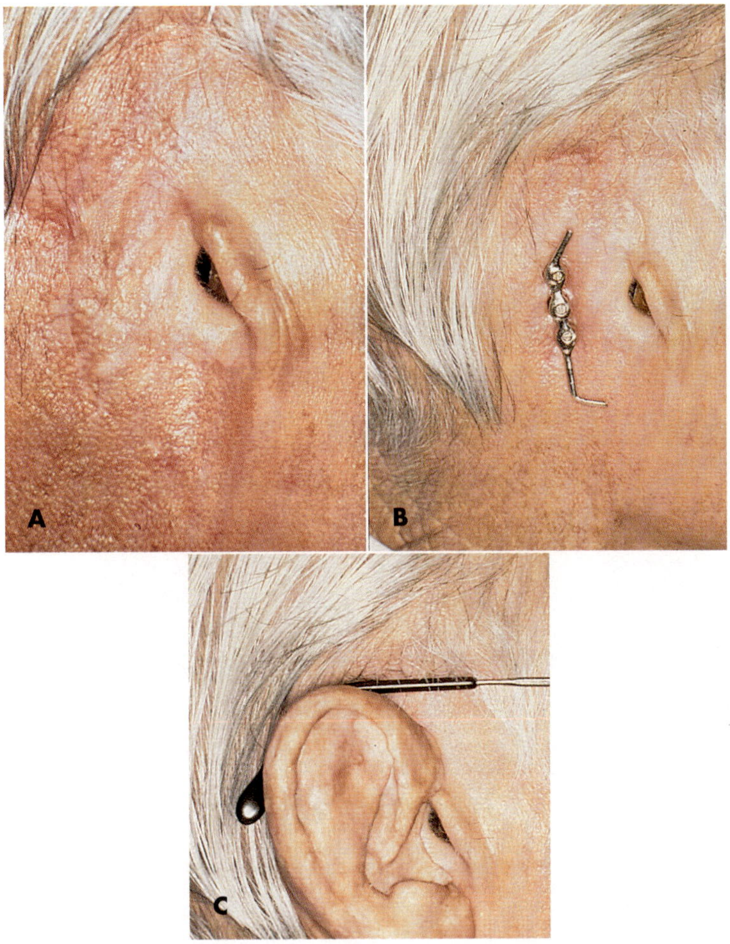

Figure 19–10. Excellent result following auriculectomy with a skin graft. *A*, Skin graft and tragus; radiation therapy port stopped at the level of the external auditory meatus. *B*, Implants and gold bar. *C*, Prosthesis clipped in place.

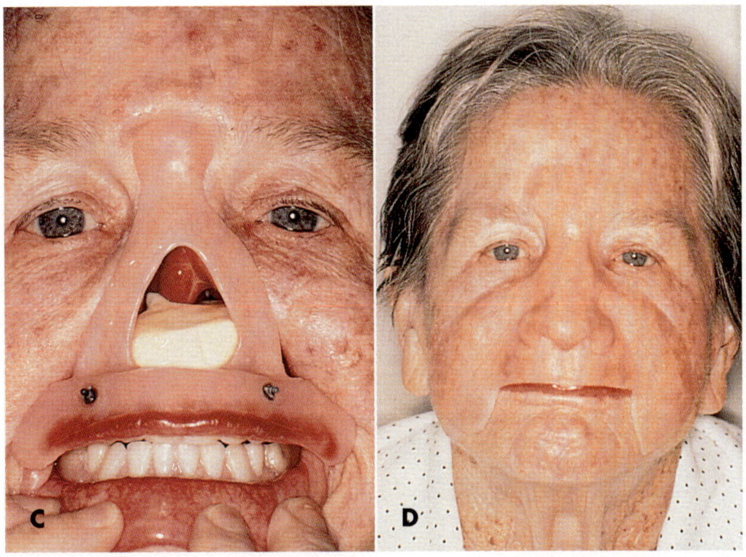

Figure 19–12. Bilateral maxillectomy, rhinectomy, and removal of the upper lip. *C*, Obturator in the patient's mouth; note the two horizontal projections and upper lip in acrylic to support the silicone facial prosthesis. *D*, All prostheses in place.

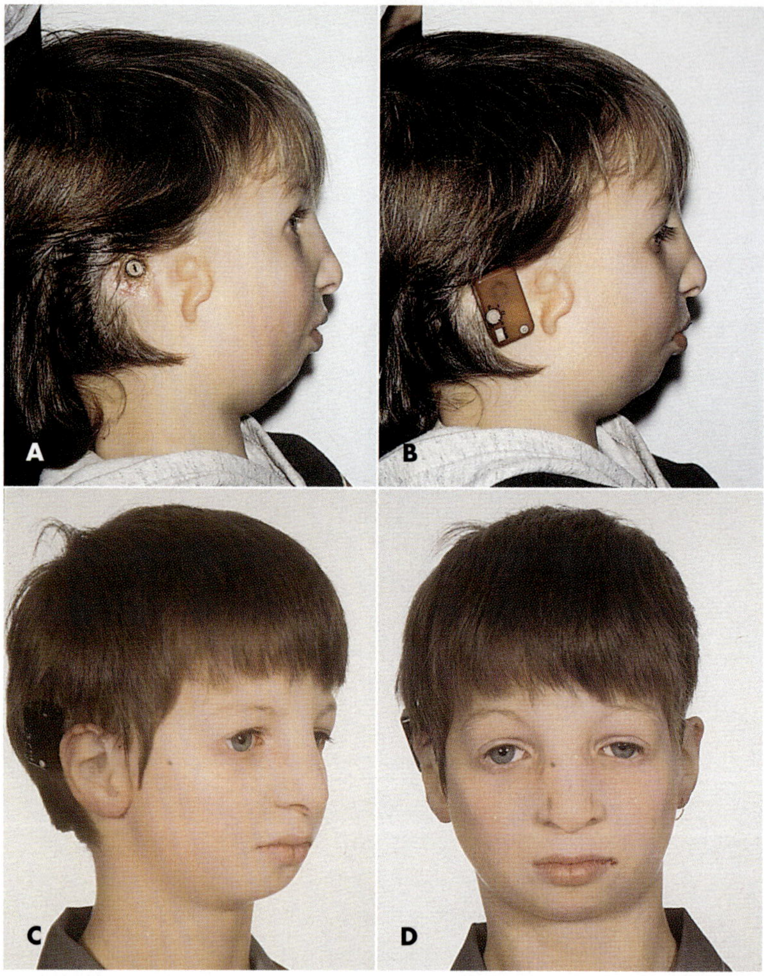

Figure 20–2. Case 2: Treacher Collins syndrome. *A*, Bone-anchored abutment. *B*, Bone-anchored hearing aid. *C*, Auricular prosthesis and bone-anchored hearing aid. *D*, Full-face view of bilateral auricular prosthesis.

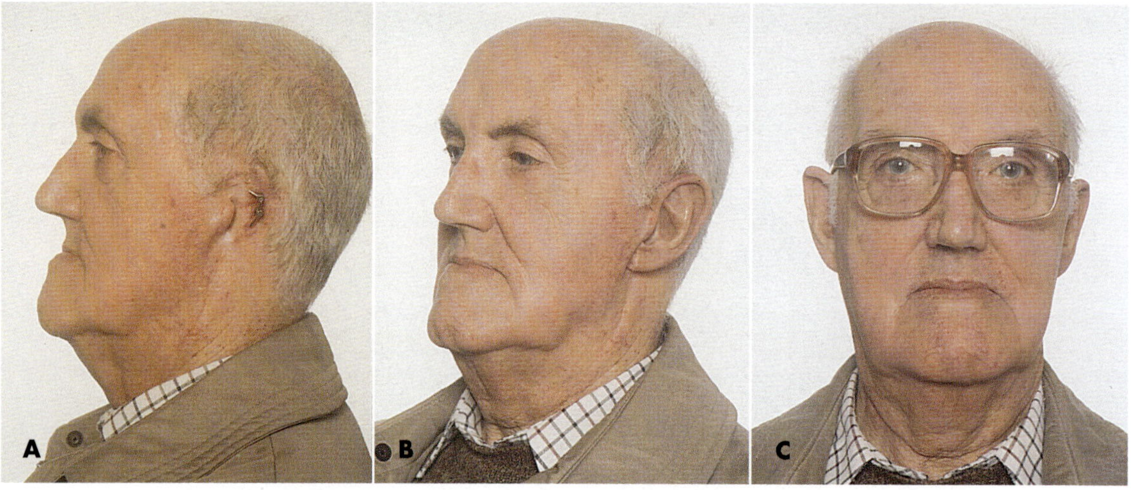

Figure 20–4. Case 4: Single-stage auricular replacement following a nonirradiated pinnectomy. *A*, Fixtures and bar following single-stage osseointegration procedure. *B*, Auricular prosthesis in place. *C*, Full-face view of prosthesis supporting spectacles.

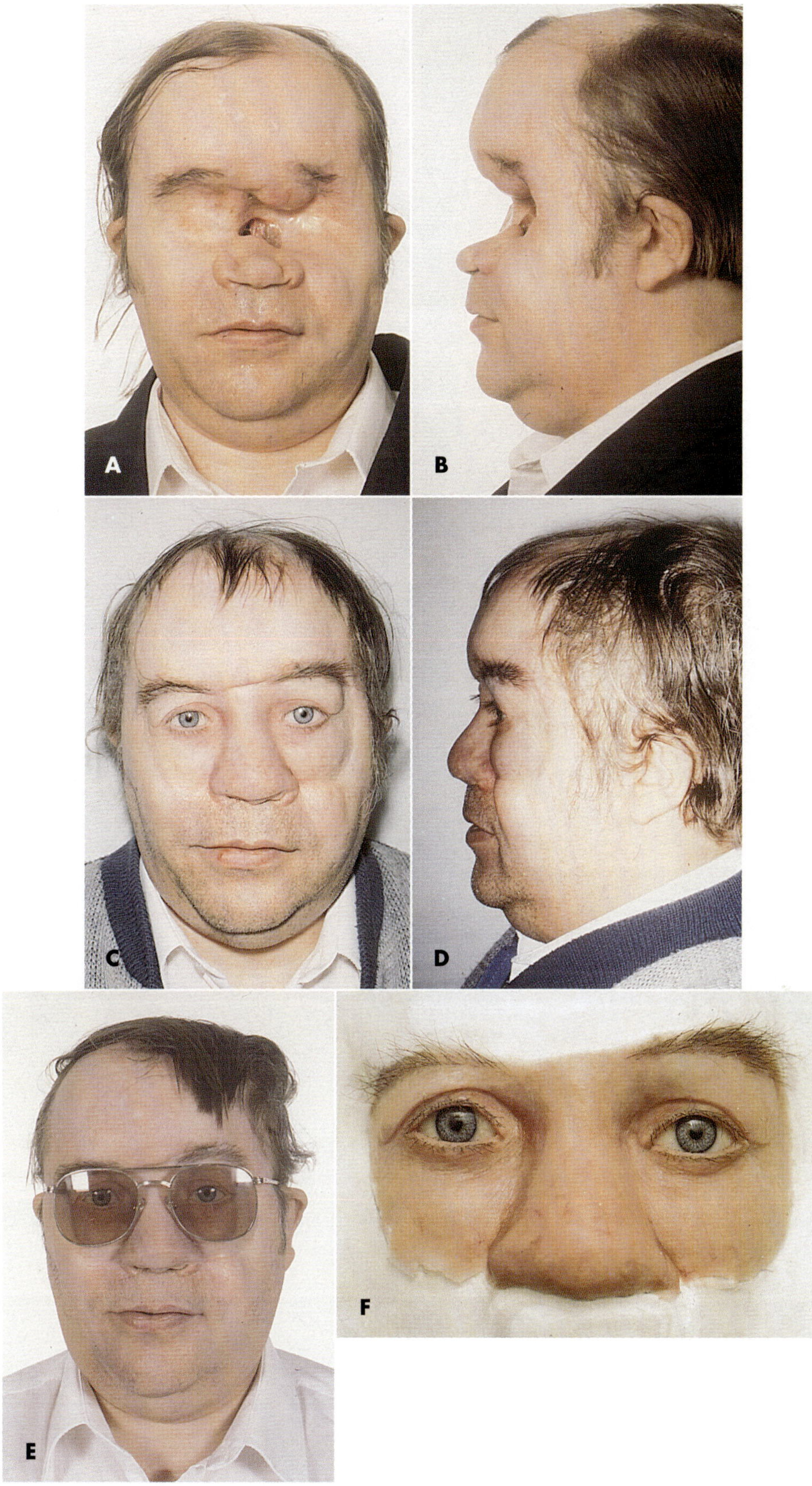

Figure 20–6. Case 6: Bilateral orbital and nasal loss due to gunshot wound. *A*, Preoperative frontal view. *B*, Preoperative lateral view. *C*, Postoperative frontal view. *D*, Postoperative lateral view. *E*, Postoperative view with spectacles. *F*, Midface prosthesis.

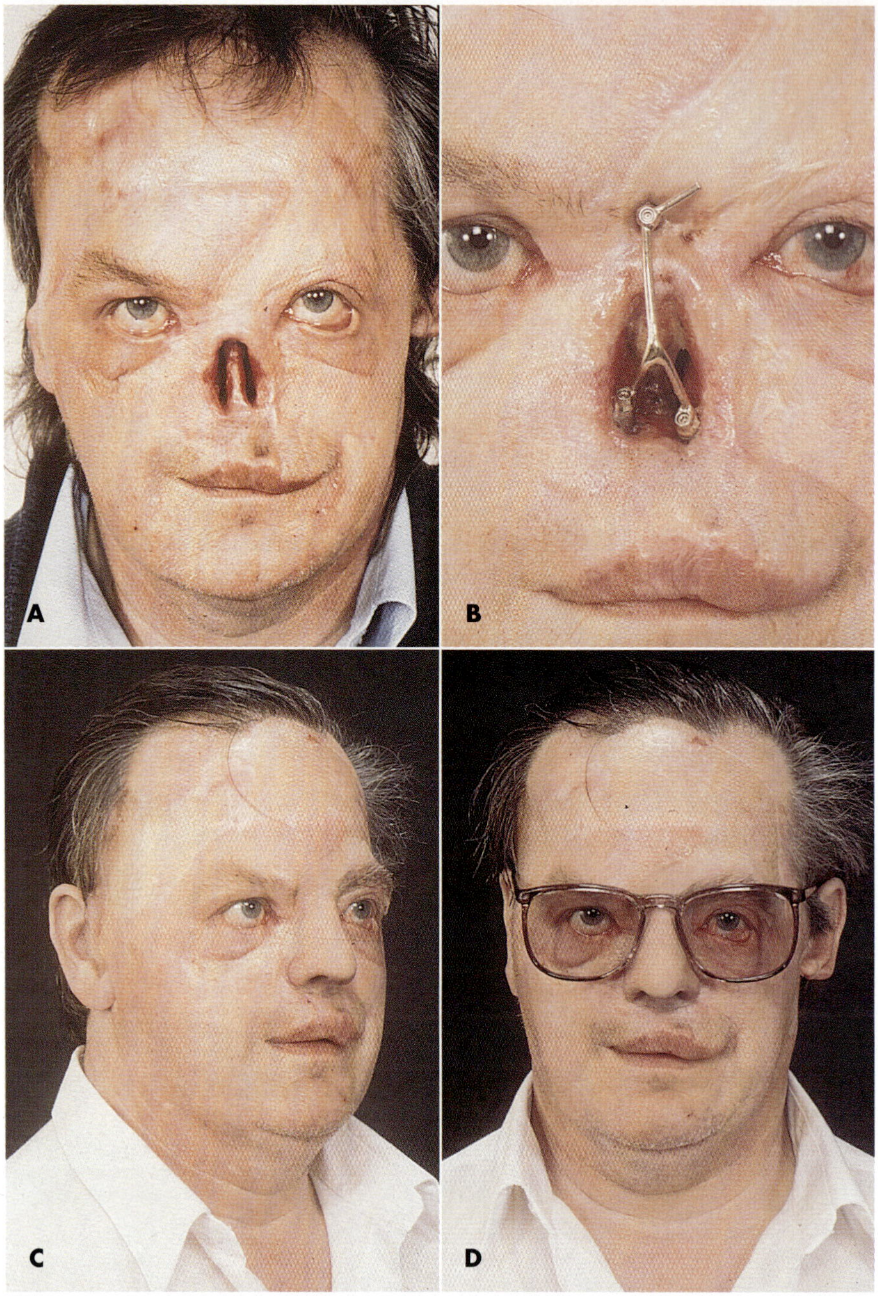

Figure 20–9. Case 9: Facial injuries due to dog attack. *A*, View of patient several weeks following injury and completion of plastic surgery procedures. *B*, Three-point fixation and bar for nasal prosthesis. *C*, Patient filled with right auricular and nasal left brow prosthesis. *D*, Full-face view. Spectacles disguise the scars and margins of the nasal prosthesis.

CHAPTER 1

History of Reconstructive and Cosmetic Septorhinoplasty

Anthony J. Maniglia, M.D.,
Taraneh Azar, M.D.,
Jeffrey S. Masin, M.D.,
David W. Stepnick, M.D.

ANCIENT INDIAN, ROMAN, AND MEDIEVAL PERIODS

The nose, the most prominent anatomic structure of the face, has always taken a beating on the battlefield and in peace due to injuries and disease. The first plastic surgery operations on the nose were performed to recreate noses that had been amputated or badly damaged. In ancient India, nasal amputation was a common punishment for adulterers and thieves. As early as 600 BC, the *Sushruta Samhita* described nasal reconstruction using cheek flaps.[1] This classic text also described the midline forehead flap, which is still known as the Indian flap. This reconstructive technique was employed by the Koomas caste, potters by trade, to reconstruct missing noses.

These techniques were apparently known to the Romans around the first century AD. At that time, Rome was a medical center where tissue transplantation techniques as described by the Indians were practiced. In the first century AD Celsus wrote *De Medicina*, which described tissue transplantation.[2] Galen, writing in the second century AD, described techniques used to repair defects of the nose, ears, and mouth.[3] His descriptions were considered authoritative, although many of them were unscientific and incorrect. Nevertheless, because his influence was so great, these writings contributed to the lack of advancement of medical science for many centuries. After the fall of the western Roman Empire (476 AD), very little, if any, medical or surgical progress occurred for centuries. Rome was ransacked by barbarians from the east, and much of the art and science accumulated by the Romans was destroyed. In the thirteenth century, Pope Innocent III forbade the performance of any surgical procedures. During the Middle Ages, physicians stopped performing surgery because it was considered manual labor and thus beneath them. It was not until the Renaissance, during the fifteenth and sixteenth centuries, that the art of nasal reconstruction was described and again practiced in Europe.

THE RENAISSANCE

Pietro Ranzano (1420–1492), the Bishop of Lucera, Sicily, mentioned in the eighth volume of his *Annals of the World* that Gustavo Branca and his son Antonio, from Catania, Sicily, had reintroduced the Indian method of nasal reconstruction to Europe in 1442.[4] They initially used cheek and forehead flaps to reconstruct noses; however, Antonio later began using skin from the medial aspect of the arm to avoid the additional scarring of the face that resulted when skin was harvested from the forehead. This technique of using medial forearm skin was then passed either directly from the Brancas or from their students to other groups of surgeons by word of mouth. In 1456, Bartolomeo Fazio (about 1400–1457) described the Brancas' technique in a pamphlet, *De Viris Illustribus*, but his work was not published for three centuries. Alessandro Benedetti (about 1445–1525), a professor of anatomy and surgery at Padua University, was the first to describe the Brancas' technique in a published article, *Anatomia, sive Historia Corporis Humani (Anatomy, Or the History of the Human Body)*, in 1502. The raw surfaces of the medial forearm were placed on the nose, and the arm was bound to the face until the flap was revascularized by the facial vessels; then the pedicle was cut, and the nose was shaped. Later, around 1549, two brothers in southern Italy, Pietro and Paolo Vivaneo, barber surgeons in Tropea, Calabria, became known for using the pedicled arm flap.[5] However, the person who is usually given credit for developing the "Italian" forearm flap method of nasal reconstruction is Gaspare Tagliacozzi.

Gaspare Tagliacozzi (1544–1599), who was a professor of anatomy and medicine at the University of Bologna, described this method of nasal reconstruction nearly 100 years after Benedetti had written about it in 1502. Tagliacozzi's book, *De Curtorum Chirurgia per Insitionem, Libri Duo; Additis Cutis Traducis Instrumentorum Omnium atque Deligationum Iconibus et Tabulis*,[6] was published in Venice in 1597 after 10 years of preparation. Tagliacozzi personally supervised all the illustrative plates and each step of the publication process (Figs. 1–1 to 1–4). He was later criticized for not giving credit to surgeons who had used similar surgical techniques before him.

Tagliacozzi was born into a family of silk merchants. He began medical school in Bologna at age 19 and became an instructor of anatomy by age 23. Dedicating his short career to reconstructive surgery of the nose, lips, and ears, he refined the methods practiced by the Brancas and Vivaneos and transformed surgical work into an art form that was accepted at the academic level. His work was known around Europe but was regarded by many as unnecessary. He was chastised most severely for reconstructing noses by those who used silver or gold prostheses. The famous Fabrizio, professor of anatomy and surgery at Padua, was among his strongest opponents.[7] Ambroise Paré and Gabriele Falloppio also condemned his method.

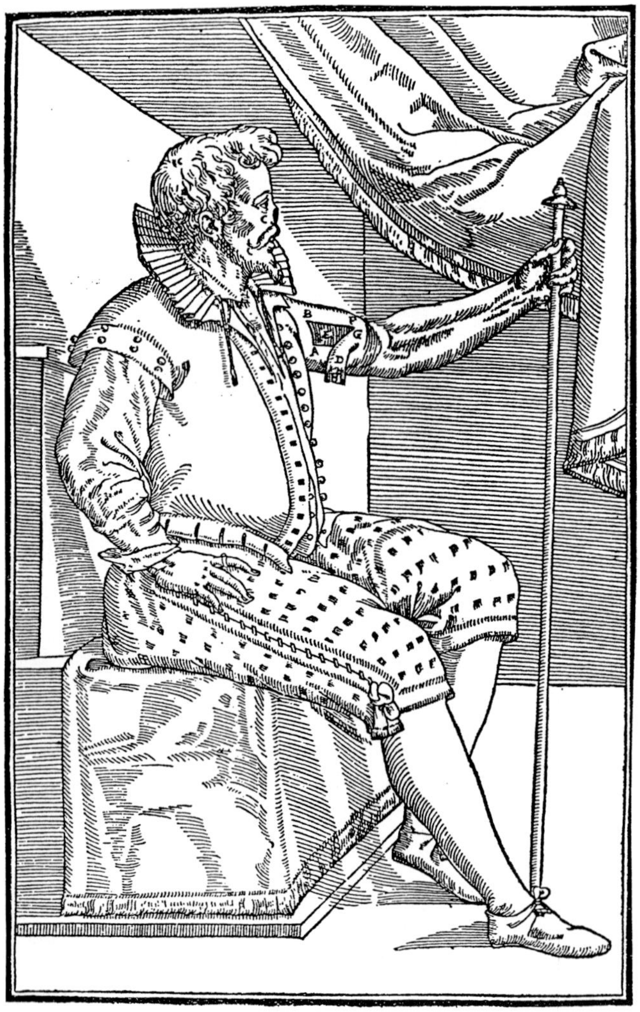

FIGURE 1–1. Creation of the medial forearm flap as depicted by G. Tagliacozzi in his book, De Curtorum Chirurgia (1597). (From Gnudi MT, Webster JP: The Life and Times of Gaspare Tagliacozzi, Surgeon of Bologna, 1545–1599. New York, Reichner, 1950.)

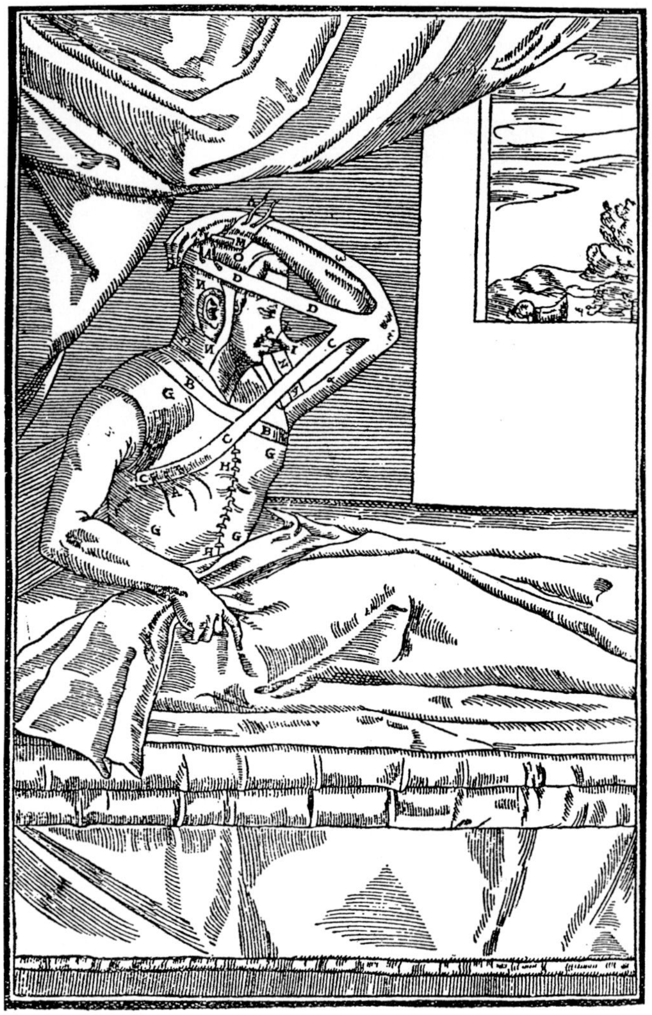

FIGURE 1–2. The arm bound to the face to allow revascularization of the skin flap by the facial vessels in Tagliacozzi's technique. (From Gnudi MT, Webster JP: The Life and Times of Gaspare Tagliacozzi, Surgeon of Bologna, 1545–1599. New York, Reichner, 1950.)

During the late sixteenth century, deformities were considered the will of God, and therefore attempts to reconstruct them were thought to be heresy. The theologians of the time attributed Tagliacozzi's success to intervention from the "evil one," and accordingly, he was persecuted for his work while he was alive. Tagliacozzi died in November 1599 and was buried according to his wishes in the church of San Giovanni, a chapel in a convent in Bologna. Rumors were

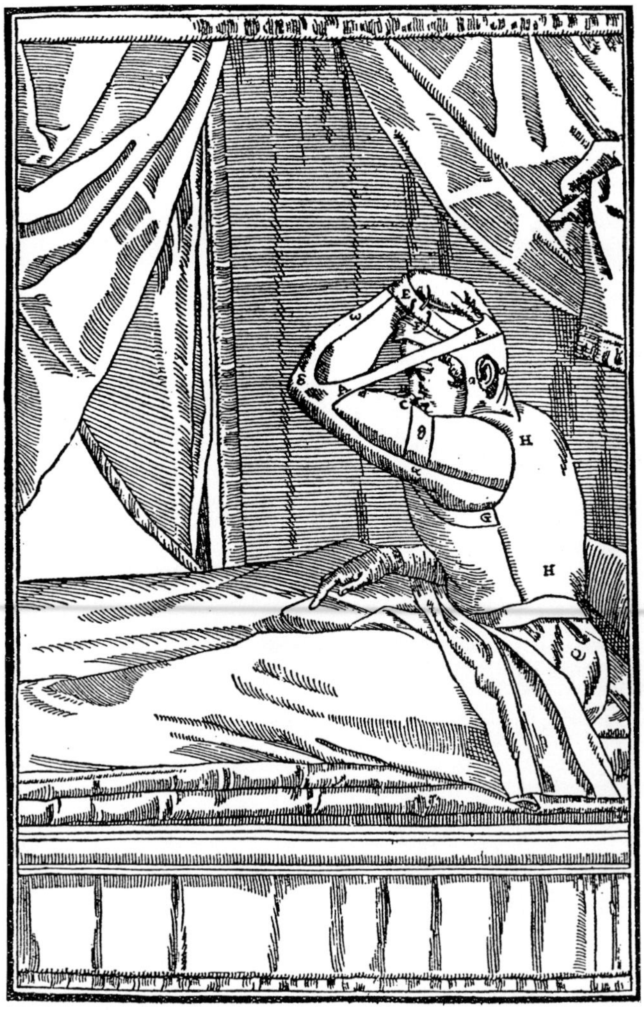

FIGURE 1–3. Lateral view of the arm bound to the face. (From Gnudi MT, Webster JP: The Life and Times of Gaspare Tagliacozzi, Surgeon of Bologna, 1545–1599. New York, Reichner, 1950.)

circulated by the nuns in the convent that the area was haunted and that voices proclaimed that Tagliacozzi was condemned to eternal hell for his works on earth. Consequently, his body was exhumed and reburied outside the city. It took two resolutions by the church to rehabilitate his memory and legacy. Finally, Tagliacozzi's remains were again exhumed and reburied in his original tomb. The precise location has been lost because the chapel's records were destroyed.[7]

EARLY MODERN PERIOD

After his death, Tagliacozzi's work largely died with him. It was rediscovered from time to time by other European surgeons such as Cortesi of Messina (1625) and Graffon of Lucerne, but otherwise it was mostly forgotten. It was not until an English surgeon, Joseph Carpue, saw an article in *Gentleman's Magazine* in October 1794 that rhinoplasty and nasal reconstruction were permanently reintroduced into Western medicine and surgery. That article was a reprint of an article published in the *Madras Gazette* in 1793 entitled, "Cowasjee, A Mahratta of the Cast of the Husbandmen." Cowasjee was a bullock driver with the English army in 1792. He was captured and imprisoned by a man who subsequently cut off Cowasjee's nose and one of his hands. He lived without a nose for almost a year until his nose was reconstructed by a Mahratta surgeon at Kumar. The article described the Indian method of nasal reconstruction. After reading this article, Carpue was convinced that this technique would work in his hands (Fig. 1–5). He reported the results of a successful operation performed at St. Bartholomew's Hospital in London in 1814.[8] This event caught the attention of King George III, who then commanded Carpue to take on the case of Captain Latham, a military hero whose nose had been amputated in 1810. The surgery on Captain Latham also had a successful outcome. Due to these two successes, especially the highly visible surgery on Captain Latham, rhinoplasty regained legitimacy as a surgical procedure. Carpue had recognized the need for some kind of supportive

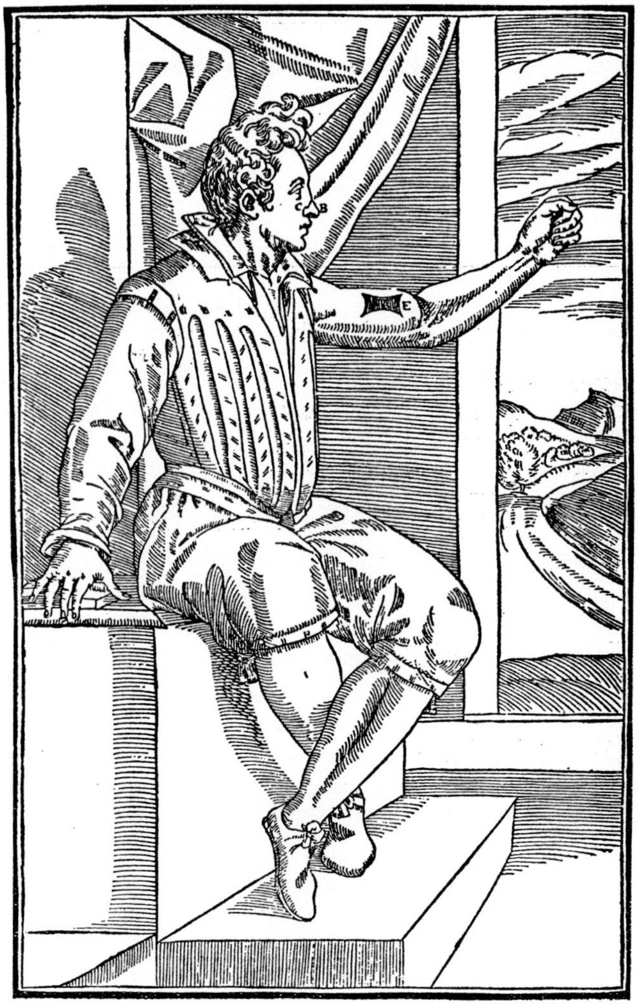

FIGURE 1–4. Healing of the forearm skin wound and shaping of the nose. (From Gnudi MT, Webster JP: The Life and Times of Gaspare Tagliacozzi, Surgeon of Bologna, 1545–1599. New York, Reichner, 1950.)

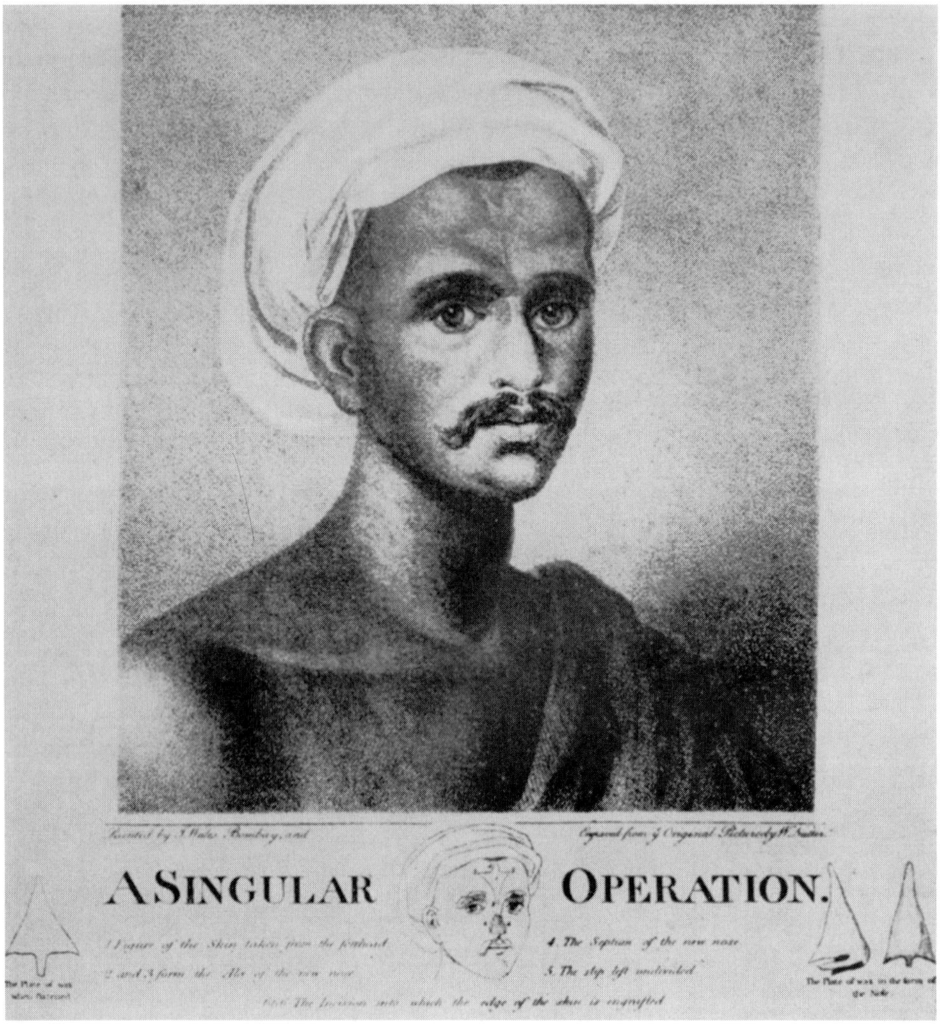

FIGURE 1–5. Indian forehead flap for nasal reconstruction. The drawings show the technique and the result after the midline forehead flap has been severed. (From Brown JB, McDowell F: Plastic Surgery of the Nose. Courtesy of Charles C Thomas, Publisher, Springfield, Illinois, 1951, 1965.)

framework under the forehead flap. Subsequently, rhinoplasty as a technique was brought to Germany by von Graefe in 1816 and by Dieffenbach in 1829.[9] Delpech, in 1828 in France, also contributed to the rhinoplasty technique.[10] Warren introduced it to the United States in 1837.[11]

J.F. Dieffenbach, in 1845, was probably the first surgeon to describe nasal reduction operations that were performed primarily for cosmetic reasons. During the midnineteenth century he described various methods of reducing nostril size by removing conical pieces of skin and cartilage from the columella and alar rims. In addition, he used external incisions to remove sections of skin and subcutaneous tissue to reduce the size of a large nose and to straighten a twisted nose. In 1860, Linhart improved on Dieffenbach's technique for reducing nostril size by using elliptical incisions rather than conical ones. In 1884, Lossen described a technique of straightening crooked noses by employing a device that applied external pressure.[12]

Meanwhile, although cosmetic rhinoplasty with internal incisions was not yet performed, advances in reconstructive rhinoplasty continued to be made. Rousseet pointed out in his 1828 Paris thesis that reconstructed noses often collapsed.[13] Many substances, including precious metals, animal bones, and amber, were used by nineteenth century surgeons to provide supportive scaffolding. All of them worked temporarily, but eventually almost all extruded.

The first person to use autogenous bone for support in a rhinoplasty procedure was Ollier, who in 1864 transposed a forehead flap that contained not only skin but also a piece of frontal bone.[14] In 1875, Hardie used the first and second phalanges of a person's finger to correct a saddle nose deformity.[15] In 1886, Konig further refined Ollier's composite flap by incorporating a large piece of the outer cortex of the frontal bone into a forehead flap when the nasal dorsum of the patient needed substantial reconstruction.[16] Further advances in using free tissue grafts to create or augment the nasal dorsum were made when Israel transferred a section of anterior tibia in 1896,[17] and von Mangold transferred autologous ribs in 1900.[18] Also in 1900, Keegan recognized the importance of providing an internal lining that prevents contraction of the forehead flap.[19] This increased concern for the final aesthetic appearance of the reconstructed nose paralleled an increased interest in and development of cosmetic rhinoplasty.

MODERN DEVELOPMENT OF COSMETIC RHINOPLASTY

True cosmetic rhinoplasty began in 1887 when an otolaryngologist from Rochester, New York, named John Orlando Roe published a paper in *The Medical Record* entitled, "The Deformity Termed 'Pug Nose' and its Correction, by a Simple Operation."[20] In this paper, Roe somewhat loosely described a tip-plasty performed entirely through intranasal incisions. His tip-plasty was achieved by removing excess soft tissue and, when necessary, cutting the alar cartilages in "different places" until the nasal tip became the desired shape. He helped the nose maintain that shape by placing silver tubes inside the nostrils and molding a saddle or splint over the exterior. In 1891, Roe published another important paper, "The Correction of Angular Deformities of the Nose by a Subcutaneous Operation."[21] Here he described the correction of bony and cartilaginous humps through intranasal incisions. In 1908, Roe, Joseph Beck, and Harmon Smith discussed the new techniques in nasal reconstruction at the fourteenth annual Triological Society Meeting. Beck was one of the first to document with photographs the preoperative appearance and the postoperative results.[22]

However, it is Jacques Joseph, a general and orthopedic surgeon from Berlin, who is considered the father of cosmetic rhinoplasty. He published his first paper in 1898 in a German language journal, where he described his technique of reduction rhinoplasty: cartilage, bone, and mucosa were removed through a V-shaped external skin incision on the nasal dorsum. The classic steps have undergone few changes to this day. Joseph published his results of the correction of nasal deformities using external incisions with skin excisions in 1902.[23] Despite the continued successful results reported in America by Roe using intranasal incisions, Joseph did not admit until 1904 that intranasal incisions produced better cosmetic results.[24] In 1907, Joseph published his extensive treatise in rhinoplasty;[25] overall, he published more than 12 articles dealing with different aspects of rhinoplasty.[26] Joseph also devised many surgical instruments that are still used in nasal surgery.[26]

In Berlin, Joseph kept his surgical technique a secret; he operated behind closed doors and charged students and observers a high price to attend. Two students of his, Joseph Safian and Gustave Aufricht, brought Joseph's techniques and knowledge to New York City in the 1930s.[27] Joseph, a Jew, committed suicide in 1939 because he was allegedly persecuted by the Nazis.

Advances in reconstructive rhinoplasty continued in the twentieth century. John Marquis Converse, an otolaryngologist who trained at the Massachusetts Eye and Ear Infirmary and also worked under Kasanjian, professor of oral-maxillofacial surgery at Harvard, introduced the forehead scalping flap for nasal reconstruction in 1942. He also advocated the use of iliac crest bone grafts for dorsal support in the third stage of nasal reconstruction after the lining and return of the forehead flap had been completed.[28] In 1966, Millard established the principle of the cantilevered bony support using rib grafts secured by wires.[29] These grafts were inserted during the first stage of nasal reconstruction, which was a great innovation. The major problem associated with rib and iliac crest grafts was their tendency to resorb with time because they are composed of cancellous bone. Also, there is loss of tip support.

Maniglia worked under Converse at the Manhattan Eye, Ear, and Throat Hospital in the late 1960s and early 1970s. He used Converse's technique of the forehead scalp flap and iliac bone grafts for support. In 1989, he began to use cantilevered parietal bone grafts fixed rigidly with titanium plates to provide dorsal support. The plates provide longer-lasting support than previously described materials.[30] He used either the remnant of nasal skin or a nasolabial flap for the inner lining. Both the horizontal forehead flap based on the superficial temporal artery, as described by McGregor, and the vertical midline and paramedian forehead flaps based on the supra- and infratrochlear arteries were used as supportive covering for parietal bone grafts during the first stage of the procedure.[30]

Finally, Burget has contributed to precise reconstruction of the cartilaginous supporting structures of the nose by using nasal septum and/or conchal cartilage.[31] He combined this principle with the paramedian forehead flap (Indian flap) and has produced excellent results after multistage procedures.

Alloplasts including those made of silicone, Supramid, Gore-Tex, and hydroxyapatite have been used to reshape the nose for the last several decades.[32] Overall, for good long-term results, autologous tissues are preferable.

SUMMARY

Rhinoplasty is a surgical procedure that was first performed by Indian tradesmen more than 2500 years ago after the nose had been traumatically amputated. Today, cosmetic and functional septorhinoplasties are performed by otolaryngologists, head and neck surgeons, plastic surgeons, and oral-maxillofacial surgeons. Numerous practitioners have contributed to the development and finesse of such surgical procedures, but a detailed historical review is not within the scope of this chapter. Because the nose is a prominent and noticeable feature of the face and attracts attention, the cosmetic implications of the use of flaps, the complexity of the nasal anatomy and nasal dynamics, and problems associated with long-term healing and fibrous tissue contraction make reconstructive rhinoplasty one of the most challenging surgical procedures. Staged procedures are necessary to achieve good, lasting results. Nevertheless, reconstructive rhinoplasty can be a rewarding experience for both the patient and the surgeon.

REFERENCES

1. Sushruta S: English translation of Sushruta Samhita based on original Sanskrit text. Edited and published by Kaviraj Kunja Lal Bhishagratna. Bose, Calcutta, India, 1907–1916.
2. Celsus AC: De Medicina. Cambridge, Harvard University Press, 1971.
3. Mumford JG: Surgical Memoirs, and Other Essays. New York, Moffat, Yard & Co, 1908.
4. Ranzano P: Annals of the World. 1492.
5. Furlan S, Mazzola RF: Alessandro Benedetti, a fifteenth century anatomist and surgeon: His role in the history of nasal reconstruction. Plast Reconstr Surg 96(3):739–743, 1995.
6. Tagliacozzi G: De Curtorum Chirurgia per Insitionem, Libri Duo. Venetiis, Apud Gasparem Bindonum, juniorem, 1597.
7. Bernardelli JC, Zini C: Las ciencias medicas Italianas en el desarrollo de la otorrinolaringologia. Anal Otorrinolaringol Mex 42:47–62, 1997.
8. Carpue JC: An Account of Two Successful Operations for Restoring a Lost Nose from the Integuments of the Forehead. London, Longman, Hurst, Rees, Orme and Brown, 1816.
9. Dieffenbach JF: Die Operative Chirurgie. Leipzig, FA Brockhaus, 1845.
10. Delpech JM: Sur l'operation de rhinoplastique. *In* Delpech JM: Chirurgie Clinique de Montpellier, Vol. II. Paris, Gabon, 1828, p. 221.
11. Warren JM: Rhinoplastic operation. Boston Med Surg J 16:69, 1837.
12. Lossen H: Hueter-Lossen's Grundriss der Chirurgie, Vol. 2. Leipzig, FCW Vogel, 1884.
13. Nelaton C, Ombredanne L: La Rhinoplastie. Paris, G Steinheil, 1904.
14. Ollier L: De l'osteoplastie appliquee a la restauration du nez. Gaz Hop (Paris) 37:349, 1864.
15. Hardie J: On a new rhinoplastic operation. Br Med J 393, 1875.
16. Konig F: Eine neue Methode der Aufrichtung ein-gesunkener Nasen. Arch Klin Chir 34:41, 1886.
17. Israel J: Zwei neue Methoden der Rhinoplastik. Arch Klin Chir 53:255, 1896.
18. von Mangold: Hilung der Sattelnase durch Knorpelübertragung. Chir Kongr Verhandl 1900.
19. Keegan DF: Rhinoplastic Operations with a Description of Recent Improvements in the Indian Method. London, Bailliere, Tindall and Cox, 1900.
20. Roe JO: The deformity termed pug nose and its correction by a simple operation. Medical Record 31:621, 1887.
21. Roe JO: The correction of angular deformities of the nose by a subcutaneous operation. Medical Record 40:57, 1891.
22. Crumley R: Turn of the century facial plastic surgeons and The Laryngoscope. Laryngoscope 106:1199–1203, 1996.
23. Joseph J: Ueber die operative Verkleinerung Nase (rhinomiosis). Berl Klin Wochenschr, p. 851, 1902.
24. Joseph J: Intranasale Nasenhockerabtragung. Berl Klin Wochenschr, p. 650, 1904.
25. Joseph J: Beitrage zur Rhinoplastik. Berl Klin Wochenschr, 44:470, 1907.
26. Rodgers BO: Early historical development of corrective rhinoplasty. *In* Symposium on Corrective Rhinoplasty, Vol. 13. St. Louis, Mosby, 1976, pp. 18–31.
27. Safian J: Corrective Rhinoplastic Surgery. New York, Paul B. Hoeber, 1935.
28. Converse JM: New forehead flap for reconstruction of the nose. J Laryngol Otol 57:508, 1942.
29. Millard DR: Total reconstructive rhinoplasty and a missing link. Plast Reconstr Surg 37:167–183, 1966.
30. Maniglia AJ: Reconstructive rhinoplasty. Laryngoscope 99:865–867, 1989.
31. Burget GC, Menick FJ: Aesthetic Reconstruction of the Nose. St. Louis, Mosby, 1994.
32. Byrd HS, Hobar PC: Alloplastic nasal and perialar augmentation. Clin Plast Surg 23(2):315–326, 1996.

CHAPTER 2

Cartilage Grafts in Nasal Reconstruction

Fred J. Stucker, M.D.
Robert F. Aarstad, M.D.

Cartilage is one of the most versatile grafting materials available for tissue transfer procedures. It is readily available from the patient's own tissue, or it can be kept on hand in the form of irradiated homograft chondral cartilage (IHCC). Cartilage can be easily sculpted and has a low rate of rejection. It can provide structural and architectural support or can serve as an augmentation material. The authors' bias is overwhelmingly in favor of the use of autogenous cartilage because of its universal success and its adaptability and ready availability. In those rare instances in which it is unavailable, irradiated homograft material can be employed, but this is clearly an inferior choice.

Cartilage is avascular and is nourished only by tissue fluid diffusion; therefore it has a very low metabolic rate—1:100 to 1:500 that of other tissues.[1] Chondrocytes are very sparse but continually produce chondromucoprotein, elastin, and collagen that generate the more abundant surrounding matrix. As long as living chondrocytes remain they will reproduce the matrix, thus maintaining the graft's bulk. Dead chondrocytes result in reabsorption of the cartilage, which is usually replaced by fibrous tissue.[2] Chondrocytes originate from the perichondrium by apositional growth. The inclusion of perichondrium with the cartilaginous graft helps to ensure its mechanical strength and enhances and speeds its healing to the surrounding tissues.[3] Perichondrium that remains in the donor site has the potential to originate new cartilage growth by new chondrogenesis.[4–6]

The cartilage matrix contains a fibrous network whose fiber type determines the properties of the matrix and ultimately the specific type and function of the cartilage. Depending on the type of fiber weaving through the matrix, the cartilage can be classified as hyaline, elastic, or fibrous cartilage. This fibrous weaving immersed in the ground substance of the cartilage gives the cartilage its memory for shape and tension as well as its recoil ability. This is especially true of rib cartilage. In costal cartilage, the tight, dense outer subperichondrial cartilage layer helps to prevent the main loose inner mesh from expanding and becoming distorted.[7] Thus, removal of this subperichondrial layer may explain the undesirable warping and twisting that many of these cartilage grafts undergo.

Cartilage has been regarded as an immunologically privileged tissue that possesses little or no antigenicity. This concept leads to the hypothesis that cartilage allografts fare nearly as well as autografts. Cartilage appears to be immunologically privileged early on; however, numerous studies have shown that this is not the case in the long term. The paucity of chondrocytes and the thick surrounding matrix retard the antigenic response, but nonetheless, relentless resorption does occur.[8]

HISTORICAL ASPECTS OF CARTILAGE GRAFTS

The first recorded use of cartilage grafts was in an animal experiment performed by Leopold in 1881, who demonstrated that cartilage homografts lived longer than any other homograft tissue.[9] Koenig was the first to transplant an autograft of living cartilage in humans in 1896.[10] Friedrich von Mangoldt in 1900 is credited with the first free cartilage transplant to the nose. He used costal cartilage to reconstruct a saddle deformity of the nose through a glabellar incision.[11] In 1913, Davis and Gibson reported that there was essentially no difference between autografted and homografted rib cartilage in an animal experiment.[12]

Little work was done during the first third of the twentieth century because of the prevailing view that a cartilage graft would not survive transplantation. In the 1930s, costal cartilage autografts were again introduced. Eventual failure secondary to cartilage warping occurred after the initial success of these grafts. This failure led to the use of preserved cartilage homografts, which resisted warping but resulted in delayed and unpredictable resorption.[13]

Peer's work during the 1950s with nasoseptal, conchal, and costal cartilage grafts showed that both autografts and homografts could remain viable without resorption.[14, 15] The notion that a homograft cartilage graft remains intact following transplantation has subsequently been questioned.[16] Since that time, many articles have dealt with the technical aspects of using cartilage grafts for nasal reconstruction. These uses range from nasal dorsum augmentation and tip refinement to alar cartilage replacement and total nasal reconstruction.

AUTOGENOUS GRAFTS

Two cartilage grafts are commonly employed for nasal reconstruction at the present time. The most commonly used is the autogenous cartilage graft, which is, by all accounts, the most successful. These grafts are commonly harvested from three sites: the nasal septum (septal cartilage), the ear (auricular or conchal cartilage), and the rib (costal cartilage).

Septal Cartilage

The nasal septum is made up of hyaline cartilage; it gives structural support to the dorsum of the nose and separates the nasal cavities. It is the most common source of autogenous cartilage graft material for most surgeons practicing nasal reconstruction. It is easily and readily available during the course of nasal surgery, and there is little morbidity if both a dorsal and a caudal strut of the septum are left intact. A subtotal submucous resection can be performed to obtain a large portion of graft material. Thicker cartilage grafts can be obtained from the posterior ventral aspect of the septal cartilage, and thinner pieces are harvested from the anterior dorsal areas. Septal pathology can frustrate these selective needs.

Septal cartilage can be used cosmetically for columellar struts, shield grafts, and fillers in various areas about the nose. It can be stacked or tiered and used for significant dorsal augmentation. Septal cartilage grafts can also be used in such functional roles as battens or spreader grafts when repairing a valve or alar collapse.

Auricular (Conchal) Cartilage

The auricle is made up of elastic cartilage that can be used by itself or as a composite graft with the perichondrium attached or with both the perichondrial and cutaneous portions attached. It is readily available through a posterior or, more appropriately, an anterior approach to the concha. As mentioned, it can be and universally is harvested with the perichondrium attached. Both skin and perichondrium may be attached to the cartilage depending on the required need. When skin is attached, the donor site is closed using a postauricular interpolated skin island flap from behind the ear (flip-flop flap).[17]

Conchal cartilage is the most common cartilage graft material used in nasal reconstruction by the senior author (FJS). In cases requiring major support tissue, conchal cartilage is available in the required amounts more often than septal cartilage, which is often absent or available in scant amounts due to previous nasal surgery. Septal cartilage is superior to conchal material for pure structural support but is quite inferior for reconstruction of the upper or lower lateral cartilages. Auricular cartilage is available through a traditional postauricular approach, but it can be harvested more expediently through an anterior approach to the concha (Fig. 2–1). The conchal cartilage graft is routinely harvested with the perichondrium attached to the cartilage. When a perichondrial cutaneous or a composite (cartilage and skin) graft is harvested, the defect is closed with a postauricular interpolated skin island flap (flip-flop flap).[17]

One distinct advantage of the chonchal cartilage graft is the almost assured posterior attachment of the posterior perichondrium. This adherent perichondrium increases the likelihood of rapid and complete assimilation of the graft in the new host site.

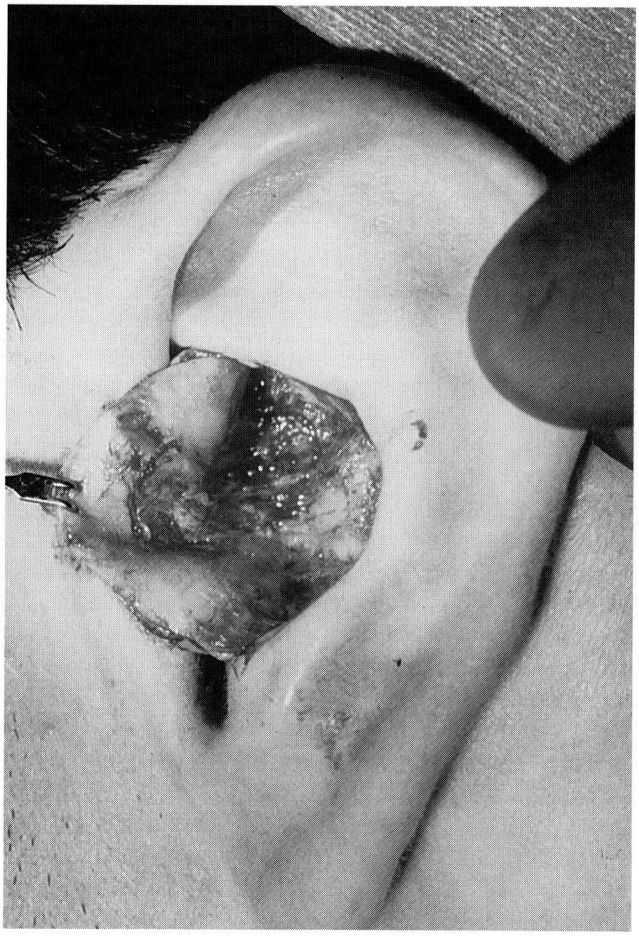

FIGURE 2–1. Harvest of conchal cartilage through an anterior approach. Note the adherent perichondrium, which ensures rapid assimilation in host site.

The elasticity and curvature of conchal cartilage make it ideal in grafting lateral alar components of the nose. In cases of valve or alar collapse, especially from iatrogenic or traumatic causes, a conchal-perichondrial graft may be used as a cap or hood over the septum. This recreates the rigid side-to-side structure or the bilateral integrity of the upper lateral cartilages, which are coapted to the graft with mattress sutures and ultimately heal to it. This conchal graft is placed through an open rhinoplasty approach to position the graft precisely and ensure a cosmetic and functional reconstruction (Fig. 2–2).

Conchal-perichondrial or conchal-perichondrial-cutaneous grafts are also used to reconstruct the structural and functional components of the lower lateral cartilages[18] (Fig. 2–3). Auricular composite grafts can also be used to reconstruct full-thickness defects of the nasal ala.

As previously stated, most facial plastic surgeons employ septal cartilage far more often than auricular cartilage for nasal reconstruction. The senior author uses conchal (auricular) cartilage approximately two or three times more often than septal cartilage for this purpose. Because this practice tends to be against the conventional thinking, it is perhaps wise to explain this aberration. It is also important to describe some technical aspects of the harvesting and use of conchal cartilage that simplify what may appear to be a much more complex technique. It is actually just as expedient to harvest and close conchal cartilage donor site defects as it is those of the septum.

First, one must realize that in patients requiring more complicated nasal surgery for reconstruction following ablation or revisional nasal surgery, in which much of the architectural cartilage of the nose has been removed, septal cartilage is often not present in sufficient amounts to be a viable alternative. On the other hand, this is rarely the case with auricular cartilage; with the exception of congenital absence or facial burns, it is always available. It is also important to understand that in general, auricular cartilage is more adaptable to more nasal reconstruction needs than septal cartilage. No one disagrees that septal cartilage is much preferred for columellar struts, spreader grafts, and tip grafts, but apart from these three uses, auricular cartilage is usually equally or better adapted to most other nasal architectural needs. Surgeons who employ a large number of tip grafts and struts as in a cosmetic practice will undoubtedly use a far larger percentage of septal grafts. The patient requiring cosmetic surgery is also more likely to have an intact and rather straight cartilaginous septum as a source of host tissue, which is ideally suited, as previously stated, for struts, spreader grafts, and tip grafts. On the other hand, in many of our revision septorhinoplasties, the patient's previous procedure or procedures have involved significant resection of septal cartilage, and there is little septal cartilage remaining for reconstructive purposes. Similarly, in patients in whom nasal reconstruction follows resection for neoplasia or avulsion losses secondary to trauma, the septum may be unavailable because of the pathology. With the exception of structural support, which is the primary role of septal cartilage, auricular cartilage may be better suited for most cartilage replacement needs in nasal reconstruction.

Physiologically, conchal cartilage is well suited for nasal reconstruction. The posterior perichondrial attachment ensures a more predictable assimilation in the new host site. The mere fact that perichondrium is universally present in the transplanted auricular cartilage and is equally absent from septal cartilage is in large measure responsible for this. Auricular cartilage has curves that are ideally suited to replacement of the alar cartilages and the upper lateral cartilage. Most replacement parts can be fashioned by using a sharp knife blade and can be further refined and precisely feathered by using a rotating diamond fraise (Fig. 2–4). The concha can be thinned with remarkable ease with the drill. This technique is used to fashion conchal cartilage with attached perichondrium to be used in a sandwiched graft repairing a septal perforation (Fig. 2–5).

Rib (Costal) Cartilage

Costal cartilage is a source of large quantities of hyaline cartilage, which is mainly used for dorsal augmentation in large saddle nose deformities. There are many who believe that the increased morbidity and amount of surgery involved in harvesting autogenous costal cartilage are not practical when irradiated homografted costal cartilage is so readily available. Postoperative morbidity is directly related to the amount of cartilage removed. Thus, proper planning to use the minimal resection necessary and tailoring the rib contour to the graft requirements are most beneficial.

HOMOGRAFTS

The only nonautogenous cartilage graft material currently used in the United States is irradiated homografted costal cartilage. Xenografts have fallen from favor owing to their rather rapid and complete resorption, among other factors. Preserved banked homografted cartilage is no longer used owing to the risk of human immunodeficiency virus (HIV) and other communicable diseases. Lyophilized cartilage is popular in Europe, where it is used to augment numerous sites on the face including the nose. It as well as cryopreserved frozen cartilage can be obtained at the University of Miami Tissue Bank. Although these transplants have not been demonstrated to transmit HIV, concerns about this possibility remain, and therefore it is not widely used.

Irradiated homografted costal cartilage is procured from donors who are screened for systemic or local infectious processes, metastatic cancer, and intravenous drug abuse. The cartilage blocks are stored in saline solutions and then exposed to 18,000 to 23,000 Gy of gamma radiation using a cobalt-60 source. Doses above 25,000 Gy cause the grafts to become brittle. Grafts are then stored in the saline-filled jars at room temperature; they have a shelf life of up to 4

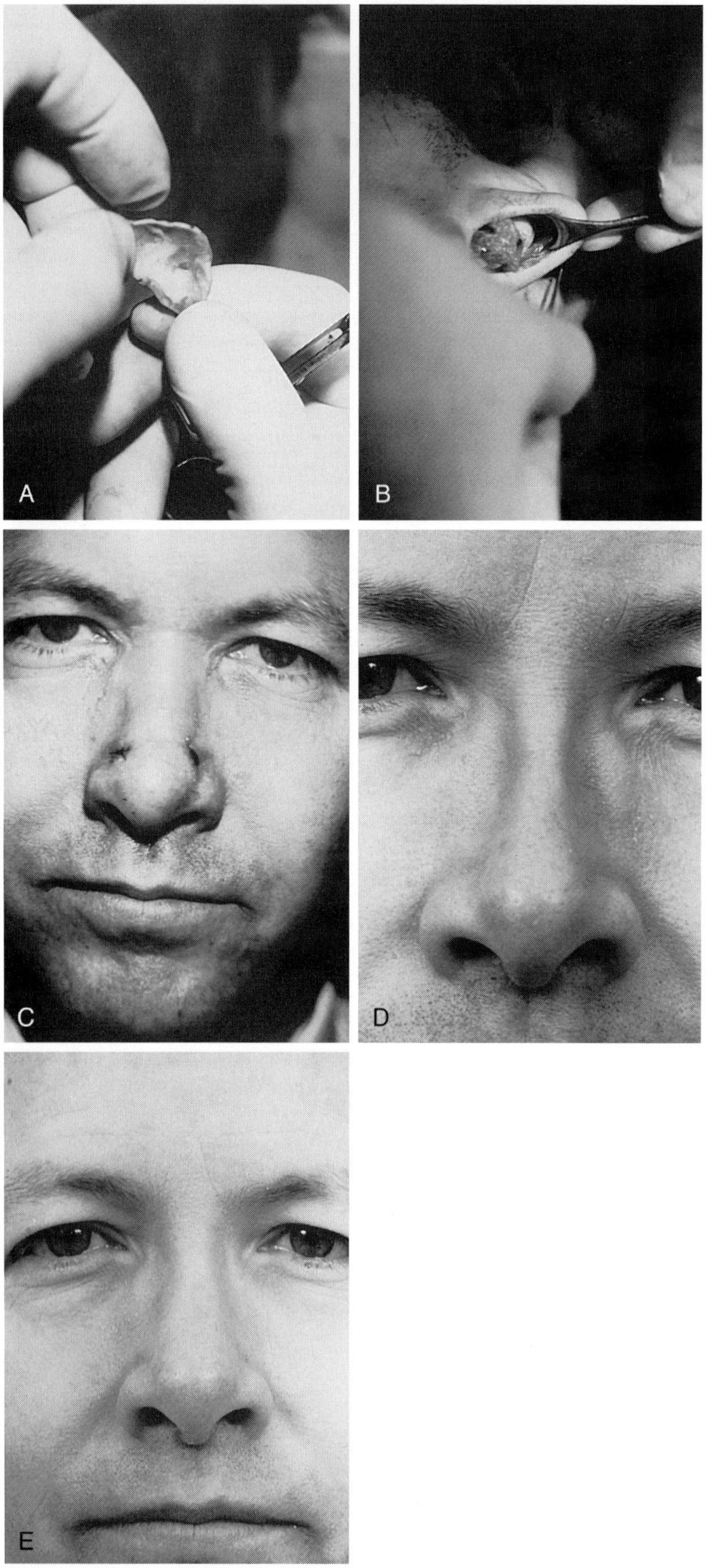

FIGURE 2–2. *A*, Conchal cartilage has a remarkable similarity to intact upper lateral cartilages. *B*, Placement of conchal graft over septum and cephalad to lower lateral cartilages. *C*, Mattress sutures sandwich the conchal graft between the mucosa of the valve apex, the upper lateral cartilages, and the dorsal skin. *D*, Patient shown in *C* had a history of three previous nasal procedures and bilateral complete nasal obstruction. *E*, Appearance of conchal graft 2 years after surgery in patient shown in *C* and *D*.

years. These grafts are relatively inexpensive and can be kept readily available in the operating room. Their other advantages include resistance to infection, extrusion, and warping. Animal studies have conclusively shown that irradiated homografted costal cartilage is largely absorbed over a long-term period. Similar absorption rates have been shown to occur in humans in smaller studies.

Clinically, the correction or augmentation is maintained to a large extent depending on the site of the graft. Graft locations that show minimal clinical absorption rates include the dorsum of the nose and other areas not subjected to regular muscular activity or significant overlying pressure. If indeed long-term IHCC resorption is inevitable, then proportionate fibrous tissue replacement must be responsible for the evident clinical successes. The actual amount of histologic resorption should not be a factor in recommending augmentation nasal surgery, if the overall cosmetic and functional results are preserved.[20]

Complications associated with IHCC include mainly graft-related infections and do not differ significantly from complications noted with autografts. Long-term complications other than resorption are mainly associated with warping, which occurs much less often with IHCC than with autografts. In short, autografted costal cartilage and IHCC have offsetting advantages and disadvantages depending on the papers read and a particular surgeon's bias. The choice should be made based on a physician's own experience.

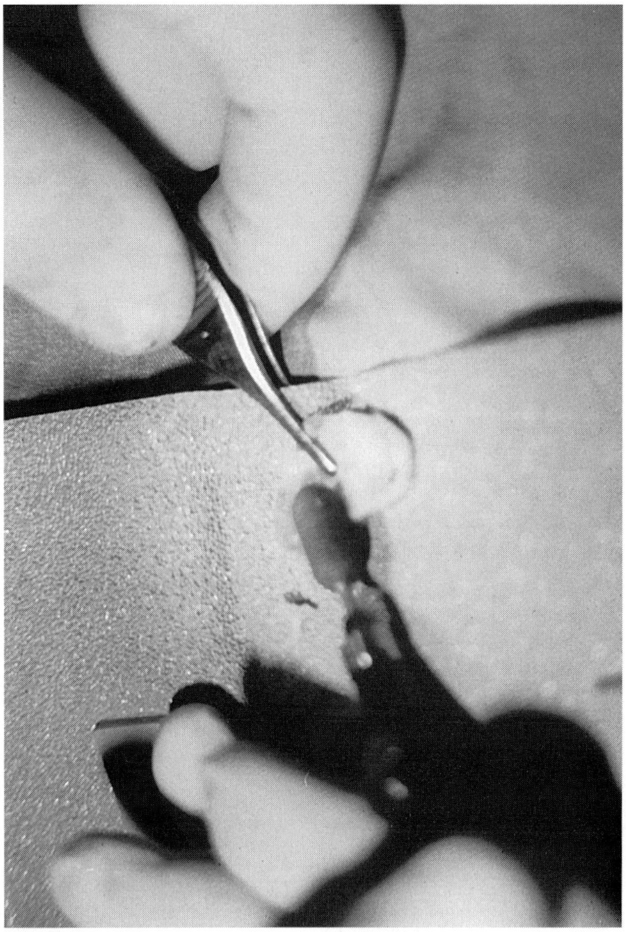

FIGURE 2–4. Conchal cartilage graft is fashioned and refined using a rotating drill with a diamond fraise.

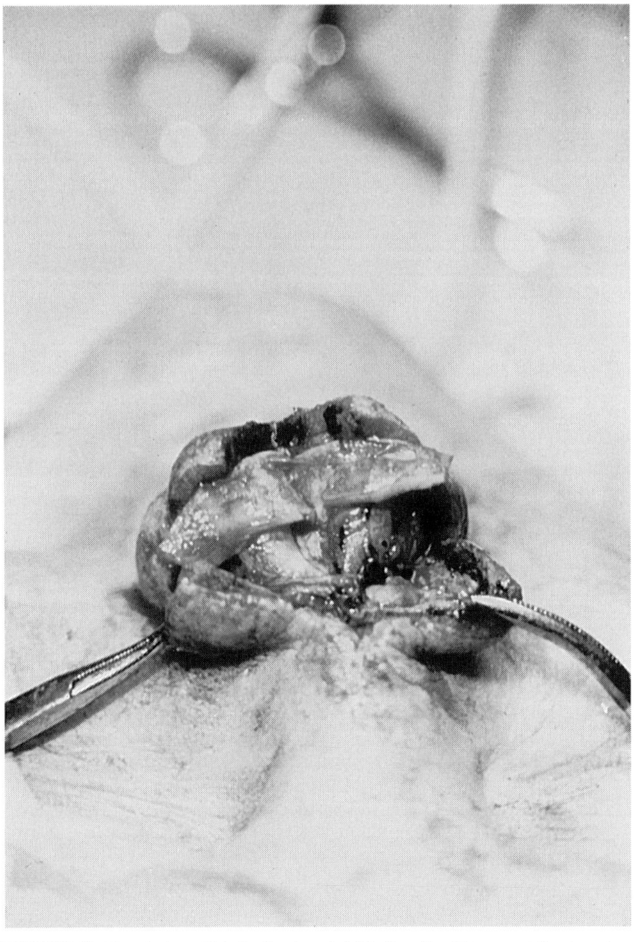

FIGURE 2–3. Conchal graft is incised and folded on itself to provide structural support and replacement of the lower lateral cartilage.

SUMMARY

The primary consideration for employing any graft material must be success. This mandates that the material must survive with minimal complications while serving the purpose for which it was intended. The overwhelming preference among most surgeons for structural support in nasal reconstruction is autogenous cartilage. There is room for discussion concerning the site and type of cartilage used. In the absence of autogenous material or when extenuating circumstances exist, other alternatives may have to be employed.

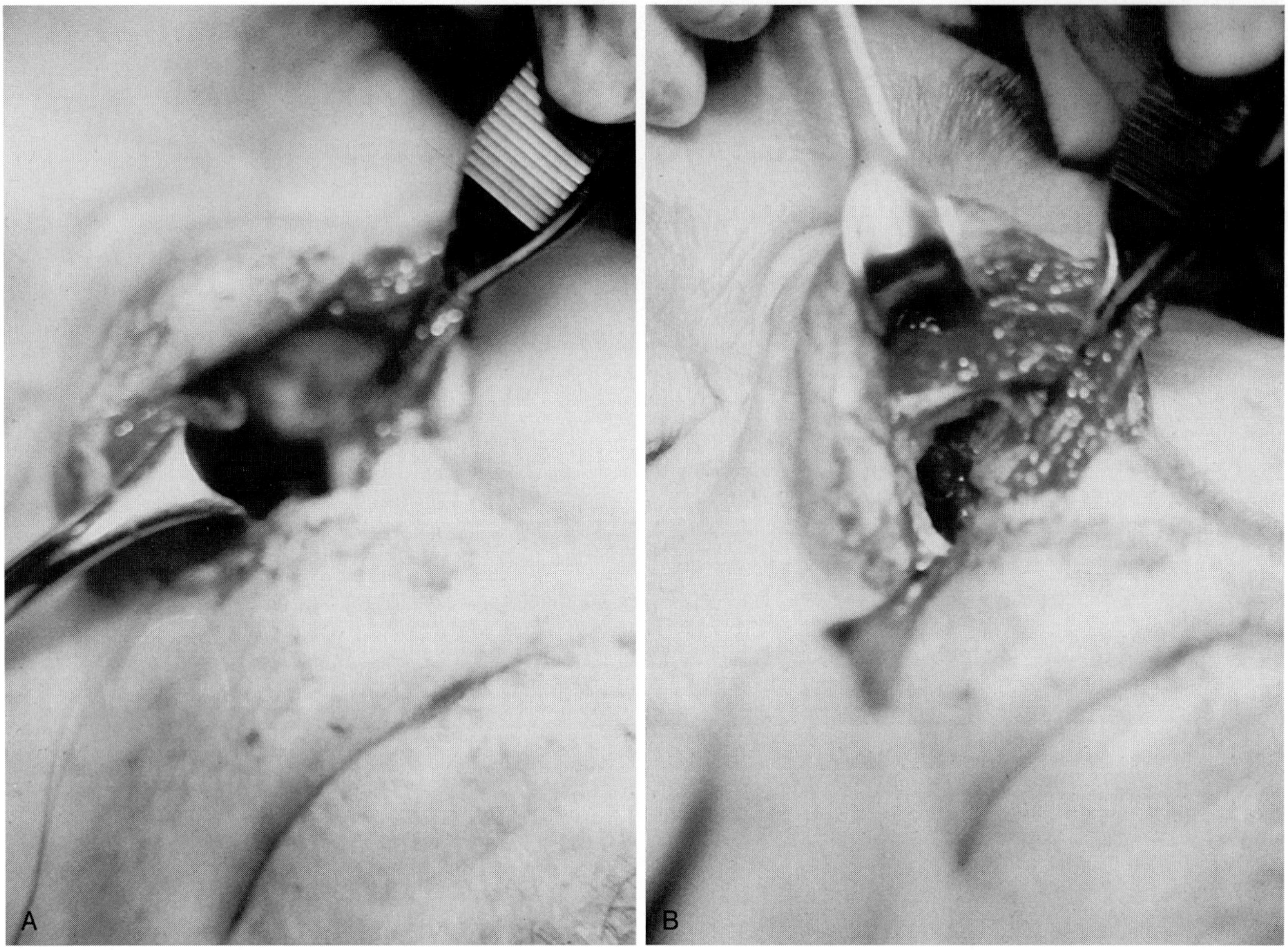

FIGURE 2–5. *A*, A septal perforation. *B*, Closure following inferior flap on right and superior flap on left advanced over paper-thin conchal graft (using diamond fraise) and septal whip stitch.

REFERENCES

1. Hagerty RF, Calhoon TB, Lee WH, Cuttino JT: Human cartilage grafts stored in air. Surg Gynecol Obstet 110:442, 1960.
2. Thomas L: Reversible collapse of rabbit ears after intravenous papain and prevention of recovery by cortisone. J Exp Med 104:245, 1956.
3. Duncan MJ, Thompson HG, Mancer JF: Free cartilage grafts: The role of perichondrium. Plast Reconstr Surg 73:916, 1984.
4. Stucker FJ: Cartilage regeneration: A clinical and experimental study. Ophth/Oto 83:785–790, 1976.
5. Skoog T, Ohlsen L, Sohn SA: The chondrogenic potential of the perichondrium. Chir Plast 3:84, 1975.
6. Brent B, Ott R: Perichondro-cutaneous graft. Plast Reconstr Surg 62:1, 1978.
7. Gibson T, Davis WB: The distortion of autogenous cartilage grafts: Its cause and prevention. Br J Plast Surg 10:257, 1958.
8. Brent B: Repair and grafting of cartilage and perichondrium. *In* McCarthy JG (ed): Plastic Surgery. Philadelphia, W.B. Saunders, 1990.
9. Leopold G: Virchow Arch Pathol Anat 84:283, 1881.
10. Koenig F: Reaktion des Knorpels auf Trauma. Langenbach Arch Klin Chir 124:1, 1923.
11. Von Mangoldt F: Reconstruction of saddle nose by cartilage overlay. Plast Reconstr Surg 46:498, 1970.
12. Davis WB, Gibson T: Absorption of autogenous cartilage grafts in man. Br J Plast Surg 9:177, 1956.
13. Arden RL, Crumley RL: Cartilage in open rhinoplasty. Facial Plast Surg 9(4):285, 1993.
14. Peer LA: Cartilage grafting. Surg Clin North Am 24:404, 1944.
15. Peer LA: Transplantation of Tissue. Baltimore, Williams & Wilkins, 1955.
16. Dupertuis SM, Musgrave RH: Experiences with reconstruction of the conger. Plast Reconstr Surg 23:361, 1959.
17. Stucker FJ, Shaw GY: The perichondrial cutaneous graft. Arch Otolaryngol Head Neck Surg 118:287, 1992.
18. Stucker FJ, Hoasjoe DK: Nasal reconstruction with conchal cartilage. Arch Otolaryngol Head Neck Surg 120:653, 1994.
19. Burget GC, Menick FG: The subsurface framework. *In* Burget GC, Menick FG (eds): Aesthetic Reconstruction of the Nose. St. Louis, Mosby–Year Book, 1994, pp. 157–204.
20. Allcroft RA, Friedman CD, Quatela VC: Cartilage grafts for head and neck augmentation and reconstruction. Otolaryngol Clin North Am 27(1):69, 1994.
21. Kridel WH, Konior RJ: Irradiated cartilage grafts in the nose. Arch Otolaryngol Head Neck Surg 119:24, 1993.

CHAPTER 3

Aesthetic Subunits of the Nose and Reconstructive Application

Frederick J. Menick, M.D.

When a facial feature such as the nose has been destroyed by trauma or ablated in treatment for cancer, most patients desire both a healed wound and the appearance they had before the injury. They wish to look normal and feel right.

Newborn infants recognize a "beautiful" face, and the daily observation of normal faces reinforces these innate standards of "normal." Throughout life, our eyes consciously "see" the unexpected but tend to disregard whatever is normal or simulates normal. We rapidly recognize a feature as familiar but are repelled by the unexpected, distorted, or grotesque. A facial reconstruction will not draw attention if the basic components of the facial part are restored and the number of deficiencies minimized. Most important, any jarring abnormality must be avoided. Although the telltale signs of surgery may remain, a reconstructed nose need not evoke horror and can even be beautiful at speaking distance.

REGIONAL FACIAL UNITS

The face is characterized by adjacent topographic areas of characteristic skin qualities (color, texture, thickness, and hairbearing capacity), two-dimensional outline, and three-dimensional surface contour. These regional units[1] of the face include the forehead, eyelids, nose, cheeks, upper and lower lips, chin, and submental area (Fig. 3–1).

The forehead and cheeks are peripheral units. They are flat, and their peripheral outlines vary from person to person during facial expression and with aging. Only part of these units can be seen in any facial position. No contralateral comparison is available for critical analysis in the frontal view. In facial reconstruction they are of lesser priority and need not be restored with exacting care. In contrast, the nose and upper lip are central facial units that are seen in primary gaze. Their outlines and landmarks are fixed. The opposite, or contralateral, side of each unit (e.g., the ala or philtrum column) is visible for easy comparison, as are abnormalities in three-dimensional surface. They must be restored with exactness and precision if they are to appear normal.

The external surface of the nose is crossed by ridges and valleys that separate the nasal unit into subunits.[2] The tip, dorsum, columella and paired sidewalls, alae and soft triangles are the nasal subunits (Fig. 3–2*A* and *B*). They are defined by gradations of light and shadow that are reflected from the nasal surface and are determined by the underlying contour of the hard and soft tissues.

Too frequently, a facial defect is seen as a "hole to be filled" (i.e., as the absence of a facial part). The mind's eye becomes absorbed in examining the crater rather than in visualizing the three-dimensional subunits that should be present. If part or all of the nose is missing, the surgeon must provide the basic elements that comprise the nose while

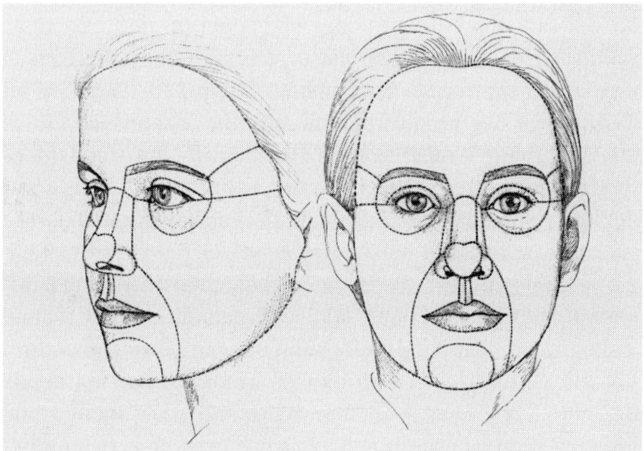

FIGURE 3–1. The facial units are adjacent topographic areas defined by skin quality (color, texture, thickness, and hair-bearing quality), two-dimensional outline, and three-dimensional contour. (From Menick FJ: Facial reconstruction in regional units. Perspect Plast Surg 8:104, 1994.)

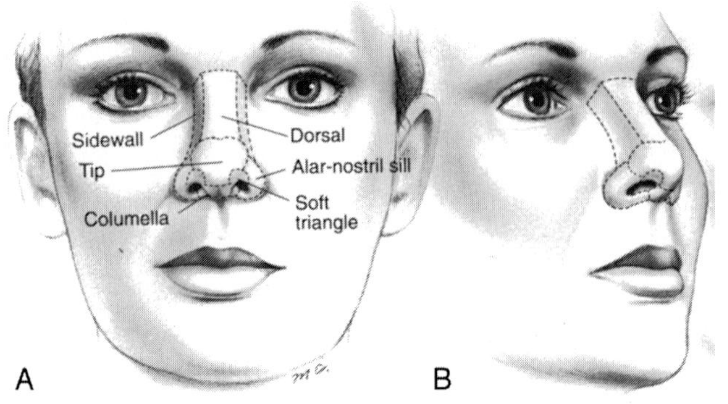

FIGURE 3–2. *A* and *B,* The surface of the nose is made up of adjacent areas of characteristic skin quality, outline, and contour. (From Burget GC, Menick FJ: Aesthetic Reconstruction of the Nose. St. Louis, Mosby–Year Book, 1994.)

minimizing deficiencies and avoiding jarring abnormalities. Specifically, the goal of reconstruction must be to restore the expected regional skin quality, outline, and contour that characterize each nasal subunit. The normal nose, which is the desired result, must be visualized during planning and execution. In an aesthetic nasal reconstruction, each nasal defect must be analyzed in terms of anatomic loss (cover, lining, and support) and aesthetic loss (subunit characteristics).

But wounds vary in size, site, outline, and depth. They may encompass one or more facial units or part of one or more regional subunits (for example, a defect may involve part of the nasal tip, dorsum, and sidewall subunits with extensions onto the adjacent cheek and lip facial units). The anatomic requirements of cover, lining, and support vary within the defect, as do the aesthetic requirements of skin quality, unit outline, and contour. Different defects require different planning methods and techniques, which will vary from unit to unit and within a single subunit if the unique character of each facial feature is to be restored. If a large defect is simply filled with one large skin graft or flap, the peripheral scars will often be obvious because rarely are they fortuitously hidden in contour lines. Equally important, the delicate three-dimensional character of multiple units cannot be replaced by one flat or concave shiny graft patch or a single contracted hemisphere of flap soft tissue. A set of priorities for reconstruction must be established. Each unit and subunit must be reconstructed to the standard of "normal." The central facial features, because of their complexity, symmetry, and visual importance, define the face and must be restored most accurately.

The regional unit theory in facial reconstruction is important because, although surgeons cannot control wound healing to prevent the development of scars, they can control the color, texture, and thickness of the donor materials used.[12–14] They can also control the site, size, shape, and direction of the incisions and excisions used, thus manipulating the scars they produce. They can choose to make defects that fit the outline of topographic units and use materials and methods designed to restore nasal contour.

RECONSTRUCTIVE APPLICATIONS: RESTORING SKIN QUALITY

Anatomically, the normal nose is composed of thin vascular lining, sculptured alar tip cartilages, bone and cartilage braces that buttress the dorsum and sidewalls, and a canopy of thin skin that matches the face in color, texture, and hair distribution. The skin of the adult nose is divided into zones of thin, smooth skin and thick, pitted skin.[3] The skin of the dorsum and sidewall is thin, smooth, pliable, and mobile. The skin of the columella, alar margins, and soft triangles is also thin and pliable, although it is relatively fixed to the underlying tissues. The zone of thick skin is finely pitted with sebaceous glands and lies over the nasal tip and ala. These zones of thin and thick skin describe areas of skin quality within the nasal unit (Fig. 3–3).

Small superficial defects of the nose are defects that are less than 1.5 cm in diameter and those that consist only of skin and a superficial layer of subcutaneous tissue that does not bare the underlying normal cartilage framework. Large and deep defects are defects that are greater than 1.5 cm in size or in which the underlying cartilage is exposed or missing; sometimes the lining is also absent. To rebuild a nose so that it looks normal, absent skin must be replaced with skin of a similar color, texture, thickness, and hair distribution. The surgeon must remember that the color and character of such replacement skin is determined by the character of the donor site from which it is taken and by the method of tissue transfer. In the past, the emphasis has traditionally been placed on the survival of the transplanted tissue—the vascular ability of the recipient bed to accept a skin graft or the vascular supply to a pedicle flap—rather than on the aesthetic result. Often forgotten are the effects of tissue transfer on wound healing.

Because of temporary ischemia, the quality of the skin transferred as a skin graft is unpredictable. Skin grafts usually appear shiny, atrophic, and irregularly pigmented; however, although they may shrink, they rarely form a "pincushion." In contrast, skin flaps maintain the characteristics of

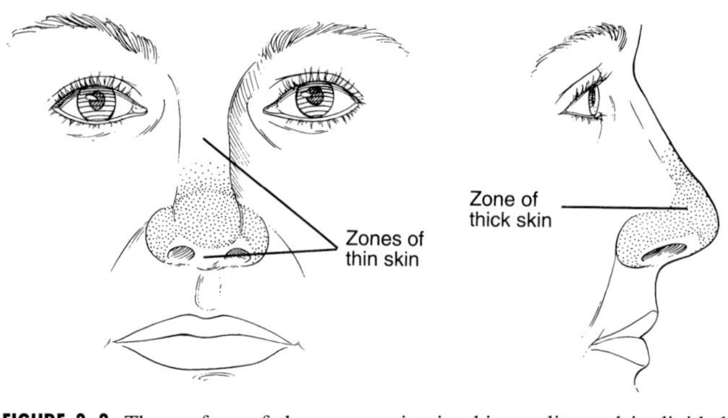

FIGURE 3–3. The surface of the nose varies in skin quality and is divided into zones of thin and thick skin. (From Burget GC, Menick FJ: Aesthetic Reconstruction of the Nose. St. Louis, Mosby–Year Book, 1994.)

the donor skin but have a tendency to form pincushions and become elevated above the surface of the defect, appearing as a bulge above the adjacent intact skin surrounding the original defect. Thus, a small defect in the normal shiny, flat nasal sidewall can be successfully resurfaced with a shiny skin graft, whereas the round, rough-textured ala or tip is best resurfaced with a flap.

Reconstructive options for a nasal surface defect include full-thickness skin grafts, local flaps, nasolabial flaps, and forehead flaps. The following rules for subunit reconstruction should be considered:

1. All full-thickness grafts appear somewhat thin and atrophic postoperatively. A graft will work well for superficial defects of the thin-skinned zone but will look like a depressed, shiny, off-colored patch if it is placed in the thick sebaceous skin of the tip or ala. Single-lobed transposition flaps also work well in thin-skinned zones because the adjacent skin of the dorsum and sidewall is mobile and lax, providing available tissue for transfer.

2. Small, superficial defects in the zone of thick sebaceous skin should be resurfaced with local adjacent skin[4, 5] because a skin flap will restore the specialized color, texture, and skin thickness characteristic of the nasal tip and ala. Geometric bilobed flaps[6, 7] are ideal for defects up to 1.5 cm in diameter in the thick-skinned zones (Fig. 3–4). However, when local flaps are used, the residual normal skin must be spread and redistributed to cover the entire nasal surface; this skin is inadequate to cover defects larger than 1.5 cm. Such defects require tissue from the cheek (nasolabial) area or forehead.

3. In patients with deeper wounds when the underlying supportive framework has been lost, cartilage must be replaced if the nasal shape is to appear normal. Under such circumstances, a skin flap must be used for cover. Local flaps are inappropriate because a delicate reconstructed cartilage framework will collapse under the tension of local skin that has been rearranged. Skin grafts will not "take" over cartilage grafts.

4. The nasolabial flap is limited in size and arc of rotation.[8, 9] However, it provides skin that is ideal for resurfacing the entire convex ala and lobule as a unit, and it replicates the rounded shape of the alar unit as the soft tissues of the flap contract (Fig. 3–5).

5. The forehead flap is large and provides an ideal match in terms of skin color, texture, and pliability. It can be used to reconstruct the tip, dorsum, large unilateral defects, or the entire nose. Well-vascularized and lying adjacent to the nose, the forehead flap[10] is acknowledged as the ideal donor site for major reconstruction of the nose because it provides skin of an almost perfect match.[11] Because adequate midline tissue can be transferred successfully as a paramedian flap, it is unnecessary to use more distant tissues to reconstruct the nose or to expand available forehead tissue.

6. Free flaps and other distant tissues provide poorly matching skin and contradict the admonition of Gillies and Millard to employ "like for like." These tissues have become invaluable bulk solutions for the salvage of life and limb but are inappropriate for facial skin resurfacing. They can, however, be employed to revascularize an area, fill a hole, or invisibly line a nasal reconstruction that can then be covered by forehead skin, which is transferred by the traditional methods.

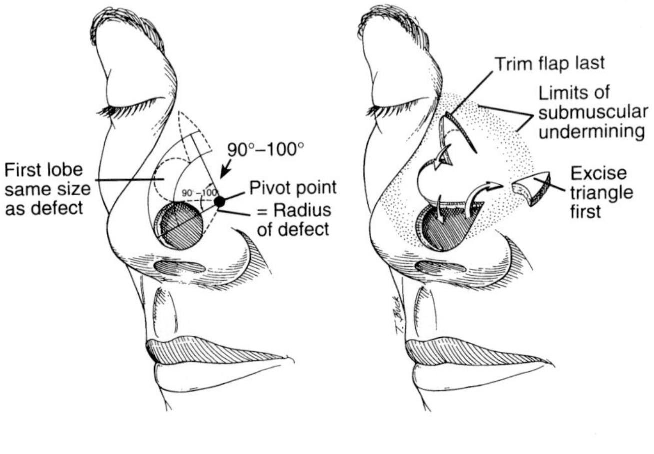

FIGURE 3–4. The geometric bilobed flap designed by Zitelli is used to transfer available loose, excess skin from the thin-skinned zone to replace small defects in the thick-skinned zones of the tip and ala. (From Burget GC, Menick FJ: Aesthetic Reconstruction of the Nose. St. Louis, Mosby–Year Book, 1994.)

RECONSTRUCTION APPLICATIONS: RESTORING A UNIT OUTLINE

Individual subunits may be exaggerated or understated in each individual, but their general outline is constant from nose to nose. Their peripheral borders mark the outer limits or boundaries between each subunit, creating a two-dimensional outcome in terms of length and width.

To restore a unit outline, the following rules[15] should be applied (Fig. 3–6).

1. The surgeon should restore the regional units, not merely fill defects. The extent of destruction does not necessarily equal the extent of reconstruction required to establish a normal appearance. Because a normal nose is defined by its regional units, the surgeon must recreate the characteristics of the unit and not simply fill the defect.

2. The wound should be altered in site, size, shape, or depth to allow reconstruction of the unit, not the defect. This means that frequently the adjacent normal tissue within a unit should be discarded, the defect enlarged, and the entire unit resurfaced rather than only the part containing the defect. This minimizes the patch-like effect that occurs when only the defect is resurfaced. As a general rule, if a defect encompasses more than 50% of a unit or subunit, the adja-

Text continued on page 20

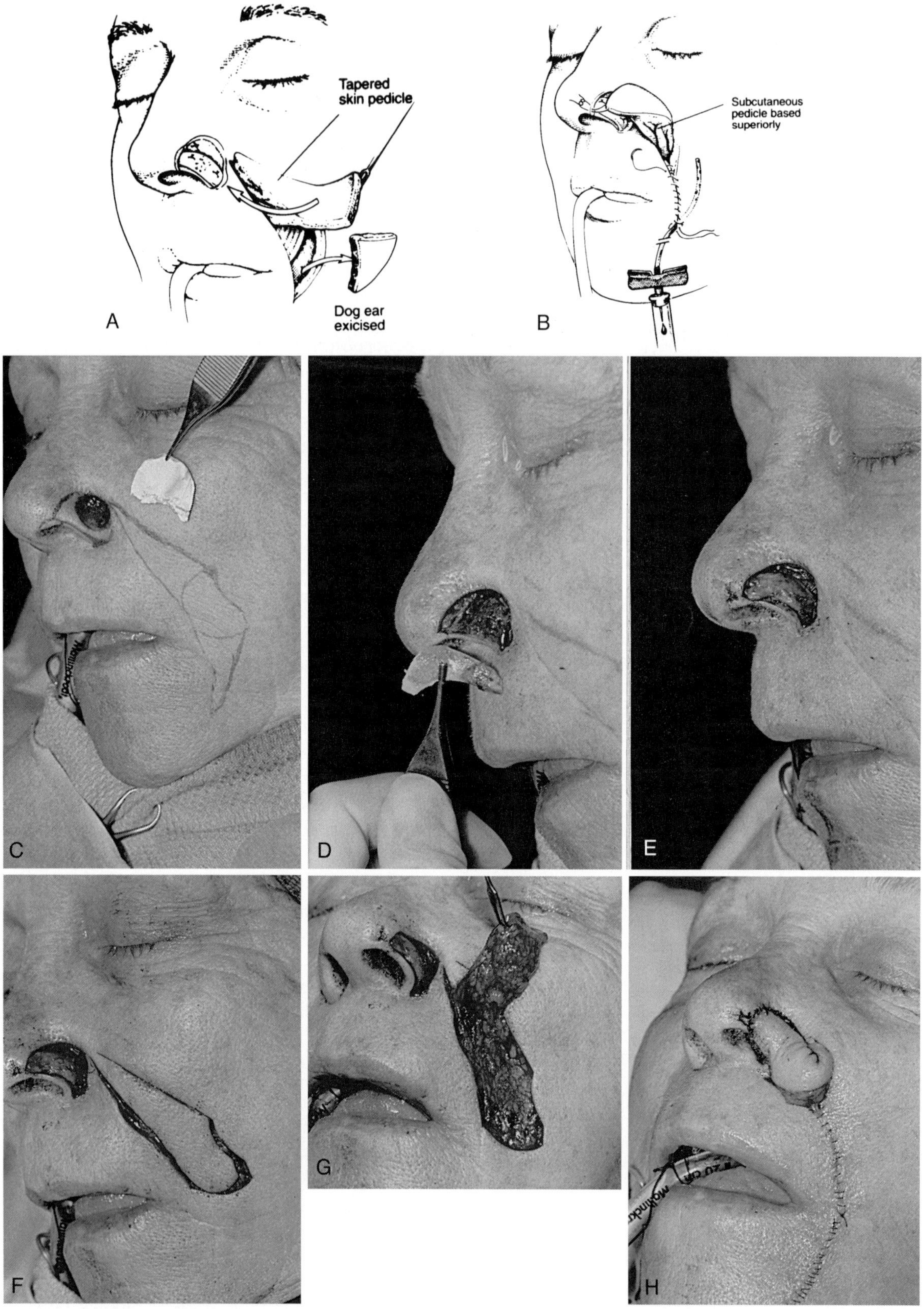

FIGURE 3–5. *A* and *B,* Excess tissue from the nasolabial fold can be transferred to repair alar defects because it is based on perforators passing vertically through the zygomatic facial muscles. *C,* A defect remains after skin cancer of the left ala has been excised. The subunit outlines of the soft triangle and alar units are marked. A foil template is cut and bent to correspond exactly to the contralateral normal right ala and is then positioned just lateral to the left nasolabial fold. The flap is tapered distally to include excision of a dog-ear and proximally to avoid extension of the late postoperative scar onto the nasal sidewall. *D,* Residual normal skin in the left alar subunit is excised, and a conchal cartilage alar batten is fashioned. *E,* With fine, nonabsorbable suture, the cartilage support batten is fixed to the residual nasal lining. *F* and *G,* The nasolabial flap is incised and elevated, maintaining the subcutaneous vertical perforators proximally. The distal flap can be thinned over its distal inset. *H,* The flap is transposed and sutured to the defect.

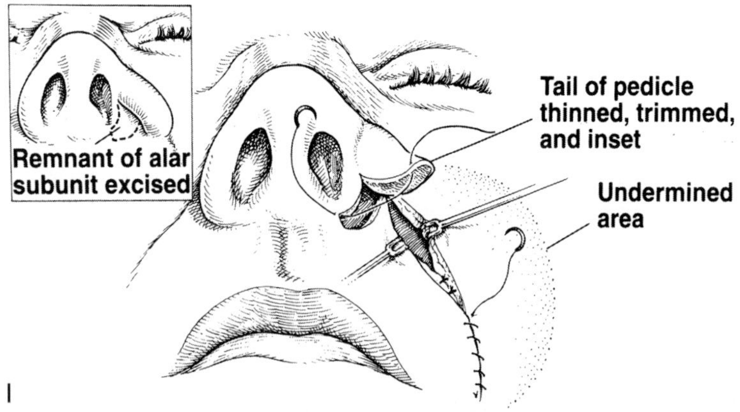

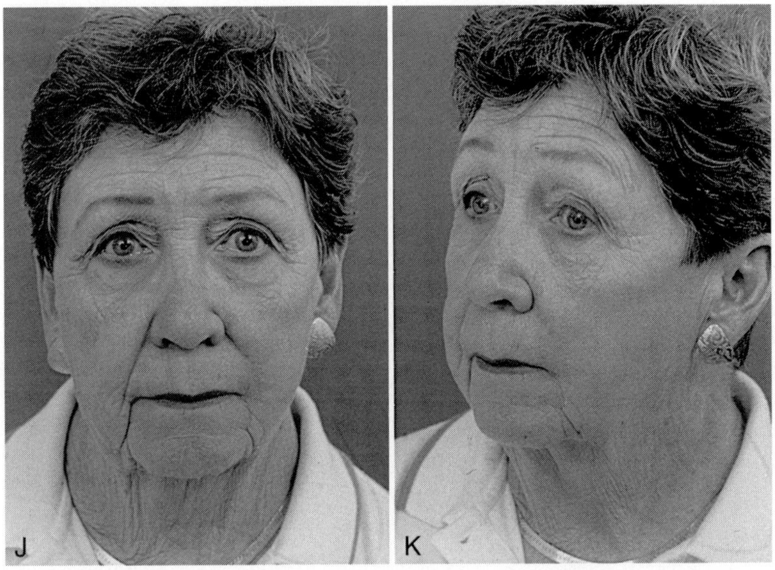

FIGURE 3–5 *Continued I,* Three weeks later, the pedicle is incised, and excess subcutaneous tissue and scar are sculpted, permitting the completion of the nasolabial flap inset into the alar base and closure of the donor site; this leaves the scar of the donor site exactly in the nasolabial fold. *J* and *K,* Postoperative result at 6 months with no further surgery. The contour and support of the left ala have been restored. The scars remain hidden in the outline border of the alar subunit and in the left nasolabial crease. (*A, B,* and *I* from Burget GC, Menick FJ: Aesthetic Reconstruction of the Nose. St. Louis, Mosby–Year Book, 1994.)

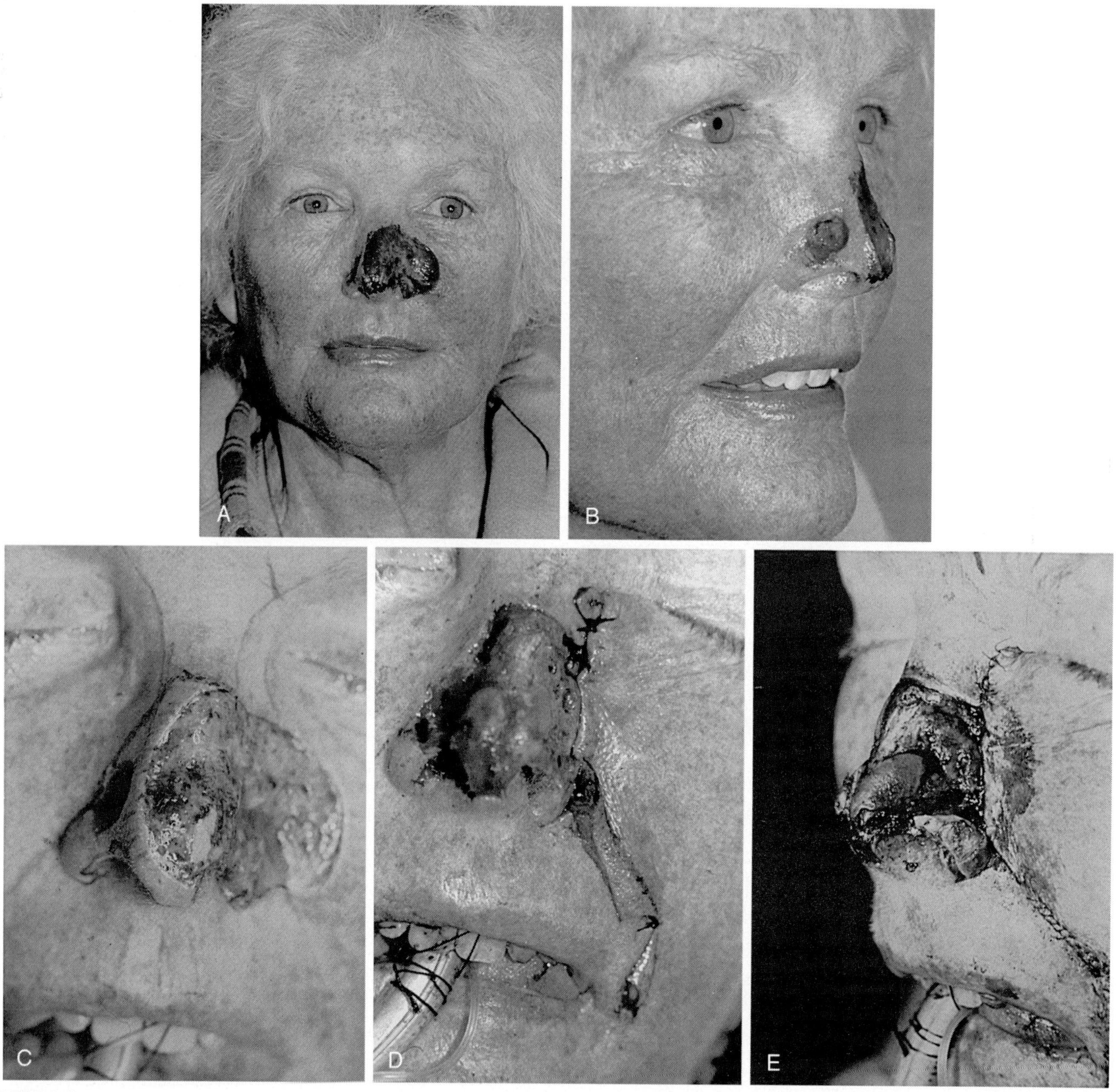

FIGURE 3–6. *A* and *B,* Nasal defects after Mohs' excision of basal cell skin cancer. A 1.3-cm defect is present overlying part of the right ala, sidewall, and tip. A larger defect extends over the tip, dorsum, left sidewall, and ala and onto the left cheek. *C,* The nasal subunits are outlined with ink on the skin surface. Residual normal nasal skin between the defects and on the tip and dorsal and left alar units will be excised. *D,* The left nasolabial fold is incised and the left cheek advanced to resurface the cheek portion of the defect with cheek skin and fat, leaving the scar within the nasal sidewall, ala, and nasolabial fold junction. *E,* A conchal cartilage graft is positioned to support and shape the left ala.

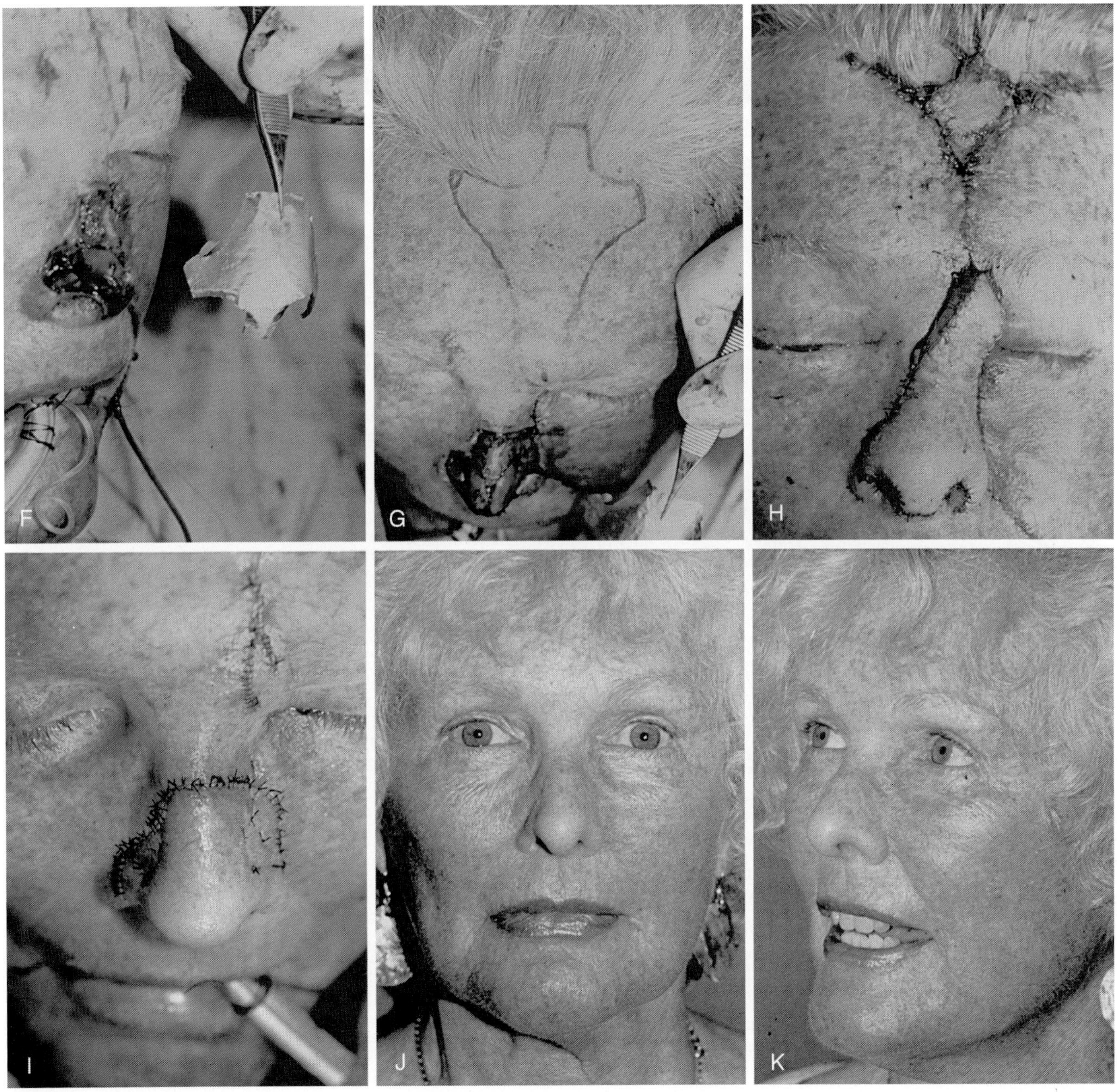

FIGURE 3–6 *Continued F* and *G,* A three-dimensional foil template is designed to replace the missing nasal covering skin exactly. It is positioned over the left supratrochlear vessels with a pedicle less than 1.2-cm wide. *H,* The forehead flap is transferred to the nose, and the 1.5- to 2.0-cm gap that remains in the forehead after partial closure of the donor site is covered with antibiotic-impregnated gauze. *I,* Three weeks later the pedicle is divided, and the distal flap is partially elevated to allow subcutaneous sculpting of excess frontalis muscle, fat, and scar. The inset of the forehead flap into the nasal defect is completed, and the proximal pedicle is trimmed and inset as a small inverted V where it simulates a glabellar frown crease. *J* and *K,* Postoperative result at 1 year. No further operations were performed. (*A* to *K* from Menick FJ: Facial reconstruction in regional units. Perspect Plast Surg 8:104, 1994.)

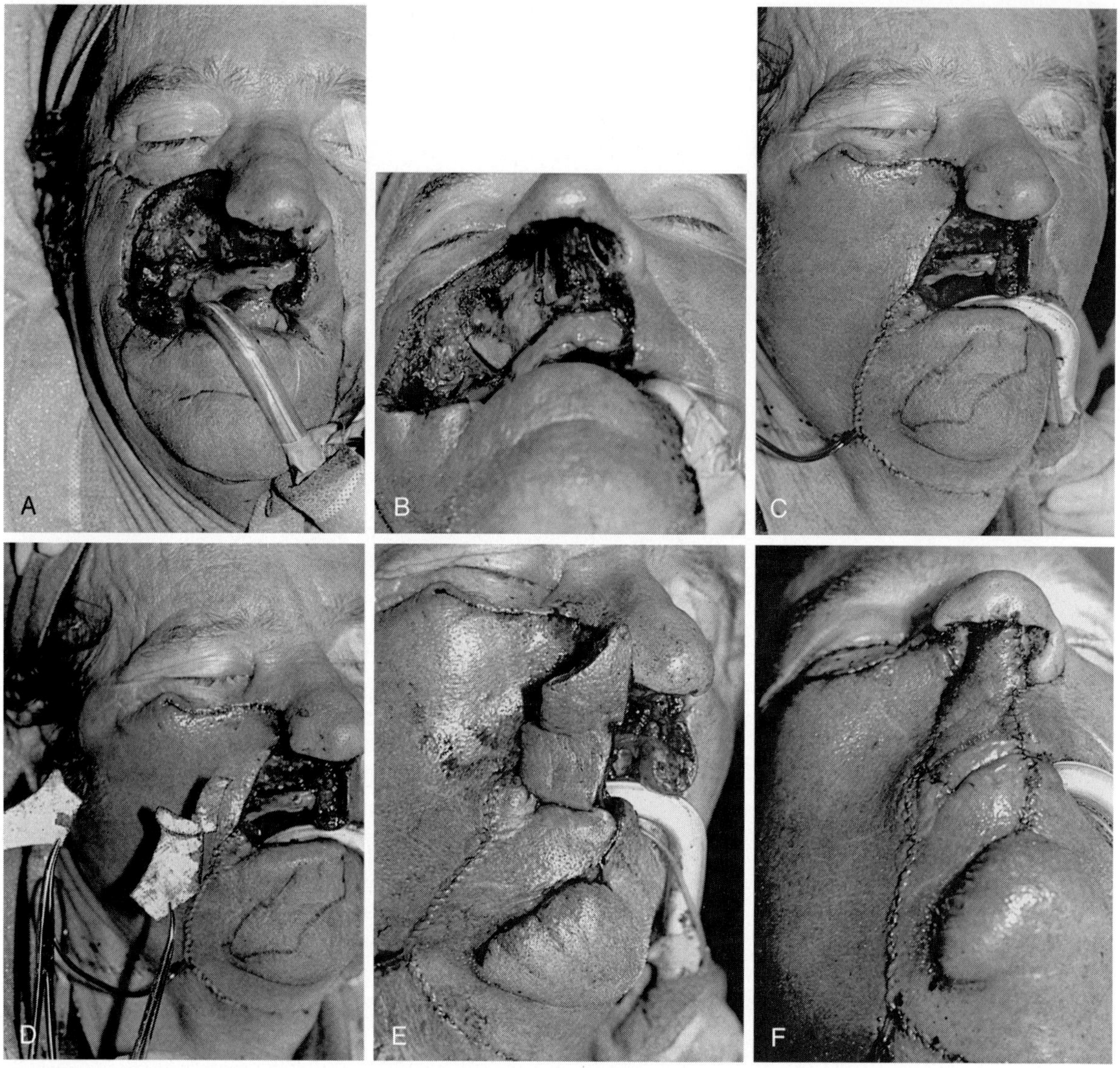

FIGURE 3–7. *A* and *B,* Defect remaining after excision of skin cancer of the right cheek, two thirds of upper lip, columella, and right ala. *C,* The cheek subunit is first restored with a superior laterally based cheek flap incised along the nasolabial fold into the submental crease. *D,* A full-thickness defect of the upper lip remains. First, using the contralateral intact left lateral upper lip unit as a pattern, a subunit template is designed and enlarged to include the missing right alar nasal sill and columella. This template is positioned in the midline of the lower lip to allow transposition of a midline subunit cross-lip Abbé flap. *E* and *F,* A composite Abbé flap of oral mucosa, muscle, and skin based on the right inferior labial artery is rotated into position to fill the upper lip defect. Closure of the donor site leaves a midline scar extending into the right mental crease.

cent normal tissue within the unit should be discarded and the wound enlarged to allow restoration of the unit and not just the defect. In other circumstances, when the defect extends over the borders of one unit to involve another, the wound edges may be advanced, creating a smaller defect that corresponds to the border between units. Frequently skin is discarded within parts of a unit, enlarging the defect, while a residual wound edge is simultaneously advanced along another of its borders, which decreases the defect. The surgeon should take charge of the wound. The defect that presents in the operating room or clinic does not correspond to the true tissue loss or to the requirements for an aesthetic restoration. It must be made to do so.

3. Scars can be raised or spread, in which case they will reflect a line of light. More often, scars are depressed and cast a linear shadow. If a line of light or shadow crosses a smooth surface where it is not expected, it will be noticed at a glance. However, if the scar is placed between topographic subunits, where it lies within the join of normal lighted ridges and shallow valleys, it will be seen as normal. Scars can be strategically placed to camouflage their borders. Border scars are best positioned so that they resemble the ridges and valleys of normal facial units and subunits. A "good" scar remains hidden from view because it is perceived visually as a "normal" facial fold or contour line. A good scar is not just a fine scar or one without suture marks, or necessarily one related to resting skin tension lines.

Equally important, the bulge of a unit flap caused by

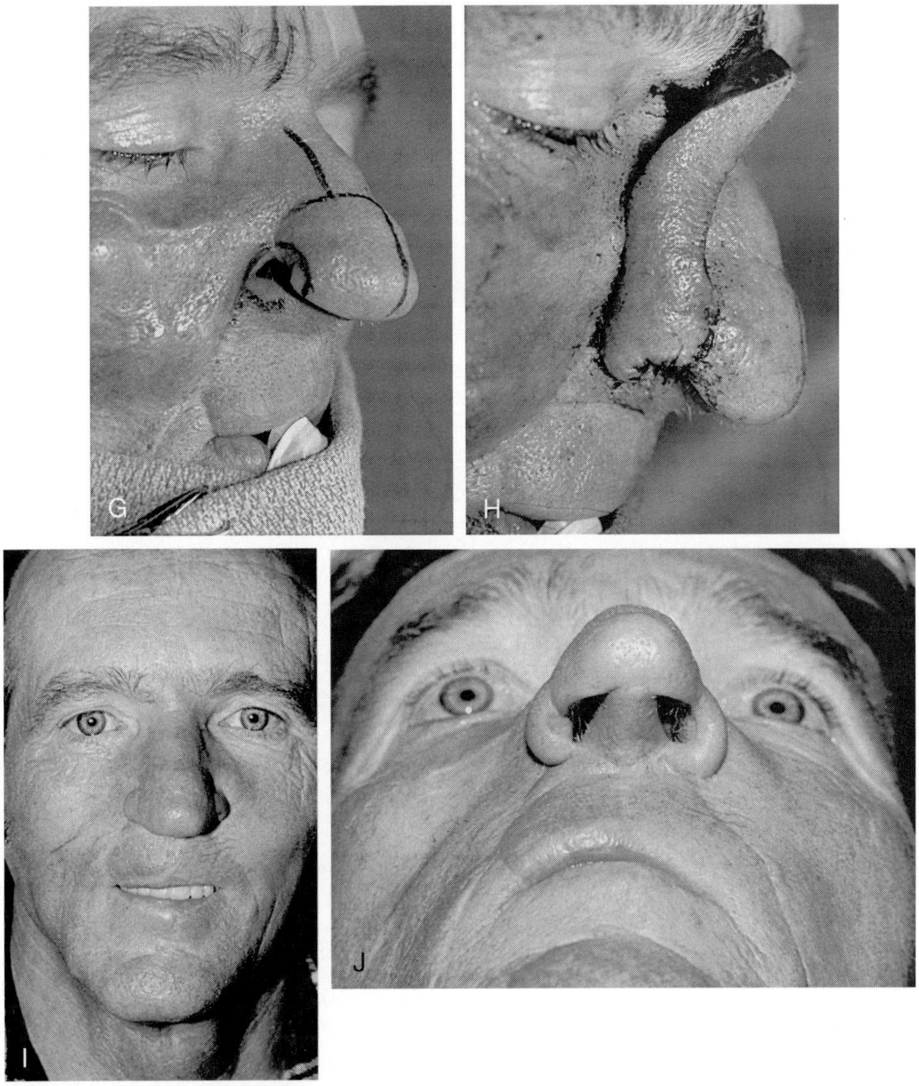

FIGURE 3–7 *Continued G* and *H,* Six weeks later, after the cheek and cross-lip Abbé flap have healed, a stable platform has been positioned for reconstruction of the full-thickness alar defect. A forehead flap that has been previously lined with a skin graft is transposed to reconstruct the missing right ala as a unit. The leaves of the forehead flap and skin graft are partially split to allow placement of a conchal cartilage graft when the forehead flap is transferred. *I* and *J,* Postoperative result 1 year after reconstruction of a massive midfacial defect following full-thickness excision of the right cheek, two thirds of the right upper lip, columella, and ala, using a cheek flap, subunit midline cross-lip Abbé flap, and a forehead flap. No further surgery was performed. (From Menick FJ, Burget GC: Nasal reconstruction: Creating a visual illusion. *In* Habal M (ed): Advances in Plastic Surgery, vol. 6. St. Louis, Mosby–Year Book, 1989.)

trapdoor contraction, which has been positioned to resurface an entire unit rather than only the part encompassed by the original defect, will mirror the normal contour of a convex subunit such as the nasal tip, ala, or dorsum. Resurfacing an entire subunit rather than part of a subunit with a flap harnesses the processes of soft tissue contraction to the advantage of the surgeon, helps ensure uniform skin quality over the entire unit, and hides scars in the unit borders.

Most often, the soft tissue defect is first modified to correspond to a unit design, and a graft or flap is then positioned within the wound, which has been enlarged by excision of the remaining skin to fit a unit outline. In other circumstances, when adjacent residual normal tissues are mobile or contain vital landmarks, a unit graft or flap is designed first and then positioned within the defect, effectively repositioning the residual soft tissues around the defect and reestablishing symmetry and the correct location of abutting landmarks. An example would be an exact unit-designed tip flap for the nose, or a philtral-shaped cross-lip Abbé flap for the upper lip that simultaneously restores the nasal tip or philtral unit while positioning the adjoining ala and lateral lip elements in their correct locations (Fig. 3–7).

4. If the exact outline and dimensions are to be reestablished, skin must be supplied to resurface the unit exactly. Replacement skin must be perfectly tailored to fit the unit defect. If a skin flap is too tight, it will cause the underlying nasal framework to collapse. If it is too large, later postoperative contraction will obscure the detail provided by primary cartilage grafts. Too little or too much skin will also distort the expected unit outline and pull inward or push outward the landmarks that lie along the border of the unit defect.

5. Exact templates based on the contralateral normal side

or the ideal must be used as guides to determine the correct amount and the outline of the missing skin. Wound edema, local anesthesia, gravity, and resting skin tension distort a fresh wound, usually enlarging it and changing its outline. Wound contracture in an old wound shrinks its borders. The size and shape of the defect do not correspond to the dimensions of the actual tissue loss and should not be used as guides to determine the dimensions of the skin required to restore the unit to normal. Fortunately, if an ala, sidewall, or half of a nose is missing, the remaining opposite side can be used to design a template that, when inverted, will correspond exactly to the size and outline of the unit that needs replacement.

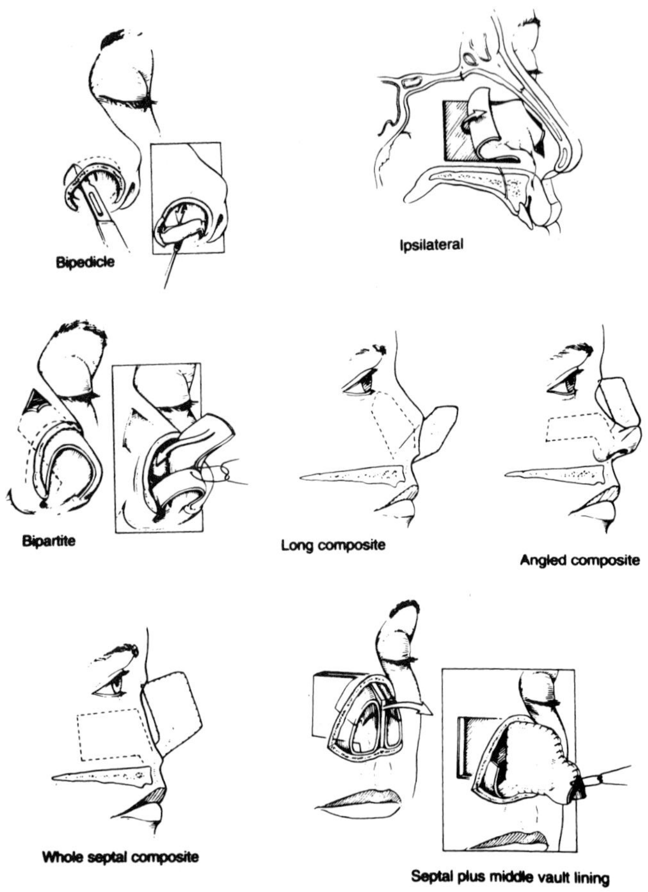

FIGURE 3–8. Residual intranasal lining based on one or both superior septal branches of the superior labial arteries can be transposed to replace missing nasal lining for various defects. (From Burget GC, Menick FJ: Aesthetic Reconstruction of the Nose. St. Louis, Mosby–Year Book, 1994.)

RECONSTRUCTION APPLICATIONS: RESTORING UNIT CONTOUR

Contour is the primary determinant of normal. Absence of scars is of lesser importance. Make-up may cover an imperfection in skin quality or scarring, but a shapeless or grotesquely distorted nose is impossible to hide. The reestablishment of correct contour must be integrated into each and every step of nasal reconstruction. Contour influences the choice of donor materials, the timing and method of framework restoration, and the sequence of surgical stages.

Cover, lining, and support materials must be thin and flexible. Only lining flaps[16, 17] taken from intranasal donor sites (vestibule, middle, vault, and septum) (Fig. 3–8) or staged sequential skin grafts (Fig. 3–9) are so thin that their bulk neither distorts the shape of the overlying cartilage and covering skin nor bulges in the airway and obstructs breathing. They are soft enough to conform to the desired cartilaginous contour, yet vascular enough to nourish primary cartilage grafts without any risk of extrusion.

The use of primary cartilage and bone grafts allows the surgeon to construct an assembly of hard tissue pieces into a nasal shape. When the nasal surface is supplied by a thin forehead flap, the shape of this cartilage construction shows through the skin, and the contour of the nose is correct from the outset. Cover and lining flaps provide the soft tissue canopy. Primary cartilage grafts provide the rigidity and resilience necessary for support, projection and space, airway patency, and a nasal shape. The new nose becomes permanently fixed by virtue of the cartilage that backs its lining. The entire soft tissue restoration is braced against the contractile effects of the wound myofibroblast.

Nasal support[18] must be supplied during construction of the soft tissue lining and cover because once soft tissue collapse occurs, it becomes fixed by constricting scars. Secondary placement of nasal support cannot fully regain what has been lost. If missing, the normal cartilaginous framework of the dorsum, tip, and sidewall should be replaced as it was before. Additionally, a narrow strip of cartilage should be placed along the new nostril margin even though the alar lobule normally contains no cartilage. This cartilage braces the alar rim and prevents contracture inward and upward and collapse during the healing phase.

Four different hard tissue grafts are required for a major nasal restoration—a buttress, a brace, a batten, and a strut. Each piece fixes the underlying mucosal lining in position, imparting shape to the overlying surface subunit (Fig. 3–10). Struts of septal or conchal cartilage 4.0 mm wide can be scored and bent to form a replacement for one or both of the alar cartilages. These alar cartilage replicas are fixed to the stump of any residual medial crura, scored and bent laterally, and sutured to the reconstructed lining of the vestibule. They support the lining of the nasal dome and recreate the shape of the nasal tip. Added tip projection can be achieved by adding one or two Peck-type grafts 4.0 × 9.0 mm wide, which are anchored to the top of these newly reconstructed cartilage domes. A sidewall brace of septal cartilage and bone can be harvested and trimmed to a trapezoidal shape. Once positioned on the nasal sidewall lining, the brace acts as a replacement for the upper lateral cartilage

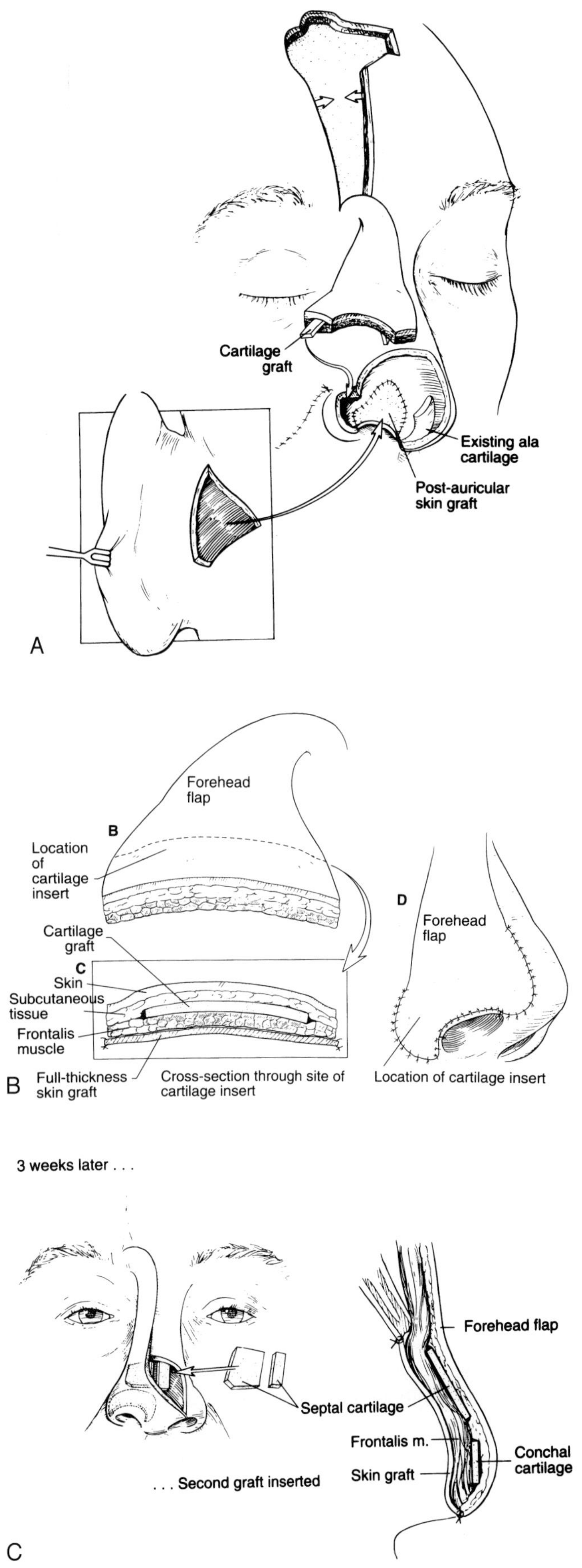

FIGURE 3–9. *A* and *B,* Because of its great vascularity, a forehead flap can be used to revascularize a full-thickness skin graft employed to line the nose at the time of forehead flap transfer. *A,* Positioned with its raw surface outward, a postauricular skin graft is used to replace the missing nasal lining. *B,* Because the forehead flap is composed of skin, subcutaneous tissue, and frontalis muscle, a primary cartilage graft can be placed in a subcutaneous tunnel between the skin and the frontalis muscle without compromising the skin graft. A supported and contoured alar rim is thus restored at the initial operation. *C,* If sidewall support is missing, a sidewall cartilaginous brace can be shaped and positioned 3 weeks later, after the skin graft has solidly healed to the adjacent normal lining and to the forehead flap. The forehead flap can then be elevated as a bipedicle flap attached at its origin at the brow and distally at the nasal tip and ala. Subcutaneous tissue, frontalis muscle, and scar are excised, exposing the now well-vascularized skin graft. A delayed primary cartilage graft support can then be positioned to brace the sidewall unit, and the forehead flap is divided or repositioned until its final division 3 weeks later. (*A* to *C* from Burget GC, Menick FJ: Aesthetic Reconstruction of the Nose. St. Louis, Mosby–Year Book, 1994.)

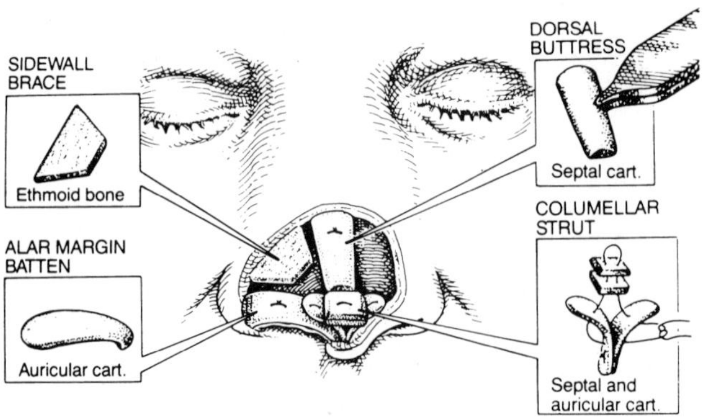

FIGURE 3–10. A cartilaginous support framework should be positioned prior to completion of wound healing to supply nasal support, a three-dimensional nasal shape, and airway patency. (From Burget GC, Menick FJ: Nasal support and lining: The marriage of beauty and blood supply. Plast Reconstr Surg 84:189, 1989.)

and nasal bone. It supports the middle vault against collapse and braces the nasal sidewall against upward contraction. An alar rim batten can be placed along the leading edge of the lining sleeve from the alar base to the nostril apex. Buried in a pocket laterally and attached medially to the tip framework, it fixes the new alar rim in position and provides a normal bulging contour to the reconstructed alar lobule. A bridge buttress of layered septal or rib cartilage can be installed along the dorsum to prevent upward contraction and postoperative shortening of the nose. In this position, it gives shape and projection to the nasal bridge and reconstructs the form of the dorsal subunit. The surgeon, after analyzing the defect, must determine which part of this internal nasal chassis is missing and replace it as necessary.

Because the ala sits on a platform of lip and cheek in a precise facial location and angle, no attempt should be made to reconstruct the nose and lip simultaneously (see Fig. 3–9). If the lip, cheek, and ala require reconstruction, only the lip and cheek should be rebuilt initially.[19] If such multiple three-dimensional units are fabricated at one sitting, subsequent wound settling will distort the position of the newly reconstructed ala. Wound contraction shifts the lip and cheek platform, dragging the new nose inferiorly and laterally. If both the nose and lip or cheek are lost, the nose should be made at a second stage when its platform is stable.

The surgeon should not fall prey to the obvious temptation of filling the entire defect with one flap. Several unfortunate sequelae ensue if this is done. First, residual scars are more obvious because they are not placed within the normal contour lines such as the join of the ala and lip. Second, it is impossible to reproduce the delicate three-dimensional character of multiple units with a single flap. Although additional revisions to reshape and debulk the reconstruction may be planned in the hope of reestablishing the contour of the alae, lip, or sidewall junction, they most often fail or are forgotten. Third, the dorsal subunit normally has a hemicylindrical shape, and the tip and ala a hemispherical contour. Convex forms reflect visual central highlights and create peripheral shadows from which we extrapolate the nasal contour. Postoperative flap trapdoor contraction draws soft tissue into a convex shape, creating reflected highlights and shadows. If a defect involving several contoured units is filled with a single flap, a single unexpected, misplaced highlight is created rather than the expected three-dimensional subunit highlights.

Traditionally, a forehead flap is positioned, and its pedicle is divided 3 weeks later. Multiple late revisions are planned to partially elevate the borders of the transferred flap and to carve its scarred subcutaneous tissue into a nasal shape. However, both the speed of reconstruction and the aesthetic result can be improved by planning an intermediate operation (Fig. 3–11). Three weeks after the initial reconstruction, when the forehead flap is well healed to the recipient bed, it can be elevated at a superficial subcutaneous level over most of its surface, leaving it attached only along some of the alar margin and all of the columella. The vascular pedicle is not divided. Because it has a good blood supply through the supratrochlear vessels at the brow and from its distal inset at the columella, it can be safely thinned nearly to the thickness of nasal tip skin. Underlying fat, scar, and frontalis muscle can be sculpted to give the recipient bed a nasal shape. If projection is inadequate, additional shaped septal or ear cartilage grafts may be added. The flap is then reinset into its newly shaped recipient bed. Three weeks later (6 weeks after the primary operation), the proximal pedicle is divided, and the final inset into the nasal defect is completed after further soft tissue sculpturing.

SUMMARY

In summary, a number of subunit principles should be applied to the reconstruction of facial defects to create an aesthetically pleasing result.

1. The primary function of the face is to look normal. Patients desire both a healed wound and the restoration of a normal appearance.
2. Our eyes "see" the unexpected and disregard what is or simulates normal.
3. A normal facial appearance is determined by the restoration of facial contour, skin quality, and regional outline; the absence of scars is of lesser importance.
4. A facial defect must be analyzed in terms of anatomic loss and the visual subunits affected. Principles and techniques must be utilized to resupply the missing tissue components and to reestablish the visual appearance of normal.
5. The surgeon should restore units, not fill defects. The final result is determined less by what is missing than by what is replaced. Flaps are designed to replace topographic units, not defects. Flap designs are taken from the contour configurations found in every human nose and are used to camouflage the final result.
6. The wound should be altered in size, site, shape, outline, and depth to improve the result.

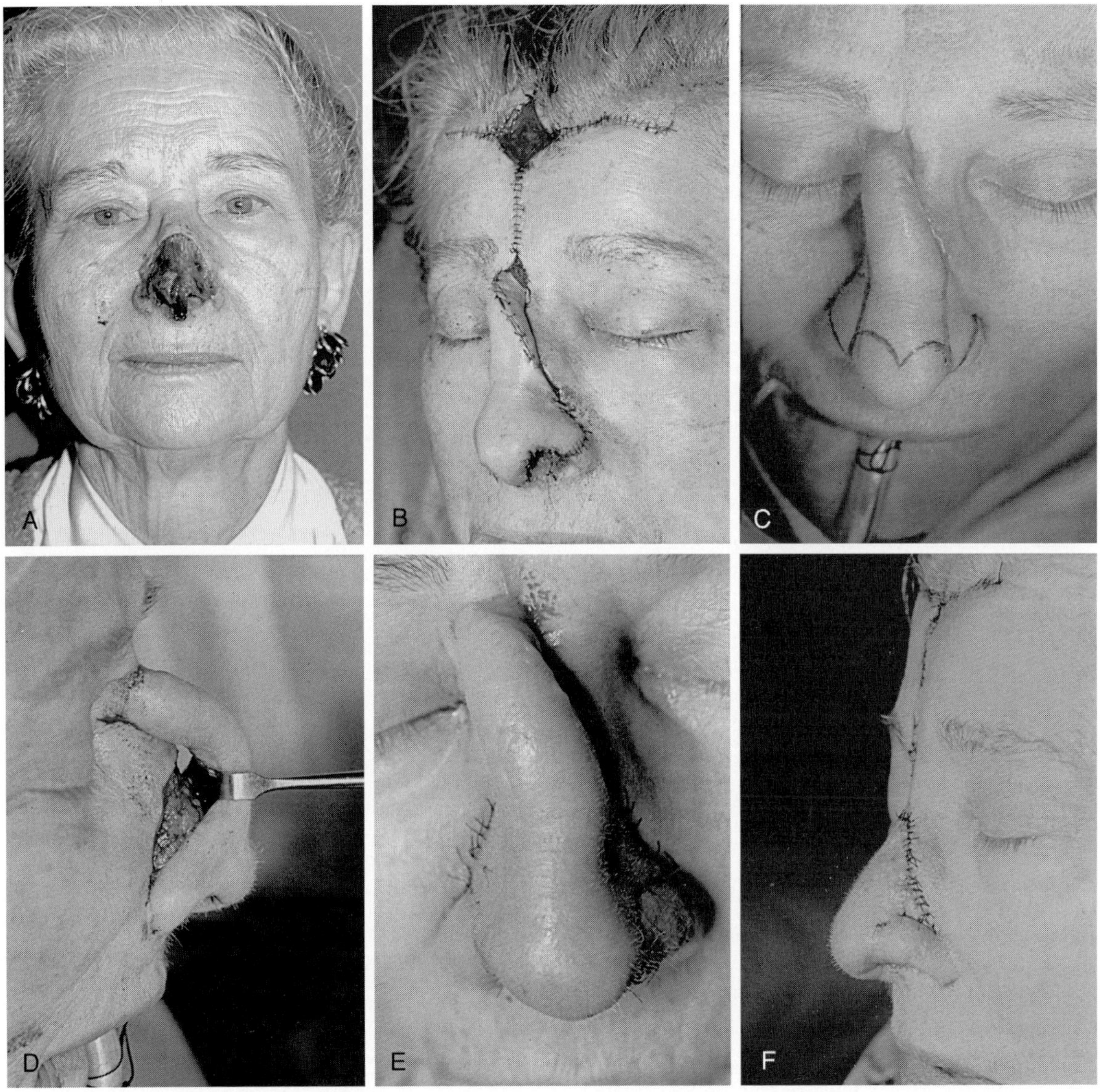

FIGURE 3–11. *A* Nasal defect encompassing the nasal tip, dorsum, sidewall, and ala after Mohs excision of skin cancer. *B,* After the necessary support grafts have been placed, a full-thickness forehead flap is designed to resurface the defect. No surgical thinning of the flap is performed. *C,* At 3 weeks, the expected unit contour lines are drawn onto the skin surface of the somewhat bulky but well-healed forehead flap. *D,* At 3 weeks, rather than dividing the pedicle, the flap is elevated as a bipedicle base flap proximally at the brow and distally at its inset into the tip, columella, and alar margin. Excessive subcutaneous tissue, frontalis muscle, and scar are excised to create an appropriate subsurface nasal shape. *E,* The forehead flap is replaced. *F,* Three weeks later (6 weeks after initiation of nasal reconstruction) the forehead flap pedicle is divided, and the inset into the nasal defect is completed.

Illustration continued on following page

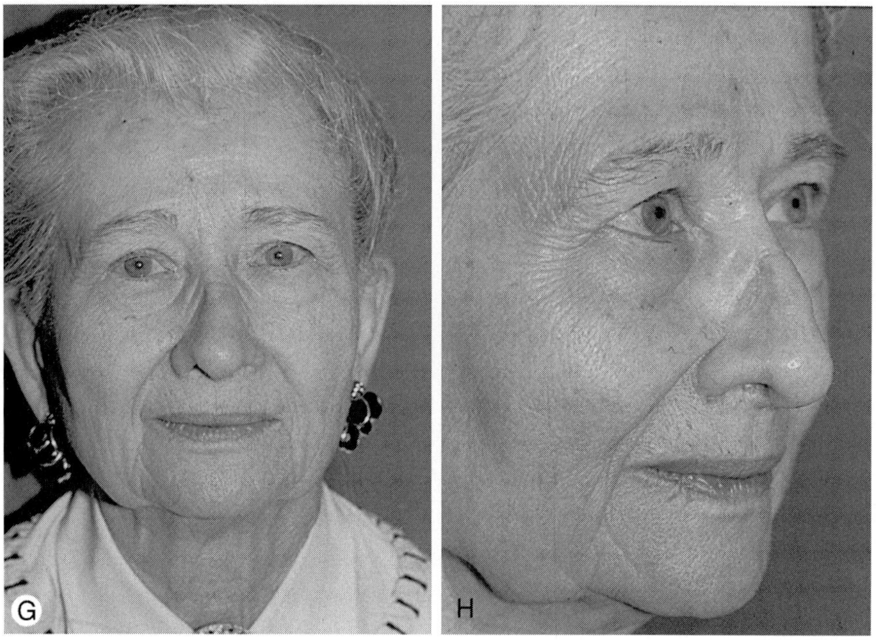

FIGURE 3–11 *Continued G* and *H,* Postoperative result at 8 months after three operations, including an intermediate operation for subcutaneous sculpturing.

7. Adjacent normal tissue should be discarded when necessary to enhance the final result.

8. Scars and normal facial folds should be positioned in contour lines to decrease their visibility.

9. The nose should be built on a stable platform.

10. One should choose ideal donor materials and methods of tissue transfer. The method of tissue transfer should be selected based on its qualities of blood supply and on the effects of wound healing on the final result. Tissue is replaced by similar tissue in three dimensions.

11. Missing tissues are replaced in exact quantities. Exact patterns are used as guides in the design of grafts and flaps.

12. The contralateral normal side or the ideal is used as a template.

13. Contour is the primary determinant of normal. It is determined by the form of the underlying hard and soft tissues and by the effects of wound healing.

14. Contour is integrated into each and every stage of reconstruction.

15. A support framework is positioned prior to the completion of wound healing. A three-dimensional reconstruction is braced against the force of the myofibroblast.

16. Recipient and donor sites must be chosen and treated aesthetically.

REFERENCES

1. Menick FJ: Artistry in aesthetic surgery: Aesthetic perceptions and the subunit principle. Clin Plast Surg 14:723–725, 1987.
2. Burget GC, Menick FJ: Subunit principle in nasal reconstruction. Plast Reconstr Surg 76:239, 1985.
3. Burget GC, Menick FJ: Aesthetic Reconstruction of the Nose. St. Louis, Mosby–Year Book, 1994.
4. Elliot RA Jr: Rotation flaps of the nose. Plast Reconstr Surg 14:723–735, 1969.
5. Rieger RA: A local flap for repair of the nasal tip. Plast Reconstr Surg 40:147, 1967.
6. Zitelli JA: The bilobed flap for nasal reconstruction. Arch Dermatol 125:957, 1989.
7. Zimany A: The bilobed flap. Plast Reconstr Surg 11:424, 1953.
8. Herbert DC, Harrison RG: Nasolabial subcutaneous pedicle flaps: 1. Observations on their blood supply. Br J Plast Surg 28:85, 1975.
9. Herbert DC: A subcutaneous pedicle cheek flap for reconstruction of alar defects. Br J Plast Surg 31:79–92, 1978.
10. McCarthy JG, Lorenc PZ, Cutting C, et al: The median forehead flap revisited: The blood supply. Plast Reconstr Surg 76:866–869, 1985.
11. Menick FJ: The aesthetic use of the forehead for nasal reconstruction—The paramedian forehead flaps. Clin Plast Surg 17:607–620, 1990.
12. Menick FJ: Principles of head and neck reconstruction. *In* Cohen M (ed): Mastery in Surgery: Plastic and Reconstructive Surgery. Boston, Little, Brown (in press).
13. Menick FJ, Burget, GC: Aesthetic reconstruction of the nose. *In* Cohen M (ed): Mastery in Surgery: Plastic and Reconstructive Surgery. Boston, Little, Brown (in press).
14. Menick FJ, Burget GC: Nasal reconstruction: Creating a visual illusion. *In* Habal M (ed): Advances in Plastic Surgery, Vol 6. St. Louis, Mosby–Year Book, 1989.
15. Menick FJ: Aesthetic restoration of the face. *In* Cohen M (ed): Problems in General Surgery. Philadelphia, J.B. Lippincott, 1989.
16. Burget GC, Menick FJ: Nasal support and lining: The marriage of beauty and blood supply. Plast Reconstr Surg 84:189, 1989.
17. Burget GC, Menick FJ: Nasal reconstruction: Seeking a fourth dimension. Plast Reconstr Surg 78:145, 1989.
18. Burget GC, Menick FJ: Restoration of nasal defects—an aesthetic viewpoint. *In* Jurkiewicz M, Krizek T (eds): Plastic Surgery—Principles and Practice. St. Louis, Mosby–Year Book, 1990.
19. Burget GC, Menick FJ: Aesthetic reconstruction of one-half of the upper lip. Plast Reconstr Surg 78:583, 1986.

CHAPTER 4

Subtotal Nasal Reconstruction

Fred J. Stucker, M.D.
Paul C. Drago, M.D.
Paul Goco, M.D.

Nasal reconstruction was first performed around 3000 BC in India.[1] The first modern forehead flap was performed in America by Warren in 1837. In 1966 Millard pioneered the concepts that set the stage for today's practice of nasal reconstruction. He described modifications in harvesting forehead flaps, the creation of an internal nasal lining with nasal skin, turn-in flaps, and the creation of dorsal and tip support with chondromucosal septal composite flaps.[2, 3] Millard also wrote about the subunit principle, which he summarized by saying that in general it is better to cover the entire half nose with a one-piece unit than to patch the whole nose.[4] Burget and Menick popularized the principles of subunit nasal reconstruction in 1985.[5] They emphasized that similar tissue should replace similar tissue. The development of their work is well illustrated through the field.[6] Adamson and others have also expanded the applications of the midline forehead flap.[7, 8]

The blood supply for the median and paramedian forehead flaps comes from the vertically oriented supraorbital and supratrochlear vessels. Classic anatomy books describe a natural dehiscence in the midline of the frontalis muscle. Thus the forehead flap has less bulk and makes more ideal flap. Burget and Menick proposed making the flap with a narrower base, which not only eases donor site closure but also facilitates rotation, which in turn results in a longer flap.[9] In 1992, Shumrick and Smith described the blood supply to the forehead flap in a cadaveric study.[10] They demonstrated that the supratrochlear artery consistently anastomoses with the angular, supraorbital, and frontal branches of the superficial temporal arteries. Doppler examination of healthy volunteers consistently showed that the supratrochlear artery lay in the paramedian position (1.5 to 2.0 cm from the midline), which corresponds roughly to the medial portion of the eyebrow. The supratrochlear artery is a branch of the internal carotid system, and the paired supratrochlear arteries freely anastomose with one another. Proximally, the supratrochlear arteries pass superficial to the corrugator muscle and deep to the orbicularis and frontalis muscles. As the arteries ascend, they perforate the frontalis muscle and travel just under the dermal plexus in the upper third of the forehead. This anatomic arrangement allows significant thinning and debulking of the flap during the primary operation.

Depending on the defect, the bony or cartilaginous skeleton may have to be reconstructed. If the bony skeleton has to be replaced, the best option is to use a split calvarial graft. This graft can be attached to the skull using miniplates or wire fixation. The parietal bone is most often chosen as the donor site. Local skin flaps can be draped over this bony support. If the cartilaginous portion of the nose needs reconstruction, the best donor sites are conchal cartilage and septal cartilage. Both are readily available and easily harvested. Percutaneous placement of sutures may be needed to align these grafts properly.

The use of cartilage composite grafts is over 100 years old. In 1887, Konig used and described the principles of composite grafting.[11] His first series of 47 cases resulted in a 53% rate of graft survival. Autogenous graft tissue is widely preferred to homografts because it has a predictable resorption rate and it avoids the potential transmission of infectious diseases.

The issue of graft survival has been the major problem when using homologous tissue. In 1986, Donald reported a rate of 87.7% resorption of irradiated cartilage in dog and sheep models.[12] However, he noted only a 43.8% resorption rate with grafts treated with thimerosal (merthiolate). Long- and short-term resorption rates are probably a multifactorial process that is intimately related to the immune system.[13] Merthiolate decreases antigenicity, therefore allowing less cellular processing of immunogenic agents and decreasing the rate of resorption. Currently, intense radiation is the preferred method of sterilizing homogeneous cartilage. It has been shown to destroy most organisms, including viruses,[14] and is widely available from tissue banks in the United States. The average dosage ranges from 1.8 to 2.3 mrad using gamma irradiation from a cobalt-60 source. Graft resorption rates vary depending on where the graft is placed on the face.[15] Grafts placed in areas of overlying muscle movement are more subject to resorption,[16] whereas grafts within the nasal framework tend to show less resorption.[17] This fact may explain the wide discrepancies in success rates that have been reported.

Graft survival, and therefore, indirectly, resorption, depends on (1) immediate serum imbibition, (2) inosculation within 24 hours, and (3) neovascularization within 3 to 5 days.[18] Early revascularization is most important to the survival of cartilage grafts, and the presence of attached perichondrium greatly enhances the likelihood of success. Other factors critical to graft survival include the size of graft, the graft harvesting technique used, preparation of the recipient site, and graft placement.[19] The use of preoperative corticosteroid therapy was deemed important in a rabbit study,[20] but postoperative corticosteroids given to animals in an attempt to salvage a composite graft proved ineffective.

The need for subtotal nasal reconstruction arises from a variety of causes. Most commonly, these causes include oncologic resection and traumatic events such as avulsion, burns, human and animal bites, industrial accidents, and altercations. Soft tissue injuries of the nose can involve one or all of the following structures: skin, subcutaneous fat, nasal musculature, and endonasal lining. Other structures that must be assessed include the nasal cartilages and fibrous attachments, the nasal bony structures, the nasal septum and its respective coverings, perichondrium, and periosteum. It is important to be aware of the type of mechanism that caused the injury and to administer the appropriate drugs (e.g., antibiotics, tetanus prophylaxis, antirabies immunoglobulin, and so on). Assessment of nasal defects is facilitated by computed tomography, fiberoptic instruments, and better illumination. In patients with traumatic injuries a formal ophthalmologic evaluation should be considered because the incidence of ocular damage associated with nasal or midface fractures has been reported to be as high as 59%.[21]

PLANNING AND DESIGN OF LOCAL FLAPS

As with any reconstruction, the adjacent tissues and their structures must be taken into account. The reconstructive surgeon must be mindful of the tissue and the defect that will result if it is used as a flap. The donor site must have an adequate blood supply to close the defect created. This closure is usually done primarily. Closure lines are optimally placed in the natural skin creases or in relaxed skin tension lines. The tension or closure should be minimized with wide undermining when appropriate. Placement of the necessary incisions, and thus the closure lines, is the critical factor and should be kept in mind when designing the flap. Ectropion, unacceptable scars, and asymmetry between the sides of the face are only a few of the complications that must be avoided. As with all incisions, the surgeon should plan for the natural process of scarring with its resulting contracture and maximum pull, and all connections should be designed to minimize these adverse effects.

SURGICAL TECHNIQUES

More than 90% of our patients who require subtotal nasal reconstruction are managed by using three workhorse local flaps and the perichondrial cutaneous graft. The three flaps are the nasolabial flap, the sliding nasal dorsal flap, and the paramedian forehead flap. Architectural design and support are provided wholly by the use of autogenous cartilage and calvarial bone grafts.

The Paramedian Forehead Flap

For unilateral defects the paramedian forehead flap is usually used, based on the supratrochlear artery contralateral to the nasal defect. Either side of the forehead can usually be used, regardless of the location of the defect, because of the narrow base recommended by Burget and Menick.[9] Either palpation or Doppler examination provides the exact location of the flap's base. The base is usually placed low to allow for maximum rotation. So consistent is the blood supply that the senior author (FJS) has not employed Doppler examination in over 200 cases and reports no failures using only clinical landmarks.

The shape of the flap is planned using a foil template or suture wrapper to correspond to the defect (Fig. 4–1). After the paramedian flap has been elevated, the midline forehead defect is closed with horizontally oriented sliding forehead advancement flaps. Not infrequently, there is a central portion of the wound that cannot be closed by this means, and this is left to heal by secondary intention. Tissue expansion has been used preoperatively for defects greater than 5 cm; however, the senior author does not find this technique particularly helpful. The flap includes skin, subcutaneous tissue, frontalis muscle, and galea aponeurotica. The average flap is 2 to 4 cm in width and 6 to 9 cm in length.[22] For resurfacing the nasal tip, the flap should be debulked, especially primarily along the random portion at its apex, to more naturally match the corresponding defect. The arc of rotation used can be up to 180 degrees. The flap is divided during a second-stage procedure, usually within 2 to 3 weeks, depending on convenience and other associated conditions of the patient, such as diabetes, prior irradiation, and the concurrent use of tobacco. This flap is the most reliable

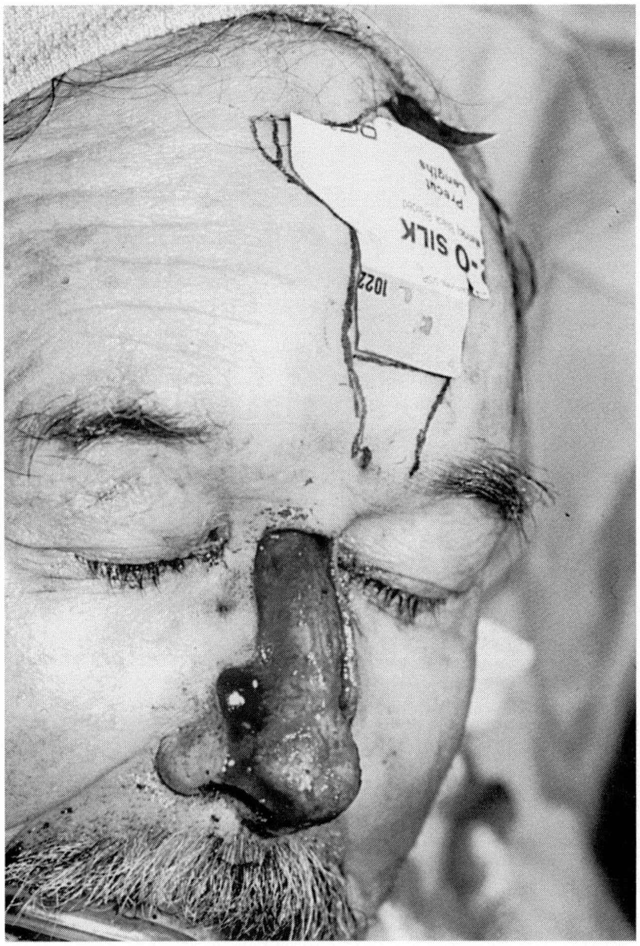

FIGURE 4–1. Template used to map defect.

of all facial flaps and is remarkable for its adaptability (Fig. 4–2).

The tip of the flap is often curvilinear. The incisions near the flap's base are made just through the skin in order not to disturb the vessels in the pedicle.

It is imperative to remember that the internal lining of the nasal defect must also be addressed. Local advancement flaps from the nasal septum or local epidermal turn-in flaps are most often used and provide excellent coverage of the internal nasal lining.[23] These epidermal turn-in flaps are thin, consisting only of skin except in the hinge, and are sutured into position. After internal lining has been provided but prior to resurfacing, the supporting tissue, usually cartilage, is placed (Fig. 4–3).

Sliding Nasal Dorsal Flap

The sliding nasal dorsal flap is an excellent flap and has been used to reconstruct full-thickness wounds of the nose that may or may not extend onto the medial canthus. It consists of a single-stage reconstructive option and produces consistently excellent results. The flap is essentially a V-Y advancement flap that takes advantage of the excess skin in the intercanthal and glabellar regions. The flap can cover defects of the lateral nose, nasal tip, and nasal dorsum. Because it is based (hinged) on one side, it slides into the defect. After the skin has been elevated, it is rotated inferiorly. The triangular defect in the glabellar region is closed primarily. Superiorly, the skin edges are closed in the standard V-Y fashion. This flap is not as reliable as the midline forehead flap, but with careful planning the outcome is regularly successful. The flap's reliability is increased when the pedicle is not narrow. This is a full-thickness flap in which the periosteum and perichondrium remain undisturbed. Because the flap does not violate the angular vessels, it is an excellent choice for the reconstruction of relatively large nasal defects. To avoid encountering the angular vessels and to ensure success, the two sides of the flap are treated differently. The base side of the flap's elevation includes everything but the periosteum and perichondrium; thus, the base is quite thick and includes the angular vessels. The free end includes only skin and thus avoids the vessels, leaving them deep and undisturbed. This flap produces excellent results if the incisions are correctly placed (Fig. 4–4).

Nasolabial Flaps

The nasolabial flap is considered the workhorse flap for nasal reconstruction, thus, it has often been overused. It is extremely dependable and reliable. This flap has been used for the repair of nasal defects since the earliest description of facial reconstruction. Several variations have been described, and the flap can be based either superiorly or inferiorly. It is a random flap that relies on the distal branches of the angular and facial vessels.

There is an abundance of mobile skin in the medial cheek area that is easily mobilized. Primary closure of the defect can be well hidden in the nasolabial cheek fold or the lateral border of the nose, producing minimal postoperative deformity.

Planning the incision for the superiorly based flap is based on the defect to be covered. Dissection and elevation are performed deep to the subdermal plexus and within the subcutaneous plane. The same plane of dissection is used in the cheek area to advance the cheek locally and close the defect primarily. The nasolabial flap can be used for endonasal lining by employing it as a turn-in flap.

The nasolabial flap can also be based inferiorly. Defects that are ideal for the inferiorly based flap include those of the floor of the nose and the columellar and alar regions. The flap length must be at least as long as the defect is tall. Careful placement of the ala at a second stage can yield excellent results (Fig. 4–5).

Perichondrial Cutaneous Graft

The perichondrial cutaneous graft (PCCG) has been used extensively for resurfacing nasal defects for nearly 20 years. The graft, which is a single-stage reconstructive procedure, is extremely reliable and predictable. The cosmetic results are consistently excellent. The graft is based on the principle

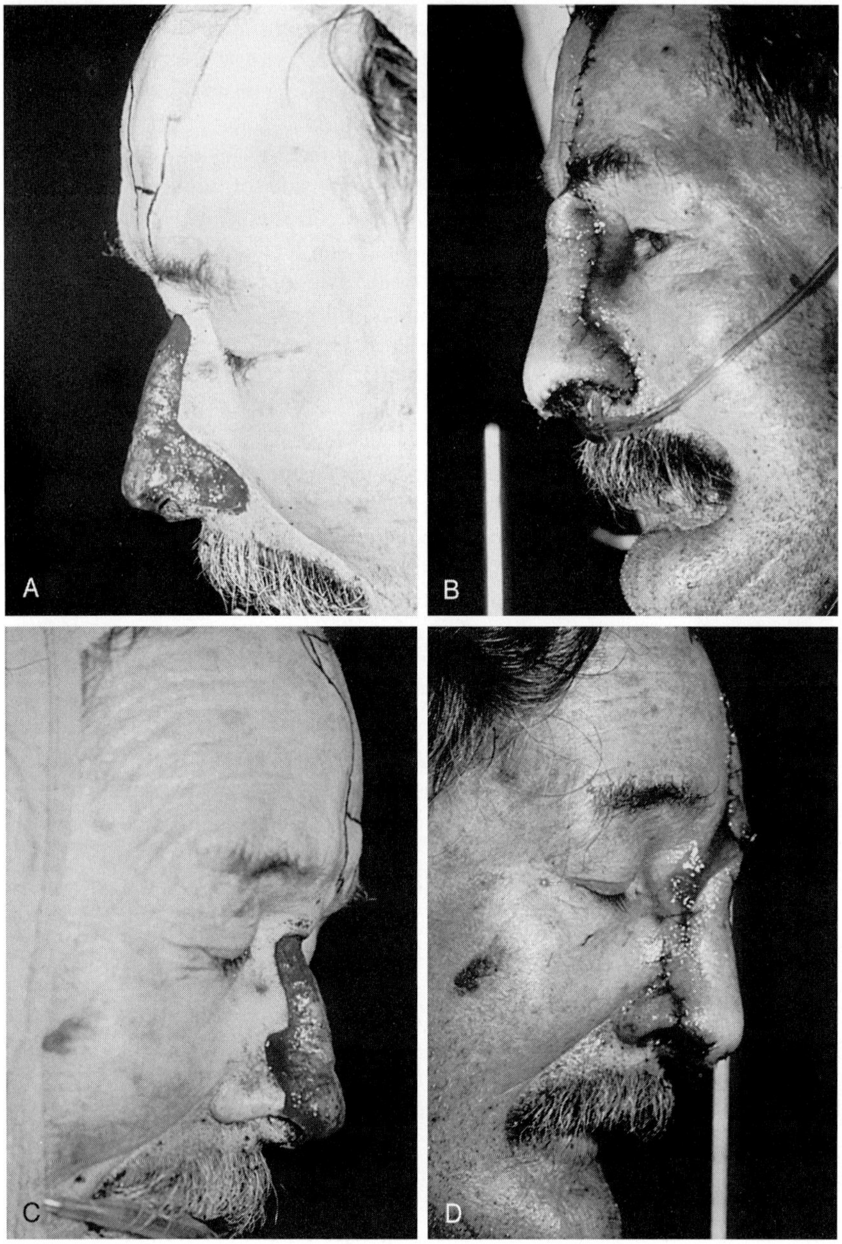

FIGURE 4–2. *A,* Area to be resurfaced on left side of nose. *B,* Paramedian forehead flap sutured in place. *C,* Area to be resurfaced on right side of nose. *D,* Paramedian forehead flap sutured in place.

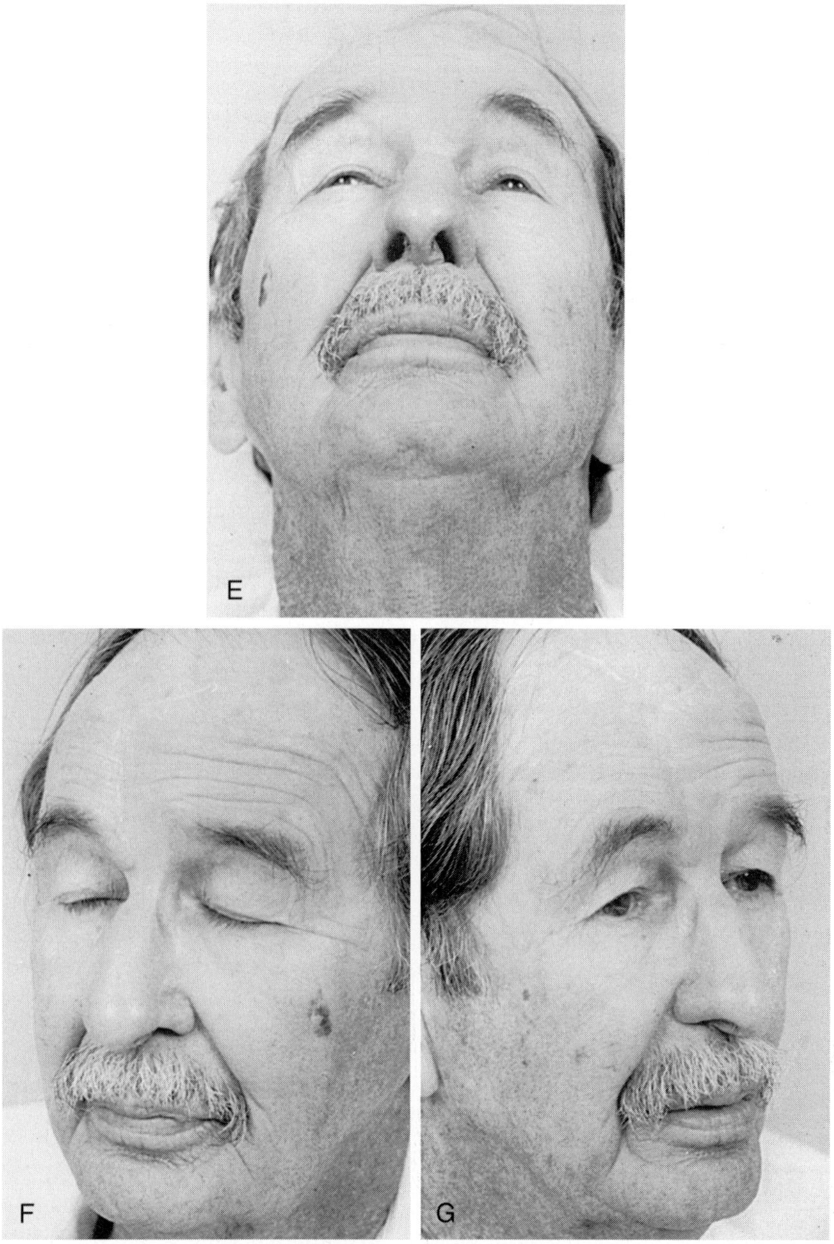

FIGURE 4–2 *Continued. E,* Submental view at 1 year. *F,* Left oblique view at 1 year. *G,* Right oblique view at 1 year.

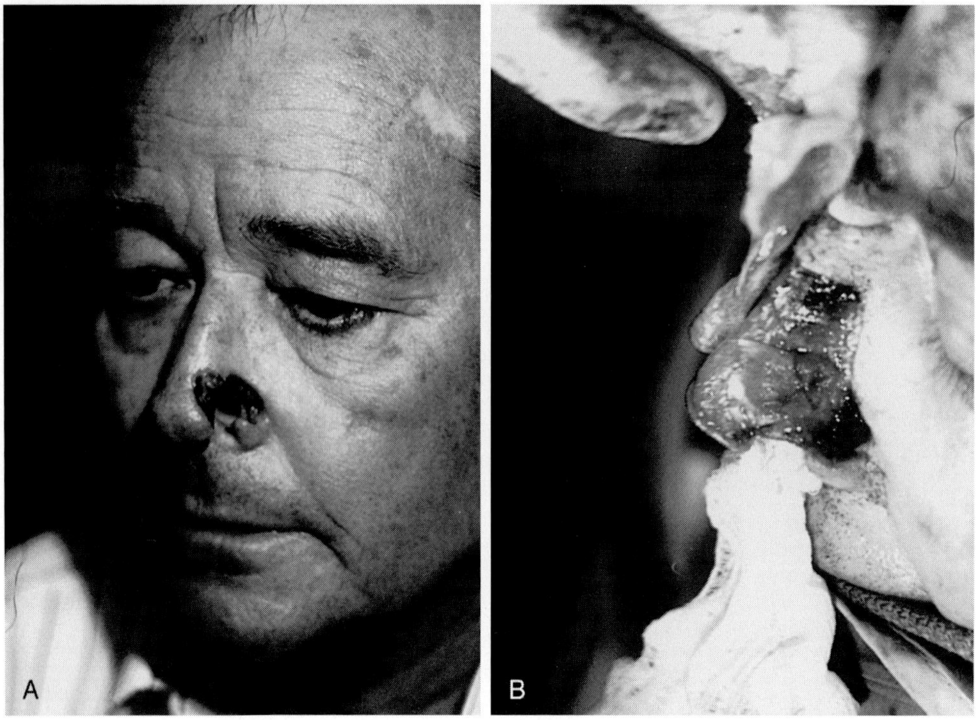

FIGURE 4–3. *A,* Full-thickness loss of left ala. *B,* Superior turn-in flap with overlying cartilage graft in place.

that the perichondrium of the conchal bowl is much more adherent to the overlying skin than to the underlying cartilage. Hydrodissection is very helpful in harvesting this graft.

Placement of the PCCG requires exact sizing because this graft does not shrink. In our hands, it is more reliable than full- or split-thickness skin grafts and produces results that are far superior, especially when placed over cartilage. Additionally, no bolster dressings are required at either the donor site or the recipient site. Strategically placed mattress sutures coapt the tissues, allowing for more precise monitoring. The donor site is closed with a "flip-flop" flap, which has been previously described (see Chapter 2).[25] Dental rolls can be used as bolsters but are not necessary. The donor site has a slightly narrower postauricular sulcus.

STRUCTURAL SUPPORT

Techniques for Harvesting the Conchal Cartilage Graft

The conchal cartilage graft (autogenous cartilage graft) is harvested after the ear has been prepared and injected with 1 to 2 mL of 1% lidocaine with 1:100,000 epinephrine. The incision is made just inferior to the antihelical rim. The skin flap includes the perichondrium of the cartilage on the anterior surface. The entire conchal cartilage is harvested to ensure adequate size,[24] since the graft must be large enough to span the entire width of the nose when it is positioned over the nasal dorsum to correct midnasal collapse. The perichondrium is left undisturbed on the posterior aspect of the cartilage. The skin is closed with a running 4–0 chromic suture. The concha is coapted to the posterior tissues with two or three vertical mattress sutures without a bolster.

The cartilage graft is fashioned using a high-speed diamond fraise and anchored into position with nonreactive sutures. The graft is placed only when there is an intact endonasal lining or after the lining has been reconstructed. The graft can be sandwiched and sutured between the endonasal lining and the paramedian forehead flap or other resurfacing tissue to provide support (Fig. 4–6). The transcutaneous sutures are removed 7 to 14 days after the procedure.

The conchal cartilage graft can be effectively feathered at its periphery using the diamond fraise and drill. This allows the surgeon to maximize aesthetic detail. This graft should not be placed without adequate endonasal lining, which must be addressed separately. The conchal cartilage graft does provide exceptional support for anchoring the flaps.

Septal Cartilage

The septum is composed of hyaline cartilage, which is the most widely used cartilage for grafting in the nose. In many subtotal nasal reconstructive procedures septal cartilage may be unavailable. When present, it can be transferred to the dorsum to provide additional height and support. It can be attached to the upper lateral cartilage or to transplanted calvarial bone. Septal cartilage is thicker and stronger posteriorly. It also can be fashioned and shaped with a diamond fraise but is more amenable to shaping with a knife. Septal cartilage has a very low resorption rate. It is an excellent source of semisolid material that is easily accessible when present.

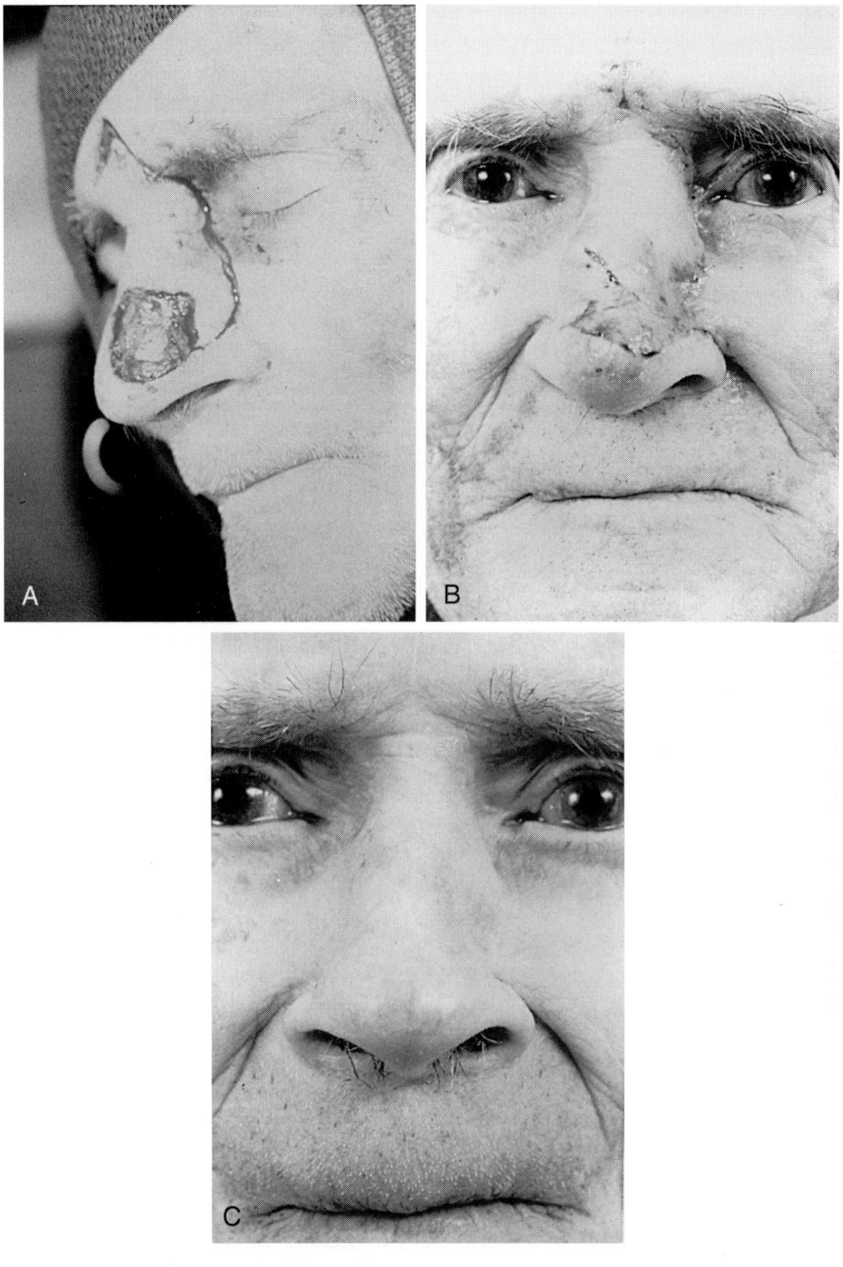

FIGURE 4–4. *A,* Outline of sliding nasal dorsal flap. *B,* One week postoperatively. *C,* Six months postoperatively.

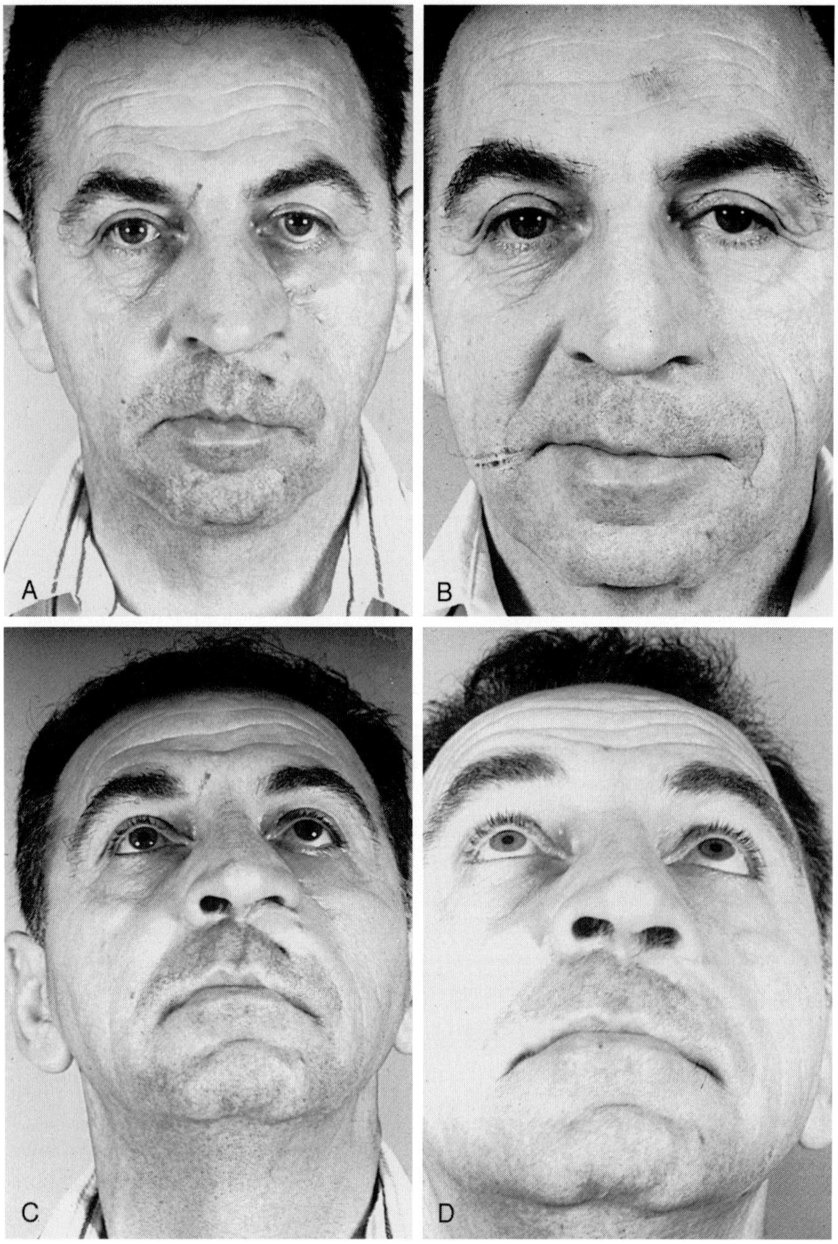

FIGURE 4–5. *A,* Inferior-based nasolabial flap employed 2 weeks ago to resurface columella floor of nose and caudal septum. *B,* One year following precise placement of alar base. *C,* Submental view following first stage of inferior-based nasolabial flap placement. *D,* One year following second stage of precisely placed ala.

Calvarial Bone Grafts

Calvarial bone grafts have been a source of controversy, but their success and the excellent results achieved support their popularity for facial reconstruction. The sites used for harvesting split calvarial bone graft material are the frontal and upper occipital bones, the squamous portion of the temporal bone, and the parietal bones. All the bones are of membranous origin. The parietal bone is the most common site of material for facial bone grafts. The intervening diploe is not completely developed until the fourth year of life.[26] The harvesting of the split calvarial bone graft should therefore be delayed until after this age. The outer surface is convex and smooth with a central tuberosity, whereas the inner surface is concave and contains grooves for the middle meningeal vessels.[27] The outer table is thicker than the inner table. The overall skull thickness ranges from 6.9 to 7.2 mm. Split calvarial bone grafts are created using a 90-degree oscillating saw to fit into the diploic gutter. The horizontal and vertical bone cuts can be made with a standard rotating bur. Generally, the 90-degree saw is used to cut the diploe around the entire perimeter of the graft; this decreases the chance of splitting and cracking the graft. Curved chisels are used to complete the osteotomy. Because of the curvature of the skull, the harvesting of the central portion of the graft is the most difficult. The danger here is the risk of completely transecting the skull and entering the cranial cavity. Bleeding from the vascular diploic space is controlled with bone wax and bipolar cautery. The defect is palpated for several months until new bone grafts fill in the area.

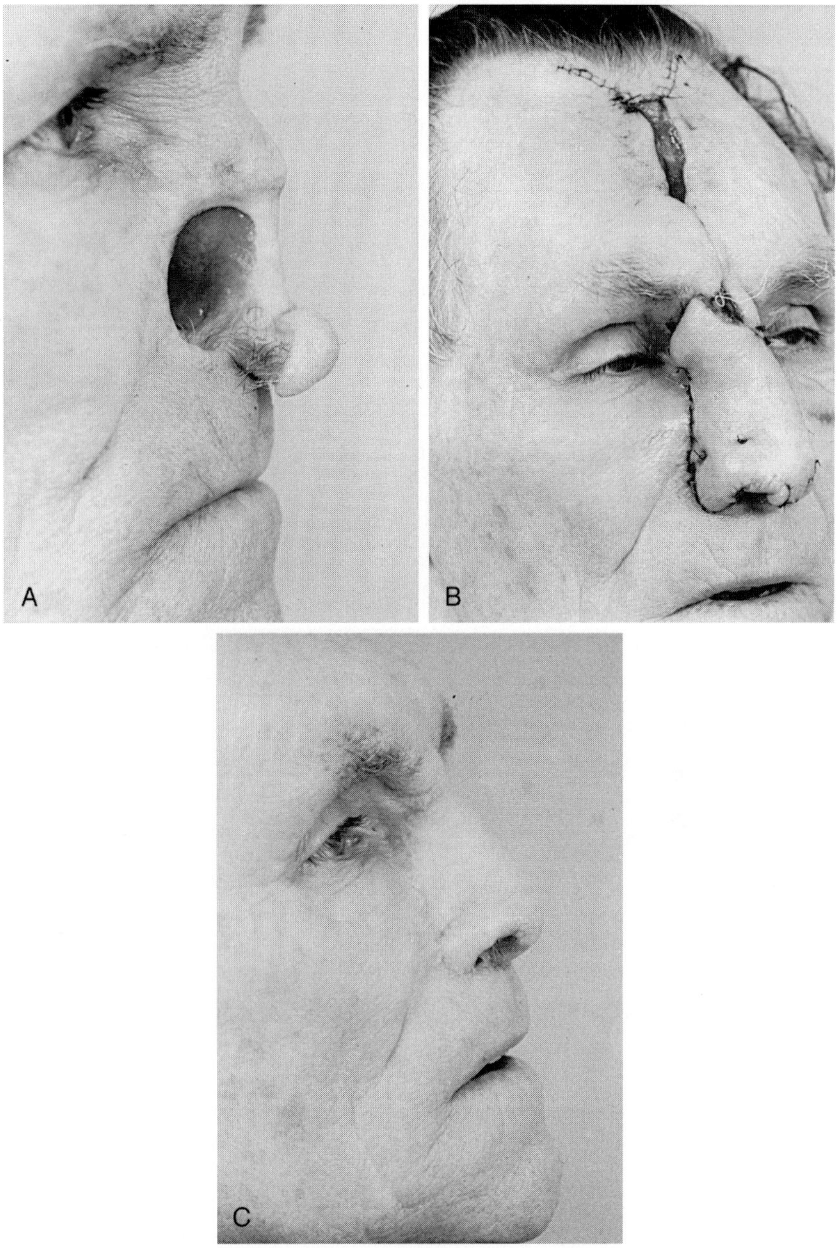

FIGURE 4–6. *A,* Right lateral view demonstrating need for endonasal lining, structural support, and external resurfacing. *B,* Paramedian flap and turn-in flaps sandwiching conchal cartilage graft used for support. *C,* Right lateral view at 6 months.

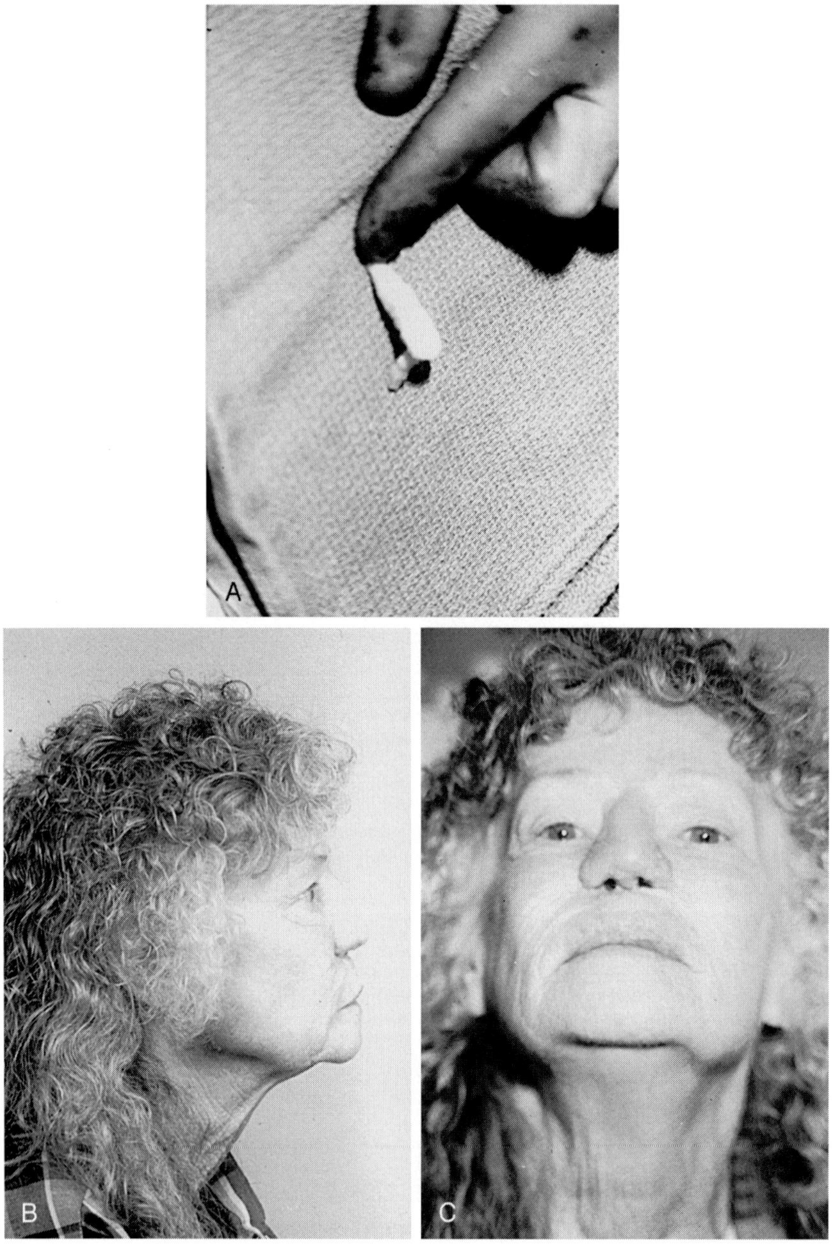

FIGURE 4–7. *A,* Calvarial bone graft for tip support doweled into another graft for dorsal support. *B,* Patient with doweled grafts at 2 years following total nasal reconstruction. *C,* Lateral view of patient 2 years following total nasal reconstruction.

TABLE 4–1. SUBTOTAL NASAL RECONSTRUCTION OPTIONS

DEFECT	OPTION
Nasal tip	Skin graft (full- or split-thickness)
	Perichondrial cutaneous graft
	Dorsal (sliding) nasal flap
	Midline forehead flap
	Local flap
	Granulation
Bridge	Glabella flap
	Nasolabial flap
	Bilobed flap
	Transportation flap
	Eyelid flap
Nasal alae	Composite graft (auricular)
	Local flap with conchal cartilage graft
	Paramedian forehead flap
Columella	Composite graft (auricular helix, rout)
	Full-thickness
	Local flap (nasolabial, lip)
Extensive	Composite grafts, bone, cartilage, skin flaps
	Prosthetic rehabilitation

Modified from Shockley WW: Special problems associated with carcinoma of the nose. Otolaryngol Clin North Am 26(2):247–264, 1993.

The split calvarial bone graft is first fashioned with a cutting bur and then refined with a diamond bur. Micro holes are placed to prepare the graft for plate and screw fixation into the frontal bone. Additionally, flaps, free or pedicled, can be used to cover the graft. The bone graft can be used to provide support for the dorsal or columellar region of the nose; in this case, they can supply the total support for the nose (Fig. 4–7). Cartilage grafts can also be used with calvarial bone grafts.

SUMMARY

When presented with a significant nasal defect, a facial surgeon can derive structural support for the nose from conchal cartilage, septal cartilage, and/or split calvarial bone grafts. Soft tissue coverage can be provided by a nasolabial flap (inferiorly or superiorly based), a sliding nasal dorsal flap, or a paramedian forehead flap.

Subtotal nasal reconstruction requires a comprehensive understanding of the extent of the primary defect and its component tissues. The armamentarium of today's facial plastic and reconstructive surgeon allows him or her to provide a tailored method of repair with minimal donor site morbidity and excellent cosmetic results (Table 4–1).

REFERENCES

1. Nichter LS, Morgan RF, Nichter MA: The impact of Indian methods for total nasal reconstruction. Clin Plast Surg 10:635–647, 1983.
2. Millard DR: Total reconstructive rhinoplasty and a missing link. Plast Reconstr Surg 37:167–183, 1966.
3. Quatela VC, Sherris DA, Round MF: Esthetic refinements in forehead flap nasal reconstruction. Arch Otolaryngol 121:1106–1113, 1995.
4. Millard DR: Hemirhinoplasty. Plast Reconstr Surg 40:440–445, 1967.
5. Burget GC, Menick FJ: The subunit principle in nasal reconstruction. Plast Reconstr Surg 76:239–247, 1985.
6. Burget GO, Menick FJ: Nasal reconstruction: Seeking a fourth dimension. Plast Reconstr Surg 78:145–157, 1986.
7. Adamson JE: Nasal reconstruction with the expanded forehead flap. Plast Reconstr Surg 81:12, 1988.
8. Kroll SS, Rosenfield L: Delayed pedicle separation in forehead flap nasal reconstruction. Ann Plast Surg 23:327, 1989.
9. Burget GC, Menick FJ: Nasal support and lining: The marriage of beauty and blood supply. Plast Reconstr Surg 84:189–201, 1989.
10. Shumrick KA, Smith TL: The anatomic basis for the design of forehead flaps in nasal reconstruction. Arch Otolaryngol Head Neck Surg 118:373–379, 1992.
11. Konig F: Eine neue Methode der Aufrichtung eingesunkener Nasen durch Bildung des Nasanruckens aus einem haut-peeriost Knocheniappen der Stim. Arch Klin Chir 34:165–169, 1887.
12. Donald PJ: Cartilage grafting in facial reconstruction with special consideration of irradiated grafts. Laryngoscope 96:786–807, 1986.
13. Bujia J, Wilmes E, Hammer C, Kastenbour E: Class II antigenicity of human cartilage: Relevance to the use of homologous cartilage graft for reconstructive surgery. Ann Plast Surg 265:541–543, 1991.
14. Lefkovits G: Irradiated homologous costal cartilage for augmentation rhinoplasty. Ann Plast Surg 25:317–327, 1990.
15. Burget GC: Aesthetic restoration of the nose. Clin Plast Surg 12:463–480, 1988.
16. Allcroft RA, Friedman CD, Quatela VC: Cartilage grafts for head and neck augmentation and reconstruction—autografts and homografts. Otolaryngol Clin North Am 27(1):69–80, 1994.
17. Kridel RWH, Koniur RJ: Irradiated cartilage grafts in the nose: A preliminary report. Arch Otolaryngol Head Neck Surg 119:24–30, 1993.
18. Smith RD, Dickinson JT, Cipcic A: Composite grafts in facial reconstructive surgery. Arch Otolaryngol 95:252–264, 1972.
19. Konior RJ: Free composite grafts. Otolaryngol Clin North Am 27 (1):81–90, 1994.
20. Aden KK, Biel MA: The evaluation of pharmacologic agents on composite survival. Arch Otolaryngol Head Neck Surg 118:175–178, 1992.
21. Holt GR: Maxillofacial trauma. *In* Cummings CW, Fredrickson JM, Harker LA, et al (eds): Otolaryngology—Head and Neck Surgery. St. Louis, Mosby–Year Book, 1986, pp. 313–334.
22. Conley JJ, Price JC: The midline vertical forehead flap. Otolaryngol Head Neck Surg 89:38, 1981.
23. Gonzales-Ulloa M, Castillo A, Stevens E, Fuertes GA, Leonell F, Ubaldo F: Preliminary study of the total restoration of the facial skin. Plast Reconstr Surg 13:151–161, 1954.
24. Stucker FJ, Hoasjoe DK: Nasal reconstruction with conchal cartilage. Arch Otol Head Neck Surg 120:653–658, 1994.
25. Stucker FJ, Shaw GY: The perichondrial cutaneous graft: A 12-year experience. Arch Otolaryngol Head Neck Surg 118:287–292, 1997.
26. Williams PL, et al (eds): Gray's Anatomy, 37th ed. Edinburgh, Churchill Livingstone, 1989.
27. Day TA, Vuillemin T, Ladrach K, Raveh J, Stucker FJ: Calvarial bone grafting in craniofacial reconstruction. Facial Plast Surg Clin North Am 3(3):241–255, 1995.

CHAPTER 5

Subtotal and Total Nasal Reconstruction—Flaps and Bone Grafts

Anthony J. Maniglia, M.D.

Autologous frontal bone grafts were first used in nasal reconstruction by Ollier in 1864.[1] Mueller[2] and Konig[3] were the first to describe the use of calvarial bone grafts in facial augmentation in 1890. In 1942, Converse introduced the forehead-scalp flap for reconstruction of the nose and also advocated the use of autologous iliac bone grafts for support after lining and covering had been completed.[4] The use of the calvarial outer table graft with periosteal attachment in craniofacial reconstruction was first reported by Santoni-Rugiu[5] in 1969. Smith and Abramson[6] in 1974 did a comparative study and reported that membranous bone affords much less resorption and maintains its original size and shape better than endochondral bone from different sources such as the iliac crest, rib, or tibia. Their experimental study was done in rabbits and showed that at least 75% of the volume of iliac bone was absorbed within 1 year. Zins and Whitaker[7] repeated similar experiments in rabbits and monkeys in 1983 and confirmed the findings of Smith and Abramson.[6]

Tessier[8] in 1982 reported on autogenous bone grafts taken from the calvarium for facial and cranial reconstruction. He advocated harvesting full-thickness cranial grafts, then splitting the graft into outer and inner tables, and reconstructing the regional graft defect with the same material. In 1987, Powell and Riley[9] recommended the use of the outer table only for craniofacial reconstruction. The outer table was harvested, leaving the inner table intact. Kusiak and colleagues[10] demonstrated the early vascularization of parietal bone. Phillips and Rahn[11] in 1988 demonstrated decreased resorption in rigid versus nonrigid fixed bone grafts in an animal model. The volume of the grafts present at 20 weeks was greater for the rigidly fixed grafts. Maniglia[12] in 1989 first reported on the use of a full-thickness parietal bone graft fixed with titanium miniplates in a patient with total nasal reconstruction following rhinectomy for malignant mucosal melanoma. The full-thickness parietal bone donor site defect was repaired using a methylmethacrylate plate wired to the outer table of the parietal bone. Table 5–1 illustrates the different types of flaps and grafts used prior to 1988 for nasal reconstruction for a variety of defects. Maniglia and Swim[13] in 1993 reported on parietal bone grafts used for reconstructive rhinoplasty in five trauma and cancer patients.

Traumatic nasal deformities may present difficult reconstructive problems. There may be loss of soft tissue as well as the supporting architecture of bone and cartilage. Ablative procedures used in the treatment of nasal carcinoma or malignant melanoma result in large defects that require staged reconstruction using regional flaps and bone and cartilage grafts to achieve a cosmetically pleasing result while maintaining a functional airway. Indeed, regional flaps and bone and cartilage grafts are excellent alternatives to plastic prostheses for cosmetic rehabilitation of such defects. Autologous iliac bone and rib grafts and homologous rib grafts are plagued by various degrees of resorption over the long term and result in lack of dorsal and tip support.[11, 12]

The purpose of this chapter is to describe our experience in correcting traumatic nasal deformities and in applying reconstructive rhinoplasty to repair defects created after ablation of malignant neoplasms. We have used autologous and homologous bone grafts from different donor sites, but membranous (parietal) bone grafts with attached periosteum is our preferred material for support.

MATERIALS AND METHODS

Reconstructive rhinoplasty for major surgical defects requiring graft support has been performed in 19 patients during the past 20 years. The patients' ages ranged from 32 to 78 years; the average age was 56. Three patients were females, and 16 were males. The types of pathology in these patients are listed in Table 5–2. The predominant pathology

TABLE 5–1. RECONSTRUCTIVE RHINOPLASTY

CASE	AGE/SEX	NASAL PATHOLOGY	RECONSTRUCTION	OUTCOME
1 (VB)	57/F	Malignant mucosal melanoma	Converse forehead scalping. Iliac bone graft	NED 8 years
2 (AC)	53/M	Malignant mucosal melanoma	Oblique seagull forehead flap. Parietal bone support	NED 8 months only. Excellent bone support
3 (GP)	59/M	Squamous cell cancer	Forehead vertical flap. Chondromucosal right-angle septal flap	NED for 2½ years. No recurrence in the nose. Died from second primary to lung. T-spine metastasis
4 (JP)	52/M	Squamous cell cancer. Radiation failure	Converse forehead scalping flap. Abbé flap. Prosthesis for support of anterior maxillectomy defect	NED 2 years. Lost to follow-up
5 (AP)	61/M	Squamous cell cancer. Radiation failure	Converse forehead scalping flap. Vertical forehead flap for lining. Iliac bone graft	NED 7 years survival
6 (AR)	78/M	Squamous cell cancer. Radiation failure	Horizontal forehead flap. Freeze-dried homologous rib	NED 5 years survival. Loss of support. Total absorption of rib
7 (RP)	52/M	Squamous cell cancer. Extension to upper lip	Horizontal forehead flap. Nasolabial flap. Cantilevered autologous rib (bone)	NED 5 years survival. Died from second primary of tongue metastasis, 8 years after nasal surgery
8 (PR)	57/M	Squamous cell cancer	Horizontal forehead flap. Cantilevered autologous rib (bone)	NED 2 years postoperative
9 (CW)	70/M	Squamous cell cancer. Extension to upper lip, maxilla, eyelid	Vertical forehead flap. Mustarde cheek flap. Skin graft. Chondromucosal nasal septal support	NED 2 years. Modified radical neck dissection and postoperative radiation therapy added
10 (GA)	33/M	Traumatic defect, 357 magnum gunshot wound	Converse forehead scalping flap. Iliac bone graft	Lost to follow-up

NED, No evidence of disease.
From Maniglia AJ: Reconstructive rhinoplasty. Laryngoscope 99:866, 1989.

was untreated squamous cell carcinoma or that following radiation therapy failure.

From 1988 to 1998, 12 of these 19 patients underwent surgical procedures using membranous parietal bone grafts with rigid fixation. Two of these patients had deformities resulting from severe nasal trauma and the loss of cartilaginous and bony support with a saddle nose. The other patients had defects secondary to ablative procedures used for the treatment of squamous cell carcinoma and malignant mucosal melanoma. The shortest follow-up was 24 months, and the longest was 10 years; the average was 53 months. Eight patients had split calvarial grafts, and four had full-thickness grafts.

Table 5–3 shows the types of flaps and skin covering used. The horizontal forehead flap was mainly used because most of these defects were very large and required a large flap for reconstruction. Table 5–4 lists the different types of bone grafts used for support. Table 5–5 lists the complications encountered. No major complications occurred, and there was no significant bone graft resorption in the group of patients with parietal bone grafts. Two patients were subsequently involved in accidents resulting in fractures of the bone grafts fixed by titanium plates. The parietal bone grafts, after being disconnected from the titanium plate, were significantly reduced in volume.

The use of parietal bone grafts fixed by titanium plates has been used for subtotal and total reconstruction in the majority of cases. In this chapter, we describe the details of this most extensive and complicated technique for total nasal reconstruction. There are two stages; stage I has six steps:

1. Formation of the lining with local skin flaps.
2. Provision of support by the autologous parietal bone

TABLE 5–2. TYPES OF PATHOLOGY IN RECONSTRUCTIVE RHINOPLASTY IN CASES OF CANCER AND TRAUMA

Squamous cell carcinoma	10
Inverted papilloma with malignant degeneration and atypia	3
Malignant melanoma	3
Mucoepidermoid carcinoma (high grade)	1
Trauma	2
Total	19

TABLE 5–3. TYPES OF FLAP AND SKIN COVERING IN RECONSTRUCTIVE RHINOPLASTY IN CANCER AND TRAUMA CASES[a]

Horizontal forehead flap	10
Preservation of skin of nasal dorsum and tip[a]	4
Converse forehead-scalp flap	3
Midline forehead flap	1
Seagull flap	1
Total	19

[a]A total of four cases had preservation of the skin of the nasal dorsum and tip: two had extensive infiltrating inverted papillomas with malignant degeneration and atypia; one had severe nasal trauma with loss of support and total septal perforation; and one had high-grade mucoepidermoid carcinoma of the nasal septum and premaxilla.

TABLE 5–4. BONE GRAFT FOR SUPPORT IN RECONSTRUCTIVE RHINOPLASTY IN CANCER AND TRAUMA CASES

Iliac bone graft	3
Freeze-dried rib (homologous)	1
Rib (autologous)	3
Parietal bone graft (autologous)	12
Total	19

graft, which is secured with rigid titanium plates to the frontal bone.

3. Preparation of the horizontal forehead flap, or midline or paramedian vertical or oblique forehead flap for covering.
4. Transfer, tapering, and sculpting the flap used in No. 3 to the shape of the nose; this flap is then sutured to the flap used for the lining (in No. 1).
5. Reconstruction of the columella with the tip of the forehead flap and buccal mucosal flap from the upper lip.
6. Placement of supraclavicular full-thickness skin graft to cover the forehead defect, or direct closure of the midline or paramedian vertical flap of the forehead.

Stage II takes place ideally after a period of 3 weeks and involves return of the flap to the forehead. A delay of even 1 additional week results in increased contraction of the flap, and surgery needed to cover the donor area is more difficult. There are three steps:

1. Division of the forehead flap.
2. Return to the donor area of the proximal end of the forehead flap.
3. Proper tailoring of the remainder of the newly vascularized distal portion of the forehead flap used for covering to complete the reconstruction of the newly formed nasal pyramid.

Cosmetic and functional refinements can be accomplished in subsequent stages. Refinements include serial resection of the full-thickness skin graft of the forehead with advancement of the forehead flap. Scar revisions or defatting of a portion of the flap are other techniques that may be used. Conchal cartilage grafts are also useful as implants to improve cosmesis and add rigidity to the newly formed alae and nostrils, thereby improving the airway.

TABLE 5–5. COMPLICATIONS IN RECONSTRUCTIVE RHINOPLASTY IN CANCER AND TRAUMA CASES

1. Flap failures (minor, tip only, mainly detachment from lip structures)	
a. Converse flap	1
b. Seagull flap	1
2. Partial support resorption	
a. Iliac bone graft (autologous)	3
b. Rib (partial, homologous)	1
c. Rib (partial, autologous)	2
d. Parietal bone graft	0
3. Infection of flap, bone graft, or titanium plate	0
4. Fracture of parietal graft secondary to trauma	
a. Truck accident	1
b. Blow to the nose	1

CASE 1

The first case illustrates the cantilevered rib graft technique. We no longer use this technique because the fixation with stainless steel wire is semirigid, and it resulted in partial rib resorption. Several important technical points are demonstrated in this case, as is the long-term follow-up showing resorption of the rib support and flap shrinkage. A 57-year-old white man was referred to us after undergoing an ablative procedure for removal of a squamous cell carcinoma of the nose. The patient was left with a floppy piece of lateral nasal skin that was reserved for future lining material during the reconstructive technique. Part of the nasal bone was also removed, as was the cartilaginous nasal septum. All surgical margins were found to be free of malignancy. Preoperative photographs are shown in Figure 5–1. Four months had elapsed from the time of the initial surgical procedure until the reconstruction began.

Stage I

1. The lining is formed with local skin flaps (Fig. 5–2). The rib graft is harvested and sculptured using a round bur.
2. Support is provided by the autologous cantilevered rib bone graft technique and secured in the nasal bone with 24-gauge stainless steel wire (Fig. 5–3). Nasal dorsum and tip support is provided by two separate pieces of rib wired together.
3. A horizontal forehead flap with extension is used to reconstruct the columella. This distal third of the flap is elevated with no muscle attachment. A rectangular buccal mucosal upper lip flap based superiorly is outlined, raised, and transferred through a puncture incision in the upper lip (Fig. 5–4).
4. This flap is transferred, properly tailored, and sculptured to cover the cantilevered rib graft.
5. The columella is reconstructed using the tip of the forehead and upper lip mucosal flaps (Fig. 5–5*A* and *B*).
6. A supraclavicular full-thickness skin graft is used to cover the forehead defect (see Fig. 5–5*B*). Figure 5–6 illustrates the flap and skin graft healing after 3 weeks.

Stage II

1. The forehead flap is divided (Fig. 5–7*A*).
2. The proximal end of the forehead flap is returned to the donor site (Fig. 5–7*B*).
3. The distal end of the forehead flap is tailored to complete reconstruction of the newly formed nasal pyramid.

Figure 5–8 shows the result 1 year following the second stage reconstruction.

Figure 5–9 illustrates the postoperative result 9 years after the reconstruction. The patient shows no evidence of disease (9-year survival) and is very well adjusted socially. He declined any other revision of the reconstruction. He has developed a second primary (prostate cancer), but his condition has remained stable. Long-term follow-up revealed the obvious disadvantages of rib bone graft with semirigid fixation; we observed marked loss of volume of the dorsum and tip support as well as further contraction of the distal segment of the forehead flap used for covering.

Comments

Millard[14] was the first to report the rib cantilever technique in which the rib graft is fixed semirigidly with stainless steel wiring. It would be helpful to know

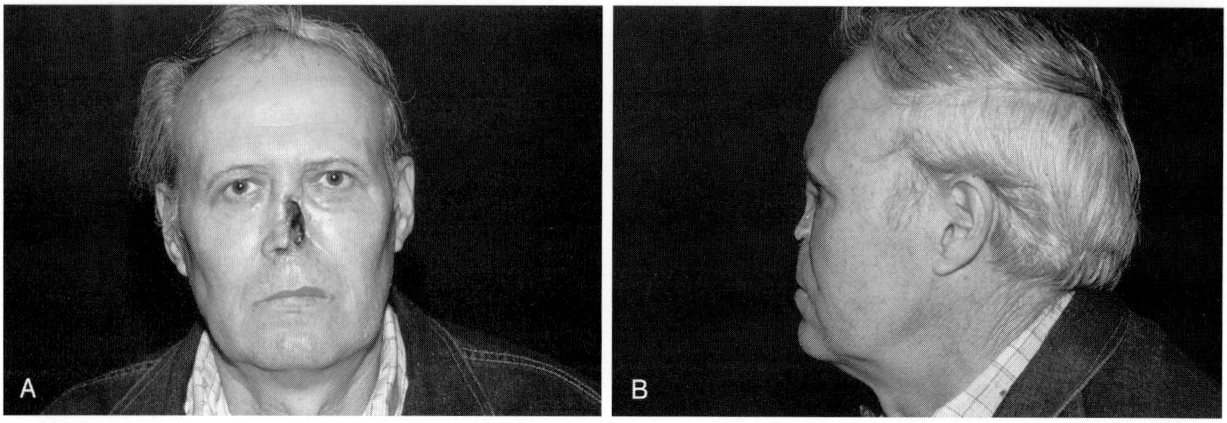

FIGURE 5–1. *A* and *B,* Preoperative photographs. The cartilaginous nasal septum has been totally removed, and there is no nasal support.

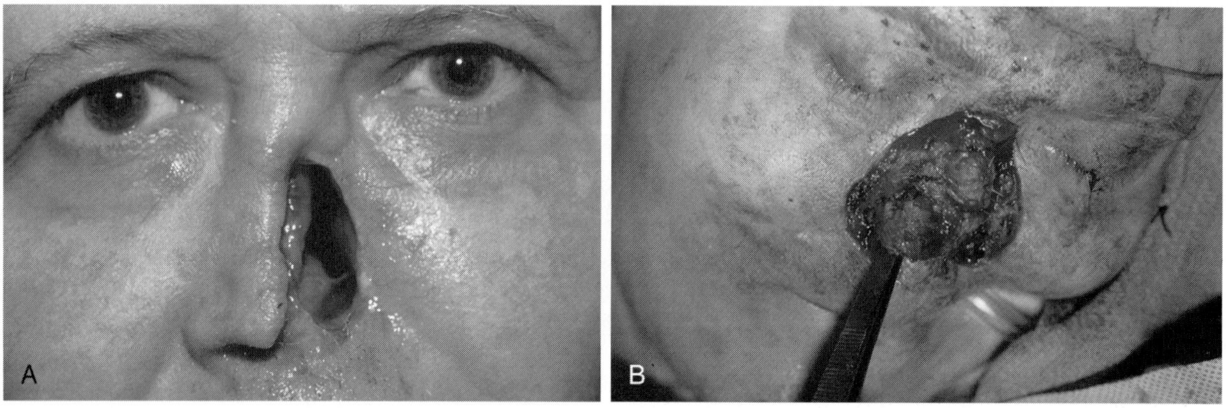

FIGURE 5–2. *A,* Close-up front view showing the remnant of the nasal septum and the turbinates. *B,* Incisions were made to circumscribe the defect, and the local skin flaps are turned in to form a lining and prepare a bed for the bone graft.

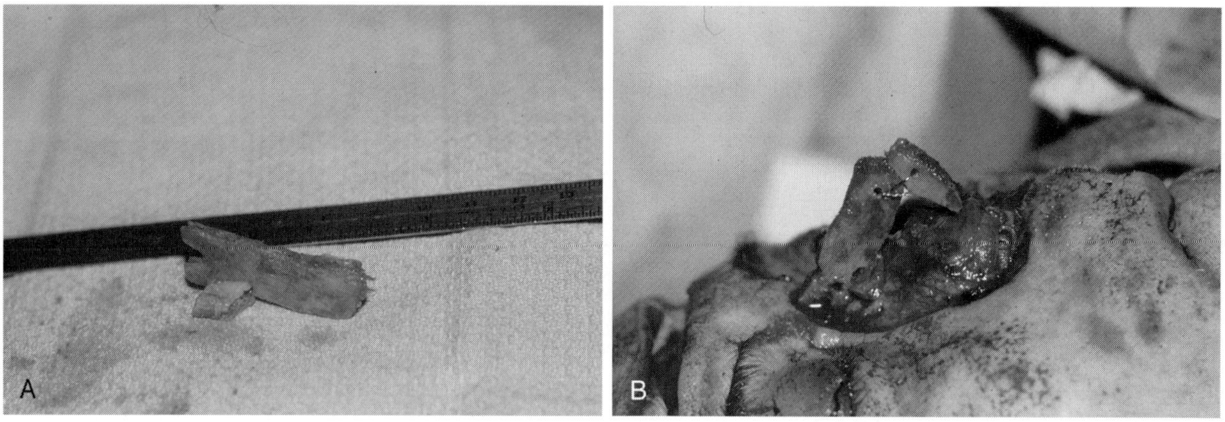

FIGURE 5–3. *A,* Rib (bone) is harvested and sculptured in a tongue-and-groove configuration to fit on the nasal bone. *B,* A cantilevered autogenous rib bone is anchored to the nasal bone and properly wired to the frontal process and proximal nasal bone (with two 24-gauge wires). For better tip support, another piece of rib is wired to the tip distal portion of this bone graft.

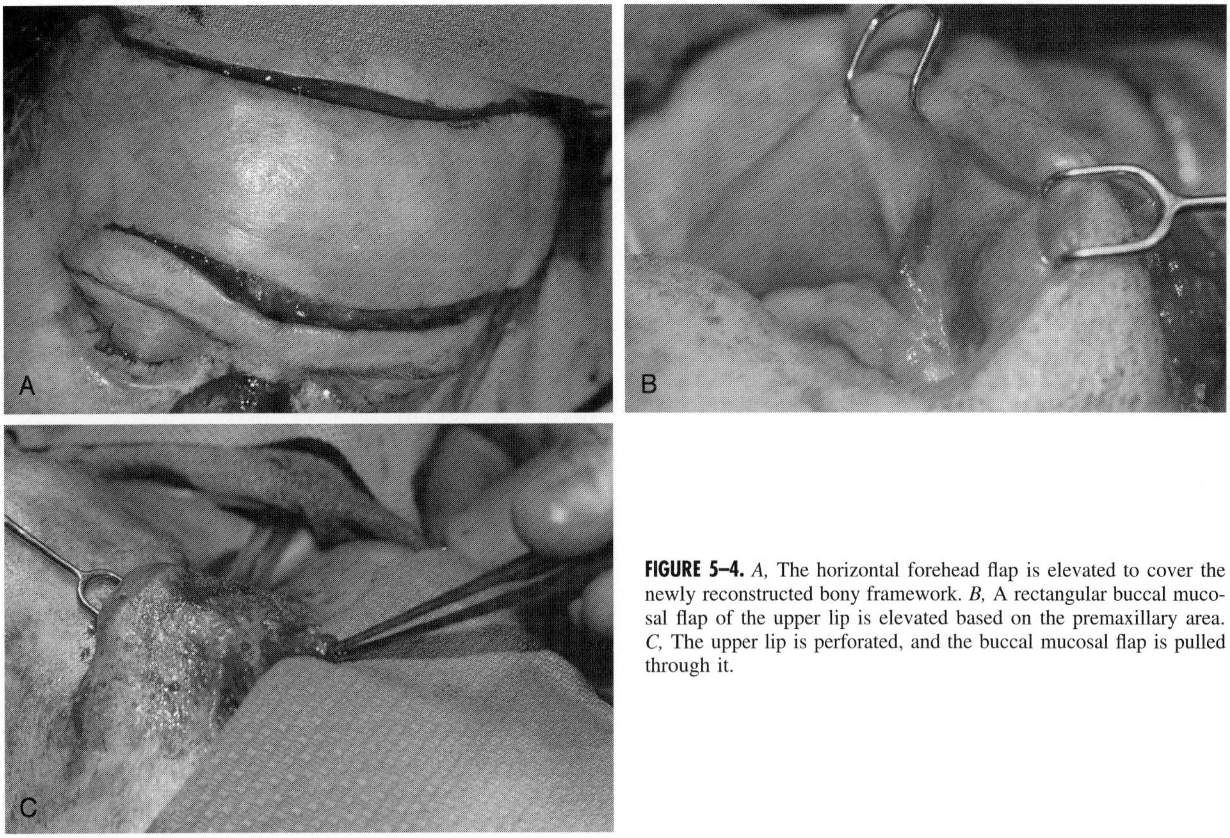

FIGURE 5–4. *A,* The horizontal forehead flap is elevated to cover the newly reconstructed bony framework. *B,* A rectangular buccal mucosal flap of the upper lip is elevated based on the premaxillary area. *C,* The upper lip is perforated, and the buccal mucosal flap is pulled through it.

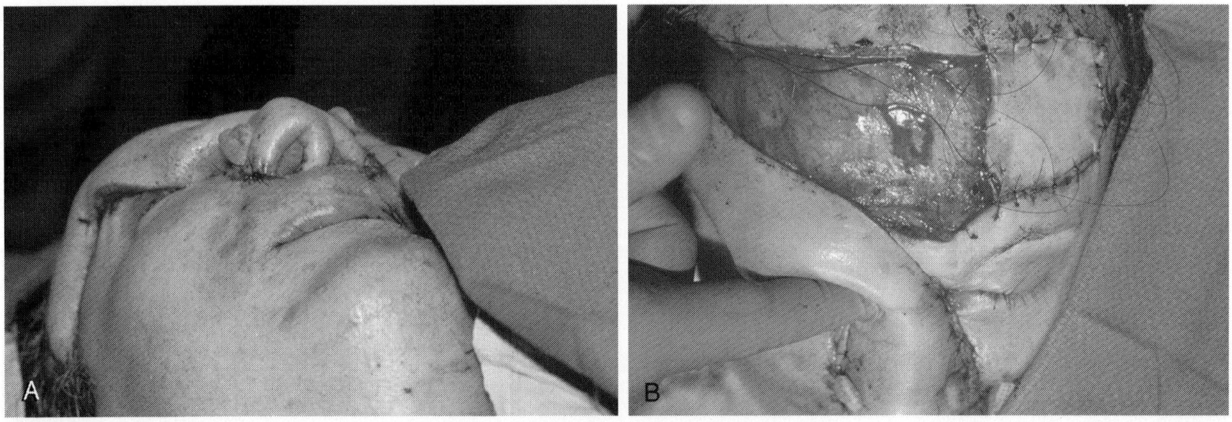

FIGURE 5–5. *A,* The forehead flap is used to cover the bony framework. It is based laterally and supplied by the superficial temporal artery. *B,* The nasal tip and columella are reconstructed. The bony framework is totally covered with flaps as previously described. Packing (gauze and antibiotic ointment) is used for hemostasis.

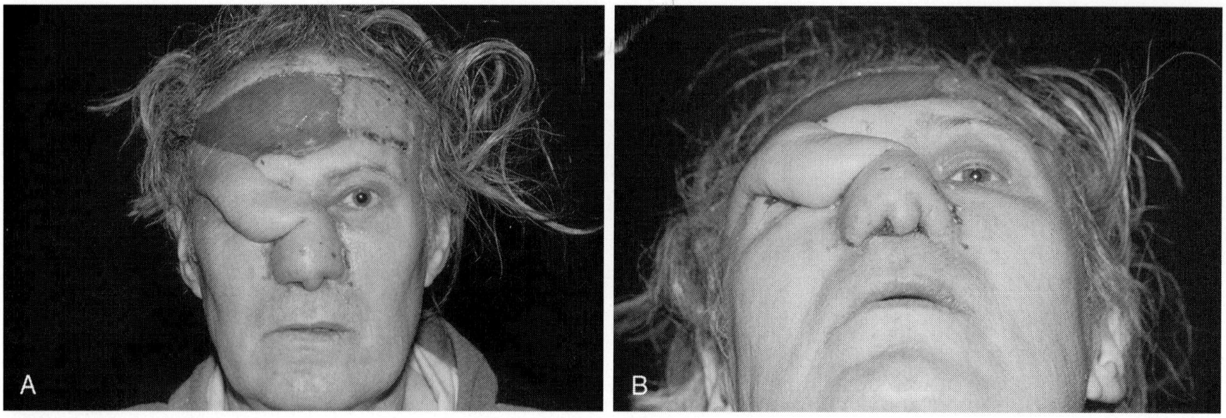

FIGURE 5–6. *A,* Front view of the patient 3 weeks postoperatively. *B,* Basal view of the patient showing the reconstructed tip, which is still very edematous.

the results of long-term follow-up of his cases and the alternative choices used to improve cosmesis and function as the support of the nasal pyramid is lost and the flap used for the primary reconstruction contracts further. The rib cantilever technique has fallen into disfavor among many surgeons who accept the challenge of reconstructive rhinoplasty.

CASE 2

The second case is rather complex and involved the repair of ablative defects following cancer resections (for two different primary neoplasms). The patient was a 64-year-old white male with a history of well-differentiated squamous cell carcinoma of the nasal septum and lower and upper lateral cartilages (Fig. 5–10). He had completed a full course of radiation therapy 1 year prior to our evaluation. Then he developed a recurrent lesion in the same area and was advised to undergo ablative surgical resection and be fitted with a plastic nasal prosthesis (anaplastology). He came to us for a second opinion, and other alternative options were presented to him. These included (1) resection and immediate reconstruction if the surgical margins were free of lesion; (2) resection and observation for a period of 6 to 12 months if warranted. The patient chose option 1 and underwent extensive rhinectomy with preservation of the nasal bone and frontal process of the maxilla. Multiple frozen sections showed ample free margins; therefore, immediate reconstruction was undertaken, and a horizontal forehead flap was selected (Figs. 5–11 and 5–12). The surgical reconstruction consisted of two stages.

Stage I

1. The lining is formal from local skin flaps from skin overlying the nasal bone, frontal process of the maxilla, and short nasolabial flaps.
2. Support is provided by an autogenous (full-thickness) parietal bone graft fixed with titanium plates to the frontal bone (Fig. 5–13).
3. A horizontal forehead flap with extension is elevated to reconstruct the nose and columella. The distal third of the flap is elevated with no muscle.
4. The flap is transferred, tailored, and sculpted to cover the parietal bone graft and titanium miniplate.
5. The columella is reconstructed with a flap from the tip of the forehead and a mucosal flap from the upper lip.
6. A supraclavicular full-thickness skin graft is used to cover the forehead defect. Figures 5–14 illustrates the patient's appearance 3 weeks postoperatively; he is now ready for the second stage. (See Color plate.)

Stage II

Stage II was performed 3 weeks after stage I.

1. The forehead flap is divided.
2. The proximal end of the forehead flap is returned to the donor site.

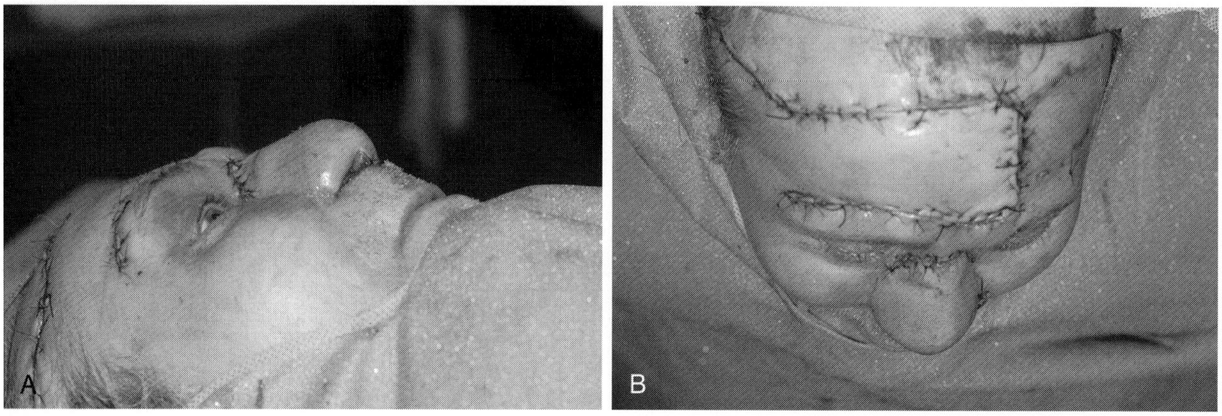

FIGURE 5–7. *A,* Three weeks later, the forehead flap is sectioned and returned to the donor site. *B,* Profile of the nasal reconstruction right after the flap return and tailoring.

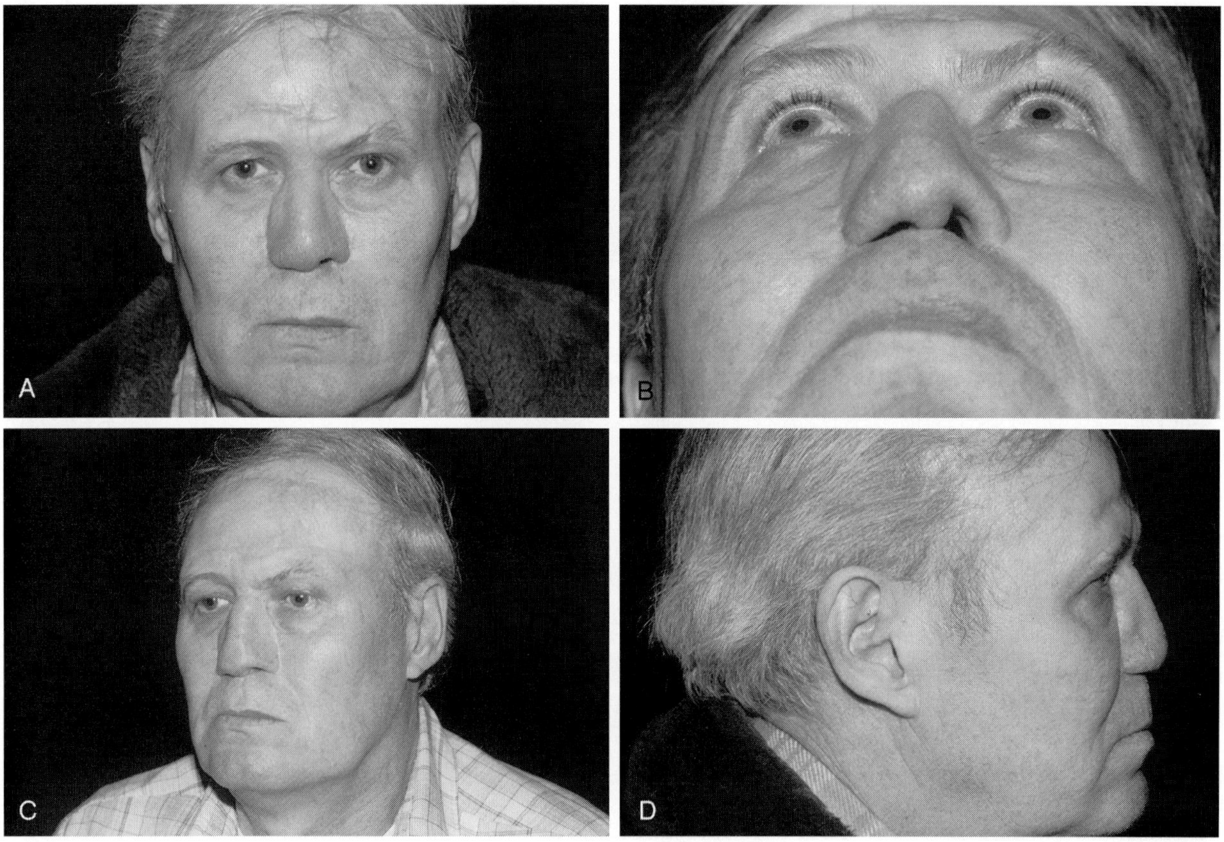

FIGURE 5–8. Front (*A*), basal, (*B*), three-quarter (*C*), and lateral (*D*) views 1 year postoperatively. Lack of tip support is already evident. (See also Color plate.)

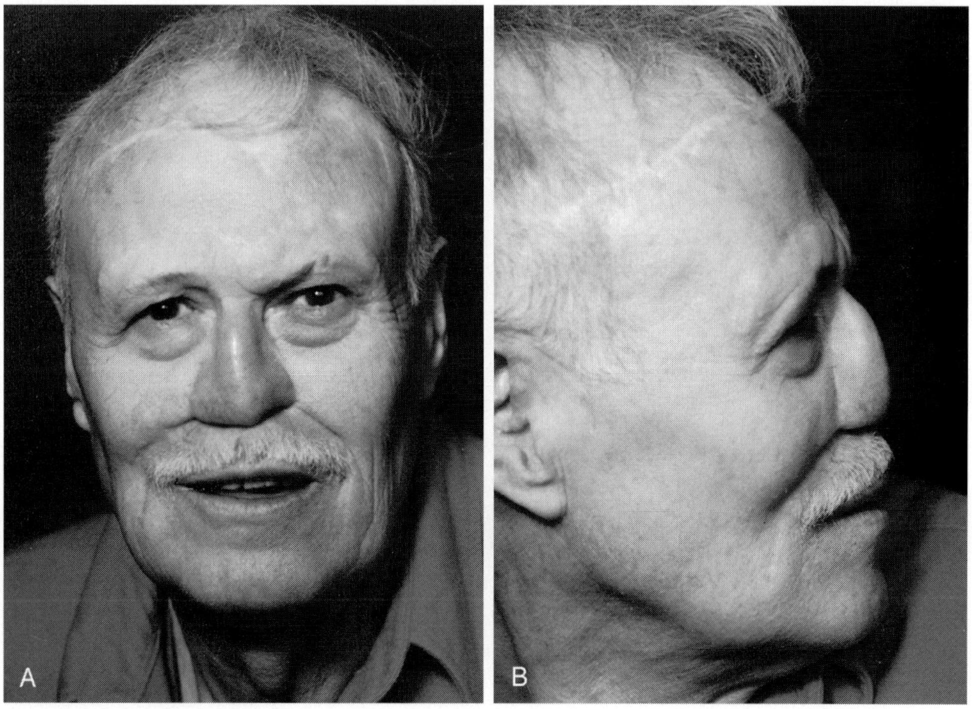

FIGURE 5–9. *A* and *B,* Front and lateral views, 9 years postoperatively. The patient has no evidence of disease. Resorption of rib graft is very noticeable on the inferior aspect of the reconstructed nasal pyramid.

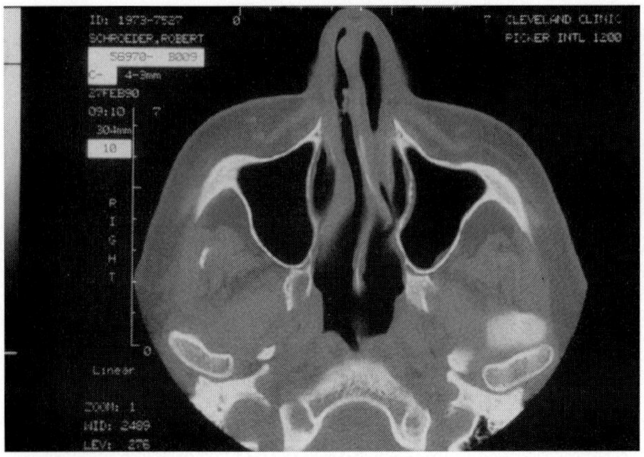

FIGURE 5–10. CT scan, axial cut, shows recurrent tumor involvement on the right side of the nasal septum. The maxillary sinuses are clear.

3. The distal end of the forehead flap used for covering is tailored to complete the reconstruction of the newly formed nasal pyramid (Fig. 5–15). (See Color plate.)

Figures 5–16 and 5–17 illustrate the status of the patient about 3 months after the second stage. The patient underwent two serial excisions of the supraclavicular full-thickness skin graft under local anesthesia that resulted in further improvement of his appearance (Fig. 5–18). Three years later, a second primary neoplasm was diagnosed; this was located on the lacrimal sac and left inner canthal area (mucoepidermoid carcinoma, low grade). This tumor was excised, and free surgical margins were obtained. Six months after excision, the surgical defect was smaller, and there was no evidence of any recurrence of this lesion. The patient was then ready for reconstruction of the defect (Fig. 5–19). The defect was reconstructed using the following technique (reported by Maniglia previously).[15] A myocutaneous upper eyelid flap based medially was used to line and reconstruct the defect (Figs. 5–20 and 5–21). A full-thickness skin graft of the opposite eyelid was used to line the nonepithelial underface of the flap, which faces anteriorly (Fig. 5–22). Ten years after the initial resection, the patient had no evidence of disease (NED). External appearance and nasal function remained satisfactory. Excellent nasal support has been sustained. Despite implantation into a heavily irradiated field, the parietal bone graft (initially implanted 10 years previously) showed insignificant resorption, which has been documented by periodic plain radiographs and postoperative photographs (Figs. 5–23 to 5–26). (See Color plate.)

Comments

The patient in Case 2 is NED (10-year survival). He is very pleased with the cosmetic and functional results. He follows the recommended daily toilet consisting of washing the large epithelial-lined nasal cavity using a WaterPik and a homemade saline solution (1 liter of boiled water, 2 teaspoons of table salt, plus 2 tablespoons of over-the-counter hydrogen peroxide). This twice-daily toilet (morning and evening) by and large keeps the cavity clean and free of epithelial and mucous debris. At follow-up visits the interior of the very large nasal cavity, which has no septum, can be thoroughly inspected with the use of the microscope or endoscope, paying special attention to the turbinates, cribriform plate, and inferior aspect of the anterior skull base.

DISCUSSION

Converse once said, "Only God can make a perfect nose and a perfect auricle."[16] Nasal reconstruction for very large defects (soft tissue, cartilage, and bone) presents difficult challenges to many head and neck surgeons.

The three-dimensional anatomy is complex, and important cosmetic and functional considerations are of concern. Congenital, traumatic, or ablative defects are readily visible to observers because the nose commands attention. Traumatic and congenital deformities often have structural and soft tissue deficiencies requiring augmentation and resculpturing. Massive defects secondary to surgical treatment of malignant

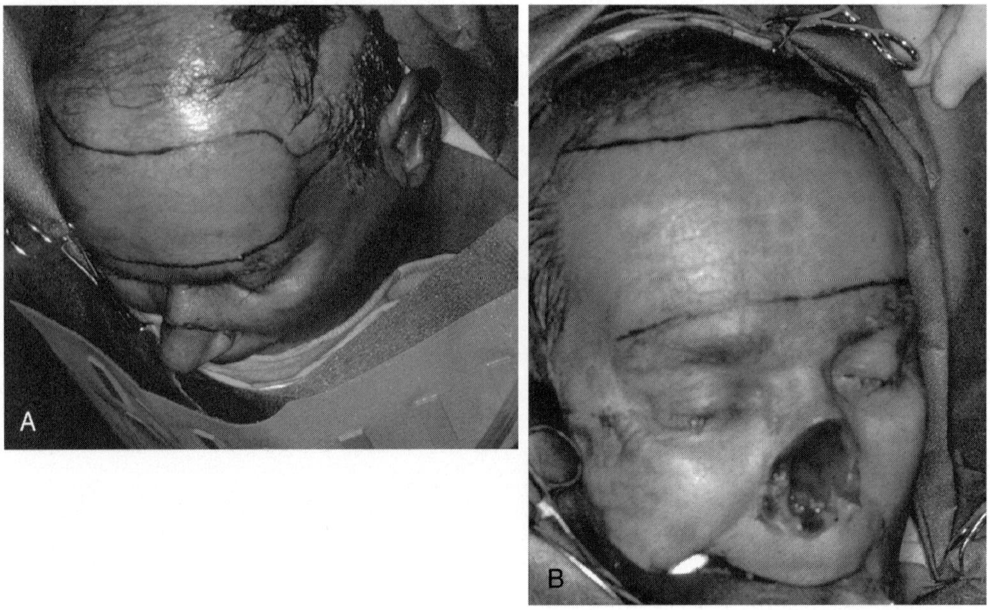

FIGURE 5–11. *A,* Surgical view of the patient outlining the horizontal forehead flap and nasal resection. *B,* Another view after the gross specimen had been surgically removed. (See also Color plate.)

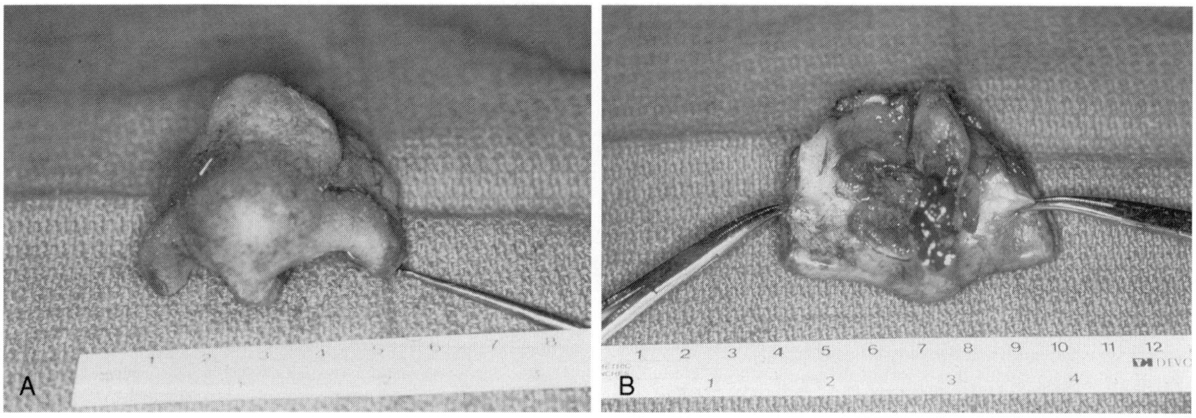

FIGURE 5–12. *A*, Gross specimen, lower nasal pyramid. *B*, Inner aspect of gross specimen, posterior view, showing the extensive infiltration of the recurrent squamous cell carcinoma. (See also Color plate.)

neoplasms present the most challenging problems. Many centers throughout the world prefer to use anaplastology (noses made of silicone or plastic materials) rather than surgical reconstruction, often with results that are satisfactory to patients. One of the main problems with prostheses is fixation. Tissue glues or cements so far remain unsatisfactory. Titanium screws or magnets also often fail in the nose. Osseointegrated titanium implants frequently extrude because the bone is rather thin and are especially troublesome when vascularity is very poor, as it often is in patients who have been treated with full-course radiation therapy.

Autogenous bone grafts have been used for many years and offer advantages over other homologous or plastic materials for augmentation. Homologous bone grafts are more likely to be resorbed owing to immunologic rejection. Autogenous grafts are often readily available, and there is a lesser potential chance for rejection or infection. Traditionally, iliac bone and rib or tibia were the grafts previously used for nasal reconstruction. The disadvantages of these grafts are significant resorption over a long period of time, resulting in loss of architecture and support with consequent functional and cosmetic problems.

Smith and Abramson[6] demonstrated decreased resorption of membranous bone compared with endochondral bone in 1974. They postulated that the cancellous portion of the endochondral bone might very well lead to early revascularization and more resorption compared with membranous bone. Kusiak and colleagues[10] proved this to be incorrect in 1985, demonstrating earlier revascularization in membranous bone than in endochondral bone in a rabbit model. They speculated that the osteogenic cells in membranous bone may be different from those in endochondral bone, and the early revascularization may be an important factor in preventing resorption. However, in 1988, Phillips and Rahn[11] showed that rigid fixation may be one of the critical factors in preventing resorption. They demonstrated that decreased resorption occurred in rigidly fixed bone grafts compared with nonfixed bone grafts in a sheep model. The volume of graft present at 20 weeks was statistically significantly greater for the fixed grafts. Nonfixed membranous grafts showed much less resorption than nonfixed endochondral grafts.

Membranous bone, especially parietal bone, is readily available. Harvesting of the outer table alone provides a split graft that is sufficient to provide excellent support for the nose with rigid fixation using titanium miniplates. The tech-

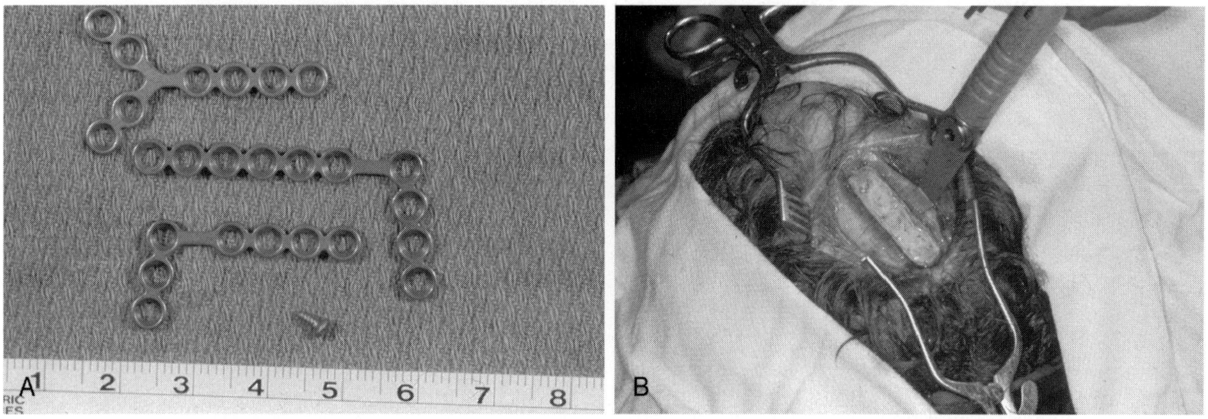

FIGURE 5–13. *A*, Mini-plates made of titanium alloy of different configurations. *B*, Donor site of parietal area shows the bone graft being harvested. The angulated reciprocating saw is helpful in removing the outer table only, when this is indicated. (See also Color plate.)

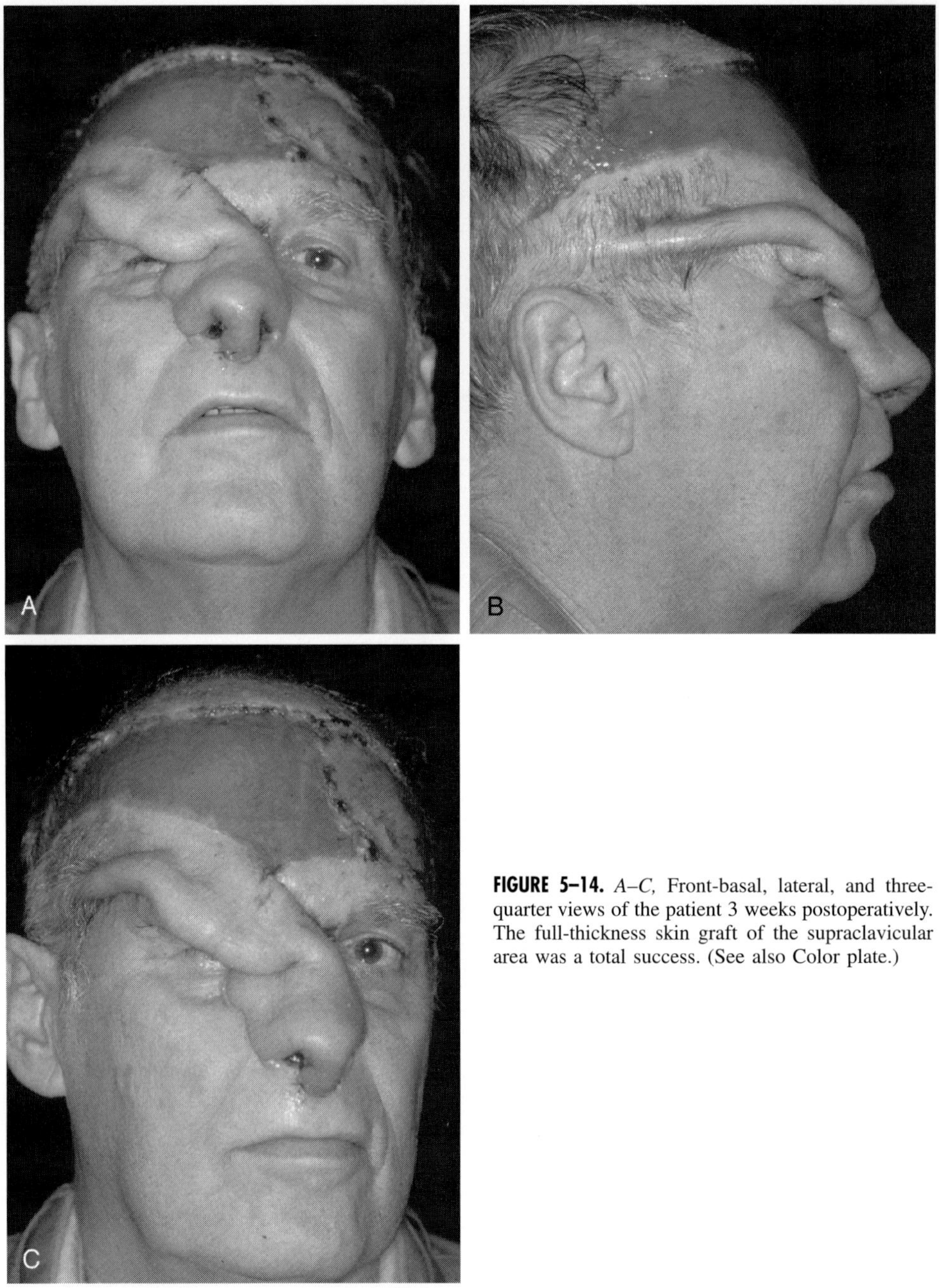

FIGURE 5–14. *A–C,* Front-basal, lateral, and three-quarter views of the patient 3 weeks postoperatively. The full-thickness skin graft of the supraclavicular area was a total success. (See also Color plate.)

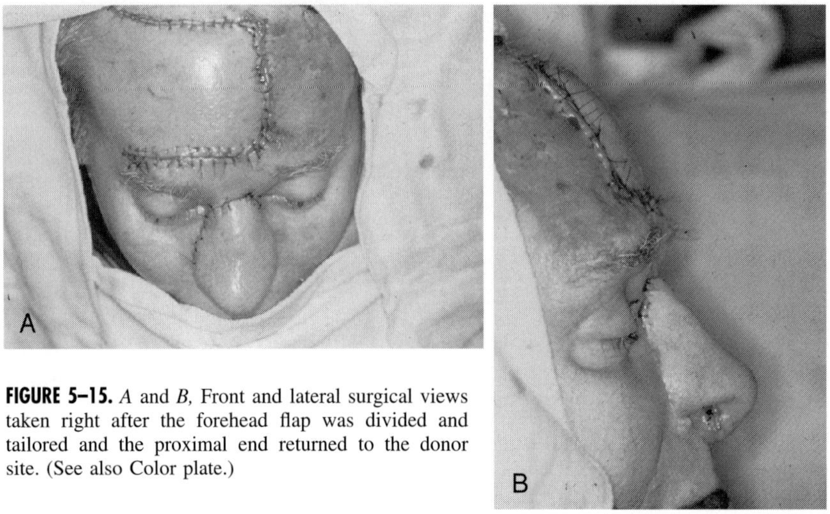

FIGURE 5–15. *A* and *B,* Front and lateral surgical views taken right after the forehead flap was divided and tailored and the proximal end returned to the donor site. (See also Color plate.)

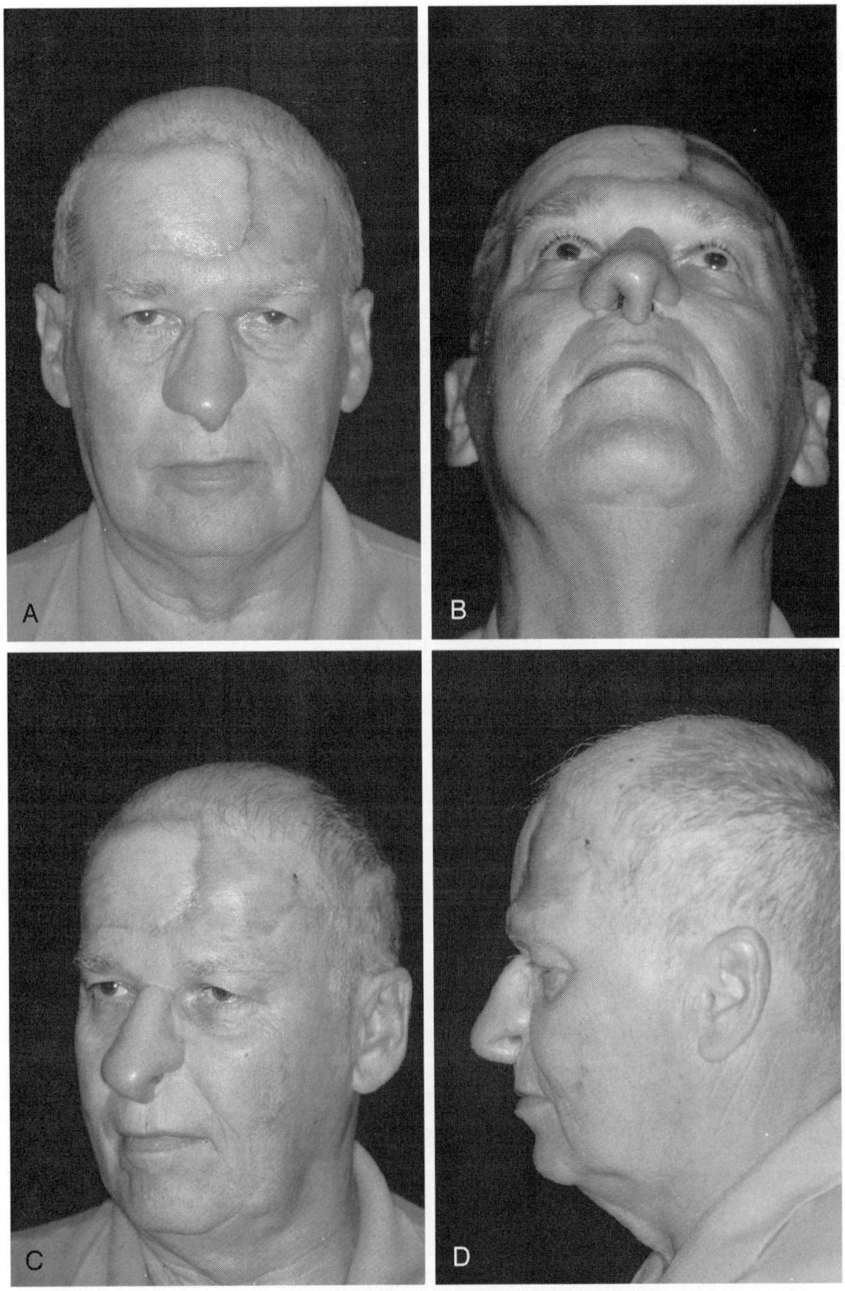

FIGURE 5–16. *A–D,* Front, basal, three-quarter, and lateral views of the patient taken 3 months after the second stage of the procedure. (See also Color plate.)

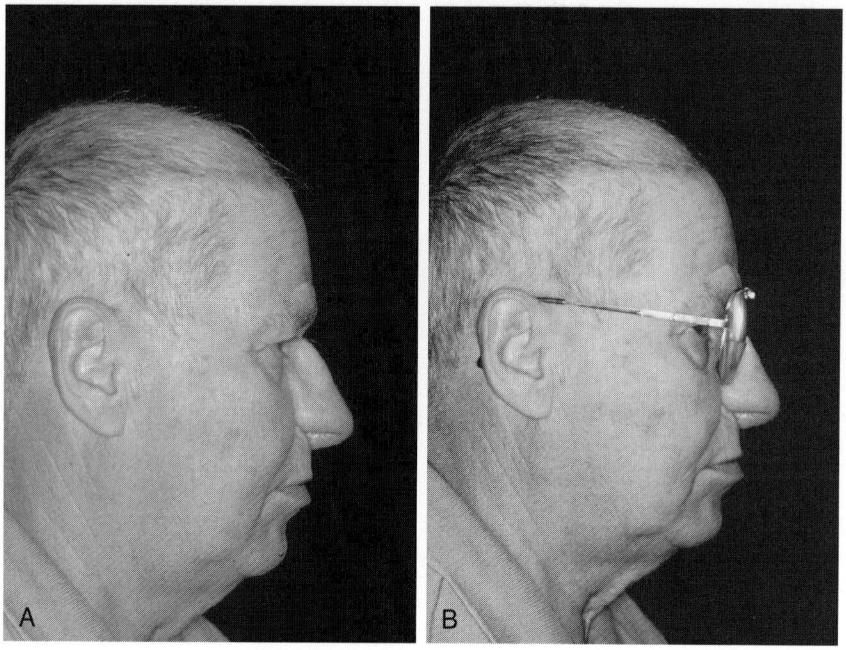

FIGURE 5–17. *A* and *B*, Profile views taken 3 months postoperatively. The eyeglasses help to camouflage the scars. (See also Color plate for Fig. 5–17*A*.)

nique is done using a round bur, a right-angle reciprocating saw, and a curved sharp osteotome. When properly done, the inner table is not violated, and no dural tear occurs. Bleeding at the donor site is controlled with bone wax and suction drains. Leaving the periosteum attached to the bone graft offers excellent conditions for early revascularization. Donor site morbidity is minimal, and the scar is well hidden above the hairline. Unless a full-thickness graft is removed, there is no need for any other tissue or plastic material to reconstruct the donor site defect created by the harvesting of the outer table of the parietal bone. The cosmetic result in our patients so far has proved to be very satisfactory. The amount of parietal bone resorption in all cases has been insignificant over a follow-up period of up to 10 years. One patient with malignant melanoma showed no evidence of any local recurrence after 7 years but died of metastases in the brain and lung. The rigid fixation employing titanium plates and screws remains stable and is well integrated biologically into the parietal bone graft and frontal bone. The titanium alloy used has the advantage of excellent bio-integration and tissue compatibility.

Based on our experience, our patients, even those who wore prostheses temporarily before reconstruction, prefer a nose made of flesh, titanium, and bone rather than a nose made of plastic. There are, however, definite indications for prosthetic devices, especially in patients who are poor surgi-

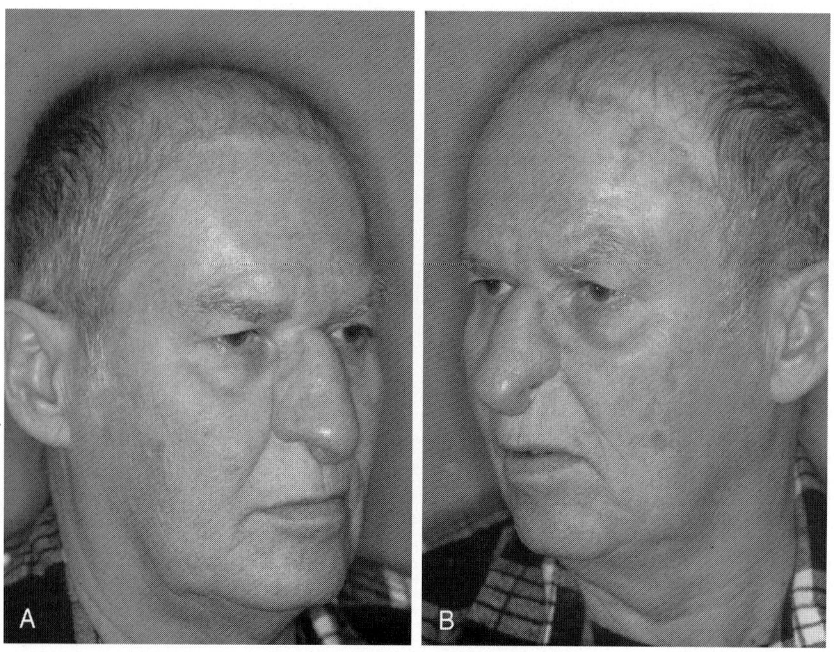

FIGURE 5–18. *A* and *B*, Three-quarter views of the patient taken after some defatting and partial excision of the full-thickness skin graft of the forehead. (See also Color plate for Fig. 5–18*A*.)

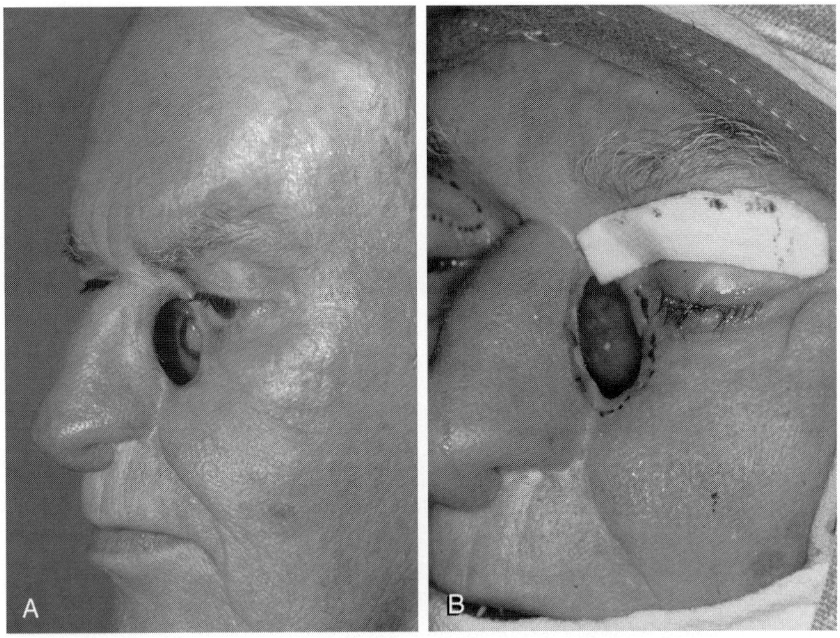

FIGURE 5–19. *A,* The surgical defect 6 months following excision of a second primary malignancy. *B,* Telfa pad outlines the myocutaneous upper lid flap that will be rotated inferomedially to reconstruct the defect.

cal risks, have a poor prognosis, or who dread the need for at least a two-stage surgical procedure for reconstruction. Recurrent basal cell carcinomas or other neoplasms with deep infiltration should be excised and reconstruction delayed 6 to 12 months to detect any possible recurrence. Also, if the surgical margins are close or involved, primary reconstruction should be avoided. Surgical resections should always be generous to ensure good margins. There can be no compromise on resection to favor easier reconstruction. Postoperative radiation therapy may be necessary. The parietal bone graft with titanium plate fixation tolerates radiation therapy very well with no significant resorption or loss of structural stability. Three of our patients had radiation therapy postoperatively. The two patients who suffered fractures of the parietal graft due to severe trauma were not previously irradiated. In these patients, after the the titanium plate that was fixing it rigidly was detached, the resorption of the parietal bone graft was obvious.

Stanley and Olsen[17] in 1988 reviewed the Mayo Clinic's 20-year experience of 51 patients treated with total rhinectomy for malignant disease. Basal or squamous cell carcinomas (86%) were the most common histopathologic diagnosis. Only 12 of their patients had had a true surgical nasal reconstructive procedure. Five patients had had reconstructive rhinoplasty with a forehead flap. These authors noted:

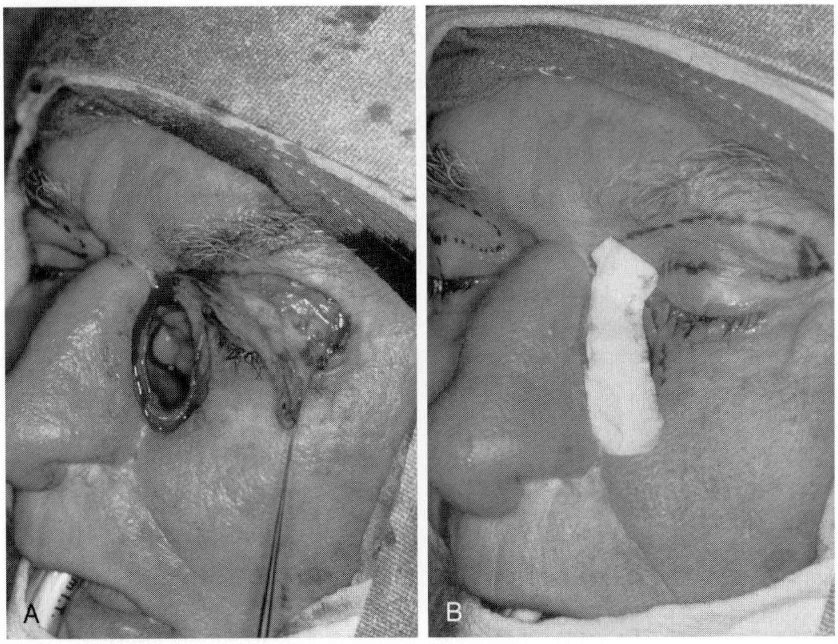

FIGURE 5–20. *A,* The Telfa pad is rotated. It is 10% to 20% larger than the defect to allow for contraction. *B,* A circumferential incision is made on the edges of the defect, and the myocutaneous flap, based medially, is raised.

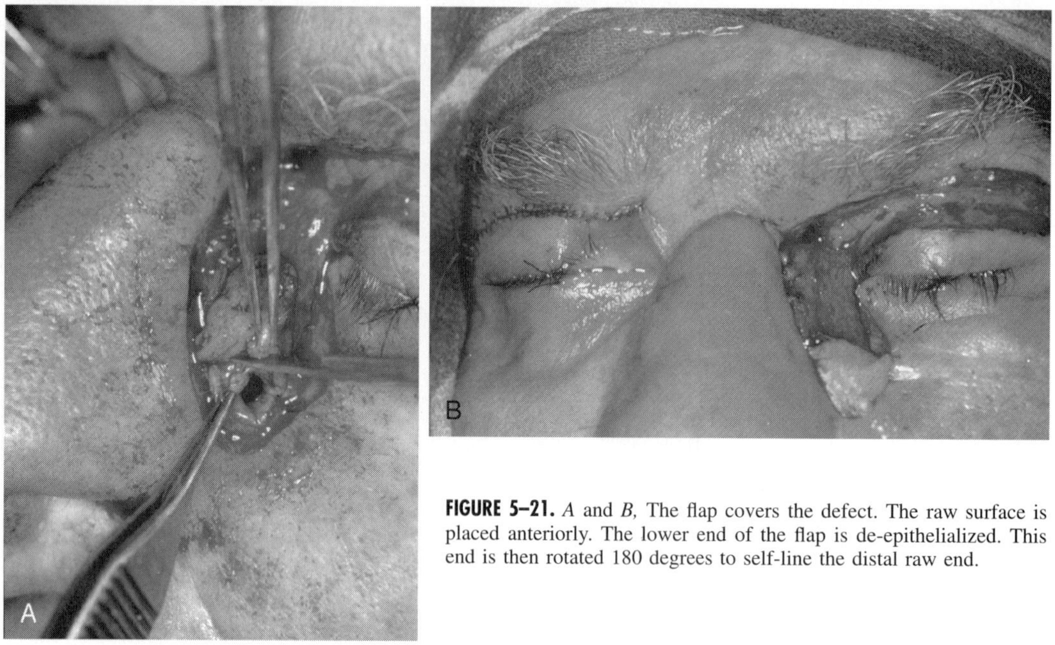

FIGURE 5–21. *A* and *B,* The flap covers the defect. The raw surface is placed anteriorly. The lower end of the flap is de-epithelialized. This end is then rotated 180 degrees to self-line the distal raw end.

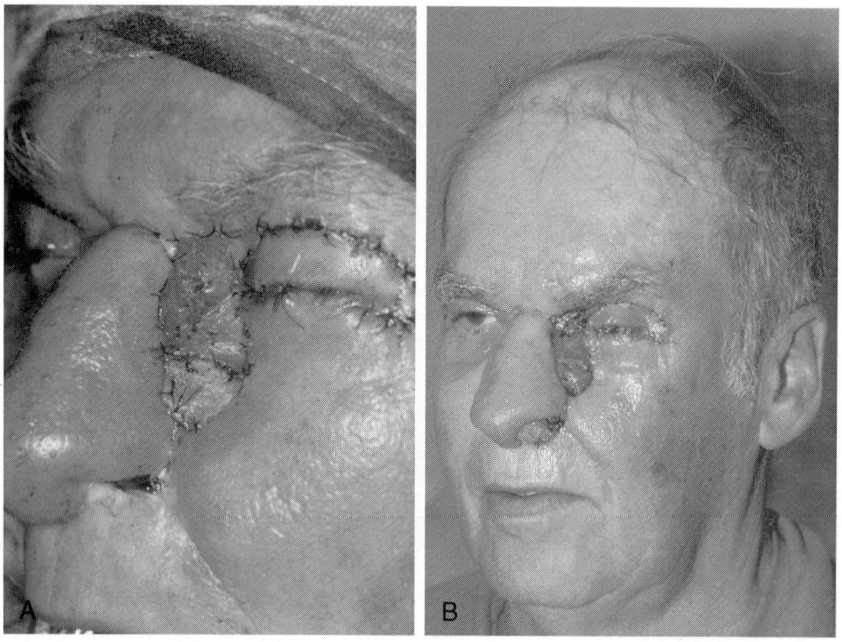

FIGURE 5–22. *A,* The upper lid defect is approximated, and the remaining portion of the myocutaneous flap is lined with full-thickness skin graft of the opposite upper eyelid. *B,* One week postoperatively, the skin graft looks dark, but it survived well, especially with cotton and ice saline cooling during the first 48 hours.

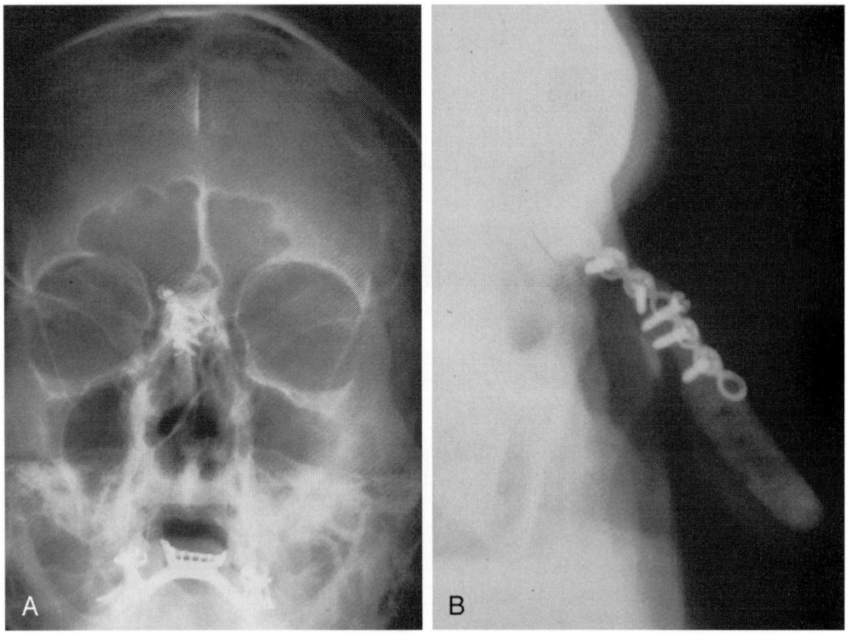

FIGURE 5–23. *A* and *B,* Plain x-rays showing the full-thickness parietal bone graft, the titanium plate, and the anchoring screws (2 mm in diameter by 6 mm long).

These were satisfactory in only one patient, failed after development of local recurrence in one patient and partially failed initially in one patient in whom recurrence later developed. The fifth flap survived, but several local flaps and split thickness skin grafts were needed later to correct airway obstruction.

Two out of four patients with scalping flap nasal reconstruction had multiple combined procedures, and each had a satisfactory result. They recommended nasal prostheses for most of their patients, stating that a prosthetic nose looks better than one reconstructed by even the most artistic and gifted surgeon. They admit that the prostheses do tend to fall off at most inopportune times because of problems with the skin-prosthesis cements or glues used for retention. Skin reactions, leakage of air and secretions, and a poor skin color match are the problems encountered. The Mayo Clinic report does not address osseointegrated implants and magnets for retention of nasal prostheses. Proops[18] in 1996 and 1997 stated that usually these do not work well, especially in irradiated patients, even with hyperbaric oxygenation. Although they are artistically sculpted, the prostheses never

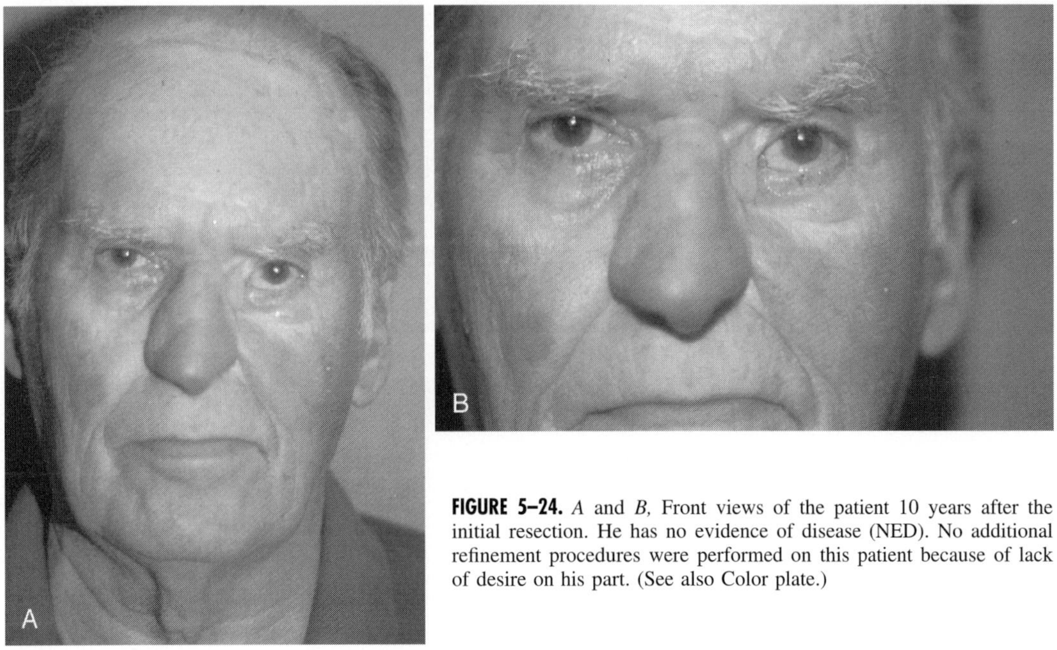

FIGURE 5–24. *A* and *B,* Front views of the patient 10 years after the initial resection. He has no evidence of disease (NED). No additional refinement procedures were performed on this patient because of lack of desire on his part. (See also Color plate.)

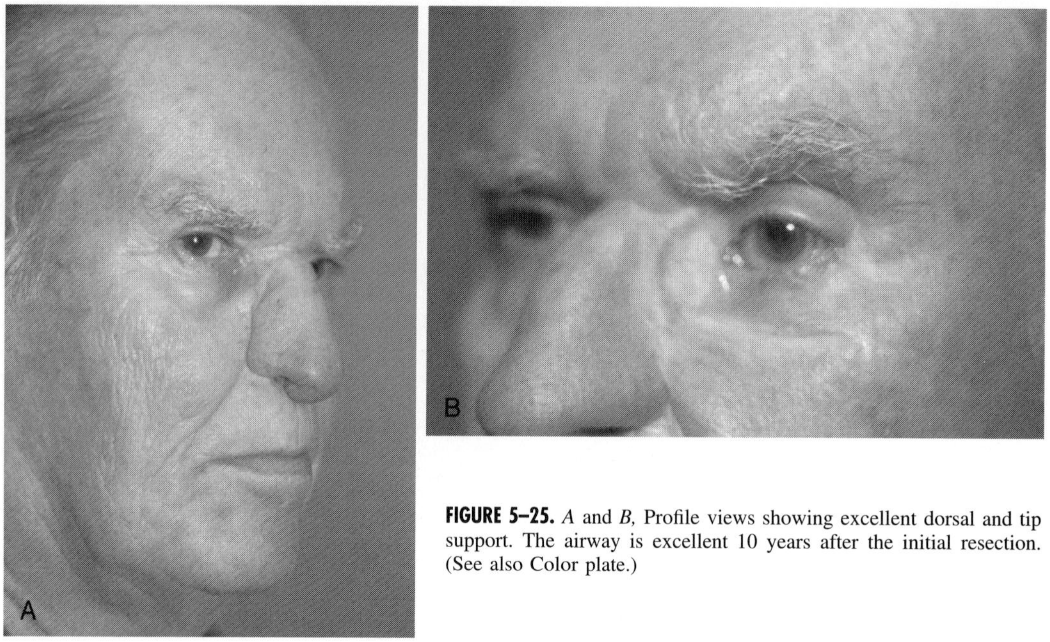

FIGURE 5–25. *A* and *B*, Profile views showing excellent dorsal and tip support. The airway is excellent 10 years after the initial resection. (See also Color plate.)

look "natural."[17] Eyeglasses are helpful in camouflaging the facial skin-prosthesis interface.

However, although nasal reconstruction is challenging, Burget, Menick, and many others[4, 12, 13, 14, 15, 19] have achieved very good results using different methods of reconstructive rhinoplastic techniques. These techniques do need multiple stages and refinements. But if the patient is well informed about alternative management approaches, understands the efforts and challenges needed, and accepts the discomfort involved in undergoing multiple surgical procedures, reconstructive rhinoplasty is worthwhile because it can be very satisfactory to both patients and surgeons and can produce permanent results.

SUMMARY

1. Based on our experience, the forehead flap (horizontal, vertical, or seagull-shaped) offers the best technical advan-

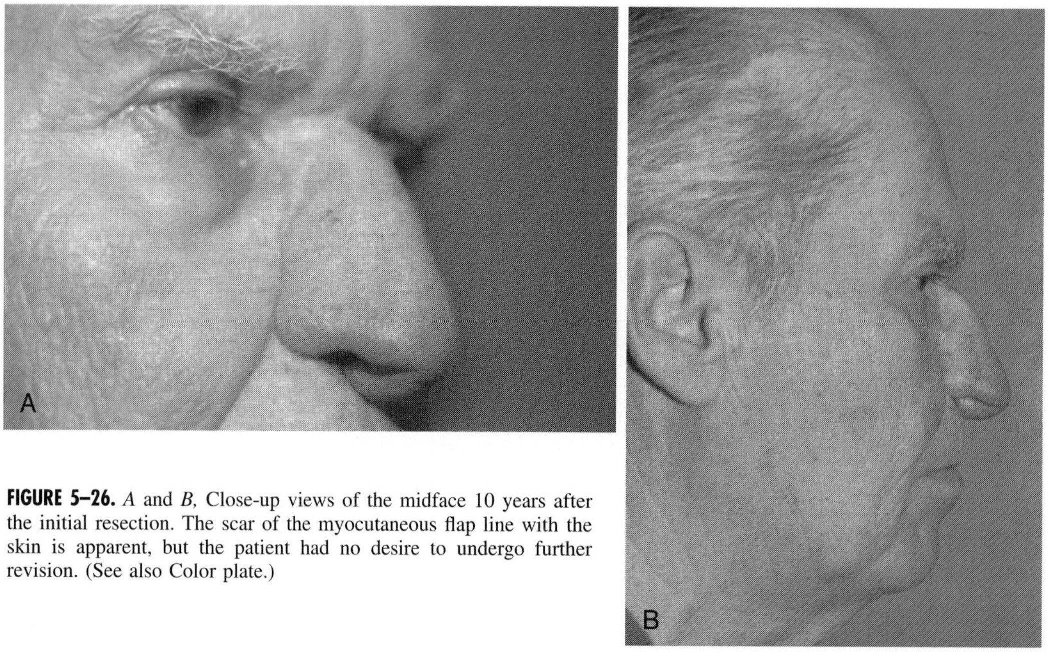

FIGURE 5–26. *A* and *B*, Close-up views of the midface 10 years after the initial resection. The scar of the myocutaneous flap line with the skin is apparent, but the patient had no desire to undergo further revision. (See also Color plate.)

tages, especially when it is combined with nasal dorsum support provided by parietal bone grafts fixed with rigid titanium plates.

2. Autologous parietal bone grafts appear to undergo the least amount of resorption. Long-term follow-up, even in patients requiring preoperative or postoperative radiation therapy, reveals that this material provides the best support and stability because resorption is insignificant compared with autologous rib or iliac bone grafts.

3. Membranous calvarial bone grafts are near the nasal and forehead surgical field and are convenient for harvesting with minimal donor site morbidity, especially when the outer table only is removed.

4. Rigid fixation with titanium plates and screws appears to offer precise, long-lasting fixation of the bone graft. It should be done during the first stage of reconstructive rhinoplasty and is followed by covering with the flap. This type of fixation helps to minimize further contraction of the soft tissues.

5. The advantages of using bone grafts for support during the first stage of reconstructive rhinoplasty are apparent. It is safe, and based on our experience, there is no incidence of postoperative infection, even when metal plates are used. The facial blood supply is generous and very helpful.

6. The parietal bone graft technique appears to offer the best cosmetic and functional results.

7. No significant donor site morbidity of the parietal bone graft occurred, such as hematoma, excessive pain, or infection. There were no intracranial complications.

8. Longer-term follow-up is needed to study further the effects of rigid fixation and loss of graft volume and architectural support, especially in irradiated patients.

9. Many patients can benefit from the use of nasal prostheses and can be reintegrated into society by this means. However, for a select group of patients, reconstructive rhinoplasty can accomplish satisfactory cosmetic and functional results that may very well be lasting and trouble-free.

REFERENCES

1. Ollier: De l'osteoplasie appliquée à la restauration du nez. Gaz Hôp Paris 37:349, 1864.
2. Mueller W: Zur Frage der temporaren Schadelresektion der Trepanation. Zentralbl Chir 17:65, 1890.
3. Konig F: Eine neue methode der Aufrichtung gesunkener nasen. Arch Klin Chir 34:41, 1890.
4. Converse JM: New forehead flap for reconstruction of nose. Proc R Soc Med 35:811, 1942.
5. Santoni-Rugiu P: Repair of skull defects by outer table osteoperiosteal free grafts. Plast Reconstr Surg 43:157, 1969.
6. Smith JD, Abramson M: Membranous vs. endochondral bone autografts. Arch Otolaryngol 99:203, 1974.
7. Zins JE, Whitaker LA: Membranous versus endochondral bone: Implications for craniofacial reconstruction. Plast Reconstr Surg 72:778, 1983.
8. Tessier P: Autogenous bone grafts taken from the calvarium for facial and cranial applications. Clin Plast Surg 9:531, 1982.
9. Powell N, Riley R: Cranial bone grafting in facial aesthetic and reconstructive contouring. Otolaryngol Head Neck Surg 113:713, 1987.
10. Kusiak JF, Zins JE, Whitaker LA: The early revascularization of membranous bone. Plast Reconstr Surg 76:510, 1985.
11. Phillips JH, Rahn BA: Fixation effects on membranous and endochondral onlay bone graft resorption. Plast Reconstr Surg 82:872–877, 1988.
12. Maniglia AJ: Reconstructive rhinoplasty. Laryngoscope 99:865–870, 1989.
13. Maniglia AJ, Swim S: Parietal bone graft and titanium plate fixation in nasal reconstruction. Laryngoscope 103:1066–1072, 1993.
14. Millard DR: Total reconstructive rhinoplasty and the missing link. Plast Reconstr Surg 37:167–183, 1966.
15. Maniglia AJ, Megerian CA: The medially based myocutaneous upper eyelid flap for lateral nasal defect reconstruction. Am J Otolaryngol 17(2):118–121, 1996.
16. Converse JM: Personal communication, 1971.
17. Stanley RJ, Olsen KD: Rhinectomy for malignant disease. Arch Otolaryngol Head Neck Surg 114:1307–1311, 1988.
18. Proops D: Personal communication, 1996; and paper presented at Osseointegrated Implants for Hearing and Craniofacial Rehabilitation, Symposium at Case Western Reserve University School of Medicine, Department of Otolaryngology-Head and Neck Surgery, co-sponsored by Nobel Biocare. Cleveland, Ohio, February 14–15, 1997.
19. Burget GC, Menick FJ: Aesthetic Reconstruction of the Nose. St. Louis, Mosby, 1994.

CHAPTER 6

Midfacial Degloving for Nasal, Sinus, and Skull Base Lesions

Anthony J. Maniglia, M.D.
João J. Maniglia, M.D.
J. Victor Maniglia, M.D.
David A. Phillips, M.D.
Robert C. Sprecher, M.D.
David W. Stepnick, M.D.
James E. Arnold, M.D.

Lesions involving the paranasal sinuses, nose, and skull base in adults and children are rather unusual. Neoplasms of the nose and paranasal sinuses are uncommon, accounting for only 0.3% of all cancers.[1] Because of this, most practitioners have a limited experience in managing these lesions. Compounding this limited experience is the insidious nature of the disease and its late diagnosis. Nasal and paranasal sinus neoplasms originate in air-filled cavities, and thus significant growth may occur prior to the development of signs and symptoms. When symptoms do occur, they may mimic benign processes such as rhinosinusitis, and the patient commonly complains of only obstruction or rhinorrhea. Symptoms such as nasal obstruction or purulent discharge may even respond temporarily to treatment with antibiotics or decongestants. Thus, often neither the patient nor the physician are alarmed by the seemingly benign nature of the disease process, and the tumor continues to grow until alarming symptoms and signs such as bleeding indicate that more invasive disease has developed. The average delay between the first symptoms and the diagnosis is 6 to 8 months. Although the maxillary sinus is involved in 80% of cases, disease limited to this sinus occurs in only 25% of patients,[1] owing in part to the ease with which tumors can spread between the sinuses. These factors all contribute to the advanced stage and poor prognosis of nasal and sinus neoplasms at diagnosis.

The etiology of these tumors is varied, and many are related to occupational exposure to various substances. Nickel workers have a higher incidence of squamous cell carcinoma,[2] whereas woodworkers are at increased risk for adenocarcinoma.[3] Additional occupations at risk are leather, mustard gas, and isopropranol workers.

The presenting symptoms depend on the site of origin as well as the extent of disease.[2] Nasal examination may reveal unilateral obstruction, purulent discharge, or benign polyps.[4] Examination of the oral cavity may reveal loose teeth, malocclusion, or trismus. Orbital examination may reveal erosion through the floor of the orbit, which may lead to proptosis, diplopia, decreased visual acuity, ophthalmoplegia, or cranial nerve deficits. Facial symptoms may include cheek swelling, numbness in the distribution of the infraorbital nerve, and widening of the nasal dorsum. Although the first echelon of nodes for posterior nasal and sinus tumors is the retropharynx, the neck should be carefully examined for cervical metastases.

Patient evaluation should include a complete history, examination of the head and neck, and evaluation of the cranial nerves. In the past, radiographic evaluation frequently began with plain sinus films. These are not particularly useful in defining the extent of a tumor. Computed tomography (CT) and magnetic resonance imaging (MRI) have revolutionized the ability to evaluate sinus tumors. Many tumors, both benign and malignant, can involve the lateral nasal wall and ethmoid sinuses or even invade the orbit and skull base.

Various surgical approaches to the midfacial structures have been developed in an attempt to resect these neoplasms adequately while leaving an acceptable cosmetic result. These include the lateral rhinotomy, the extended lateral rhinotomy or Weber-Ferguson incision, the total rhinotomy, and the midfacial degloving approach. A sublabial approach has been employed but offers limited exposure, especially when treating malignant disease. The disadvantages of the lateral and total rhinotomy are the facial incisions and the unilateral approach. The transpalatal approach also yields only limited access to the nasal and paranasal structures. The first documented sublabial approach for the treatment of nasal or paranasal disease was by Portmann and Retrouvey,[5] who in 1927 described a sublabial-transoral radical maxillectomy for the treatment of cancer. The technique of rhinoplastic release coupled with a sublabial incision as used today was presented by A.J. Maniglia and Joseph Arigo to the New York Academy of Medicine in 1971, and a 15-year experience was published in 1986.[6, 7] At that time, they reported a total of 30 cases for the surgical management of benign and malignant diseases. Conley and Price[8] have employed this approach since 1969, and in 1979 they reported their experience in the management of nasal and paranasal tumors using this technique. Allen and Siegel[9] reported four cases in 1981 and described their use of this technique since the 1960s.

The technique of midfacial degloving is also very useful in the pediatric patient. As in adults, excellent exposure of the midface and paranasal sinuses can be achieved with minimal morbidity and excellent cosmesis. The approach can be extended to a lateral ethmoidectomy approach if needed. Because of the shorter length of the midface in children, even lesions high in the nasal vault can still be successfully resected through this versatile approach. The soft tissues of the midface may be dissected and elevated even above the level of the glabella. In some instances, however, the midfacial degloving approach can be more difficult in pediatric patients because of the relatively small nasal vestibules, which make intranasal incisions as well as closures more difficult. In such cases, postoperative nasal stenosis could occur.

INDICATIONS

Indications for the degloving approach to the midfacial structures are varied. Because of the low morbidity and excellent exposure associated with this technique, the approach has been employed for benign as well as malignant processes. When indicated, benign lesions such as osteomas and fibromas can be exposed well and resected without difficulty. Adequate exposure to the anterior skull can also be obtained for the management of more aggressive benign neoplasms, including inverted papilloma, angiofibroma, and ameloblastoma, among others.

Malignant processes, most commonly squamous cell carcinoma, can also be adequately managed via a midfacial degloving approach. Resections such as medial maxillectomy, total maxillectomy, and maxillectomy with orbital exenteration can all be employed. Midfacial degloving can also be combined with craniofacial resection for the excision of benign and malignant lesions. In children, a wide variety of congenital and acquired lesions can be resected using this approach.

Benign lesions that can be approached include juvenile nasopharyngeal angiofibroma, nasal dermoids and gliomas, encephaloceles, chordomas, hemangiopericytomas, angiomas, fibrous dysplasia, ossifying fibromas, schwannomas, and extensive nasal polyps. Malignant lesions that can be resected include rhabdomyosarcomas, osteosarcomas, chondrosarcomas, and low-grade minor salivary gland tumors. High-grade salivary gland tumors can be resected through this approach only if they are limited to the anterior or inferior maxillary sinus.

Cosmetic and reconstructive procedures can be performed through the midfacial degloving approach. These include the treatment of midfacial fractures, midfacial osteotomies for advancement procedures, and augmentation procedures with onlay grafts.

This approach is contraindicated in the following situations: large malignant neoplasms, small tumors accessible by less invasive procedures, and inflammatory processes amenable to standard operations. Patients whose surgical risk is poor can be approached with another procedure or an alternative treatment, such as radiation as indicated.

SURGICAL TECHNIQUE

General anesthesia is administered through an oral endotracheal tube. The endotracheal tube is secured to the chin either in the midline or on the side opposite the pathologic findings. The patient is placed in the supine position, and the oropharynx and hypopharynx are packed with gauze. The eyelids are temporarily sutured together with 6.0 silk for corneal protection. Topical cocaine solution (4%) is applied intranasally via cotton pledgets. Lidocaine (1%) with epinephrine (1:200,000) is then infiltrated in the maxillary gingivobuccal sulcus, canine fossae, and the greater palatine foramina, bilaterally. The nose is injected in a fashion similar to that used for septorhinoplasty. After the patient has been prepared and draped and at least 5 minutes have elapsed to allow for vasoconstriction, four incisions are made. These include (1) bilateral intercartilaginous incisions, (2) septocolumellar-complete transfixion incision, (3) bilateral sublabial incisions from maxillary tuberosity to tuberosity, and (4) bilateral pyriform aperture incisions extending to the vestibule (Fig. 6–1). As in septorhinoplasty, the soft tissue of the nasal dorsum is then elevated and released. The periosteum of the maxilla is also elevated bilaterally, taking care to identify and preserve the infraorbital nerves. Any connections from the nasal soft tissue to the bony framework of the midface are sharply released; then two wide Penrose drains are placed through the nostrils, brought out through

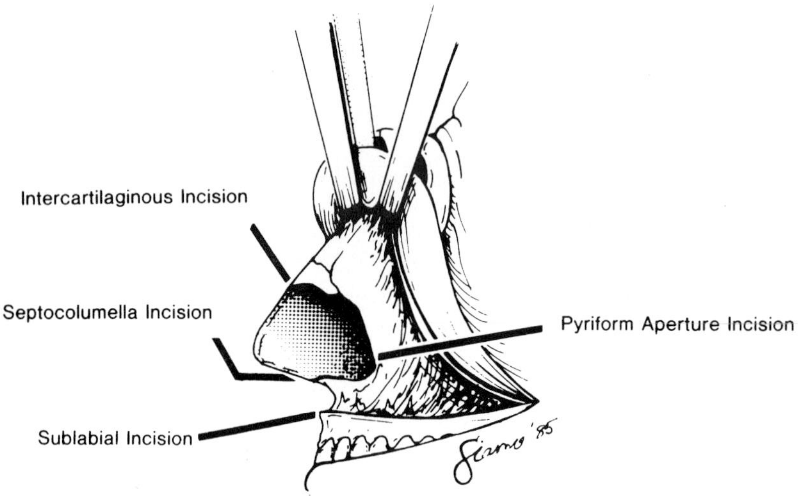

FIGURE 6–1. Illustration of four incisions made. (From Maniglia AJ: Indications and techniques of midfacial degloving: A 15-year experience. Arch Otolaryngol Head Neck Surg 112:750–752, 1986; copyright 1986, American Medical Association.)

the sublabial incisions, and secured with Kelly clamps to the drapes at the head of the table. The drains are then used to self-retract the midfacial soft tissues to the level of the glabella and orbits (Fig. 6–2).

The area of the pathologic process is then exposed. The ipsilateral antrum is usually entered using a gauge and widened using a Kerrison forceps. The anterior face of the maxilla is then removed to the frontal process of the maxilla. If the area of the nasofrontal duct or cribriform plate is involved, medial, lateral, and superior osteotomies are performed to allow retraction of the nasal bone or frontal process of the maxilla (Fig. 6–3). The orbital floor can be explored by retracting the periorbita superiorly. Lateral extension of the periosteal elevation also yields good exposure of the zygoma. Access to the pterygopalatine and infratemporal fossa is also possible. Depending on the need for visualization of the nasopharynx, the nasal septum and turbinates may be released, retracted, or even resected, and the posterior wall of the maxillary sinus may be removed to expose the pterygoid plates and skull base anteriorly. This technique may be combined with a frontal sinus osteoplastic flap or frontal craniotomy to manage processes involving the frontal sinus, cribriform plate, or anterior cranial fossa. Thus, by employing this procedure, the surgeon may perform a medial or radical maxillectomy, ethmoidectomy, or sphenoidectomy, or may gain access to the skull base. Also, the maxillary artery can be initially ligated to control bleeding, preferably using the extramaxillary transoral buccal mucosal approach.[10]

After removal of the lesion, hemostasis is obtained with bipolar cautery and Surgicel gauze packing. For extensive resections, a 15- or 30-mL Foley catheter is used to control posterior bleeding. The nasal tip is repositioned, and packing is placed in the nasal cavity and maxillary antrum. Incisions 2, 3, and 4 are reapproximated with 3.0 chromic catgut sutures. Incision 1 (the intercartilaginous incision) is not sutured to allow drainage of blood. Finally, paper tape and an Aquaplast splint are applied to provide immobilization and reduction of postoperative edema and hematoma formation. High-dose dexamethasone (40 mg) is used periop-

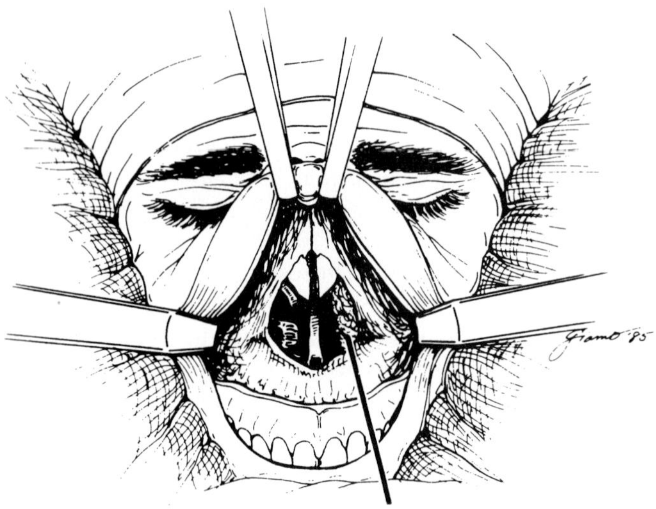

FIGURE 6–2. Degloved midface is retracted to level of the glabella and orbits. (From Maniglia AJ: Indications and techniques of midfacial degloving: A 15-year experience. Arch Otolaryngol Head Neck Surg 112:750–752, 1986; copyright 1986, American Medical Association.)

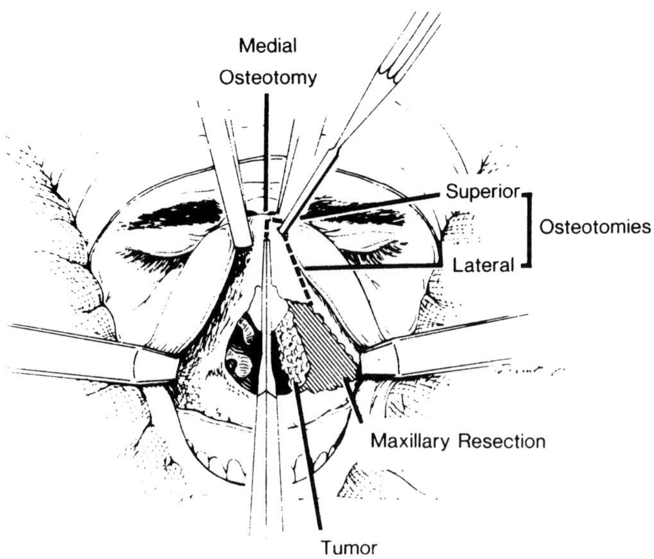

FIGURE 6–3. Lateral, medial, and superior osteotomies for exposure of nasofrontal duct and cribriform plate areas. (From Maniglia AJ: Indications and techniques of midfacial degloving: A 15-year experience. Arch Otolaryngol Head Neck Surg 112:750–752, 1986; copyright 1986, American Medical Association.)

eratively, followed by 60 mg in divided doses over the first 24 hours postoperatively. In children, the dose is 0.5 mg/kg per 24 hours. Perioperative antibiotics (cephazolin and metronidazole) are also employed and are continued by mouth for the first 10 days postoperatively in adults. Ampicillin/sulbactam is given intravenously in children for 3 to 4 days, followed by ampicillin/clavulanic acid by mouth for 7 days. Packings are left undisturbed for a period of at least 3 to 4 days.

CLINICAL MATERIAL

A total of 174 cases comprise our combined series of patients from the United States of America and Brazil. In 1986, A.J. Maniglia reported a series of 30 patients treated with the midfacial degloving approach since 1969 (Table 6–1).[6] He introduced the technique at University Hospitals of Cleveland in 1985. From 1986 to 1997, 36 more adult patients have undergone the procedure for disease ranging from benign neoplasms to squamous cell carcinoma. Table 6–2 reviews the histopathology of disease in these 36 adult patients. Only three complications were noted on review of these 36 patients. Severe epistaxis requiring transfusion and posterior nasal packing occurred in one patient. A persistent oroantral fistula was noted in a second patient. This patient had undergone a maxillectomy for squamous cell carcinoma and had had a persistent oroantral fistula on the opposite side while undergoing radiation therapy. The fistula healed spontaneously at the conclusion of the radiation therapy. Mild stenosis of the nostril occurred in another patient who

TABLE 6–1. PATHOLOGY OF CASES TREATED WITH MIDFACIAL DEGLOVING PROCEDURE

PATHOLOGY	NO. CASES
Angiofibroma	6
Inverted papilloma	8
Glioma of olfactory groove, nasal cavity	1
Extensive intracranial and extracranial mucocele	1
Large septal perforation	1
Squamous cell carcinoma of inferior turbinate posterior tip (radiation failure)	1
Squamous cell carcinoma of maxilla	8
Malignant melanoma, nasal septum	1
Adenocarcinoma, nasal cavity	1
Adenoid cystic carcinoma of hard palate	1
Malignant fibrohistiocytoma of maxilla	1
Total	30

was asymptomatic and desired no further treatment. Other postoperative sequelae included moderate nasal crusting and infraorbital paresthesias. The crusting was easily managed with saline irrigations, and the paresthesias resolved spontaneously within 1 to 2 months. There were no deaths in the combined series of 66 patients.

Rainbow Babies and Childrens Hospital of University Hospitals of Cleveland Experience

During the last ten years (1987–1997), 16 pediatric patients underwent midfacial degloving for the treatment of a variety of disease processes. The histopathology of lesions treated in this pediatric age group, varying from 6 months to 16 years of age, is illustrated in Table 6–3. One procedure was a revision performed to correct severe vestibular stenosis that occurred following a midfacial degloving procedure done at another institution.

Of the patients undergoing primary procedures at this institution, 2 of the 16 children had mild vestibular stenosis postoperatively, which was corrected with a simple Z-plasty. One patient had a persistent encephalocele, which was re-excised through a midfacial degloving approach.

TABLE 6–2. HISTOPATHOLOGY OF TUMORS TREATED WITH MIDFACIAL DEGLOVING IN ADULT PATIENTS, 1986–1997

PATHOLOGY	NO. CASES
Inverted papilloma	14
Squamous cell carcinoma	10
Angiofibroma	1
Hemangioma	1
Cementifying fibroma	1
Plasmacytoma	1
Hemangiopericytoma	2
Cavernous hemangioma	1
Mucosal melanoma	1
Chondrosarcoma	1
Adenoid cystic carcinoma	1
High-grade mucoepidermoid carcinoma	1
Ameloblastoma	1
Total	36

TABLE 6–3. HISTOPATHOLOGY OF LESIONS TREATED WITH MIDFACIAL DEGLOVING IN PEDIATRIC AGE GROUP PATIENTS, 1986–1997

PATHOLOGY	NO. CASES
Nasal dermoid	6
Angiofibroma	3
Encephaloceles	2
Glioma	1
Chordoma	1
Neuroectodermal neoplasm	1
Rhabdomyosarcoma	1
Revision vestibular stenosis	1
Total	16

From 1969 to 1997, A.J. Maniglia and co-workers accumulated an experience consisting of 82 cases, with no mortality. The complications (seven cases [8.5%]) were minor in nature, consisting mainly of bleeding problems, stenosis of the nostril, and oroantral fistula. The youngest patient was 6 months old and the oldest was 79 years.

Brazilian Experience

A.J. Maniglia trained J.J. Maniglia in New York City in the late 1960s. He also trained J.V. Maniglia at the University of Miami in the late 1970s. Both of them became familiar with the technique of midfacial degloving and went on to practice in Brazil and teach in Brazilian academic medical centers. Brazil, Mexico, and Egypt have a very high incidence of juvenile angiofibroma, unlike North America.

Table 6–4 illustrates the combined experience of J.J. Maniglia (Curitiba, Parana) and J.V. Maniglia (Rio Preto, S. Paulo), a total of 92 cases. The majority of lesions (47) were juvenile angiofibromas (51%), mainly in children under 18 years old (age range, 6 to 22 years; average, 14 years). Ten of such cases were surgically treated for angiofibromas with skull base extension, lesions similar to that in case No. 8 reported in this paper. The complications were similar to those previously reported, with no mortality whatsoever.

TABLE 6–4. HISTOPATHOLOGY OF LESIONS TREATED WITH MIDFACIAL DEGLOVING IN BRAZIL

PATHOLOGY	NO. CASES
Juvenile nasopharyngeal angiofibroma	47
Inverted papilloma	9
Osteoma	8
Fibrous dysplasia	6
Osler-Weber-Rendu (septal dermoplasty)	2
Septal tumors—neurogenic tumor	1
Septal tumors—hemangiopericytoma	1
Malignant fibromatosis	1
Trigeminal neuroma	3
Clival chordoma	1
Chondroma	1
Clival chondrosarcoma	6
Aneurysmatic bone cyst	1
Clival giant cell tumor	1
Branchial hypertrophic myositis of masticator muscles	1
Aesthesioneuroblastoma	3
Total	92

CASE REPORTS

Midfacial Degloving for Benign Disease and In Situ Carcinoma

Medial Maxillectomy for Recurrent Inverted Papilloma in a Pediatric Patient

The first case includes long-term follow-up of an 11-year-old boy in whom an intranasal procedure was performed to remove an inverted papilloma involving the lateral wall of the right nasal cavity. The lesion recurred 6 months postoperatively. A midfacial degloving with extended unilateral medial and lateral osteotomy of the nasal bone and frontal process of the maxilla was performed to allow access to the nasofrontal duct area. An extended medial maxillectomy was necessary to allow complete removal of the neoplasm (Fig. 6–4). In a 15-year follow-up the patient has had no recurrence of the neoplasm, and the midface has developed normally.

Medial Maxillectomy for Ameloblastoma

The second case is that of a 50-year-old white man who presented with left-sided nasal obstruction. Examination revealed complete obstruction of the left nasal passage. Ameloblastoma was diagnosed by biopsy. A preoperative CT scan revealed that the mass filled the left nasal passage and left maxillary sinus and extended to the nasopharynx (Fig. 6–5). A medial maxillectomy through a midfacial degloving approach was employed (Fig. 6–6). The entire lesion was resected, and the patient did well postoperatively and suffered no complications. He has had no recurrence of the disease through 10 years of follow-up.

Bilateral Medial Maxillectomy and Rhinectomy for Massive Inverted Papilloma with In Situ Carcinoma

The third case is that of a 62-year-old white woman who had previously undergone a lateral rhinotomy for treatment of an inverted papilloma. She presented 1 year later with nasal obstruction due to a cold septal abscess, mainly due to tumor necrosis. After drainage of the abscess, intranasal examination revealed recurrent papilloma involving the lateral nasal walls bilaterally with extension to the nasal septum. The patient underwent bilateral extended medial maxillectomies with a subtotal rhinectomy through a midfacial degloving. Both nasal bones, frontal processes of the maxilla, upper lateral cartilages, and nasal septum were removed. Only the nasal skin and tip were preserved. The nose was reconstructed using a parietal bone graft with titanium plate fixation (Fig. 6–7*A*). Her postoperative course was complicated by severe epistaxis requiring posterior packing and transfusion. The patient did well after the hemorrhage was controlled. Squamous cell carcinoma in situ and early focal invasion were documented on histopathologic examination.

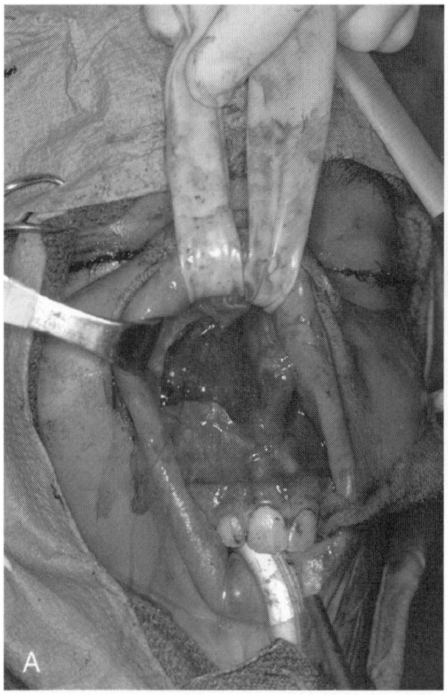

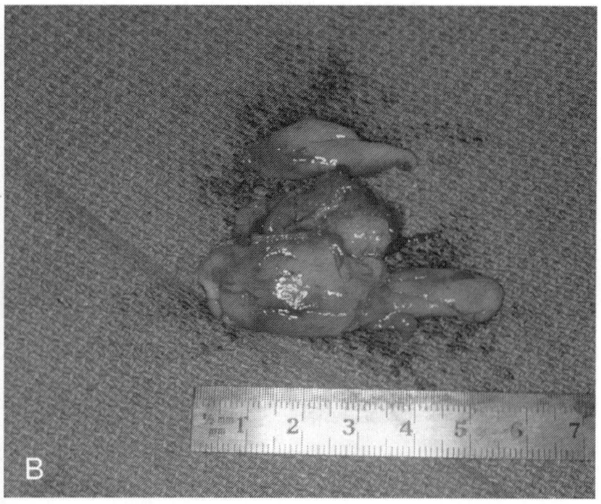

FIGURE 6–4. *A,* Midfacial degloving exposure in a pediatric patient. Note the wide Penrose drains for self-retaining retraction. *B,* Surgical specimen of the medial maxillectomy.

A full course of postoperative radiation therapy was given. However, even after radiation therapy, a localized recurrence had to be dealt with by local excision; this again showing proved to be carcinoma in situ in an inverted papilloma. Three-year follow-up after the initial excision showed no evidence of disease, and the patient maintained her excellent cosmetic result. No resorption of the parietal bone graft has been detected (Fig. 6–7*B* and *C*). Her nasal breathing is satisfactory. She uses daily nasal irrigations for toilette.

Radical Maxillectomy for Cementifying Fibroma

The fourth patient was a 39-year-old woman who presented with a 4-month history of a right cheek mass and palatal bulge. Two weeks prior to presentation, she reported onset of diplopia. Physical examination revealed right cheek swelling, a bulge in the right palate and alveolar ridge, and complete obstruction of the right nasal passage. CT scan revealed a radiopaque expansile maxillary sinus lesion extending to the orbit and nasal cavities (Fig. 6–8*A* and *B*). A cementifying fibroma was diagnosed by biopsy. Because this was a benign lesion, it was initially managed by shelling it out through a midfacial degloving procedure with a partial maxillectomy and external ethmoidectomy. However, the lesion rapidly regrew and the patient then underwent a radical maxillectomy with orbital preservation, again through a midfacial degloving approach. Figure 6–9 shows the specimen and temporary bolster employed in the reconstruction. Six years after the second resection, the patient has had no postoperative complications or recurrence of disease.

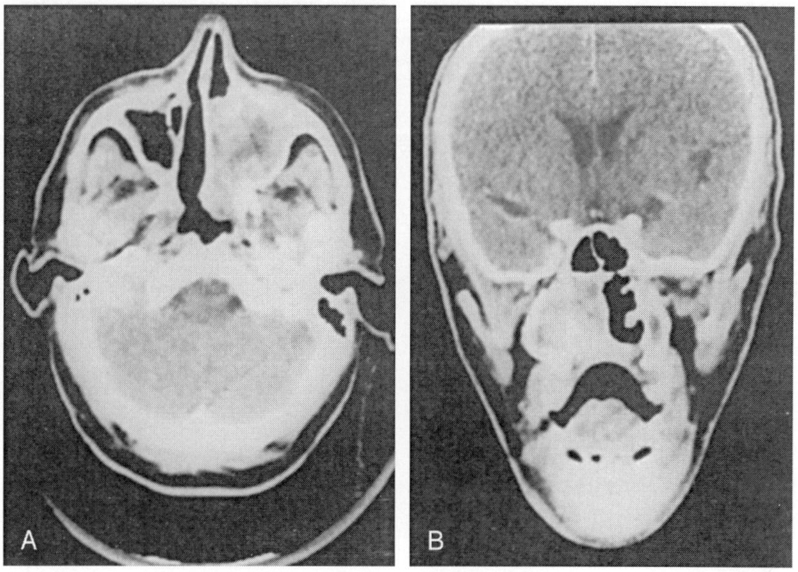

FIGURE 6–5. *A,* Preoperative axial CT scan of patient with an ameloblastoma involving the left maxillary sinus with intranasal extension. *B,* Preoperative coronal CT scan of patient with ameloblastoma. (From Maniglia AJ, Phillips DA: Midfacial degloving for the management of nasal, sinus, and skull-base neoplasms. Otolaryngol Clin North Am 28(6):1127–1143, 1995.)

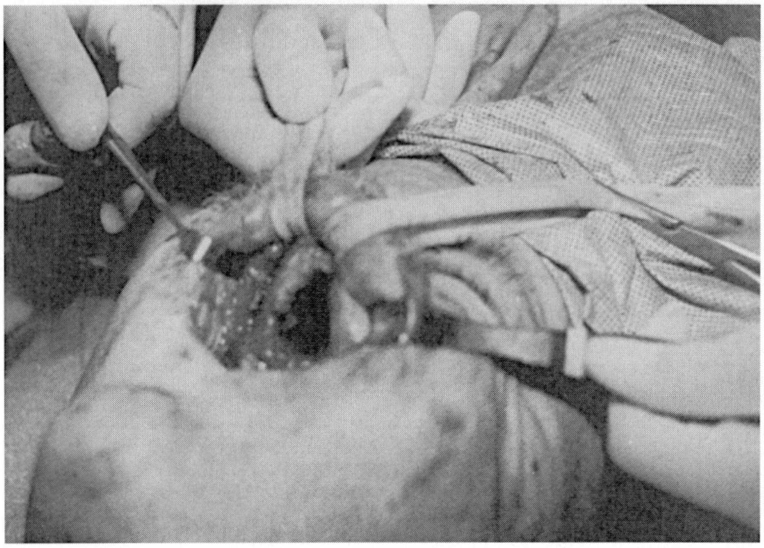

FIGURE 6–6. Midfacial degloving for medial maxillectomy and resection of ameloblastoma. (From Maniglia AJ, Phillips DA: Midfacial degloving for the management of nasal, sinus, and skull-base neoplasms. Otolaryngol Clin North Am 28(6):1127–1143, 1995.)

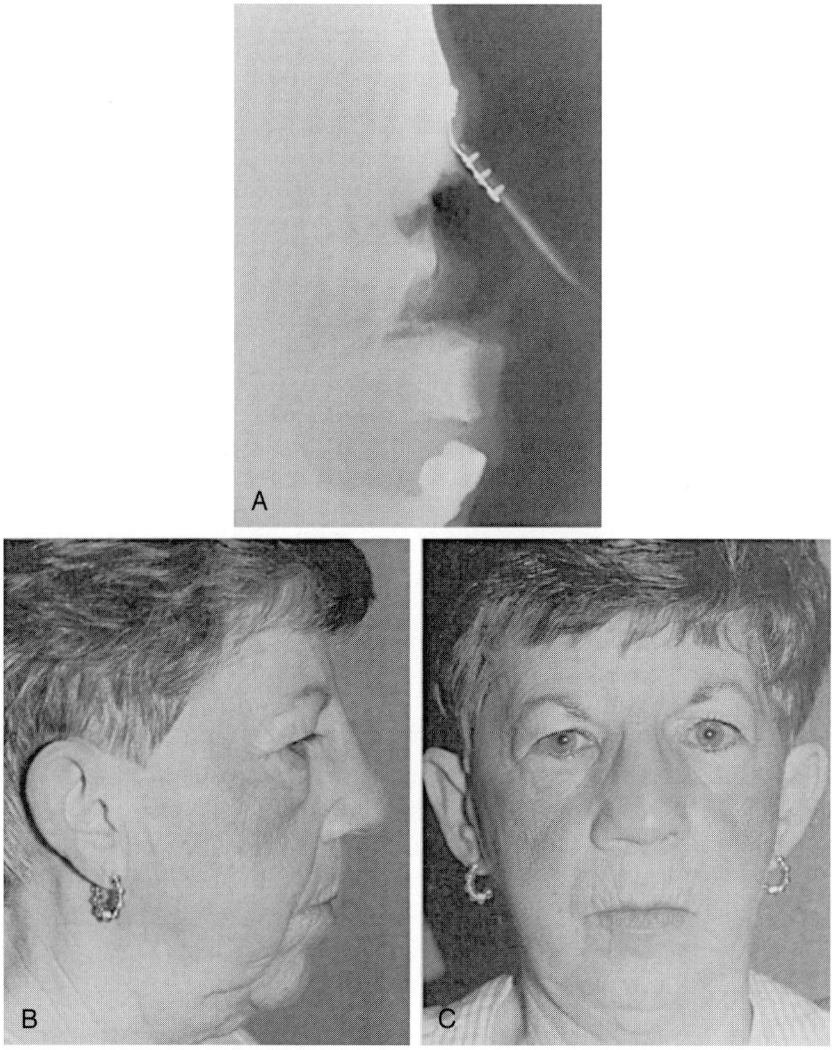

FIGURE 6–7. *A,* Lateral plain film demonstrating a parietal bone graft fixed with a titanium plate for reconstruction of the nasal dorsum in a patient who had undergone a subtotal rhinectomy. *B* and *C,* Front and lateral views of same patient at 3-year follow-up after radiation therapy. No evidence of parietal bone resorption. (From Maniglia AJ, Phillips DA: Midfacial degloving for the management of nasal, sinus, and skull-base neoplasms. Otolaryngol Clin North Am 28(6):1127–1143, 1995.)

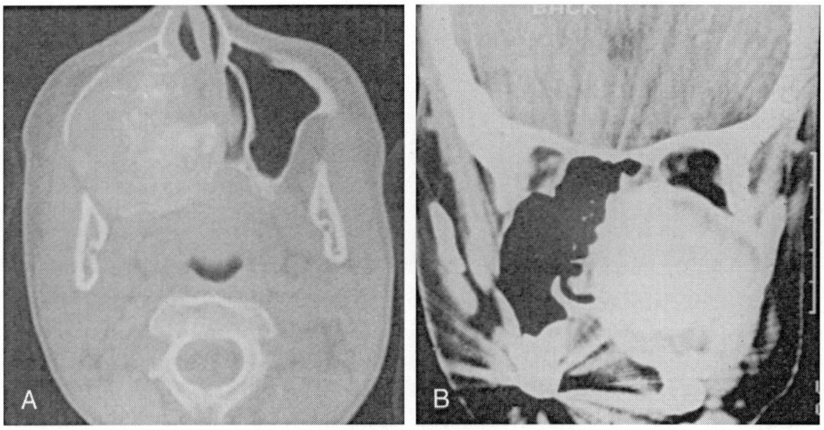

FIGURE 6–8. *A,* Axial CT scan demonstrating a cementifying fibroma involving the right maxillary sinus with extension to the nasal cavity. *B,* Coronal CT scan in same patient demonstrating extension to the palate. (From Maniglia AJ, Phillips DA: Midfacial degloving for the management of nasal, sinus, and skull-base neoplasms. Otolaryngol Clin North Am 28(6):1127–1143, 1995.)

Midfacial Degloving for Malignant Diseases

Septectomy and Premaxillectomy for Carcinoma

The fifth case is a 67-year-old white man with a history of a 6-week duration of recurrent episodes of epistaxis and a burning sensation inside the right nasal cavity. Anterior rhinoscopy revealed a 2- × 1-cm lesion involving the nasal septum with extrusion toward the nasal floor. On biopsy the lesion was reported as mucoepidermoid carcinoma high grade. A midfacial degloving with septectomy, turbinectomy, and premaxillectomy was performed. The cartilaginous septal support was lost entirely, and the nose was reconstructed with a parietal bone graft with titanium plate fixation, a technique similar to that used in Case 3. Also, a full course of postoperative radiation therapy was added after 3 to 4 weeks. The patient shows no evidence of disease after 6 years. The parietal bone graft has survived well with no significant resorption (Fig. 6–10).

Bilateral Radical Maxillectomy for Inverted Papilloma with Squamous Cell Carcinoma

The sixth case is a 62-year-old white man who had a 3-month history of maxillary sinusitis treated with multiple courses of antibiotics. After the symptoms failed to resolve, the patient underwent a left Caldwell-Luc procedure elsewhere. Frozen section of a suspicious lesion at the time of surgery revealed squamous cell carcinoma. The CT scan showed opacification of the left maxillary sinus with deviation of the septum of the right side and involvement of the hard palate bilaterally. There was no orbital or pterygoid involvement (Fig. 6–11). The patient underwent a left radical maxillectomy and an extended right maxillectomy with preservation of the second and third molars only (Fig. 6–12*A*). Prosthodontic rehabilitation was achieved, with excellent cosmetic and functional results (Fig. 6–12*B*). Figure 6–13 shows two views of the prosthesis-obturator. The final pathology report noted that the squamous cell carcinoma arose from an inverted papilloma. The patient did well postoperatively and suffered no complications. He was treated with a full course of postoperative radiation therapy and has had no evidence of disease at 9-year follow-up.

Radical Maxillectomy with Orbital Exenteration

The seventh case is a 65-year-old white woman who complained of right nasal obstruction for 4 months. She also reported otalgia and rhinorrhea and was noted to have proptosis of the right eye. A CT scan revealed a massive lesion of the right maxillary sinus with extension to the orbit and pterygoid plates (Fig. 6–14*A*). Biopsy revealed poorly differentiated squamous cell carcinoma. The patient underwent a radical maxillectomy with orbital exenteration through a midfacial degloving approach (Fig. 6–14*B*). She

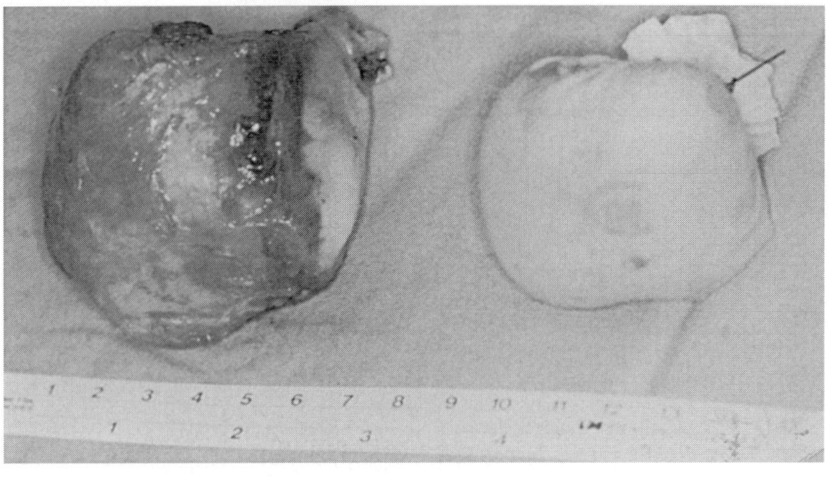

FIGURE 6–9. Radical maxillectomy specimen and bolster employed to support the skin graft after resection of the cementifying fibroma. (From Maniglia AJ, Phillips DA: Midfacial degloving for the management of nasal, sinus, and skull-base neoplasms. Otolaryngol Clin North Am 28(6):1127–1143, 1995.)

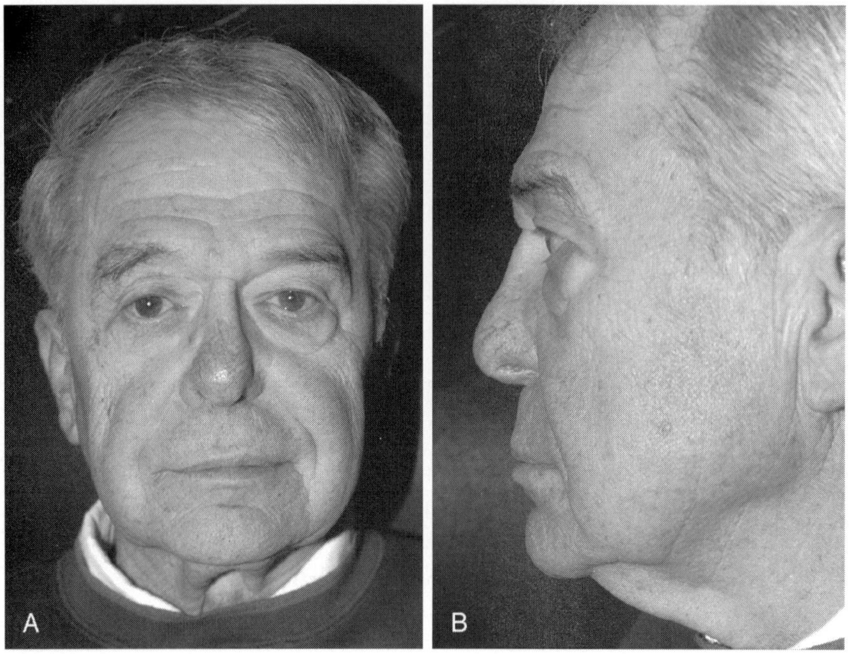

FIGURE 6–10. *A* and *B,* Front and lateral photographs of the same patient showing excellent support (6-year follow-up).

was treated with a full course of postoperative radiation therapy and has shown no evidence of disease after 5 years of follow-up.

Midfacial Degloving for Lesions Involving the Anterior Skull Base

Angiofibroma

The eighth case is a 20-year-old white man who presented with a history of nasal obstruction and epistaxis for 1 year.

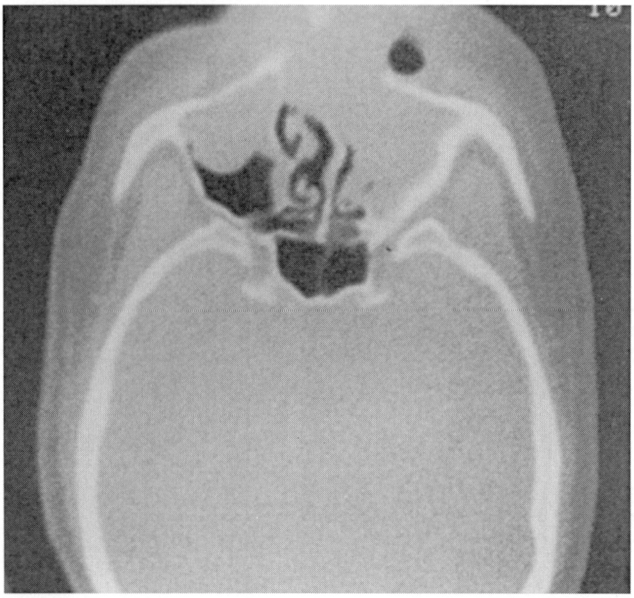

FIGURE 6–11. Axial CT scan demonstrating bilateral maxillary involvement by an inverted papilloma with squamous cell carcinoma. (From Maniglia AJ, Phillips DA: Midfacial degloving for the management of nasal, sinus, and skull-base neoplasms. Otolaryngol Clin North Am 28(6):1127–1143, 1995.)

A CT scan revealed a nasopharyngeal lesion with skull base destruction and extension to the left cavernous sinus and extradural compression of the temporal lobe. MRI further delineated the extent of the lesion (Fig. 6–15). A blush in the region of this mass was subsequently demonstrated by carotid angiogram (Fig. 6–16). The lesion was thought to be most consistent with angiofibroma, and the patient underwent a transantral ligation of the maxillary artery, medial maxillectomy, ethmoidectomy, and excision of the angiofibroma through a midfacial degloving approach. Using the microscope, the skull base extension of the lesion was removed and proved to be entirely extradural. The arterial feeder branch coming from the internal carotid artery was treated with bipolar coagulation. No neurosurgeons were involved in the resection, although preoperative consultation was obtained. Postoperatively, the patient suffered no complications, and the wound healed well with a good cosmetic result. No radiotherapy was given postoperatively, and there has been no evidence of recurrence at 7-year follow-up.

Cavernous Hemangioma

The ninth case is a 54-year-old white woman who presented with a 1-year history of right-sided headaches. Her evaluation included an MRI scan, which revealed a lesion lateral to the sphenoid sinus and posterior to the right pterygoid plate (Fig. 6–17). The patient underwent a midfacial degloving procedure with a transantral approach to the pterygomaxillary fossa and skull base, and the tumor was completely excised. The final pathology proved to be cavernous hemangioma. The patient did well postoperatively with no complications and reported resolution of her headaches.

Hemangiopericytoma

The tenth case is a 67-year-old white man who underwent a septoplasty for septal deviation at another institution. On

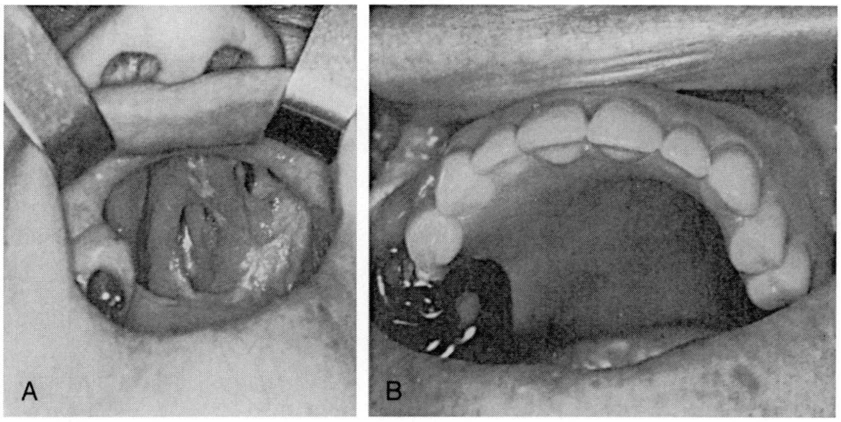

FIGURE 6–12. *A,* Postoperative view showing surgical defect after bilateral maxillectomy in patient with inverted papilloma and squamous cell carcinoma. *B,* Same patient with prosthesis in place. (From Maniglia AJ, Phillips DA: Midfacial degloving for the management of nasal, sinus, and skull-base neoplasms. Otolaryngol Clin North Am 28(6):1127–1143, 1995.)

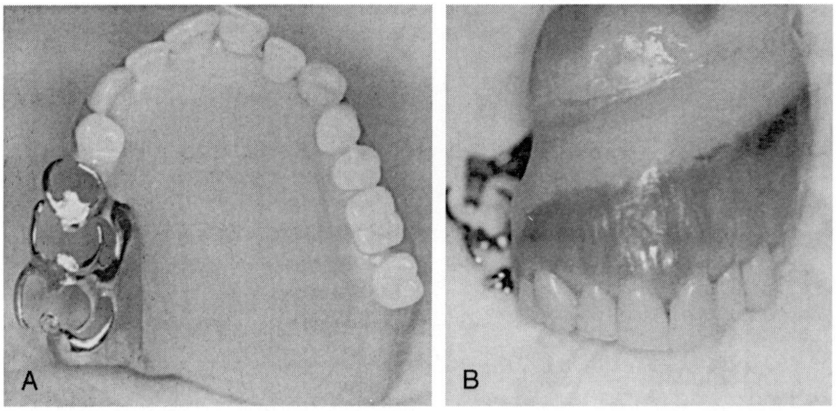

FIGURE 6–13. *A* and *B,* Prosthesis used for bilateral maxillary reconstruction. (From Maniglia AJ, Phillips DA: Midfacial degloving for the management of nasal, sinus, and skull-base neoplasms. Otolaryngol Clin North Am 28(6):1127–1143, 1995.)

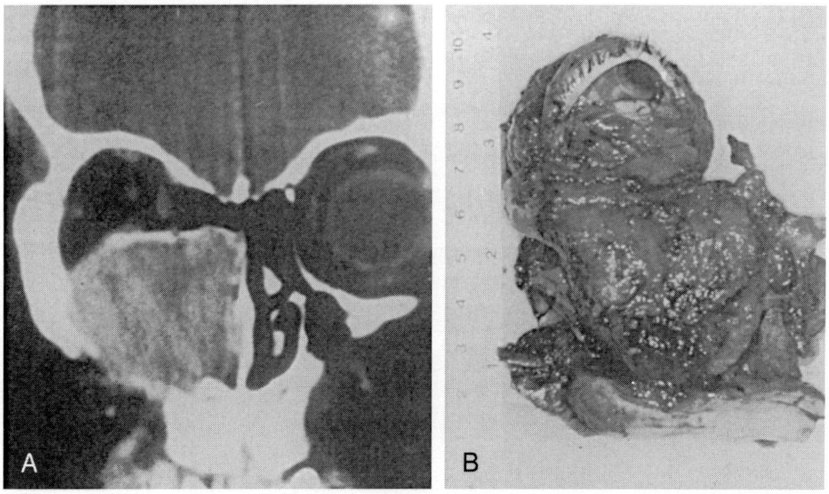

FIGURE 6–14. *A,* Coronal CT scan of patient with squamous cell carcinoma in the right maxillary sinus extending to the right orbit. *B,* Surgical specimen from right maxillectomy and orbital exenteration. (From Maniglia AJ, Phillips DA: Midfacial degloving for the management of nasal, sinus, and skull-base neoplasms. Otolaryngol Clin North Am 28(6):1127–1143, 1995.)

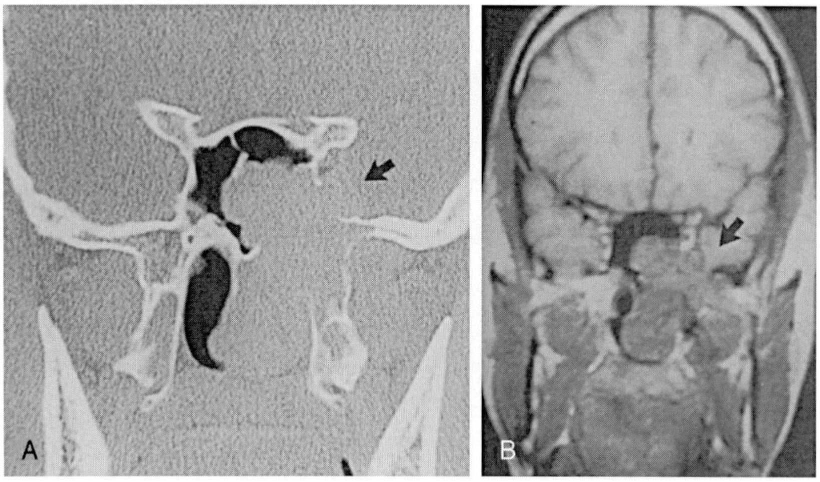

FIGURE 6–15. *A,* Coronal CT scan demonstrating right nasopharyngeal, sphenoid, and pterygoid involvement by angiofibroma. Bone destruction of middle cranial fossa is also seen (*arrow*). *B,* Coronal magnetic resonance image (MRI) (T1 imaging) of patient with an angiofibroma invading the middle cranial fossa and pushing the anterior horn of the temporal lobe (*arrow*). (From Maniglia AJ, Phillips DA: Midfacial degloving for the management of nasal, sinus, and skull-base neoplasms. Otolaryngol Clin North Am 28(6):1127–1143, 1995.)

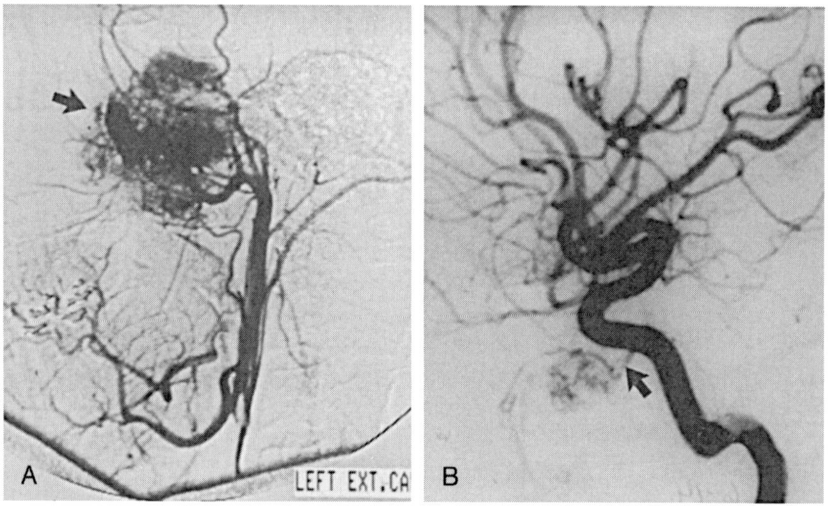

FIGURE 6–16. *A,* Carotid arteriogram revealing a vascular neoplasm that was found to be an angiofibroma (*arrow*). *B,* angiofibroma fed by a vessel coming from the internal carotid artery (*arrow*). (From Maniglia AJ, Phillips DA: Midfacial degloving for the management of nasal, sinus, and skull-base neoplasms. Otolaryngol Clin North Am 28(6):1127–1143, 1995.)

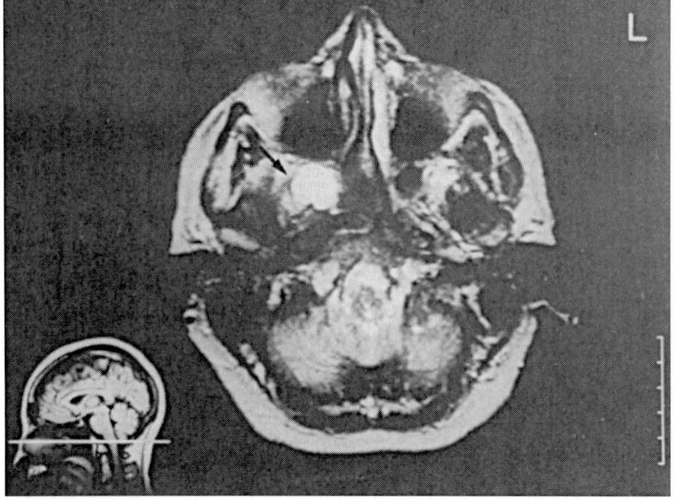

FIGURE 6–17. Axial MRI image of a cavernous hemangioma in the right pterygomaxillary space (*arrow*). (From Maniglia AJ, Phillips DA: Midfacial degloving for the management of nasal, sinus, and skull-base neoplasms. Otolaryngol Clin North Am 28(6):1127–1143, 1995.)

pathologic analysis the specimen was noted to be consistent with hemangiopericytoma. Postoperatively, the patient suffered from intermittent epistaxis. A CT scan revealed involvement of the left sphenoid and ethmoid sinuses in addition to changes consistent with chronic sinusitis. The patient underwent a left medial maxillectomy through a midfacial degloving approach with bilateral endoscopic ethmoidectomies and a left sphenoidotomy for resection of the hemangiopericytoma. Postoperatively he did well and suffered no complications. A routine examination at the 1 year follow-up revealed a 5- × 5-mm recurrent lesion under the nasal bone. Laser excision was employed, and the patient has had no other recurrence. Because of the noninvasive nature and histopathology of the lesion, no radiation therapy was added postoperatively.

Craniofacial Resection for Recurrent Inverted Papilloma with Atypia

The eleventh case is a 30-year-old black woman who had had a long history of recurrent inverted papilloma. Four years prior to this presentation, while pregnant, she had undergone a lateral rhinotomy for inverted papilloma, but she frequently failed to keep her follow-up appointments. She also had multiple transnasal laser excisions of the neoplasms. When she finally returned, she complained of bilateral nasal obstruction, and an extensive recurrent lesion was noted involving both orbits and nasal bones. MRI revealed that the lesion involved the ethmoid sinuses and skull base and had also extended intracranially (Fig. 6–18). The patient underwent a subtotal rhinectomy, bilateral medial maxillectomy, orbital explorations, and external ethmoidectomies through a midfacial degloving approach as well as a craniofacial resection in conjunction with the neurosurgery service. The nose was reconstructed with a parietal bone graft and titanium plate fixation. Histopathologic examination showed atypical cells. Evaluation of the papilloma revealed human papilloma virus (HPV) types 6 and 11; thus it had a low risk for malignancy. Because of the multiple recurrences and aggressive invasive growth of this disease with atypia, postoperative radiation therapy (5000 cGy) was instituted. The patient has had no recurrence at 3-year follow-up.

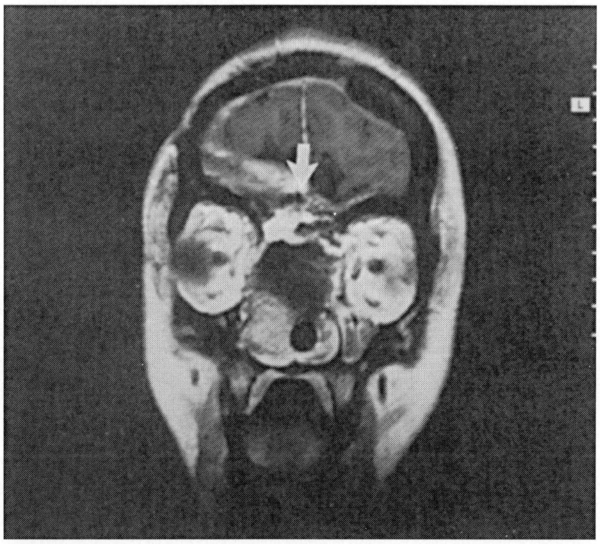

FIGURE 6–18. Coronal MRI image (T1 image) of a patient with an inverted papilloma involving the orbit and ethmoid sinuses with skull base erosion and extension to the anterior cranial fossa. (From Maniglia AJ, Phillips DA: Midfacial degloving for the management of nasal, sinus, and skull-base neoplasms. Otolaryngol Clin North Am 28(6):1127–1143, 1995.)

DISCUSSION

The midfacial degloving approach to the midfacial structures is a versatile procedure. As demonstrated by the reported cases, there is a low complication rate when the procedure is employed for a variety of lesions. For short-duration procedures in a suitable patient, local or general anesthesia may be used. Large septal perforations and benign neoplasms as well as invasive malignant carcinomas can all be managed with this approach. It provides excellent access for a wide range of resections from medial maxillectomy to radical maxillectomy with orbital exenteration. Neoplasms involving the nasopharynx and skull base can also be treated using this approach. When there is invasion of the orbit, the external ethmoidectomy approach is necessary to allow possible preservation of the orbital contents. Midfacial degloving can also be combined with craniofacial resection for lesions involving the cribriform plate and anterior cranial fossa. It yields bilateral exposure, and there is a low postoperative complication rate. Problems such as postoperative bleeding, vestibular stenosis, and oroantral fistula are infrequently encountered. Extensive resections with large cavities result in nasal crusting that requires saline irrigation. Paresthesias may be encountered; however, these frequently resolve in 2 to 3 months. Because the sublabial incisions are usually performed bilaterally, patients rarely complain of annoying, persistent paresthesias. In addition, the cosmetic result is very good because there are no external midfacial incisions. This is especially important in women, public figures, and children, because facial scars are less acceptable by these patients. As demonstrated in the illustrative cases, if a subtotal rhinectomy is necessary, the nose can be reconstructed with excellent cosmetic results using a parietal bone graft with titanium plate fixation.[11–13] In such cases, when the nasal skin is the only structure available, the parietal bone graft with titanium plate fixation is used with periosteum on one side, opposite the graft facing the nasal skin of the dorsum. No skin graft is necessary for lining. The graft periosteum heals well, forming a mucosal layer that totally covers the parietal bone. Even with full-course postoperative radiation therapy, the bone grafts survive well with minimal resorption problems during long-term follow-up. No intranasal exposure of the nasal bone was noted in these cases.

SUMMARY

In conclusion, the midfacial degloving procedure is an excellent approach for many pathologic processes, and can be combined with other procedures for more extensive lesions. Although it is not meant to totally replace the external approaches, it should be incorporated into the surgical armamentarium of the otolaryngologist or head and neck surgeon and used whenever possible to avoid external facial scarring. Other head and neck specialists, such as general plastic surgeons and oral and maxillofacial surgeons, could use this approach as well.

REFERENCES

1. Harrison DF: The management of malignant tumors of the nose and paranasal sinuses. Otolaryngol Clin North Am 4:159, 1971.
2. Barton RT: Nickel carcinogenesis of the respiratory tract. J Otolaryngol 6:412, 1977.
3. Acheson ED, Cowdell RH, Hadfield E, et al: Nasal cancer in woodworkers in the furniture industry. Br Med J 2:587, 1968.
4. Batsakis JG: Cancer of the nasal cavity and the paranasal sinuses. *In* Batsakis JG (ed): Tumors of the Head and Neck, 2nd ed. Baltimore, Williams & Wilkins, 1979, pp 177–187.
5. Portmann G, Retrouvey H: Le cancer du nez. Paris, Gaston Doin et Cie, 1927.
6. Maniglia AJ, Arigo J: Sublabial rhinotomy for the treatment of angiofibroma. Otolaryngology Section Meeting, New York Academy of Medicine, November, 1971.
7. Maniglia AJ: Indications and techniques of midfacial degloving: A 15-year experience. Otolaryngol Head Neck Surg 112:750–752, 1986.
8. Conley J, Price JC: Sublabial approach to the nasal cavity and nasopharyngeal cavities. Am J Surg 38:615–618, 1979.
9. Allen GA, Siegel GJ: The sublabial approach for extensive nasal and sinus resection. Laryngoscope 91:1635–1640, 1981.
10. Stepnick DW, Maniglia AJ, Bold EL, et al: Intraoral-extramaxillary sinus approach for ligation of the maxillary artery: An anatomic study with clinical correlates. Laryngoscope 100:1166–1170, 1990.
11. Maniglia AJ: Reconstructive rhinoplasty. Laryngoscope 99:865–870, 1989.
12. Maniglia JJ, Ramina R: Facial degloving approach in skull base surgery. *In* Donald P (ed): Skull Base Surgery. Philadelphia, Lippincott-Raven, 1998, pp 195–206.
13. Radkowski D, McGill T, Ohlms L, Jones DT: Angiofibromas. Changes in staging and treatment. Arch Otolaryngol Head Neck Surg 122:122–129, 1996.

CHAPTER 7

Concepts in Orbital Reconstruction and Optic Nerve Decompression

Gene Howard, M.D.
J. David Osguthorpe, M.D.

The diagnosis and surgical management of orbital disease often requires interaction among several specialties. The coordinated efforts of otolaryngologists, ophthalmologists, neurosurgeons, plastic surgeons, and prosthodontists can be essential to the rehabilitation of patients who have suffered facial trauma or the extirpation of neoplasms. This article provides a review and update for the diagnosis of orbital disease as well as a practical approach to the treatment of several orbital reconstructive problems. Information is provided on anatomic considerations and radiologic studies that assist the surgeon in developing an appropriate surgical plan. Specific attention is paid to the areas of cutaneous grafting, muscular and myocutaneous grafts, osseous reconstruction, plating techniques, and dacryocystorhinostomy. Additional attention is directed toward orbital decompression for Graves disease and optic nerve decompression for acute compressive neuropathy after trauma.

ANATOMIC CONSIDERATIONS

A standard physical examination of patients with an orbital mass lesion or injury can indicate the need for further diagnostic testing and may alert the physician to the need for urgent treatment. An ophthalmologic examination starts with an assessment of visual acuity. Acute visual loss may herald trauma to the globe (hyphema, retinal disruption, globe perforation), or, if this is intact, an optic nerve pathway injury; the latter is likely if an afferent pupillary defect is present. Traumatic optic neuropathy with afferent defects is seen not only with avulsion or transection of the optic nerve but also with nerve compression due to hematoma, bone fragments, or edema.[6, 24, 40] Lesser optic pathway injuries may be manifest as visual field losses, which can occur without an afferent defect, although they are more common in patients with long-standing compressive phenomena such as orbital tumors or Graves disease.[33]

Limitations in movement of the globe are frequent in patients with traumatic injuries because fractures of the orbital walls can entrap or otherwise restrict the extraocular muscles, especially in orbital floor fractures.[20, 23] Entrapment of the fibrous septa around the orbital fat may occur in the absence of muscle displacement into the maxillary or ethmoid sinuses.[34] This is important because coronal computed tomography (CT) scans may disclose no gross muscle entrapment. Further complicating this picture is the possibility that intramuscular hematoma due to blunt trauma may mimick entrapment. Performance of a "forced duction test" can be more helpful than a CT scan in separating restrictive entrapment from muscular hematoma or cranial nerve palsy. This test requires anesthetizing the inferior bulbar conjunctiva of both eyes with 4% topical lidocaine. The conjunctiva in the appropriate fornix and the adjacent Tenon's capsule of the uninjured eye are grasped with a toothed forceps and moved in the direction opposite the restriction. This maneuver is then repeated on the injured side. Limitations in movement strongly suggest entrapment. Most restricted muscles demonstrate some voluntary movement opposite an entrapped or otherwise traumatized muscle, unlike a nerve palsy, which exhibits no voluntary movement. To detect this possibility using the forced duction test, the patient is asked to look in a specific direction. If no movement or tug is felt, a nerve palsy is likely.

Injuries to cranial nerves III, IV, and VI are ruled out by normal results on a motility examination. Subjective complaints of diplopia may be helpful in alert, articulate patients. Cranial nerve V is tested by gently touching the cornea with a few strands of a cotton-tipped applicator and comparing the evidence of sensation to that on the contralateral side, and by palpating the appropriate facial dermatomes. Cranial nerve VII is tested by observing the patient's facial movements.

Globe position is an important diagnostic tool in orbital injury and disease. Anteroposterior (AP) malpositioning can be appreciated if there is a difference of more than 2 mm between the positions of the two eyes. More subtle changes require exophthalmometry for detection. Normal ranges of symmetrical protrusion have been suggested and vary based on sex and race.[7] In general, exophthalmometry readings are higher in males and blacks. Asymmetry in AP globe position represents proptosis or enophthalmos with the notable exceptions of axial myopia and buphthalmos.[24] Proptosis is secondary to a retrobulbar mass effect and has many causes, including thyroid disease, intraconal and extraconal masses, hematoma or edema, traumatic bony displacement, forward or downward movement of the intracranial contents, infectious and inflammatory processes, and congenital malformations.[13, 14, 44] The causes of enophthalmos are more limited and include phthisis bulbi, orbital fracture, previous trauma or surgery with atrophy of orbital fat, and scirrhous carcinoma of the breast.[11, 28] Pseudoproptosis occurs when enophthalmos is overlooked and the examiner assumes that the normal eye is proptotic. Vertical and horizontal malposition of the globe can be demonstrated with a McCoy facial trisquare. Lateral displacement is seen in patients with congenital hypertelorism and ethmoid sinus disease. Telecanthus, when not congenital, indicates traumatic detachment of the medial canthal tendon with or without a nasoethmoid or LeFort bony disruption. In the appropriate clinical setting, inferior globe displacement can represent a roof fracture, meningioma, lymphoproliferative disorder, frontal mucocele or lacrimal gland mass. Upward displacement of the globe is most common in patients with maxillary sinus disease or invasive carcinoma of the lower eyelid or cheek.

Palpation of the orbit and orbital rims can assist in localizing an irregularity or mass. Osseous step-offs herald orbital rim fractures. Inferolateral displacement of the zygoma in a patient with trauma is a well-known sign of a tripod (trimalar) fracture. Osteomas and meningiomas may be palpated along the orbital rim. Lacrimal gland tumors, lymphoproliferative masses, mucoceles, and cutaneous carcinomas are often palpable in the anterior orbit. The technique of using retropulsion (i.e., pushing backward on the globe) and comparing the resistance felt on both sides is of limited diagnostic value because it provides no information to distinguish among the possible causes of retrobulbar pressure. Auscultation over the globe with a stethoscope may, however, identify the bruit of a cavernous sinus fistula.

Other important parts of the examination include observation of the eyelid position. Ptosis or eyelid retraction can indicate various orbital disease processes including trauma, inflammation, thyroid disease, and oculomotor nerve dysfunction. Examination of the periocular skin is helpful in assessing vascular tumors, cutaneous carcinoma with orbital invasion, and plexiform neurofibromatosis.

A complete head and neck examination is appropriate for a patient who has sustained significant trauma to any portion of that region. The examination starts with an assessment of possible cervical spine injury because trauma that has caused periorbital bony disruption may transmit sufficient force to disrupt the spine. The possibility of spinal injury increases with the severity of bony head fractures, and hence skull or LeFort fractures have the highest probability of being associated with cervical disruption. In patients with mild to moderate soft tissue injuries and isolated or minor periorbital fractures such as malar arch or nasal fractures, it is sufficient to question the patient about neck pain and assess his or her discrimination of peripheral strength and sensory stimuli. For patients with skull and LeFort fractures, plain radiographic assessment of the cervical spine is prudent.

Examination of the stability and position of the maxillary, malar, nasal, and frontal bones is the key to assessment of periorbital fractures.[23] Starting inferiorly, malocclusion or paresthesias of the maxillary teeth and gum herald a LeFort fracture. LeFort II and III fractures both involve the orbit, the former involving the medial orbital rims, nasolacrimal drainage systems, and anterior nasoethmoid regions, and the latter involving potentially all of these structures plus the malar bones. Infraorbital hypesthesia indicates a fracture of the orbital floor or inferior rim, either isolated or in combination with a LeFort II or III fracture. Epiphora may result from orbital edema, but the possibility of a LeFort or nasoethmoid fracture must be ruled out. Supraorbital hypesthesia suggests a fracture of the orbital roof (i.e., frontal bone) or greater wing of the sphenoid (i.e., superior orbital fissure). The source of any epistaxis must be ascertained and can range from minor trauma to the anterior septum to ethmoidal artery hemorrhage resulting from medial orbital disruption of a LeFort II or III fracture or a nasoethmoid fracture. If ethmoidal artery disruption causes intraorbital extravasation of blood rather than epistaxis, the expanding orbital hematoma will cause anterior and lateral globe displacement and may result in a rapid increase in intraorbital pressure and compromise of visual acuity. This situation requires emergent ophthalmologic consultation and administration of intravenous steroids, acetazolamide, and mannitol to diminish intraocular pressure.[33] Lateral canthotomy allows anterior expansion of the orbital contents and time to prepare the operating room and the patient for an orbital exploration if the hematoma continues to expand. Most surgeons favor an external ethmoidectomy approach (Lynch incision) to gain quick access to the ethmoidal arteries; bleeding from these vessels can be controlled with an insulated bipolar cautery. The lamina papyracea can then be removed to decrease the intraorbital pressure (an isolated medial orbital wall deficit does not cause significant enopthalmos).

RADIOLOGIC STUDIES

Computed tomography is the most common diagnostic imaging technique applied to patients with periorbital trauma. Plain facial radiographs, usually anteroposterior, lateral skull, Waters, and submentovertex views (the latter for the malar arches), will disclose gross bony disruptions, particularly defects of the thick orbital rims and malar arches. Opacification of a frontal, ethmoid, or maxillary sinus raises the level of suspicion for a minimal or nondisplaced fracture line between the orbit and the adjacent sinus or sinuses. Magnetic resonance imaging (MRI) offers superior delineation of the orbital soft tissue contents, particularly the globe and optic nerve, although keeping a post-trauma patient quiet and relatively immobile during the 30 minutes required for imaging can be a challenge. Computed tomography with bone windows will delineate all but the smallest nondisplaced fracture, and gadolinium intravenous contrast enhancement should be elected if an intraorbital or adjacent cranial hematoma or intraorbital soft tissue disruption is suspected. CT scans can be accomplished with a few minutes of patient immobility and usually preclude the need for other diagnostic imaging.

In patients with an old or complex orbital deformity after trauma or tumor surgery, three-dimensional reconstructive CT programs allow the surgeon and prosthodontist to visualize the deformity indirectly and to plan accurately, to within a few millimeters, the bony repositioning or onlay graft augmentation that is required (Fig. 7–1). This process is easier with unilateral orbital deformities because the normal anatomy (at least for that particular patient) can be assessed, but even bilateral deformities can be corrected using published norms for midfacial proportions and globe positions if good photographs taken prior to the injury are unavailable. If reconstructive software is not available, fine-cut axial, coronal, and sagittal CT scans at 3- to 4-mm intervals will depict the periorbital structures accurately enough to plan a reconstruction.

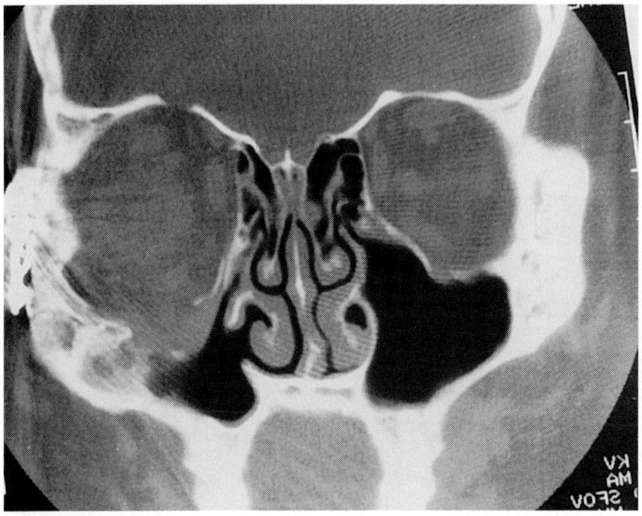

FIGURE 7–1. Computed coronal tomogram through the midface of a patient with diplopia and enophthalmos 2 weeks after open reduction of a trimalar fracture without repair of the orbital floor because the patient's globe was in a near normal position at the time of surgery (early post-trauma edema nullified the orbital volume displacement into the maxillary sinus).

SURGICAL INDICATIONS

Surgical indications in orbital surgery should be clearly identified in all cases. This seemingly obvious statement recognizes the fact that controversy exists in many cases in which indications for the same procedure seem to vary with the subspecialty. The most notable example is the treatment of medial or inferior orbital wall fractures. For some surgeons the indication for open treatment of such a fracture is simply its appearance on radiographic studies. This approach may result in unnecessary surgery and risk to ocular structures.

A more conservative approach is to limit surgical intervention to one of three circumstances, as follows.[24] Many patients present with diplopia at the time of injury. Diplopia may represent entrapment of the inferior rectus muscle, entrapment of the orbital fat, neural injury to the muscle, or simply contusion of the muscle, resulting in a temporary decrease in function. In the two latter cases, surgery will not correct the diplopia.[17] A forced duction test is helpful in identifying entrapment, especially if this is not seen on coronal CT scans. However, a hematoma in the muscle may be misinterpreted as a positive forced duction test result. Serial examinations of patients with diplopia over a 2-week period provide adequate information to resolve this dilemma. If no clear evidence of entrapment is found on radiologic studies and if diplopia improves progressively during this period, surgery should be postponed even if a small bony wall fracture exists. Conversely, if diplopia does not resolve rapidly or improvement ceases before return to baseline, surgery is indicated. This statement assumes that post-traumatic edema caused some of the diplopia but masked the full extent of diplopia caused by entrapment.

A second indication for surgery is enophthalmos. In the early post-traumatic stages the patient may have proptosis due to soft tissue swelling. As edema resolves, the orbital contents sink into the adjacent sinuses where fractures have occurred. Enophthalmos of more than 2 mm is usually noticeable by most observors and hence can be considered cosmetically disfiguring. If a patient presents with such a degree of enophthalmos or develops it during the 2-week post-traumatic timeframe, surgery is indicated. Last, surgery is indicated if a large fracture with substantial orbital soft tissue herniation is seen on CT scan. Unfortunately, there is no accepted definition of "significant herniation," although one study found that no significant enophthalmos developed in patients with orbital floor dehiscences of less than 2.5 cm^3, regardless of the soft tissue prolapse.[4]

In summary, small orbital wall fractures of the floor or lamina papyracea do not necessarily result in permanent enophthalmos or diplopia, and surgical treatment may be avoided in many patients. A 2- to 3-week period of observation after trauma is appropriate in all but the circumstances described in the preceding paragraphs. Further delay is occasionally justifiable but can be complicated by the development of fibrosis, making surgery difficult and increasing the chances of late post-traumatic enophthalmos.

SURGICAL TECHNIQUES

Cutaneous Grafts

The use of split-thickness cutaneous grafts in orbital surgery is limited to the coverage of the posterior orbital walls following exenteration.[15, 39] Spontaneous epithelialization or granulation are alternatives in the patient who has not been previously irradiated; these methods avoid donor site morbidity and the operative time required. Disadvantages include the need for multiple dressing changes during the relatively long period of reepithelialization and an increased risk of a poor cosmetic outcome, although cosmesis is usually not an issue for patients with a deep socket.[30] Patients will usually wear a prosthesis or patch regardless of the surgical approach used.

Coverage of an exenterated socket is readily achieved with a split-thickness skin graft. Meshing the graft in a 1.5:1 ratio affords safe expansion of tissue and a smaller donor site. If an eyelid-sparing exenteration is performed, the residual eyelid tissue can be folded deeply into the socket, and a skin graft is necessary for coverage of only the posterior half of the socket. Late postoperative complications include the presence of granulation tissue and the development of a fistula into the maxillary or ethmoid sinuses. Skin grafting over any bony dehiscence more than a few millimeters in width will fail and a fistula will develop. Management of a sino-orbital fistula must include the use of vascularized tissue, whether local or a distant flaps.[19, 32, 35, 38]

Muscular and Myocutaneous Flaps

Common locoregional flaps for resurfacing a major orbital defect include the paramedian forehead flap (pedicled on the contralateral surpratrochlear or supraorbital vessels), the cheek rotation flap (e.g., Mustard flap), the scalping flap (based on the ipsilateral superficial temporal vascular bundle), and the temporoparietal fascia flap (based on the ipsilateral superficial temporal vascular bundle), covered by a split-thickness skin graft or allowed to granulate.[12] Distant flaps include those from the nape of the neck, latissimus dorsi, and pectoralis major, but such may not have a sufficient pedicle to reach the orbit, and most surgeons favor free flaps such as those from the radial artery forearm distribution (Figs. 7–2 and 7–3). The latter can be bivalved to resurface any coexisting sinus or nasal wall defect. Simple obliteration of an empty orbit after exenteration can be accomplished by performing temporalis muscle transposition through the lateral orbital wall or using a thick free flap such as one of rectus muscle origin.[12]

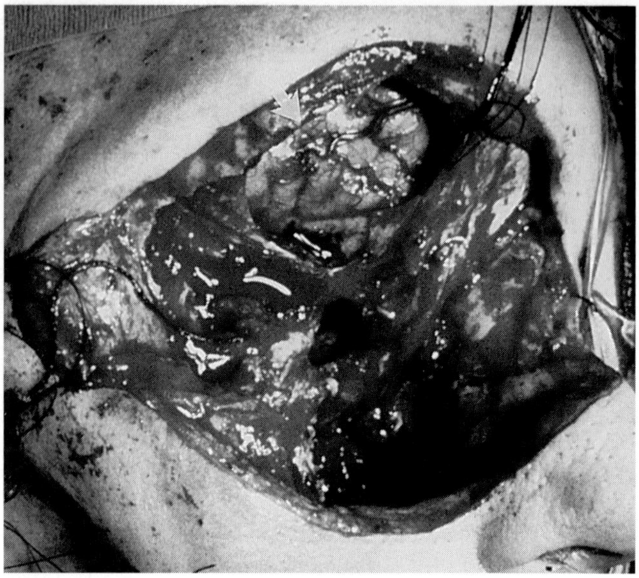

FIGURE 7–2. Periorbital and heminasal defect following wide excision of a tumor that persisted in a previously exenterated orbit (note exposed frontal lobe).

Osseous Reconstruction

There are numerous options for augmenting or repositioning the orbital walls.[12, 23] Fine kerf-cutting burs, such as those available in the Midas Rex and MedNext systems, allow the surgeon to mobilize any segment of the bony orbital rim with minimal loss of bone and hence produce a

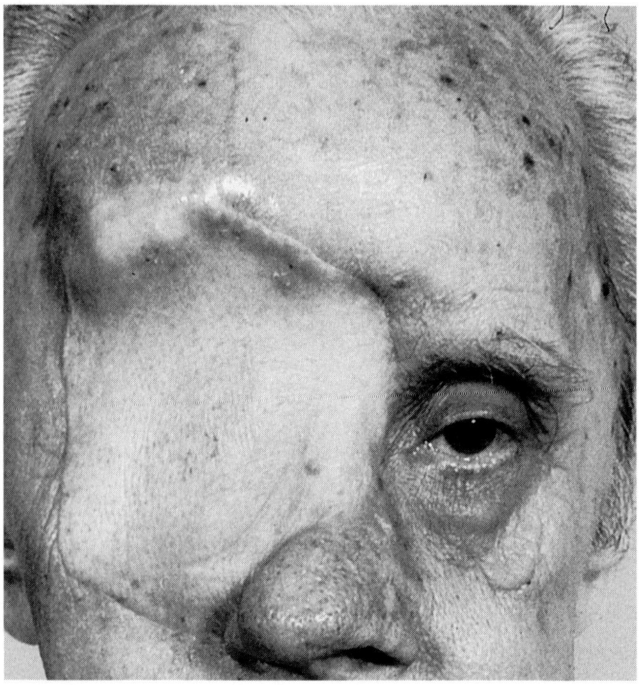

FIGURE 7–3. Same patient as shown in Figure 7–2. Defect was closed with a rectus abdominis free flap anastomosed to the facial artery and vein, its muscle portion filling the orbital cavity (and sealing the dural defect), and its cutaneous paddle bivalved to cover both the face and the ipsilateral nasal cavity.

smaller gap between repositioned segments. Fixation of larger rim segments may require the use of thicker miniplates, although in most instances microplates suffice and are less likely to be visible or palpable beneath the thin skin of the orbital rim, especially the inferolateral rim. With microplates, three or four screws are needed on each side of the defect to stabilize the bone segment sufficiently to last the 6 to 8 weeks required for bony union to occur (Fig. 7–4). Materials used for augmentation of the orbital contents, which is commonly performed to correct enophthalmos, can range from onlay bone grafts to synthetic materials such as Silastic or Teflon sheets (Figs. 7–5 and 7–6). Most surgeons favor the use of autologous bone because it avoids late problems with extrusion or infection reported with synthetic materials. The outer table of the skull, usually harvested from the parietal region through a hemicoronal incision, is the most common donor site because membranous bone from this region undergoes minimal resorption compared to free grafts from endochondral bone such as that from the rib or iliac crest. In addition, a parietal bone depression (following outer table harvest) is less obvious behind the hairline than is a frontal bone defect. One should remember to harvest bone in the parietal region no closer than 1 cm from the midsagittal, frontoparietal, and temporal suture lines because the outer and inner tables fuse in these regions, and attempts to harvest bone there will result in dural tears. Bony strips no wider than 2 cm are the norm (they can be up to 5 cm in length depending on the bony suture line positions) because right-angled sagittal saws and narrow-gauge sidecutting kerfs usually do not extend for more than 1 cm under each side of a bony donor site (Fig. 7–7). Unlike the two-point microplate fixations required for orbital rim repositioned segments/or onlay grafts, augmentation of orbital volume by placement of bone strips (characteristically three: placed along the superolateral, inferior, and medial walls) requires only a single screw or a small microplate anteriorly to prevent early extrusion prior to the expected fibrous or bony union with the orbital walls.

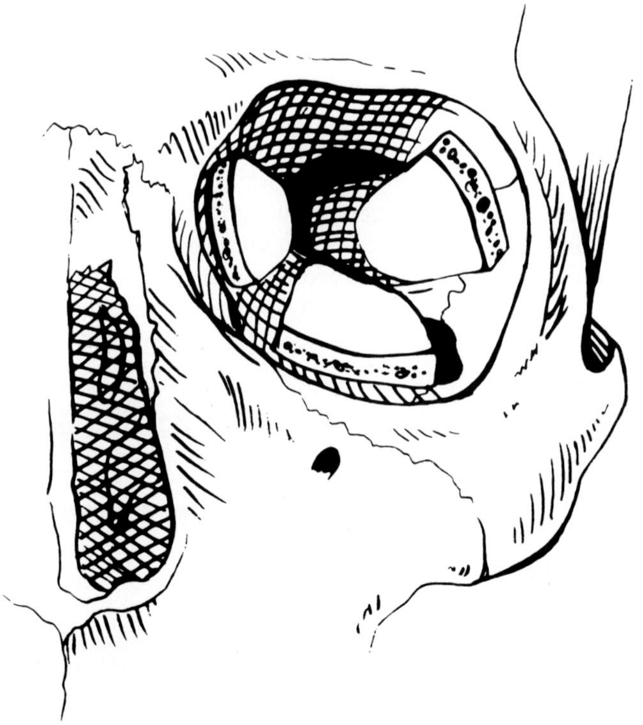

FIGURE 7–4. Common areas of placement of bone grafts for restoration of the shape and volume of the orbit. The location and size of the grafts are determined by preoperative CT scans (with three-dimensional reconstruction if available); surgical approaches include a Lynch incision for the medial orbit, a lateral brow incision for the lateral orbit (or a hemicoronal approach to gain access to both medial and lateral orbits), and a subciliary incision for the orbital floor. (From Stanley RB, Beumer J: Orbital rehabilitation: Surgical and prosthetic. Otolaryngol Head Neck Surg 21:189, 1988.)

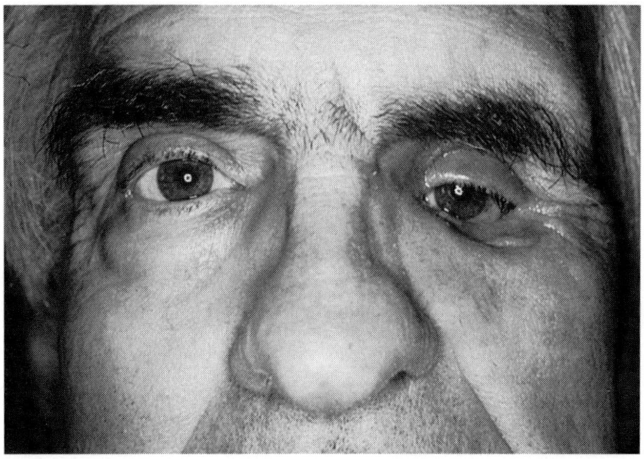

FIGURE 7–5. Patient with enophthalmos and diplopia referred 1 year after simple maxillectomy and postoperative irradiation for an antral carcinoma.

APPROACH TO THE ORBIT ACCORDING TO SITE OF LESION

The specific approach to the orbit is determined primarily by the location of the lesion or trauma. Separation of the

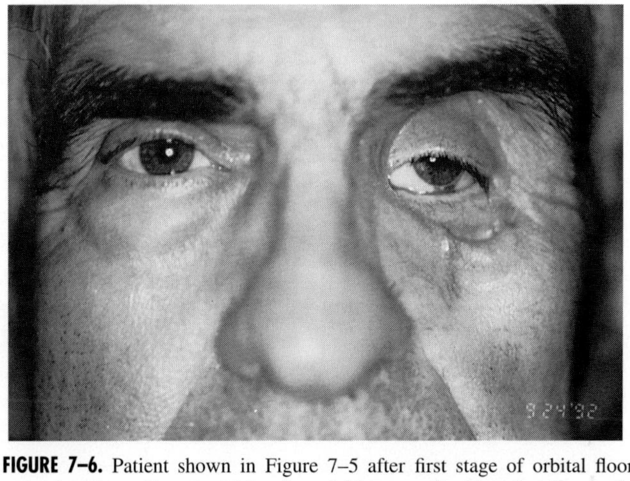

FIGURE 7–6. Patient shown in Figure 7–5 after first stage of orbital floor reconstruction with outer table of cranial bone grafts. Note that the pupils are now at the same level and enophthalmos has been corrected; eyelid repositioning and any needed extraocular muscle surgery should be performed during the final stage of rehabilitation.

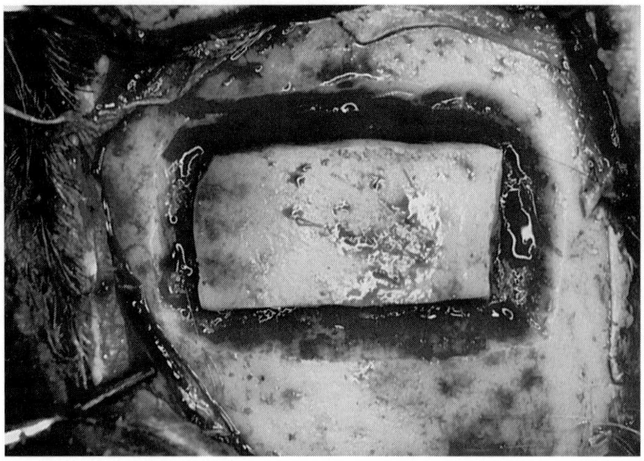

FIGURE 7–7. Harvest of outer table of parietal bone, the size of which is limited by the sagittal, temporal, and coronal bony sutures.

orbital contents into anterior and posterior compartments (to the globe equator) is one useful paradigm. Other approaches include separation into superior, medial, lateral, and inferior quadrants. Last, some practitioners would subdivide the orbit into intraconal (between the rectus muscles and behind the globe) and extraconal components. Ultimately, a combination of all these regional definitions can be used in planning the surgical approach.

Anterior approaches to the superior orbit can be made through the upper conjunctival cul-de-sac but most commonly are performed transcutaneously along an existing eyelid crease. The crease position should be 8 to 9 mm above the central lash line in men and 10 to 11 mm in women. Children have lower creases, in the range of 4 to 7 mm. When asymmetry exists between the eyelids it is preferable to match the lower crease. Careful distraction of the incision prevents unnecessary tearing of the delicate upper eyelid skin. Transcutaneous crease incisions are followed by dissection through the orbicularis oculi muscle and the orbital septum. Most anterior superior lesions are accessed by entering the postseptal compartment above the preaponeurotic fat. Another transcutaneous approach involves a sub-brow incision placed more directly over a specific lesion. This latter technique minimizes traction on the incision edges but results in a scar that is less easily camouflaged than the crease incision and may traumatize the supraorbital nerve if this nerve is not carefully dissected.

The techniques discussed above provide adequate exposure to the anterior and medial aspects of the superior half of the orbit. Posterior disease may require a coronal flap, sometimes with a craniotomy for lesions such as encephaloceles, mucoceles, osseous lesions, and frontal sinus trauma. A coronal incision can usually provide access to the lateral orbital rim, the malar arch, and the upper nasoethmoid region. Although a hemicoronal incision is adequate for malar arch and superolateral orbital rim access, full superior and any nasoethmoid access requires a bicoronal incision (Fig. 7–8). The incision is positioned across the scalp between the junctions of an anterior helices of the ears and the temples, and crosses the scalp approximately 1 to 2 cm behind the anterior hairline. Whether or not a centimeter of hair is trimmed around the incision line depends on whether a craniotomy is necessary for a neurosurgical portion of the case. (Hair trimming is unnecessary for extracranial work.) The incision line is infiltrated with an epinephrine-containing solution at least 10 minutes before the incision is made, and bleeding from branches of the superficial temporal arteries and veins laterally and from the supraorbital vascular bundles medially can usually be controlled with bipolar cautery. If a concomitant craniotomy is planned, such as for mobilizing orbital roof fragments from the anterior fossa or for patching a cerebrospinal fluid leak through the roof of the ethmoids, the scalp incision is made through the galea but not the pericranium, dissecting to the superior orbital rims in the loose connective tissue just beneath the galea.

Then the pericranium is elevated anteriorly, but it remains attached to the supraorbital vascular bundles and therefore can be used later as a vascularized flap to provide a watertight seal over the floor of the anterior fossa. If a craniotomy is unnecessary, the initial bicoronal incision can be extended directly to the skull, and a subpericranial plane can be bluntly elevated to the superior orbital rims. It should be kept in mind that terminal (frontal) branches of the facial nerve pass through the superficial temporal fascia just posterior to the superolateral orbital rims, and therefore when elevating the most lateral portion of a bicoronal flap, the plane of dissection must be deep to the superficial temporal fascia. Most surgeons prefer to incise through the fat-containing space between the superficial and deep temporal fasciae and then dissect directly through the deep temporal fascia, using the fat pad as yet another tissue barrier between the surgical field and branches of the facial nerve.

As the superior orbital rims are approached through a coronal incision, the surgeon must search for the supraorbital neurovascular bundles because keeping these intact is desirable for the cutaneous flap and essential for the viability of a pericranial flap. In about 20% of patients the supraorbital

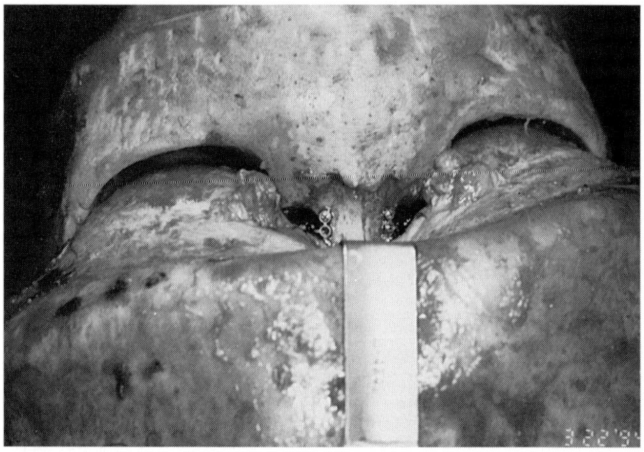

FIGURE 7–8. Bicoronal access can expose the nasal root and lacrimal fossae, supraorbital rims and superior orbits, and lateral orbital rims (note the nasion microplates used to repair the central component of a LeFort III fracture).

neurovascular bundles exit through a separate foramen up to 1 cm cephalad to the supraorbital rims. In such cases, some combination of rongeurs, drills, and the like is used to free the bundles from their canals so that they can be displaced forward with the scalp or pericranial flap during bony manipulations. Once the superior and lateral orbital rims are stripped of periosteum, bony exposure can be extended as needed to the lateral orbital rims and malar arches. Dissecting directly on these bony structures precludes injury to the facial nerve. The nasal processes of the frontal bone, along with the medial canthal ligaments, can be exposed through the central portion of a bicoronal incision by elevating the periorbita medially from the superior orbital rims and sweeping the tightly adherent periosteum from the nasal root, keeping in mind the position of the trochleas just posterior to the superomedial orbital rims. The bony integrity of the lacrimal fossa and the enclosed lacrimal sac can be assessed in this manner, although dacryocystorhinostomy requires a separate transnasal or external ethmoidectomy (Lynch) incision.

Exposure of the medial orbit is achieved by using either transcutaneous or transconjunctival approaches. A Lynch incision provides direct transcutaneous access and excellent exposure to many medial lesions. This incision is particularly helpful when treating lesions that extend from the ethmoid and sphenoid sinuses. Furthermore, exposure provided by a Lynch incision allows observation of small bone fragments in the posterior orbit that can result in optic nerve compression. Its limitations include the creation of a facial scar, the potential for damage to the lacrimal drainage system, and the need to control the ethmoid arteries. Brisk hemorrhage from the posterior ethmoid artery can be difficult to suppress owing to limited visibility and retraction of the lacerated end into the orbital fat. Hemostasis, usually achieved by bipolar cauterization of the ethmoid arteries, which are divided near the lamina papyracea to allow a stalk a few millimeters long to protrude from the periorbita, is critical because of the risk of postoperative bleeding and compression optic neuropathy. The medial orbit can also be approached by means of a transconjunctival technique, which is especially useful for foreign bodies and lesion biopsies. The medial bulbar conjunctiva is incised in a curvilinear fashion, and a dissection either medial or lateral to the medial rectus muscle is possible.

Intraconal lesions may be accessible through the Lynch incision or a medial transconjunctival approach. Inherent in accessing the intraconal area from the medial side is the need to disinsert the medial rectus muscle from the globe. While not technically difficult, this action increases the risk of globe perforation (which results from reinsertion of the muscle at the completion of the procedure) and postoperative diplopia.

Exposure of lesions due to inferior orbital disease and trauma entails a similar variety of surgical techniques. Treatment of orbital floor fractures using a transantral (Walsh-Ogura) procedure is well established in the otolaryngologic community. Visibility is excellent until one reaches the posterior wall of the maxillary sinus. Others prefer a transcutaneous subciliary incision as used in classic lower eyelid blepharoplasty. If the incision is made 2 to 3 mm below the lower eyelashes and dissection is performed carefully between the posterior surface of the orbicularis oculi and the anterior face of the tarsal plate, injury to the peripheral (lid) vascular arcade is avoided. Attempts to incise the lower lid skin along the base of the malar fold (inferior orbital rim) commonly have a poor cosmetic result, both in terms of the visibility of the scar and the increased risk of cicatricial ectropion.

Transconjunctival (palpebral) exposure of the lower orbit is technically straightforward and minimizes the risk of ectropion[22, 26] (Fig. 7–9). This technique has been popularized recently for transconjunctival blepharoplasty.[8] An incision can be made anywhere between the base of the tarsal plate and the inferior fornix (the "preseptal" approach). The advantage of the higher incision line is that the septum can be left intact because a dissection plane is created in the postorbicularis fascia. This incision also prevents billowing of the orbital fat into the surgical field during management of orbital floor fractures and orbital decompressions.

Assessment of lower eyelid laxity is an important element in preparing for any transcutaneous lower eyelid incision. A frequent complication of lower eyelid surgery is postoperative ectropion in patients with preexisting lateral canthal laxity. Diagnosis of lateral canthal laxity is easily made by

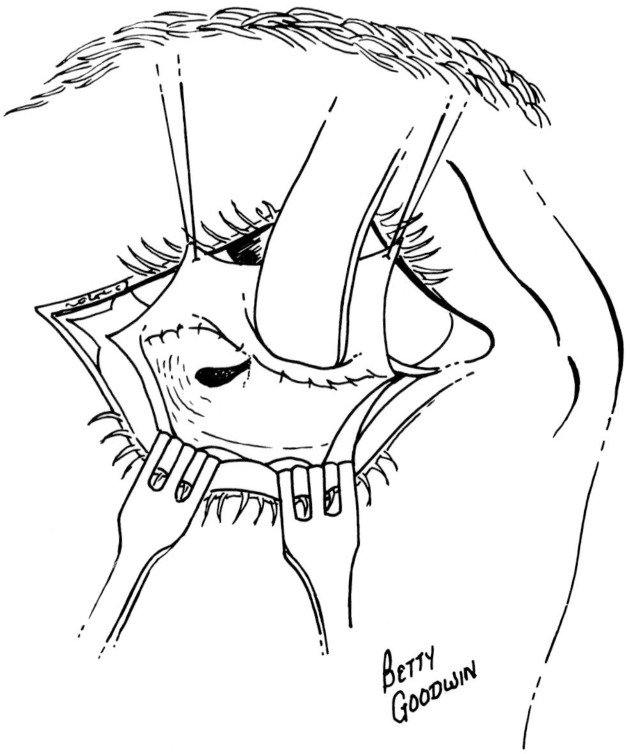

FIGURE 7–9. For inferior orbital exposure, a lateral canthotomy is performed. The lower lid is retracted inferiorly, an incision is placed through the conjunctiva just below the inferior tarsal plate, and dissection proceeds between the orbital septum and the posterior surface of the orbicularis muscle (the so-called preseptal approach) to the inferior orbital bony rim. (From Osguthorpe JD: Surgical access to primary orbital tumors. Otolaryngol Clin North Am 21:135, 1988.)

gently retracting the lower lid margin away from the globe and toward the examiner. As this tissue is released it should readily snap back to a tight position in contact with the lower portion of the globe. If contact with the globe takes seconds, occurs only after blinking, or does not occur at all, laxity is assumed and must be addressed as part of the initial surgical plan. A lateral tarsal strip resection (commonly 2 to 4 mm) and resuspension of the lower eyelid provides an excellent means for resolving this problem.

The lateral orbit can be approached with and without removing bone.[22] Transcutaneous incisions in this region are made in the lateral portion of the upper eyelid crease and the lateral canthal angle. The former incision is helpful in improving exposure in the area of the palpebral lobe of the lacrimal gland. Full exposure of the orbital portion of the lacrimal gland most likely requires removal of the lateral orbital rim. Retraction of the temporalis muscle and removal of the lateral orbital wall provide an adequate window for observation and removal of most lateral lesions. Injury to the lateral rectus muscle is minimized by passing a silk traction suture around the muscle at the point of its insertion into the globe. The suture is gently pulled away from the point of surgical entry into the posterior orbit. This prevents inadvertent rupture or splitting of the muscle that could ultimately lead to a lateral gaze palsy and allows safe entry to the lateral intraconal space. The lateral rectus muscle rarely has to be removed for exposure of a posterior or intraconal orbital mass.

ORBITAL DECOMPRESSION FOR GRAVES DISEASE

Graves' orbitopathy describes the ophthalmic manifestations of thyroid disease. It may occur in patients who are hyperthyroid, hypothyroid, or euthyroid.[1] Indeed, there appears to be some dissociation between the patient's thyroid status and the appearance of Graves' disease.[5] Although orbitopathy commonly precipitates the diagnosis of thyroid disease, it may also occur months to years after thyroid dysfunction has been diagnosed and treated. Some reports indicate that treatment with radioactive iodine can worsen the eye findings.[4]

Inflammation of the rectus muscles and deposition of glycosaminoglycans result in significant muscular enlargement, particularly in the central and posterior aspects of the muscles. Expansion of the muscle architecture in such a confined space as the orbit propels the globe forward. Normally the equator of the globe is adjacent to the anterior border of the lateral orbital wall; examination of CT scans in patients with Graves' disease usually discloses displacement of the globe equator beyond this line. Anterior displacement of the globe in conjunction with fibrosis and retraction of the levator muscle results in corneal and conjunctival exposure, which causes symptoms of foreign body sensation, tearing, photophobia, and decreased vision.[29] Untreated, such exposure can produce corneal ulceration and melting with permanent visual loss.[41] Another form of visual loss can occur in patients with a compression optic neuropathy, in which the posterior portion of the rectus muscles enlarges and surrounds the optic nerve; in such a case, a four-quadrant constriction of the visual fields can be easily documented and is a critical part of the evaluation and management of these patients.[41]

Standard initial interventions include topical lubricants, oral prednisone, and/or localized irradiation.[29] The latter two modalities are most likely to succeed during the first 6 to 12 months after diagnosis of an orbitopathy process during the inflammatory phase, characterized by lymphocytic infiltration and edematous fluid. Some of these patients may benefit from surgical intervention, but such is commonly reserved for the later fibrotic phase of orbitopathy. Intractable corneal or conjunctival exposure despite maximal medical therapy, progressive optic nerve compression during or immediately following steroid or radiation therapy, and permanently disfiguring proptosis are the usual indications for orbital decompression, which is performed prior to extraocular muscle surgery (most likely to succeed is placement of the globe in a near-normal position).

Proptosis is reduced by removing the intraorbital contents or removing or repositioning the peripheral orbital bony walls. Extensive upper and lower eyelid blepharoplasty with removal of fat deep into the extraconal space can reduce proptosis satisfactorily while minimizing the risk of postoperative diplopia.[21] Unfortunately, this approach results in a highly variable reduction in proptosis and presents a risk of postoperative hemorrhage in the orbit, which, if present, further reduces vision.[37]

Removal of orbital bone is predicated on the concept that the orbital contents will spill over into the adjacent sinuses or surgical defects, thus decreasing intraorbital pressure. Various schemes have been worked out to predict the degree of reduction in proptosis that will result depending on the number and location of the bones removed.[19, 42] A standard approach to orbital decompression is to remove the lamina papyracea below the ethmoidal foramen and the medial orbital floor. In such a case the lateral orbital floor is removed usually over to and including the canal around the inferior orbital nerve, although it can be removed as far as the junction of the lateral and inferior bony walls. Orbital floor removal must extend to the back wall of the maxillary sinus. Further removal of the lateral orbital wall may add as much as 2 mm to the reduction of proptosis, although such a modest decrease in proptosis is commonly achieved by laterally displacing the lateral orbital wall (fixing it in a new position with microplates) rather than removing it (which leads to consequent temple depression).[16, 36] Orbital roof removal has been suggested and may slightly reduce proptosis; however, this technique is not widely favored because a craniotomy is required, and without a roof, cranial pulsations may be transmitted to the orbit.

Excision of orbital bone is only part of the process of decompression. Linear incisions in the periosteum allow orbital fat to billow out of the orbital space. Chronic inflammation and fibrosis in the orbital fat decrease its pliability and may reduce its extrusion, leading to a consequent reduction in proptosis after incision of the periosteum.

DACRYOCYSTORHINOSTOMY

Dacryocystorhinostomy (DCR) is indicated in patients with obstruction of the nasolacrimal duct (NLD) in the presence of patent canaliculi. Clinical presentation usually involves chronic epiphora and mucoid discharge. Occasionally patients present with acute infectious dacryocystitis, with development of an abscess in the lacrimal fossa. Surgery in these cases is delayed until oral antibiotic treatment has largely resolved the abscess.

Nasolacrimal duct obstruction is congenital in 6% of all newborns; more than 90% of these cases resolve with conservative management by the age of 18 months.[27] A small percentage of children require a DCR after successive attempts to open the duct using probe dilation and silicone tube stents have failed. Obstruction in adults may result from trauma, lacrimal sac inflammation or tumors, contiguous nasal and sinus tumors, and primary acquired obstruction (Fig. 7–10).

Dacryocystorhinostomy can be performed with intravenous sedation augmented by local infiltration, or with general anesthesia. The former technique is well tolerated except in children. The latter technique has been noted anecdotally to result in increased intraoperative bleeding. In either case, the operation begins with packing a decongestant-saturated Cottonoid strip into the middle meatus. A cocaine solution is helpful in patients undergoing intravenous sedation but can be avoided by combining local infiltration of lidocaine with epinephrine and a decongestant such as oxymetazoline. This packing is left in position until late in the surgery and pulled only when the silicone tube is inserted (i.e., the stent).

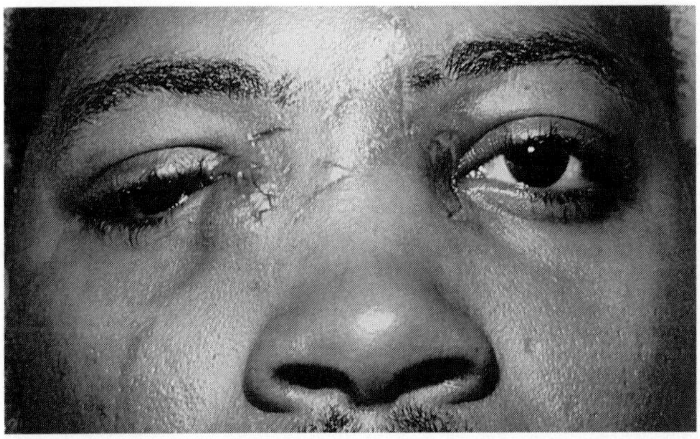

FIGURE 7–10. Lacrimal sac mucocele displaces the medial canthus in a patient who had had open reduction and intercanthal wiring to repair a nasoethmoidal fracture 3 months previously. (From Osguthorpe JD, Hoang G: Nasolacrimal injuries. Otolaryngol Head Neck Surg 24:59, 1991.)

An additional advantage of the decongestant packing is the fact that it forms a barrier to injury of the nasal septal mucosa when the lateral nasal mucosa is incised. Local anesthetic can be infiltrated directly over the medial canthus or as a regional block. It is advisable to avoid epinephrine in the anterior ethmoid block because it carries a risk of ophthalmic artery spasm.

There are two primary approaches to this surgery. The most common and probably the most successful is an external incision extending from the inferior border of the medial canthal tendon toward the base of the alae nasi. The incision is extended approximately 1.5 cm at the junction of the eyelid and nasal skin to prevent webbing at the medial canthus that would occur if the incision were made exclusively on the eyelid skin near the caruncle. Blunt or sharp dissection is carried down to the periosteum overlying the anterior lacrimal crest; care must be taken to avoid incising the angular vessels, or to maintain control of these with bipolar cautery (ligatures aggravate scarring). The periosteum can be peeled off the lacrimal crests and fossa with a Freer elevator. Infracture of the fossa can be achieved using an elevator or hemostat. The thin bone of the fossa and posterior crest is readily removed, but a ronguer may be required along the thickened anterior lacrimal crest to expose the underlying nasal mucosa.

Conventionally an osteum 1 cm in diameter is created by removing the lacrimal crests and intermediary fossa. An osteum of this size allows adequate exposure for suturing anterior or posterior flaps between the lacrimal sac and the nasal mucosa. Most such openings, however, contract to 2 mm in size over a 6-month postoperative period.[3] Creation of the osteum is followed by incising the lacrimal sac into anterior and posterior flaps. Placement of a lacrimal probe in the canalicular system and pushing it toward the medial sac wall assists in stabilizing the site of incision. Additional flaps are created in the nasal mucosa, and the packing is removed.

Controversy exists over the need to suture the flaps.[2] The basic concept is that suturing anterior and posterior flaps provides a mucosa-lined channel for the flow of tears and prevents the encroachment of scar tissue, but such sutures can be technically challenging, especially in children. Finally, silicone tubes are passed through the superior and inferior canalicular systems into the nasal cavity and retrieved through the nares (Figs. 7–11 and 7–12). The tubes are tied or tagged with hemoclips and allowed to hang adjacent to the inferior turbinate. Theoretically, these tubes prevent obstruction of the new outflow tract by scar tissue. Tears pass around the tubes by capillary action, although even modest tear production will overwhelm the drainage capacity of the narrow canaliculi filled with a solid tube, and epiphora may persist long after surgery. In most cases, the tubes are left in place for 3 to 6 months to guard against stenosis[31] (Figs. 7–13 and 7–14).

The other approach to this surgery involves a primarily intranasal procedure.[18] The mucosa is elevated for 1 cm anterior to the middle turbinate, the uncinate is removed,

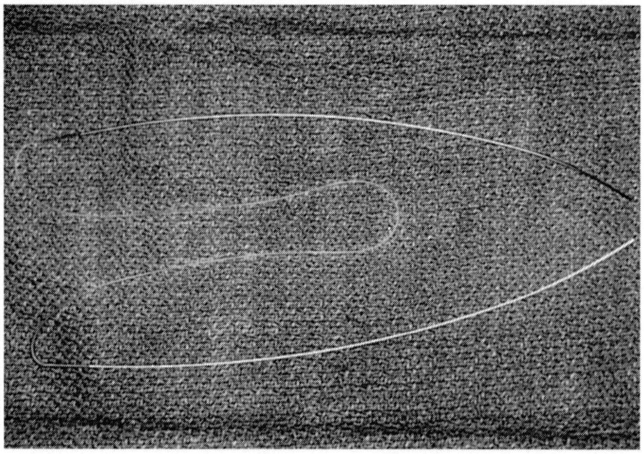

FIGURE 7–11. Hollow Silastic tube stent (1 mm in diameter) swaged onto No. 1 lacrimal probes. Common types include the Guibor and Crawford stents.

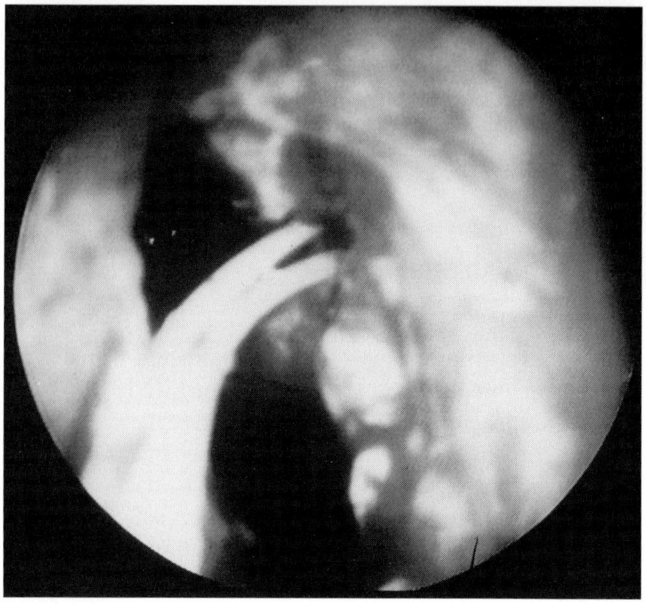

FIGURE 7–13. Endoscopic view of Silastic tube stent exiting from an open lacrimal sac (medial wall of sac was removed at dacryocystorhinostomy).

and the bony lacrimal fossa is opened with right-angled (e.g., pituitary) rongeurs or outfractured with a periosteal elevator and then removed piecemeal (Fig. 7–15). Limitations of the intranasal operation include reduced visibility, reduced hemostasis control, inability to create a mucosal channel with flaps, and comparative difficulty in visualizing the lacrimal sac to determine the need for a biopsy (approximately 2% to 4% of lacrimal obstructions in adults are caused by occult tumors).[10] Use of an endoscope can improve visualization during the surgery, but this is not required for successful completion of an endonasal DCR. Attempts to create an endonasal rhinostomy with a laser (various types have been used, most commonly the YAG) have met with limited success.[43] Long-term patency and resolution of symptoms are lower with this approach than with conventional techniques. Some surgeons postulate that the increased failure rate of the laser DCR is due to increased fibrosis resulting from laser-induced thermal effects on the bony fossa.

OPTIC NERVE DECOMPRESSION

Substantial impairment of vision occurs in 0.7% to 5% of patients with closed head injuries, and the optic nerve is the site of origin of this impairment in 0.5% to 1.5%[6, 24, 33, 40] Although the optic nerve is approximately 45 mm long in adults, it is the 5.5- to 11.5-mm portion lying within the bony confines of the optic canal that is most susceptible to trauma (Fig. 7–16). In particular, the optic foramen at the medial orbital apex is the narrowest portion of the optic pathway; it measures 4 to 6 mm in diameter and is surrounded by the thickest bone (0.6 to 0.7 mm) of the optic canal (Table 7–1). Injury to the nerve can result from a bony

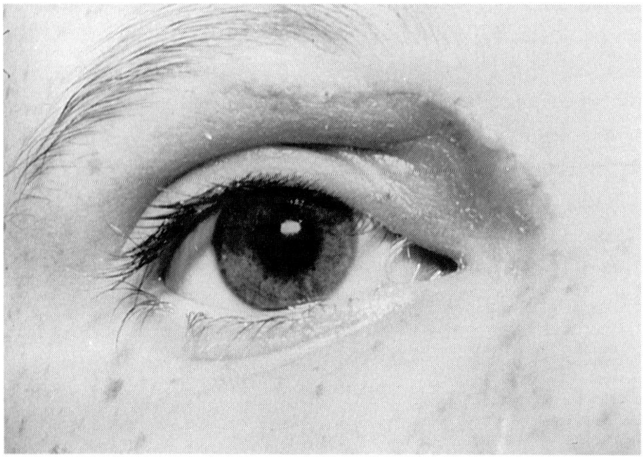

FIGURE 7–12. Loop of Silastic stent between superior and inferior lacrimal papillae; ends are tagged together with a hemaclip at the level of the superior surface of the inferior turbinate.

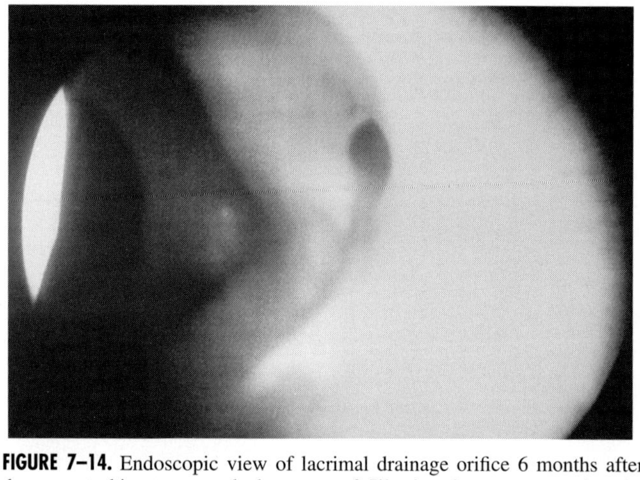

FIGURE 7–14. Endoscopic view of lacrimal drainage orifice 6 months after dacryocystorhinostomy and placement of Silastic tube stent; note that the scar characteristically heals to a lumen 2 to 3 mm in diameter within a few months after the stent has been removed. Epiphora is not a problem unless the lumen is reduced to 1 to 1.5 mm in diameter.

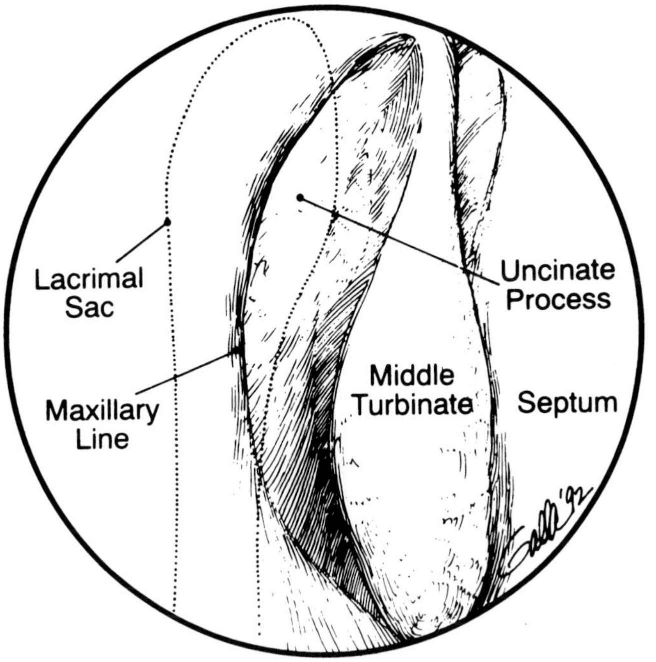

FIGURE 7–15. Schematic representation of endoscopic view of right nasal cavity demonstrating location of the lacrimal sac *(dotted outline)* underlying the lateral nasal wall; the anterior insertion of the middle turbinate is a landmark for the maxillary line and the midline of the apical portion of the sac. (From Metson R, Woog JJ, Puliafito CA: Endoscopic laser dacryocystorhinostomy. Laryngoscope 104:269, 1994.)

fracture or spicule narrowing the canal or from hemorrhage, microvascular spasm, or reactive edema from shock waves transmitted from the surrounding cranium or from the acceleration-deceleration occurring in an accident (e.g., automobile) (Figs. 7–17 and 7–18).

Loss of vision caused by gross bony displacement in the optic canal is usually immediate and total, whereas in the far more common instances of a minimally displaced fracture or nerve stretching, contusion, or concussion, the onset is delayed by many hours and is characteristically gradual in onset.[33] In a conscious patient a Snellen chart or Rosenbaum near-vision card is adequate for the assessment of gross visual acuity (the earliest changes are a diminution of red perception, for which color-coded charts are available); in a less conscious or less cooperative patient photophobia and lid closure on light stimulus indicate at least some light perception. A swinging flashlight test to detect an afferent pupillary defect (Marcus-Gunn sign) is performed in those with impaired or unknown visual acuity. Basically, with afferent compromise the pupil in the affected eye does not respond to the flashlight beam but does constrict when the beam is directed to the contralateral eye. When the flashlight is swung back and forth between the eyes, a "paradoxical dilation" occurs when the light is moved from the intact to the affected eye. Visual-evoked responses can be helpful in unconscious patients who lack consensual pupillary constriction on light stimulation. Although examination of the optic discs is always performed as part of a post-traumatic evalua-

TABLE 7–1. MEASUREMENTS OF THE MEDIAL ORBITAL WALL (196 ORBITS)

ANTERIOR LACRIMAL CREST TO:	MEAN (mm)	RANGE (mm)
Anterior ethmoidal foramen	23	20–28
Posterior ethmoidal foramen	36	29–40
Optic canal	41	37–48

Adapted from Rontal E, Rontal M, Guilford FT: Surgical anatomy of the orbit. Ann Otolaryngol 88:382, 1979; and Harrison DFN: Surgical approach to the medial orbital wall. Ann Otolaryngol 90:415, 1981.

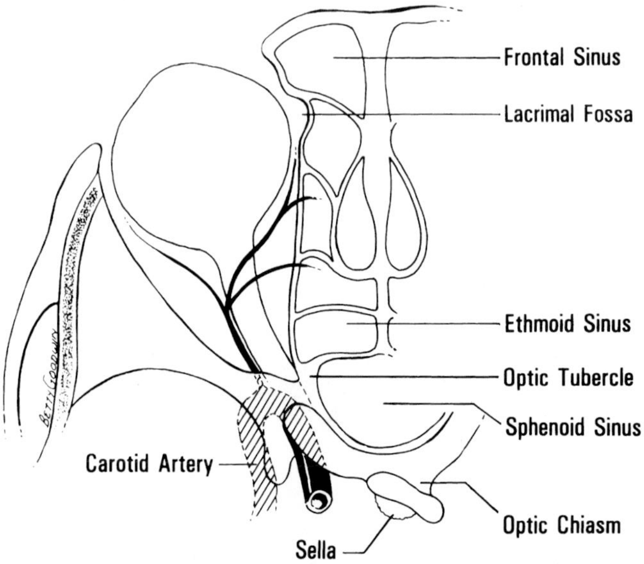

FIGURE 7–16. Schematic representation of an axial view of the orbit at the level of the optic nerve. (From Osguthorpe JD, Sofferman RA: Optic nerve decompression. Otolaryngol Clin North Am 21:155, 1988.)

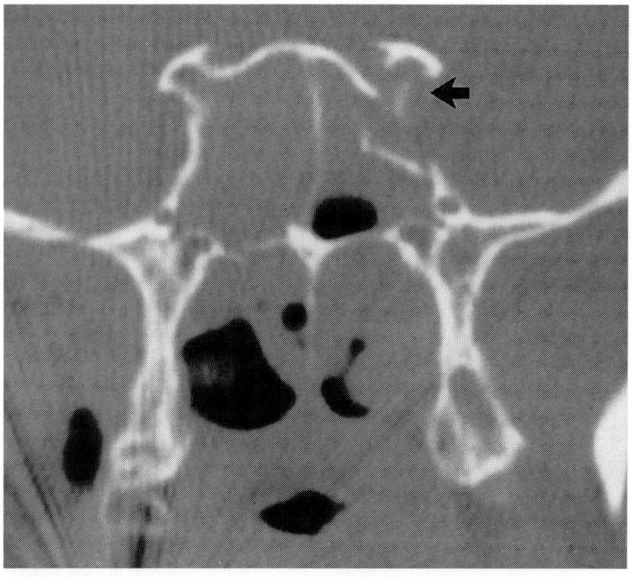

FIGURE 7–17. Computed coronal tomogram at level of anterior clinoids and optic canals; note fracture *(arrow)* of bony optic canal and adjacent lateral wall of sphenoid sinus (the sphenoid sinuses filled with blood in this patient with delayed loss of vision in one eye after LeFort III and skull base fractures).

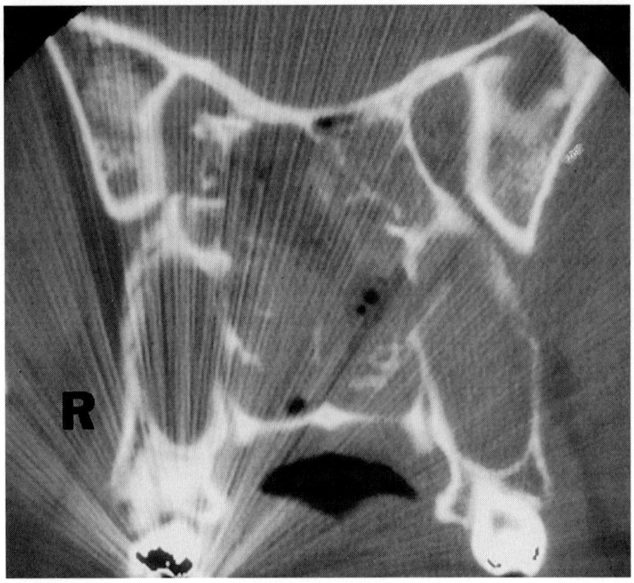

FIGURE 7–18. Computed coronal tomogram at level of posterior orbits demonstrating lateral displacement of right lamina papyracea from LeFort III fracture. Patient had delayed (by a few hours) loss of vision but immediate onset of right proptosis and diplopia.

tion of a visual decrement, gross signs of disc pallor or papilledema commonly do not develop until many hours into the post-traumatic period. If (or when) the patient is neurologically stable, an enhanced coronal CT scan of the orbits and optic canals is the best radiographic modality for evaluation of a potential optic nerve origin of a loss of vision, although the later manifestations of edema and hemorrhage in the optic nerve can be detected with MRI, a study commonly used by neurosurgeons for assessment of patients with closed head injuries.[24, 33]

Treatment of an acute and "substantial" traumatic optic neuropathy (usually defined as an ipsilateral visual acuity of 20/200 or worse, corrected in patients with preexisting myopia) is controversial, although in the past decade most data have supported the efficacy of intravenous steroids, and optic and canal decompression seems to be beneficial in many who do not respond to pharmacotherapy.[6, 24, 33] Whatever the therapy, institution of such treatment within 12 to 24 hours of the trauma improves the odds of a return to baseline visual acuity. Intravenous steroids are used in dosages comparable to those used in spinal cord injury protocols. Commonly a loading dose of methylprednisolone sodium phosphate is given; this is repeated every 6 hours for 24 to 48 hours and then tapered over 48 to 72 hours. Although most practitioners favor optic nerve decompression if an obvious narrowing of the optic canal from a bony fracture is documented on the initial radiographic studies, in the more common instance of a nondisplaced fracture or no detectable fracture, most reserve surgical intervention for patients with (corrected) acuities of less than 20/200 that have not begun to improve after the first 24 to 48 hours of treatment with megadose steroids.

The optic nerve can be decompressed by a variety of routes, including frontal or pterygonal craniotomy, and external or transnasal endoscopic or microscopic sphenoethmoidectomy. If the patient requires a craniotomy for reasons associated with a head injury, unroofing of the optic canal in question is performed through the same incision used for the craniotomy. For other patients, an external ethmoidectomy approach, which is well within the armamentarium of most otolaryngologists, is commonly selected because endoscopic techniques require special instruments and more intraoperative time.

External transsphenoethmoid decompression of the optic canal is accomplished through a Lynch incision after the patient has been premedicated with intravenous steroids and a cerebrospinal fluid-penetrating antibiotic.[24] The nose is packed with a topical vasoconstrictor, and the incision line is injected with an epinephrine-containing solution from the supraorbital notch to the medial canthus. The cornea is coated with a bland ophthalmic ointment and covered with a scleral cap. When opening the Lynch incision, the angular vessels are controlled with bipolar cautery rather than ligatures because the latter tend to enhance postoperative scarring. The trochlea of the superior oblique muscle is elevated in a subperiosteal plane to minimize postoperative diplopia, and the lacrimal sac is likewise elevated from its fossa, detaching the medial canthal ligament should such be necessary for ethmoid exposure (Fig. 7–19). The posterior lacrimal crest and the lamina papyracea are removed, controlling the anterior and posterior ethmoid arteries with the insulated bipolar cautery. The medial orbit is gently retracted laterally with a hand-held or self-retaining global retractor, the ethmoidal cells are cleared, and the anterior face of the ipsilateral sphenoid is removed.

The optic canal is located on the same plane as the ethmoid arteries and occupies the superolateral wall of the

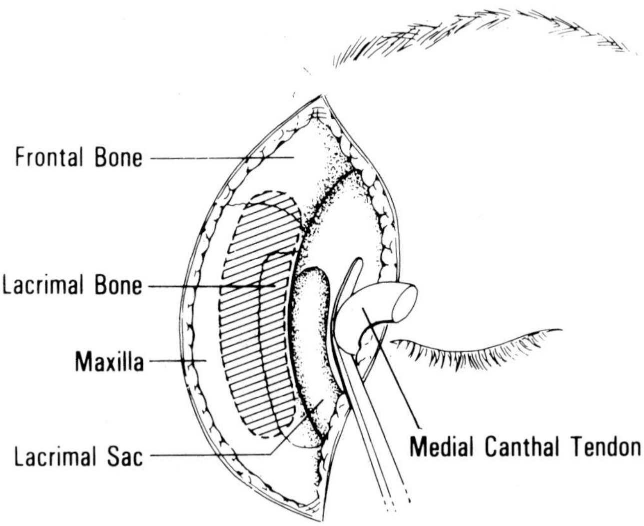

FIGURE 7–19. Schematic representation of Lynch access (via "lazy S" or gullwing variation to minimize epicanthal scar) to the lamina papyracea and ethmoid sinuses after detachment of the medial canthal tendon and lateral displacement of the lacrimal sac. (From Osguthorpe JD, Sofferman RA: Optic nerve decompression. Otolaryngol Clin North Am 21:155, 1988.)

sphenoid sinus, behind which is usually seen the impression of the internal carotid artery (Fig. 7–20). The author accomplishes sphenoethmoidectomy using headlight illumination and magnification loupes but favors an operating microscope (300-mm lens) during optic canal decompression. If there is an obvious fracture line through the optic tubercle (the name applied to the thickened anteromedial section of the optic canal), a microcurette is used to mobilize the fractured segments medially into the sphenoid sinus, where they can be removed. If the bony canal is stable, a microdrill with a long-shanked diamond bur is used to thin the optic tubercle region under continuous suction-irrigation, and then the thinned shell of bone along the medial 140 to 180 degrees or so of the optic canal is infractured with a curette. The optic canal is decompressed for at least 1 cm posterior to the optic tubercle, keeping in mind the location of the internal carotid artery.

Whether or not bony decompression is sufficient is controversial, and some favor incising the optic sheath (Fig. 7–21). Most surgeons divide the annulus tendineus (insertion of the rectus muscles, essentially a thickening of the periosteum at the orbital apex) with a sickle or similar knife but leave the optic sheath intact. The operative field is irrigated with saline, hemostasis is obtained with the insulated bipolar cautery or with neuro-Cottonoids saturated with a vasoconstrictor, and the wound is closed. If the medial canthus was mobilized for exposure, it is reapposed to the periosteum of the adjacent nasal root. A sterile rubber band can be placed along the medial orbit and brought out through the incision line, or transnasal removal of the ethmoid bulla can expose the ethmoid dissection field, allowing placement of a small collagen pack (excessive pressure on the orbit from an expanding pack should be avoided). In the immediate postoperative period, pupillary dilation, deteriorating visual acuity, or increasing orbital pain indicate a hematoma, which should be promptly evacuated. The drains or nasal packs are removed on the first or second postoperative day, the steroids are changed to oral preparations and tapered over a week, and the patient is cautioned to avoid blowing the nose for at least 2 weeks to avoid orbital emphysema. Improvement in vision can be immediate but may not become obvious for up to 2 weeks and may continue to improve slowly during the subsequent 6 to 9 months.[6, 24, 33, 40]

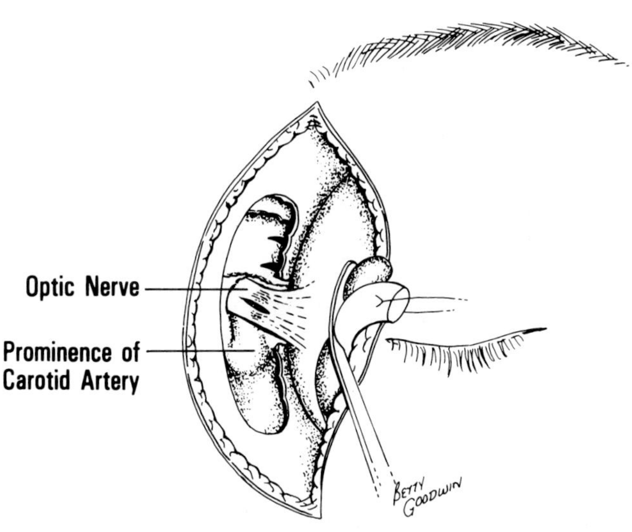

FIGURE 7–21. Schematic representation of external ethmoidectomy to gain access to the optic canal, with removal of the lamina papyracea and medial bony optic canal (superolateral wall of the sphenoid sinus). Some favor incision of the medial optic nerve sheath, but most (including the authors) incise only the dense annulus tendineus at the entrance to the optic canal in the medial orbital apex. (From Osguthorpe JD, Sofferman RA: Optic nerve decompression. Otolaryngol Clin North Am 21:155, 1988.)

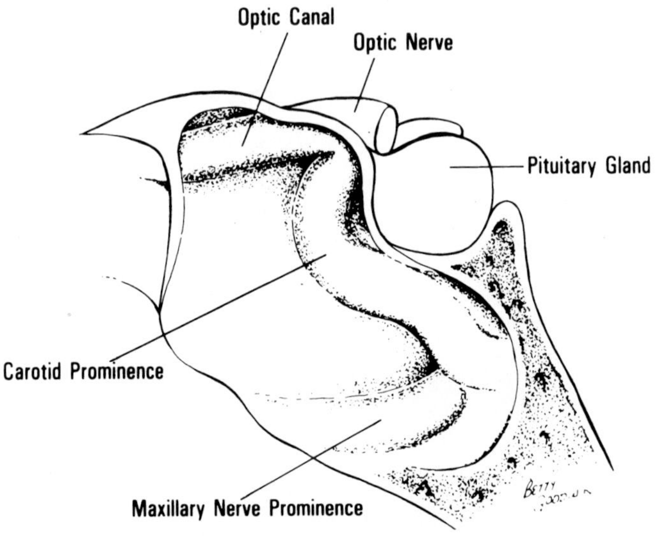

FIGURE 7–20. Schematic representation of the lateral wall of the sphenoid sinus, demonstrating the bony indentations of the optic nerve, the cavernous segment of the internal carotid artery, and the maxillary nerve. (From Osguthorpe JD, Sofferman RA: Optic nerve decompression. Otolaryngol Clin North Am 21:155, 1988.)

REFERENCES

1. Bartley GB, Gorman CA: Diagnostic criteria for Graves' ophthalmopathy. Am J Ophthalmol 119:792, 1995.
2. Becker BB: Dacryocystorhinostomy without flaps. Ophthalmic Surg 19:419, 1988.
3. Bumsted RM, Linberg JV, Anderson RL, Barretas R: External dacryocystorhinostomy. A prospective study comparing the size of the operative and healed ostium. Arch Otolaryngol 108:407, 1982.
4. Chiovato L, Santini F, Vitti P, et al: Appearance of thyroid-stimulating antibody and Graves' disease after radioiodine therapy for toxic nodular goitre. Clin Endocrinol 40:803, 1994.
5. Chopra IJ, Solomon DH: Graves' disease with delayed hyperthyroidism. Onset after several years of euthyroid ophthalmopathy, dermopathy, and high serum LATS. Ann Intern Med 73:985, 1970.
6. Cook MW, Levin LA, Joseph MP, Pinczower EF: Traumatic optic neuropathy: A meta-analysis. Arch Otolaryngol Head Neck Surg 122:1389, 1996.
7. de Juan E Jr, Hurley DP, Sapira JD: Racial differences in normal values of proptosis. Arch Intern Med 140:1230, 1980.
8. Doxanos MT: Minimally invasive lower eyelid blepharoplasty. Ophthalmology 101:1327, 1993.
9. Fatourechi V, Garrity JA, Bartley GB, et al: Graves' ophthalmology: Results of transantral orbital decompression performed primarily for cosmetic indications. Ophthalmology 101:938, 1994.

10. Gonnering RS, Lyon DB, Fisher JC: Endoscopic laser-assisted lacrimal surgery. Am J Ophthalmol 111:152, 1991.
11. Gunalp I, Gunduz K: Metastatic orbital tumors. Jap J Ophthalmol 39:65, 1995.
12. Hochman M: Reconstruction of midfacial and anterior skull base defect. Otolaryngol Clin North Am 28:1269, 1995.
13. Hurwitz JJ: Recent advances in the investigation of proptosis. Can J Ophthalmol 12:237, 1977.
14. Jacobson DH, Gorman CA: Diagnosis and management of endocrine ophthalmopathy. Med Clin North Am 69:973, 1985.
15. Kennedy RE: Indications and surgical techniques for orbital exenteration. Ophthalmology 86:967, 1979.
16. Khan JA, Wagner DV, Tiojanco JK, Hoover LA: Combined transconjunctival and external approach for endoscopic orbital apex decompression in Graves' disease. Laryngoscope 105:203, 1995.
17. Lyon DB, Newman SA: Evidence of direct damage to extraocular muscles as a cause of diplopia following orbital trauma. Ophthal Plast Reconstr Surg 5:81, 1989.
18. McDonogh M, Meiring JH: Endoscopic transnasal dacryocystorhinostomy. J Laryngol Otolaryngol 103:585, 1989.
19. McLoughlin PM, Gilhooly M, Phillips JG: Reconstruction of the infraorbital margin with a composite microvascular free flap. Br J Oral Maxillofac Surg 31:227, 1993.
20. Nathanson A, Matthis SP, Tengvar M: Diagnosis and treatment of fractures of the orbital floor. A ten-year retrospective study. Acta Otolaryngol 492 (Suppl):28, 1992.
21. Olivari N: Transpalpebral decompression of endocrine ophthalmopathy (Graves' disease) by removal of intraorbital fat: Experience with 147 operations over 5 years. Plast Reconstr Surg 87:627, 1991.
22. Osguthorpe JD: Surgical access to primary orbital tumors. Otolaryngol Clin North Am 21:135, 1988.
23. Osguthorpe JD: Orbital wall fractures: Evaluation and management. Otolaryngol Head Neck Surg 105:702, 1991.
24. Osguthorpe JD, Sofferman RA: Optic nerve decompression. Otolaryngol Clin North Am 21:155, 1988.
25. Osher RH, Shields JA, Schatz NJ: Axial myopia: A neglected cause of proptosis. Arch Neurol 35:237, 1978.
26. Palmer FR, Rice DH, Churukian MM: Transconjunctival blepharoplasty: Complications and their avoidance. Arch Otolaryngol Head Neck Surg 119:993, 1993.
27. Paul TO, Shepherd R: Congenital nasolacrimal duct obstruction: Natural history and the timing of optimal intervention. J Pediatr Ophthalmol Strabismus 31:362, 1994.
28. Pearl RM: Treatment of enophthalmos. Clin Plastic Surg 19:99, 1992.
29. Prummel MF, Wiersinga WM: Medical management of Graves' ophthalmopathy. Thyroid 5:231, 1995.
30. Putterman AM: Orbital exenteration with spontaneous granulation. Arch Ophthalmol 104:139, 1986.
31. Rosen N, Sharir M, Moverman DC, Rosner M: Dacryocystorhinostomy with silicone tubes: Evaluation of 253 cases. Ophthalmic Surg 20:115, 1989.
32. Schusterman MA, Reece GP, Miller MJ: Osseous free flaps for orbit and midface reconstruction. Am J Surg 166:341, 1993.
33. Sofferman RA: The recovery potential of the optic nerve. Laryngoscope 105 (Suppl):1, 1995.
34. Taher AA: Diplopia caused by orbital floor blowout fracture. Oral Surg Oral Med Oral Pathol 75:433, 1993.
35. Teichgraeber JF: Temporoparietal fascial flap in orbital reconstruction. Laryngoscope 103:931, 1993.
36. Tjon F, Sang M, Knegt P, et al: Transantral orbital decompression for Graves' disease. Clin Otolaryngol 19:290, 1994.
37. Trokel S, Kazim M, Moore S: Orbital fat removal. Decompression for Graves' orbitopathy. Ophthalmology 100:674, 1993.
38. Tse DT, Bumsted RM: A two-layer closure of sino-orbital fistula. Ophthalmology 96:1673, 1989.
39. Walter C: Survey of the use of composite grafts in the head and neck region. Otolaryngol Clin North Am 5:571, 1972.
40. Warner JE, Lessel S: Traumatic optic neuropathy. Int Ophthalmol Clin 35:57, 1995.
41. Wiersinga WM, Smit T, van der Gaag R, et al: Clinical presentation of Graves' ophthalmopathy. Ophthalmic Res 21:73, 1989.
42. Wilson WB, Manke WF: Orbital decompression in Graves' disease: The predictability of reduction of proptosis. Arch Ophthalmol 109:343, 1991.
43. Woog JJ, Metson R, Puliafito CA: Holmium:YAG endonasal laser dacryocystorhinostomy. Am J Ophthalmol 116:1, 1993.
44. Wright JE: Symposium on orbital tumours: Methods of examination. Transophthalmol Soc UK 99:216, 1979.

CHAPTER 8

Oculoplastic Techniques for Reconstruction of Upper and Lower Eyelids

João Jairney Maniglia, M.D.
David S. Bardenstein, M.D.
Anthony J. Maniglia, M.D.
José Victor Maniglia, M.D.
Ricardo Fabrício Maniglia, M.D.

Reconstruction of the eyelid is performed in a variety of settings, but the great majority of such operations occur following removal of a neoplasm, which is the focus of this chapter. Traditionally, surgical excision with good control of the tumor margins and functional reconstruction has been the only treatment that produces excellent prognostic results with minimal complications. More recently, this concept has been debated by radiation therapists, who, using well-controlled techniques, have claimed results similar to surgery with similar complication rates.[1]

Surgery, however, remains the treatment of choice at most centers. The eyelid poses specific challenges to the reconstructive surgeon because a delicate balance must be achieved between the needs of reconstruction, mobility, and mucous membrane function while simultaneously factoring in the effects of gravity and time (fibrosis and contraction). Gravity and time work favorably in the upper lid and unfavorably in the lower lid. A plethora of techniques have been developed by surgeons in different subspecialties who manage these patients. These approaches differ because of the diversity in training background of the head and neck oncologist, ophthalmic plastic surgeon, plastic surgeon, and dermatologist.[2–18]

This chapter illustrates some of the best surgical techniques used by us and others during the last 25 years to achieve aesthetic and functional eyelid reconstruction as well as control or cure of neoplasms. Successful eyelid reconstruction with proper control of the tumor margins can reduce the need for subsequent orbital exenteration in some cases of recurrent disease. In many of these techniques, multidisciplinary collaboration between the head and neck surgeon and the ophthalmologist is necessary to provide the optimal outcome.

EYELID FUNCTION AND ANATOMY

The eyelid protects the eyeball and maintains good vision. Mechanical protection is provided through blinking and closure. Maintenance of a clear ocular surface depends on the presence of a mucous membrane layer on the inner lid surface that is in good apposition with the globe. Eyelid position is based on a combination of several factors: tissue amount and tension, balanced muscular function of the eyelid retractors and the orbicularis oculi muscle, and intact innervation of cranial nerves III, VII (motor), and V (sensory).

The eyelid consists of four layers, which are functionally divided into the inner and outer lamellae. The outer lamella consists of the skin and muscle. The external layer is the delicate and supple skin that is loosely attached to deeper tissue. Immediately under the skin is the pretarsal portion of the orbicularis oculi muscle, which maintains resting eyelid tone and causes blinking and closure. It is innervated by branches of the facial nerve. The inner lamella consists of the tarsus, which is composed of dense collagenous connective tissue. The tarsi are 25 mm wide and 1 mm thick. The maximum tarsal height is 10 to 11 mm in the upper lid and 5 mm in the lower lid. The tarsus contains the meibomian glands and fuses with the medial and lateral canthal tendons at its margins. The innermost layer of the lid is the conjunctiva, a mucous membrane lining that reflects onto the globe and provides tear production, ocular lubrication, and free motion of the globe on the lid. The eyelid margin can be divided into the ciliary portion, which contains the lashes, and the lacrimal portion, medially, which contains the lacrimal punctum and canaliculus. The lacrimal puncta serve as the drainage point for tears through the upper and lower canaliculi to the lacrimal sac, located in the lacrimal fossa. Tear flow is based on orbicularis oculi contraction (blinking) and adequate horizontal eyelid tone. The eyelids are suspended by the medial and lateral canthal tendons and anchored by the upper and lower retractors. The lids are separated from the orbital contents by the septum orbitale and a thin layer of connective tissue. Whitnall's ligament in the upper lid and Lockwood's ligament in the lower lid stabilize the eyelid and facilitate levator and inferior retractor muscle function.

The upper lid is elevated by the levator muscle (innervated by cranial nerve III), which has complex attachments to the eyelid skin at the lid crease and the anterior surface of the tarsus and Müller's muscle, a sympathomimetic muscle originating from the lower surface of the levator and inserting into the superior tarsal border. The retractors of the lower lid, the capsulopalpebral fascia and inferior tarsal muscle (also innervated by cranial nerve III), are less robust and fuse together before inserting into the lower border of the inferior tarsus.

PATHOLOGY OF EYELID NEOPLASMS

A variety of neoplasms can involve the eyelid, but the great majority arise from the epithelium. The most frequent types of malignancy are basal cell carcinoma (90%) (Fig. 8–1), squamous cell carcinoma (<5%), sebaceous cell carcinoma (1 to 3%) (Fig. 8–2), and melanoma (1%). In a large Chinese series, sebaceous cell carcinoma was second to basal cell in frequency, comprising 32% of cases. Other rare tumors include Merkel cell tumors, adnexal carcinomas, and sweat gland carcinomas.[19]

Epithelial lesions share the etiologic factors of patient age and exposure to ultraviolet rays from sunlight. The incidence of these lesions appears to be increasing with loss of the ozone layer in the atmosphere. Because of solar exposure, epithelial lid neoplasms occur more frequently on the lower lid. Sebaceous carcinoma and Merkel cell tumors both present in the upper lid in two thirds of cases. There are rare systemic conditions such as xeroderma pigmentosum in which cutaneous cancer occurs.

TUMOR CONTROL—SURGICAL MARGINS

Control of the surgical margins is absolutely necessary if one seeks cure. There are two methods of controlling margins: (1) Mohs technique (nonchemical), the advantages of which are its minimal tissue excision in three dimensions with maximum tissue preservation. Special training and expertise of the pathologist are necessary, and close interaction between the surgeon and the pathologist is of paramount importance. (2) Standard excision with a 3 to 5 mm margin. This can be achieved in a single resection or by excision of the tumor followed by resection of separate strips of tissue representing the margins. The tissue is then placed on cardboard or paper to maintain its orientation until it is analyzed by the pathologist. Monheit and colleagues[3] believe that the standard frozen section technique, which shows a 10% tumor recurrence at 5 years, is less efficacious, whereas others have had excellent results with standard resection and frozen section control. When using standard resection, it must be

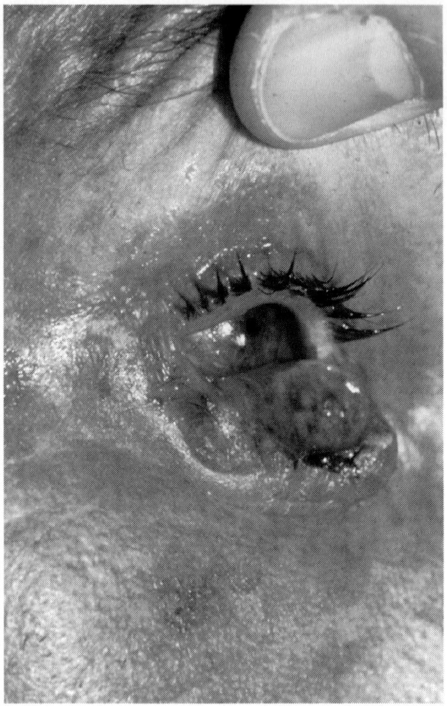

FIGURE 8–1. Very large basal cell carcinoma of lower eyelid.

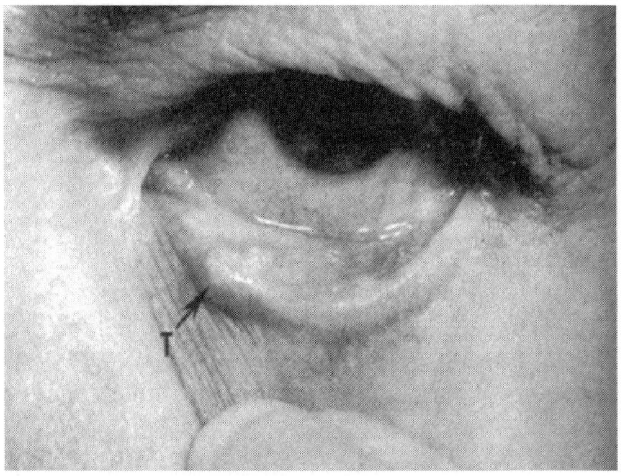

FIGURE 8–2. Meibomian gland adenocarcinoma.

assumed that a tumor involving the lid margin extends the full length of the meibomian gland, so the entire tarsal height should be resected.

The margin required for safety depends on the type of tumor. Squamous cell carcinoma, sebaceous carcinoma, and melanoma require larger margins than basal cell carcinoma, although in infiltrative or morpheaform basal cell tumors an even wider margin is desirable. Fortunately, the vast majority of eyelid malignancies are basal cell carcinomas.

PRINCIPLES OF RECONSTRUCTION

Reconstruction should be initiated only when the surgical margins are clear of tumor. If necessary, reconstruction should be delayed until definitive permanent sections have been completed or special pathologic studies have been analyzed. The surgeon should be familiar with the aesthetic units of the face and should maintain reconstruction of the eyelid and orbital tissues as one unit, being careful not to cross natural lines. Since the full extent of the tumor cannot be known until the margins have been evaluated, the decision about the type of reconstruction to be done must be made intraoperatively. Patients and families should be informed preoperatively both of this and of the spectrum of reconstructive techniques that might be employed.

Satisfactory reconstruction of the eyelid has three components—structural, functional, and cosmetic. Structurally, reconstruction requires an inner mucous membrane surface and an outer cutaneous surface. Structural support also requires either connective tissue or muscle or even scar tissue. Because reconstruction involves maintaining the continuity of the inner and outer lamellae, resections should be performed with vertical margins to allow optimal reapproximation or interposition of tissue without unsightly scars and with continuity of the lamellae and the lid margin, which itself is important functionally and cosmetically. These vertical incisions are connected with angled incisions through the adjacent soft tissue to create a pentagonal defect. As elsewhere, grafted tissue requires an adequate vasculature, so that if one lamella is reconstructed with grafts, the other must be reconstructed with vascularized flaps. In rare cases, a muscle or periosteal flap can be used to support both the mucous membrane and the outer lamellar tissue. Functional repair allows adequate eye coverage and maintenance of the tear film. Cosmetic considerations include alignment of the lid margin, matching the reconstructed tissue to the surrounding tissue, and canthal positioning. The lacrimal drainage system should be preserved when possible; if resected, it can be reconstructed primarily or secondarily.

Selection of an appropriate technique for reconstruction of the eyelid in each patient is based on consideration of a variety of factors including the size of the defect, the vascularity of the tissues, the availability of graft or flap material, the ability of the patient to undergo an operation requiring occlusion of the eye for a prolonged period, and the ultimate cosmetic result desired. Final determination of the technique used occurs intraoperatively when the position of all related structures and tissue deficits is considered. When tissue loss involves multiple aesthetic units, each unit should be repaired independently.

Direct Apposition

When possible, direct apposition of the remaining lid structures should be performed using layered closure of the tarsus and skin and carefully avoiding exposure of sutures to the ocular surface. Direct repair is applicable in cases with less than a 25% loss of the lid width. Laxity of tissue increases with age as well as with other conditions, so this method can sometimes be used in older patients with a 30% to 40% defect or in those with lax lids.

We prefer to close the tarsus first, sometimes after placing eyelid margin sutures to ensure perfect alignment. The tarsus is closed with two (lower) or three (upper) 5–0 chromic gut or Vicryl sutures, avoiding exposure on the conjunctival surface. The lid margin is closed with two or three 7–0 silk sutures as required to ensure optimal alignment. The skin is closed with 6–0 silk sutures. The 7–0 silk sutures are left long and tied to the first or second knots of the skin repair (6–0) sutures to direct them away from the ocular surface. If there are large inner lamellar gaps, additional 5–0 chromic sutures may be placed in the deep soft tissues at the level of the tarsus. Skin sutures are removed in 5 to 7 days, and the lid margin sutures are removed at 7 to 14 days.

Relaxation Techniques (Canthotomy and Cantholysis)

When direct closure is only a few millimeters short of being possible, the deficit may be closed using relaxation techniques. Lateral canthotomy and cantholysis can mobilize tissue and allow coverage of greater defects without the need for flaps in some cases. Before selecting this technique, the surgeon should exclude the use of transposition flaps and leave the canthal structures intact. The canthotomy should be performed sharply instead of with crush techniques. The inferior or superior crus of the canthal tendon is then sectioned with scissors. The canthal angle is reformed using either 5–0 chromic gut or Vicryl sutures to appose the upper and lower lids, and the knot is buried in the incision. The skin wound is closed with 6–0 silk sutures.

Special Techniques for Small Defects—Skin and Composite Grafts

Skin grafts are very useful. In some cases, a composite full-thickness eyelid graft can be placed with the advantage that tissue matching is identical and lashes are included with the graft. Such grafts should be less than 25% of the lid width to optimize survival. Lash loss is not uncommon, and the entire graft may slough. This technique is used when there is additional tissue in one of the other lids. When copious outer lamellar tissue is present, a free graft of tissue for the posterior lamella can be placed and covered with an advancement flap of adjacent outer lamellar tissue created by undermining alone.

Advancement Flaps

Multiple temporal advancement flaps exist. The principles of construction are similar in all of them. The direct temporal advancement flap can be functionally very successful, but it suffers from the cosmetic limitation of the need for two roughly parallel scars in an adjacent aesthetic unit. We prefer the semicircular rotational Tenzel flap, which achieves similar or slightly less tissue mobilization with only a single incision line that can be easily camouflaged. The details of this technique are described elsewhere, but the principles of its construction include: creation of a semicircular skin-muscle flap 10 to 20 mm in size in continuity with the line of the margin of the resected eyelid (above the canthus for lower lid repair and below it for upper lid repair), cantholysis, anchoring of the flap to the periosteum at the lateral orbital margin, and creation of a new canthal angle.

Transposition Flaps

A variety of transposition flaps have been described; they can be divided into those of the inner lamella and those of the outer lamella. Considerations include whether or not the patient's eye can be closed for extended periods of time as required with tarsoconjunctival flaps and the availability of specific tissue types of the inner and outer lamellae.

The ideal tissue for reconstruction of the inner lamella is tarsus and conjunctiva. Three to four millimeters of eyelid are needed to provide adequate support and preserve the eyelid margin in donor and host lids. This is best provided by transposition from the opposite ipsilateral eyelid. Originally described by Kollner in 1911[10] and further developed by Dupuis-Dutemps and Hughes[12] in 1937 using lid-splitting at the gray line and a full tarsal height, these techniques resulted in multiple upper lid complications (irregular margin, entropion, lid retraction). Hughes popularized the technique in the United States, and current modifications and extensions of these techniques are known eponymically as the Hughes reconstruction (tarsoconjunctival, upper to lower). Other techniques that employ multilamellar transposition of conjunctiva and tarsus with or without other tissue include the Cutler-Beard[16] reconstruction which uses a full-thickness bridge flap for lower to upper eyelid transposition, and the Hewes-Sullivan-Beard technique, a lateral-based tarsoconjunctival flap used for upper to lower transposition.[20] Tenzel, Kersten, and others have reported different eyelid reconstructive techniques.[21–25]

Hughes Technique (Modified)

The principles of the Hughes technique include creation of a tarsoconjunctival transposition flap leaving 6–8 mm of tarsus to maintain the contour of the upper lid margin and removing the retractors from the flap, suture of the flap to the lateral margins of the resected region using standard eyelid closure techniques, and coverage of the outer lamellar defect with either a full-thickness skin graft or an advancement flap. Central defects that cannot be covered with a lateral advancement flap can be covered with a flap using Bernard's triangle, an island maxillary flap, or a V-Y Dieffenbach procedure. The second stage of the reconstruction, flap severance, can be performed as early as 2 weeks after the first procedure, but we prefer to wait 6 to 8 weeks, especially in patients with larger reconstructions in which the tensile strength of the wound and the maturity of the graft are important considerations. The flap is sectioned leaving the mucosal surface higher than the skin, since the normal mucosa extends anteriorly and the line of division is curved so that it is continuous with the normal eyelid contour. Careful dissection and replacement of advanced tissues back into the upper lid at the second stage of repair minimize complications associated with upper lid retraction. Laxity of the reconstructed lid is avoided by using the smallest flap width that will fill the defect without undue tension. Shrinkage is avoided by waiting for maturation and vascularization of the flap to occur before sectioning the pedicle.

Cutler-Beard Technique

Upper lid tumors are less common than lower lid tumors and because of its greater difficulty compared to the Hughes flap, the Cutler-Beard bridge flap is less often used. It is much more straightforward than the Mustardé lid transposition procedure, in which the lower lid is transposed to the upper lid defect and the lower lid is reconstructed. Its principal features include construction of a full-thickness bridge flap that does not include tarsus, protection of the lower lid bridge by avoiding vascular compromise through suture or dressing compression, and suture reconstitution of the eyelid margin at the second stage of the procedure. This technique also requires prolonged eyelid closure.

A full-thickness flap is created, placing the upper lid margin 1 to 2 mm below the inferior border of the lower tarsus to avoid the marginal artery. The sides of the flap are made by excisions that can extend vertically 15 to 20 mm. The flap is advanced under the lower tarsal bridge and sutured in a layered fashion to the upper lid tissues. The lower edge of the bridge is not sutured, and dressings are not compressive to avoid vascular compromise. The flap is divided after 6 to 8 weeks. A mucocutaneous junction for the upper lid is created with sutures. The tissue margins of the lower lid are freshened and resutured in a layered fashion.

Hewes-Sullivan-Beard Technique

For long horizontal defects of the lower lid less than 5 mm in height, a laterally based, posterior lamellar tarsoconjunctival flap can be created. The key advantages of this repair are that the eye remains open and the posterior tissue match is excellent. The principal features of this repair are preservation of 3 to 4 mm of the tarsus of the upper lid margin, preservation of an adequate laterally based blood supply to the flap, and outer lamellar repair with full-thickness skin or a skin-muscle advancement flap. The flap base can be sectioned sharply or by cautery.

Special Techniques of Reconstruction

With larger defects, nonlid tissue must be mobilized to the defect using the Mustardé cheek rotation flap. In Mustardé's technique a cheek sliding flap with a septal cartilage graft is used for total lower lid reconstruction.[11] A.J. Maniglia in 1978[17] reported the use of a large medially based nasolabial flap and septal cartilage with perichondrium for reconstruction of total or near total lower lid defects.

SOURCES OF TISSUE FOR EYELID RECONSTRUCTION

A wide range of tissues are available for eyelid reconstruction. Ophthalmic tissues provide the best match. In situations requiring donor tissue from ocular structures, collaboration with the ophthalmologist ensures optimal protection of the donor eye. Techniques for obtaining tissues from nonophthalmic sites are well known to practitioners in other specialties.

Donor tissue for the inner lamella can come from a variety of sites. While outer lamellar tissue has one primary function, coverage, inner lamellar tissue has the dual functions of providing tensile strength and serving as a mucous membrane lining. The components required to fulfill these functions can be provided by individual tissues or, preferably, by composite grafts.

Isolated mucous membrane grafts can be provided optimally by free conjunctival grafts, but only a limited quantity of tissue is available from this site. Buccal mucosa provides excellent results with variable cosmesis, but copious amounts of it are available.

Composite grafts of connective tissue and mucous membrane can be obtained from the tarsus, nasal septum, and hard palate. Although tarsus is the ideal replacement, like conjunctiva, its quantity is limited. Mucosal grafts from the hard palate are being used with increasing frequency. The dense substantia propria of the palate is tough and firm. Inclusion of periosteum in the graft is not required. Access to this tissue is easy in most cases, and healing is rapid. Nasal septomucosal grafts can also be used. Access to this tissue is not as easy as in the other sites mentioned. In some cases, the tissue can be unduly stiff or calcified, and it conforms poorly to the curved ocular surface.

Isolated connective tissue grafts are also usable. These include grafts composed of auricular cartilage or nasal septum. These must be covered with mucous membrane. In addition, they may be rigid and require softening to conform adequately to the ocular surface. Skin grafts (full-thickness) of the eyelids and posterior auricular area are most commonly used (Table 8–1).

TABLE 8–1. SOURCES OF DONOR MATERIAL FOR EYELID RECONSTRUCTION

INNER LAMELLA
Mucous membrane
Conjunctiva
Buccal mucosa
Mucous membrane and connective tissue
Tarsus
Nasal septum-mucosal grafts
Hard palate mucosa
Dense connective tissue
Nasal septal cartilage
Auricular cartilage
OUTER LAMELLA
Other eyelid
Retroauricular skin
Supraclavicular skin
Tissue expansion

MATERIALS AND METHODS

Table 8–2 summarizes the various eyelid defects and the techniques used for reconstruction with different tissues, grafts, and flaps. Patients with different histopathological diagnoses can be treated accordingly. The following case reports illustrate a variety of surgical defects and the reconstructive techniques used to repair them.

Lower Eyelid Reconstruction

Tumors of the lower eyelid are by far the most frequent. Reconstruction of such defects is less demanding. An absent lower lid in the presence of Bell's phenomenon may cause a minor irritation, whereas a damaged upper eyelid could certainly result in loss of vision with much pain and discomfort for the patient.

Defects of Up to 25% of Eyelid

Ablation of up to 25% of the lower lid is reconstructed by primary suture (Fig. 8–3). We prefer to use the three marginal sutures technique using 6–0 silk in the gray line, the mucocutaneous junction, and the ciliary line.

After the tarsal plate has been approximated with Vicryl 5–0 sutures without closing the conjunctiva, we tie the silk knots (Fig. 8–4). They are bound to the ciliary suture and directed outward to avoid corneal injury. The skin is sutured with 6–0 silk that can be removed in 5 to 7 days. Marginal sutures may be removed in 12 days.

TABLE 8–2. SELECTION OF EYELID RECONSTRUCTIVE TECHNIQUES

	DEFECT	LAXITY	MONOCULAR	REPAIR
Upper				
	<25%	+/−		Direct closure, free skin and composite grafts
	30%–40%	+		Direct closure with cantholysis, free and composite grafts
	>50%	+/−		Tenzel flap, Cutler-Beard
	>85%			Mustardé lid transposition
Lower				
	<25%	+/−		Direct (free composite graft)
	30%–40%	+		Direct with cantholysis
	30%–40%	−	−	Tenzel flap, temporal flap, Hughes procedure
	30%–40%	−	+	Temporal flap
	>50%		−	Hughes procedure
	50%–85%		+	Tenzel flap, temporal flap, Hewes-Sullivan-Beard
	>85%			Mustardé cheek and sliding flap
				A.J. Maniglia (nasolabial flap and septal graft)

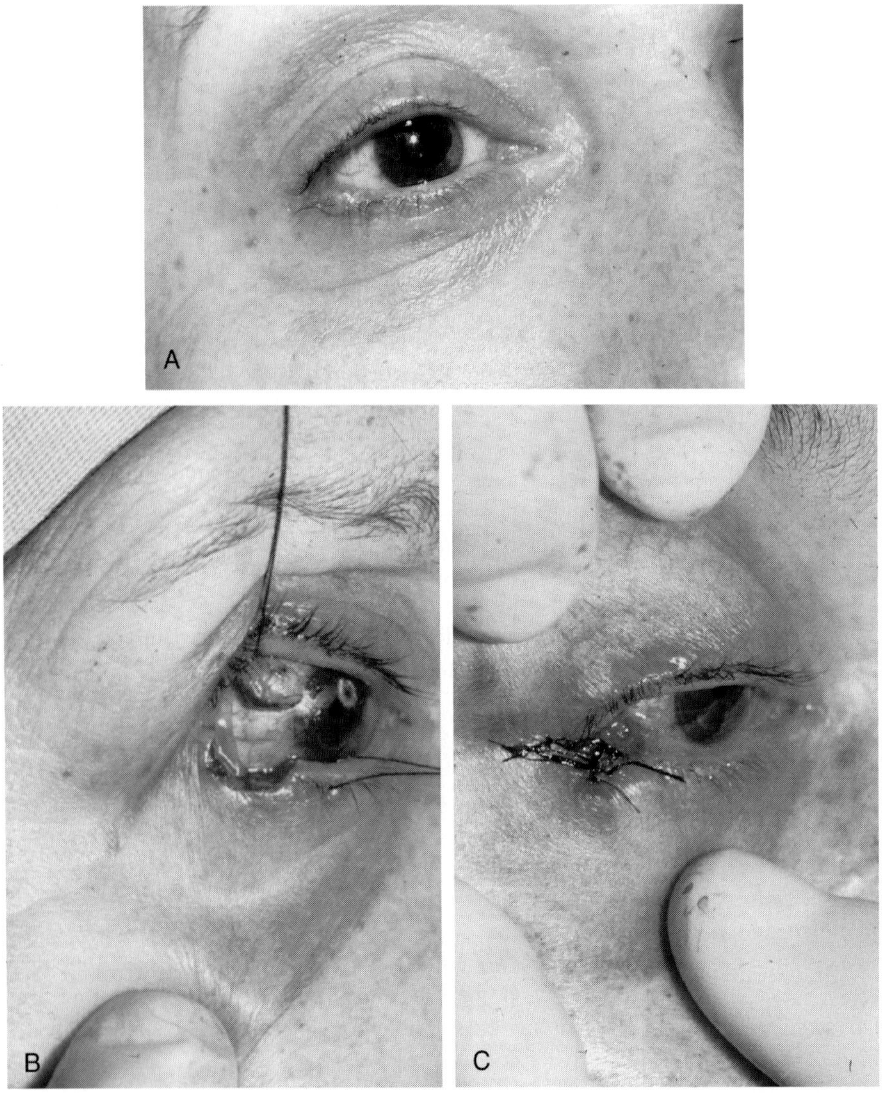

FIGURE 8–3. *A*, Basal cell carcinoma of lower lid margin. *B*, Pentagonal resection of basal cell carcinoma shown in *A*. *C*, Primary surgical closure of lid defect (shown in Fig. 8–4).

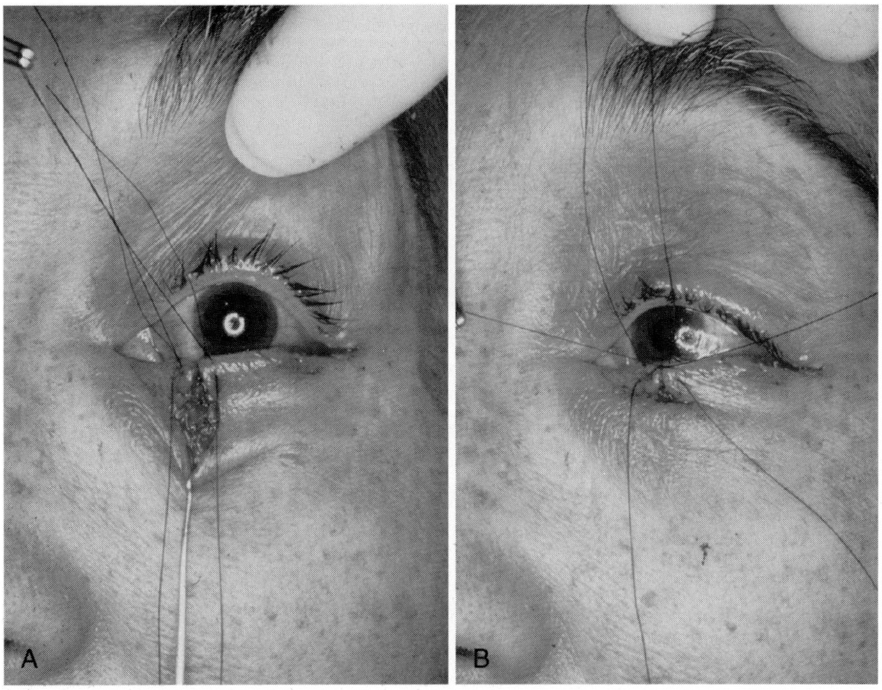

FIGURE 8–4. *A*, Three marginal suture technique. Tarsal plate closed with 5–0 Vicryl. *B*, Silk knots are tied.

Defects of 30% to 40% of Eyelid

In older people, due to lid laxity it is possible to achieve primary suture even with a 30% or 40% loss of the eyelid. If this is not possible, other procedures must be performed in a sequential fashion to avoid tension in the suture line. A lateral canthotomy and cantholysis with advancement of the lateral fornix conjunctiva may facilitate primary closure of the defect (Fig. 8–5).

Defects of Up to 50% of Eyelid

When a decision has been made to use a graft or flap, it is best not to perform a canthoplasty with cantholysis because grafts or flaps are better anchored when sutured to the remaining eyelid structures.

Temporal Defects. Temporal defects of the lower lid (Fig. 8–6*A*) can be corrected by using septal mucoperichondrial cartilage. Also, a mucoperiosteal hard palate graft may be

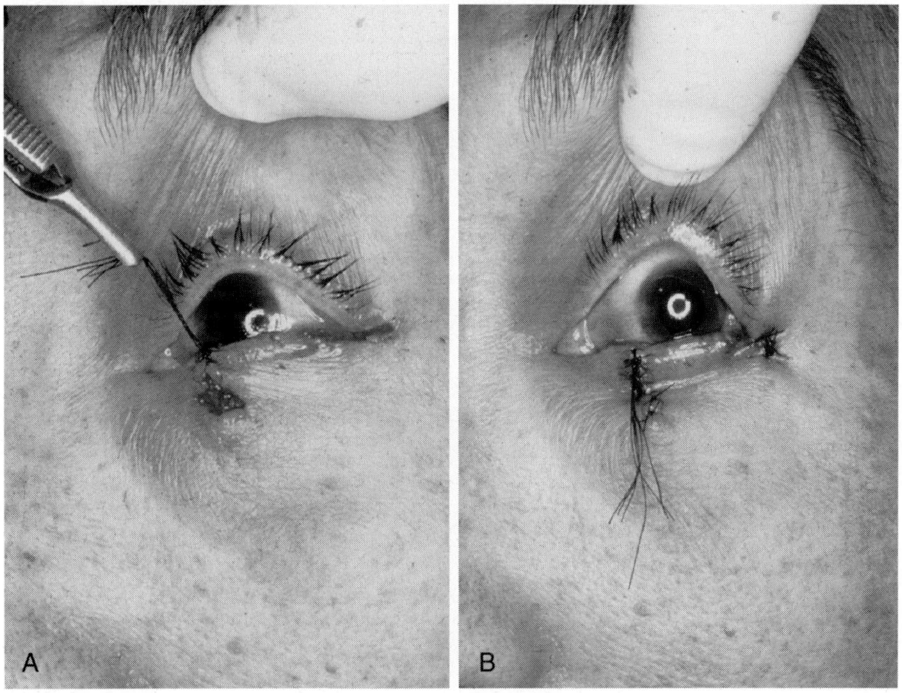

FIGURE 8–5. *A*, All marginal sutures locked to ciliary suture; note incision of canthotomy. *B*, 6–0 silk sutured to skin at surgery site and canthal area.

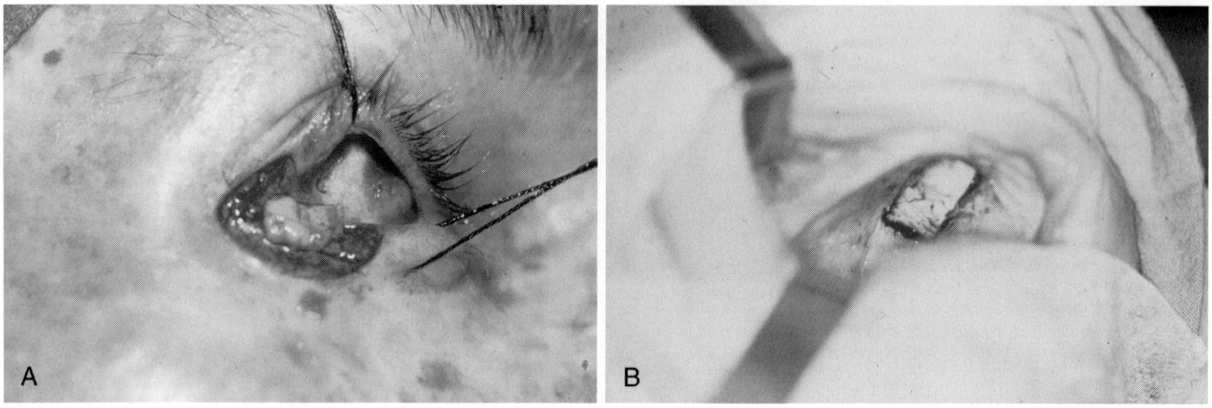

FIGURE 8–6. *A*, Lower lid temporal tumor requiring 50% reconstruction; note tumor inside the defect. *B*, Harvesting hard palate mucoperiosteum graft.

used to replace the inner layer (Fig. 8–6*B* and *C*). The graft is anchored in a periosteal flap designed to replace the tendon of the outer canthus. Skin coverage must be provided by rotating the flap (Fig. 8–7*A*), and one of the best rotation flaps is the semicircular temporal Tenzel flap. Figure 8–7*B* illustrates a bipedicled temporal flap that can also be used in similar defects.

Central Defects. In a central lower lid defect of 50% (Fig. 8–8*A* and *B*) lower eyelid remnants on both sides are present that can be used in a septal mucoperichondrial and cartilage graft (Fig. 8–8*C*). Skin coverage for the outer lamella is provided by an advancement flap from the remaining lower lid skin (Fig. 8–9*A* and *B*). If the skin excision is so large that reconstruction by flap is doubtful, a tarsoconjunctival flap from the upper lid can replace the inner lamella and provide a blood supply so that a full-thickness retroauricular skin graft in a Brown "tie-over" dressing can be used to replace the outer lamella.

Nasal Defect. The inner lamella can be replaced in the same way as described previously. The outer lamella can be reconstructed by using a rotated nasolabial flap. When a large area of skin excision precludes the use of a rotated nasolabial flap, the inner lamella should be reconstructed using an upper lid tarsoconjunctival flap, and the outer layer can be supplied by a retroauricular full-thickness skin graft. The inferior puncta and lower canaliculus can be marsupial-

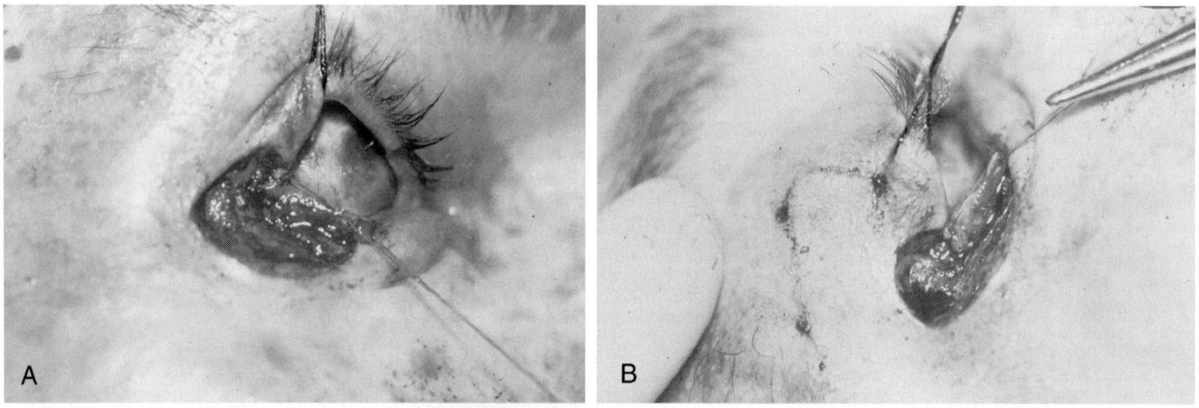

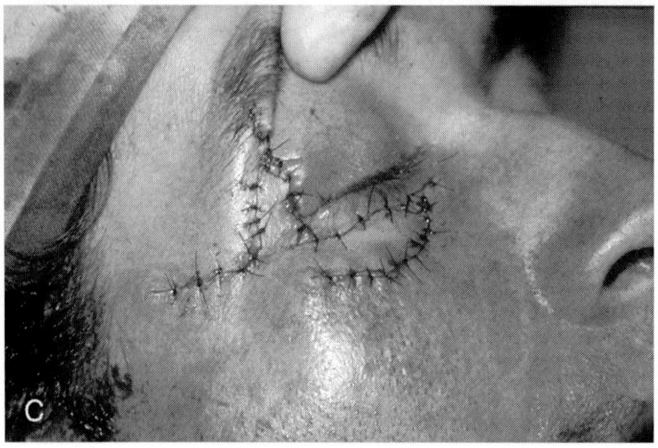

FIGURE 8–7. *A*, Mucoperiosteal graft sutured in place. *B*, Outline of rotation flap to be transferred to cover the defect. *C*, Another example of a bipedicled rotation flap to cover temporal lid skin defect.

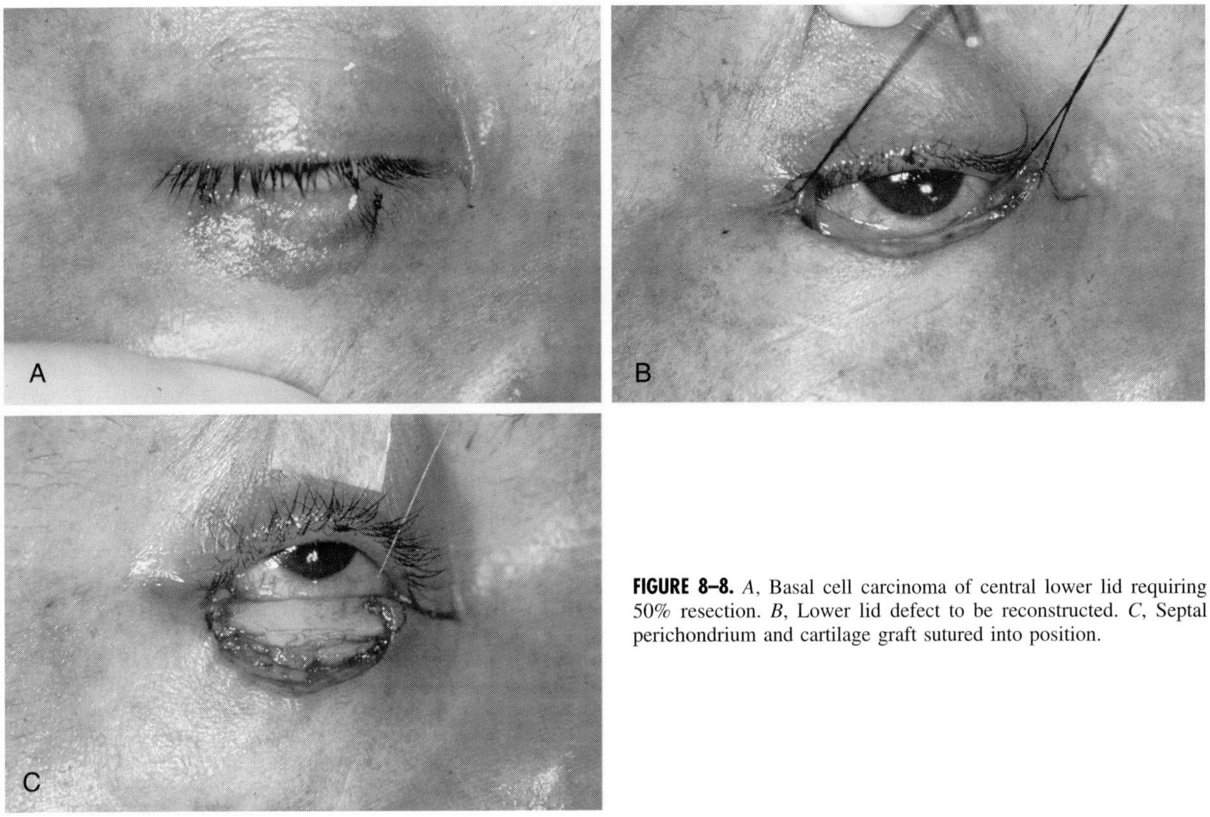

FIGURE 8–8. *A*, Basal cell carcinoma of central lower lid requiring 50% resection. *B*, Lower lid defect to be reconstructed. *C*, Septal perichondrium and cartilage graft sutured into position.

ized if necessary (Fig. 8–10). If the defect extends toward the nose or ethmoid sinus, glabellar bipedicled, forehead midline, or island flaps may have to be used.

Reconstruction of Up to 100% of Eyelid

The inner lamella can be reconstructed using a long septal cartilage mucoperichondrial or hard palate mucoperiosteal graft. Reconstruction of the outer lamella requires a lateral (Tenzel) flap associated with a medial nasolabial flap.

If the amount of resection is so extensive that it precludes the use of a skin flap, a large tarsoconjunctival flap is dissected from the ipsilateral upper eyelid (Fig. 8–11). If necessary, a buccal mucosal graft (Fig. 8–12*A*) can replace the excised bulbar and fornix conjunctiva, and the tarsoconjunctival flap is sutured to the eyelid retractors (Fig. 8–12*B*); a full-thickness retroauricular skin graft is then applied for external coverage (Fig. 8–12*C*). Rarely, older patients may present difficulty with epiphora. In these patients conjunctivorhinostomy may be done at a later time, if needed.

If the width of the tarsoconjunctival flap is not sufficient to reconstruct the defect, the temporal lower lid defect can be repaired by a palatal mucoperiosteal graft covered by a Tenzel flap. The nasal defect is reconstructed by the palatal mucoperiosteal graft covered by a nasolabial flap. The tarsoconjunctival flap is placed in the middle, covered by a retroauricular full-thickness skin graft or a central skin flap advancement.

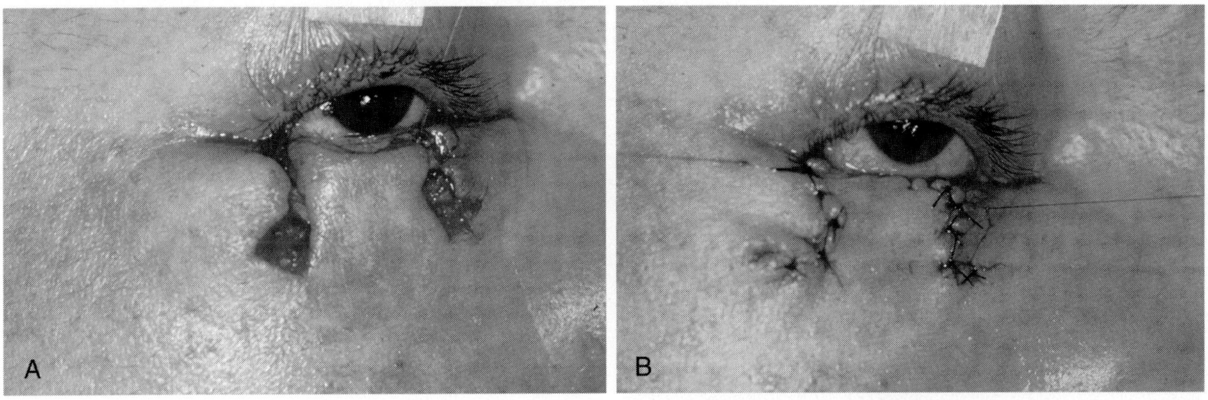

FIGURE 8–9. *A*, Advancement flap of skin with Bernard's triangle. *B*, Flap sutured in place.

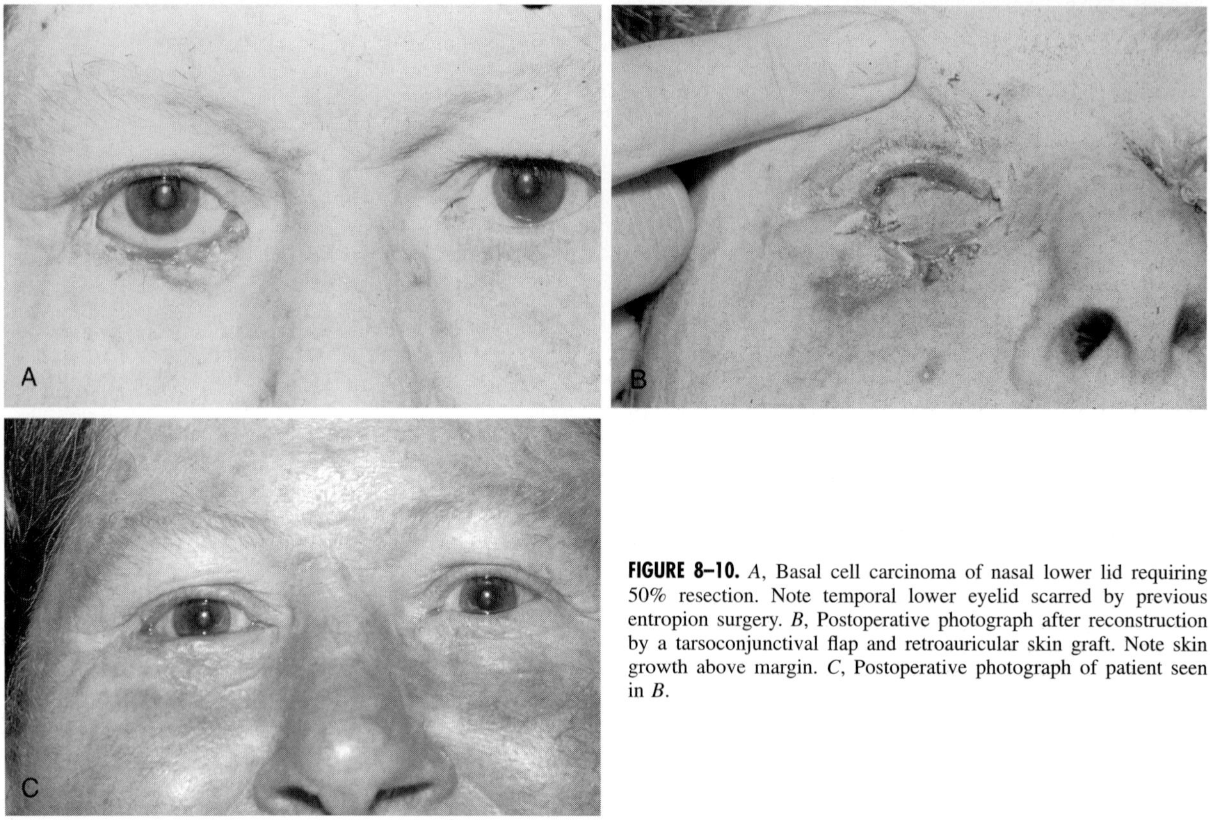

FIGURE 8–10. *A*, Basal cell carcinoma of nasal lower lid requiring 50% resection. Note temporal lower eyelid scarred by previous entropion surgery. *B*, Postoperative photograph after reconstruction by a tarsoconjunctival flap and retroauricular skin graft. Note skin growth above margin. *C*, Postoperative photograph of patient seen in *B*.

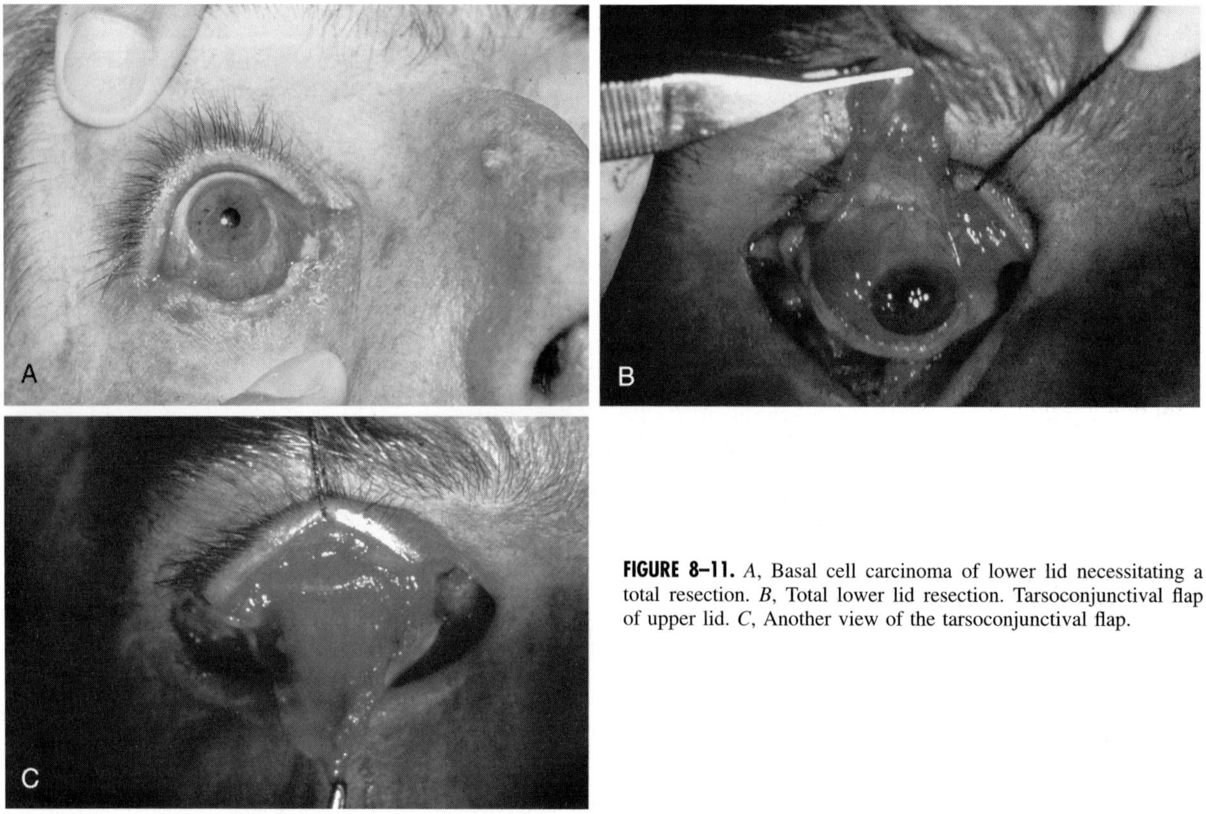

FIGURE 8–11. *A*, Basal cell carcinoma of lower lid necessitating a total resection. *B*, Total lower lid resection. Tarsoconjunctival flap of upper lid. *C*, Another view of the tarsoconjunctival flap.

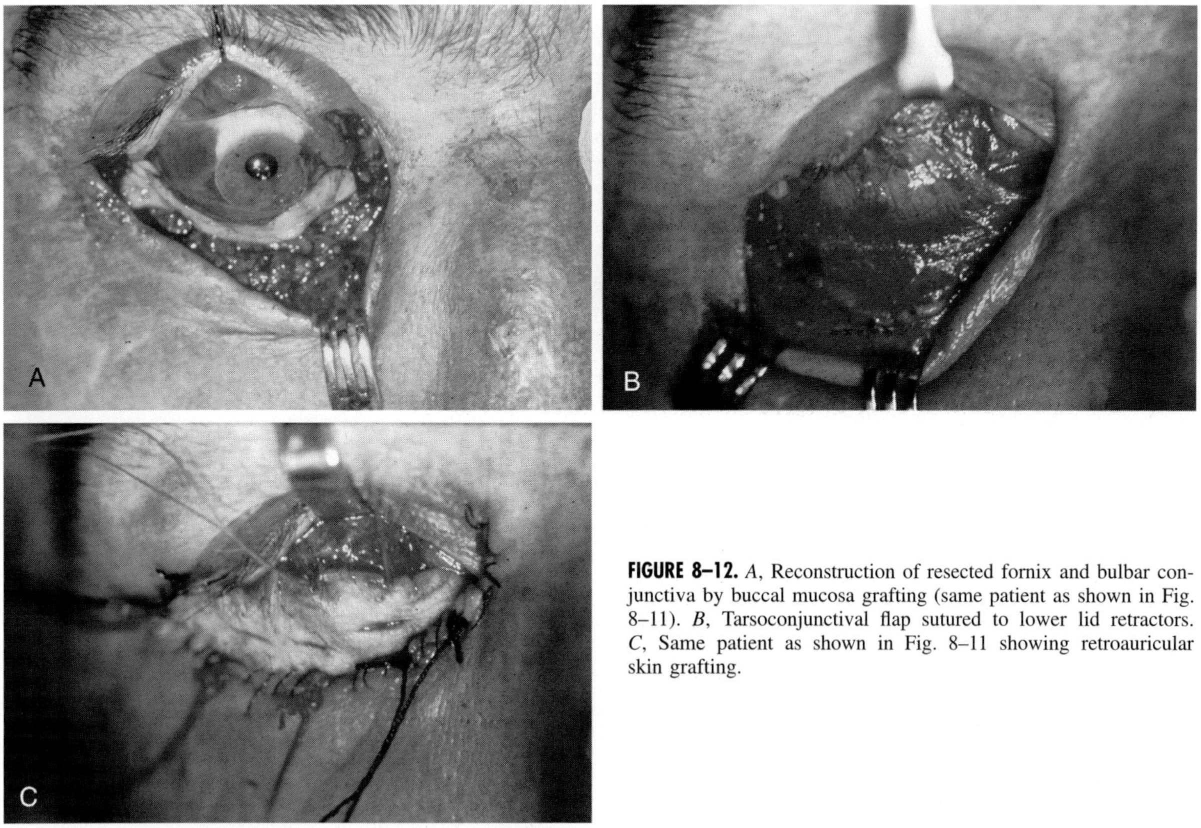

FIGURE 8–12. *A*, Reconstruction of resected fornix and bulbar conjunctiva by buccal mucosa grafting (same patient as shown in Fig. 8–11). *B*, Tarsoconjunctival flap sutured to lower lid retractors. *C*, Same patient as shown in Fig. 8–11 showing retroauricular skin grafting.

Inner Canthus Reconstruction

In the inner canthus, tumors tend to be more malignant and infiltrative. For this reason, strict control of margins must be maintained, and ample resections must be performed. If the inner canthus tendon and internal lamella as well as the periosteum can be preserved, it is possible to leave the inner canthus unreconstructed, with very good aesthetic and functional results. This technique is very good for inner canthal skin coverage but requires an intact periosteum and sutures guided toward the nasal lower and upper lids. In the same situation, a retroauricular skin graft could be used (Fig. 8–13). For larger resections, a tarsoconjunctival flap from the upper lid must be developed, and the external lamella must be provided in accordance with the size of the reconstructed area (ethmoid, lateral nasal wall).

Skin coverage may be provided from a skin graft or rotation flaps from the glabella (Fig. 8–14), forehead, or nasolabial area. The larger the defect, the worse the cosmetic result (Fig. 8–15). The lacrimal drainage system should not be repaired at this time.

Midline frontal flaps are too thick to replace the thin supple palpebral skin. In some cases the lateral nasal wall and nasal dorsum can be replaced by a midline forehead flap by excising small margins of the inner canthus eyelid (Fig. 8–16). The use of Doppler for delineation of arterial vascular

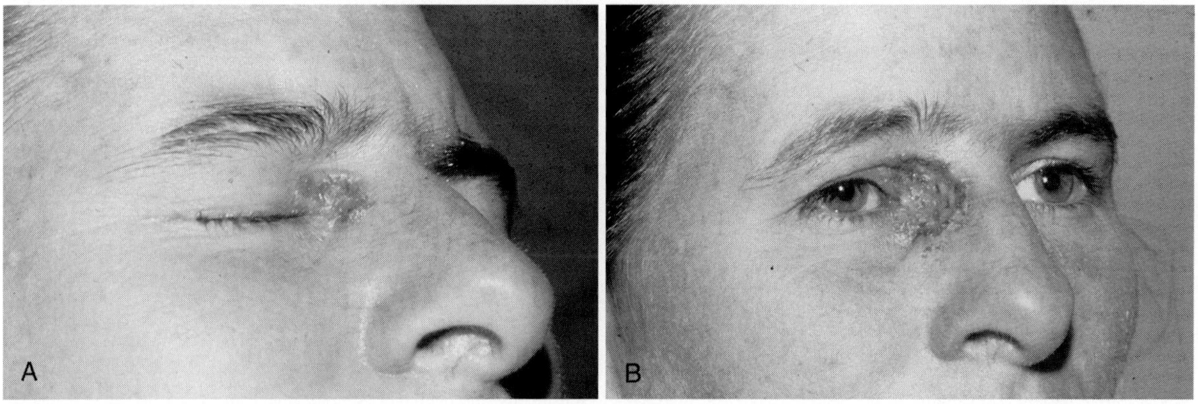

FIGURE 8–13. *A*, Inner canthus basal cell carcinoma. *B*, Reconstruction accomplished by retroauricular skin graft.

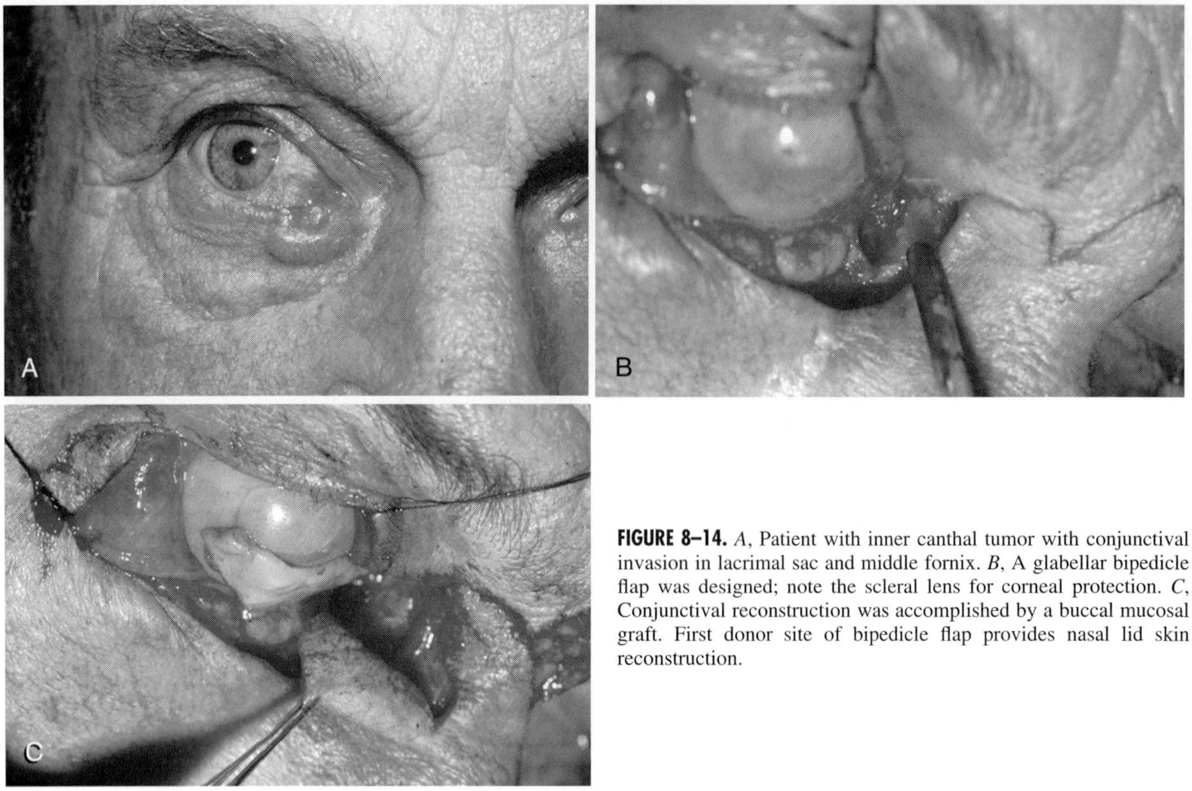

FIGURE 8–14. *A*, Patient with inner canthal tumor with conjunctival invasion in lacrimal sac and middle fornix. *B*, A glabellar bipedicle flap was designed; note the scleral lens for corneal protection. *C*, Conjunctival reconstruction was accomplished by a buccal mucosal graft. First donor site of bipedicle flap provides nasal lid skin reconstruction.

supply has made possible the use of thinner flaps, thereby producing better cosmetic results. A myocutaneous upper lid skin–orbicularis muscle flap based medially is also useful.[16]

Outer Canthus Reconstruction

Outer canthus tumors are very rare, and their resection demands reconstruction of the lower and upper lids, lateral fornix, and lateral tendons (Fig. 8–17*A*). Byron Smith[15] developed a very nice operation using a tarsoconjunctival flap from the upper eyelid anchored in a temporal periosteal flap used as a lateral tendon replacement (Fig. 8–17*B*). The upper lid remnant is sutured to the medial aspect of the newly made periosteal tendon (Fig. 8–18*A*) as well the lateral aspect of the tarsoconjunctival flap (Fig. 8–18*B*). The tip of this flap is sutured to the lateral fornix of the conjunctiva, and the lower lid is sutured to the medial aspect of the tarsoconjunctival flap. After the inner layer has been provided, skin coverage can be acquired by flap rotation, advancement (Fig. 8–18*C*), or a retroauricular full-thickness skin graft. Severance of the flap should be done in 4 weeks (Fig. 8–19).

Another case of basal cell carcinoma of the lower lid illustrates alternative techniques. After tumor-free margins were obtained, the defect included the lateral aspect of the lower lid and the lateral canthus (Fig. 8–20*A* and *B*). Because of the absence of lid laxity, it was decided to reconstruct the canthus using a periosteal flap from the lateral orbital rim.

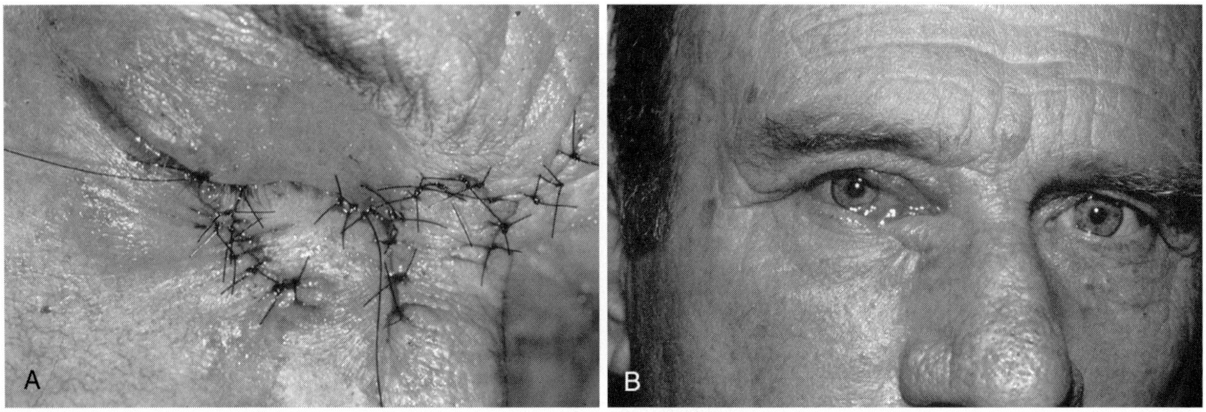

FIGURE 8–15. *A*, Same patient as in Figure 8–14. Second donor site of bipedicle flap to first donor defect. Second donor site is closed by primary suture. *B*, Patient's appearance can be improved by reoperation with hard palate mucoperiosteum to improve lid margin.

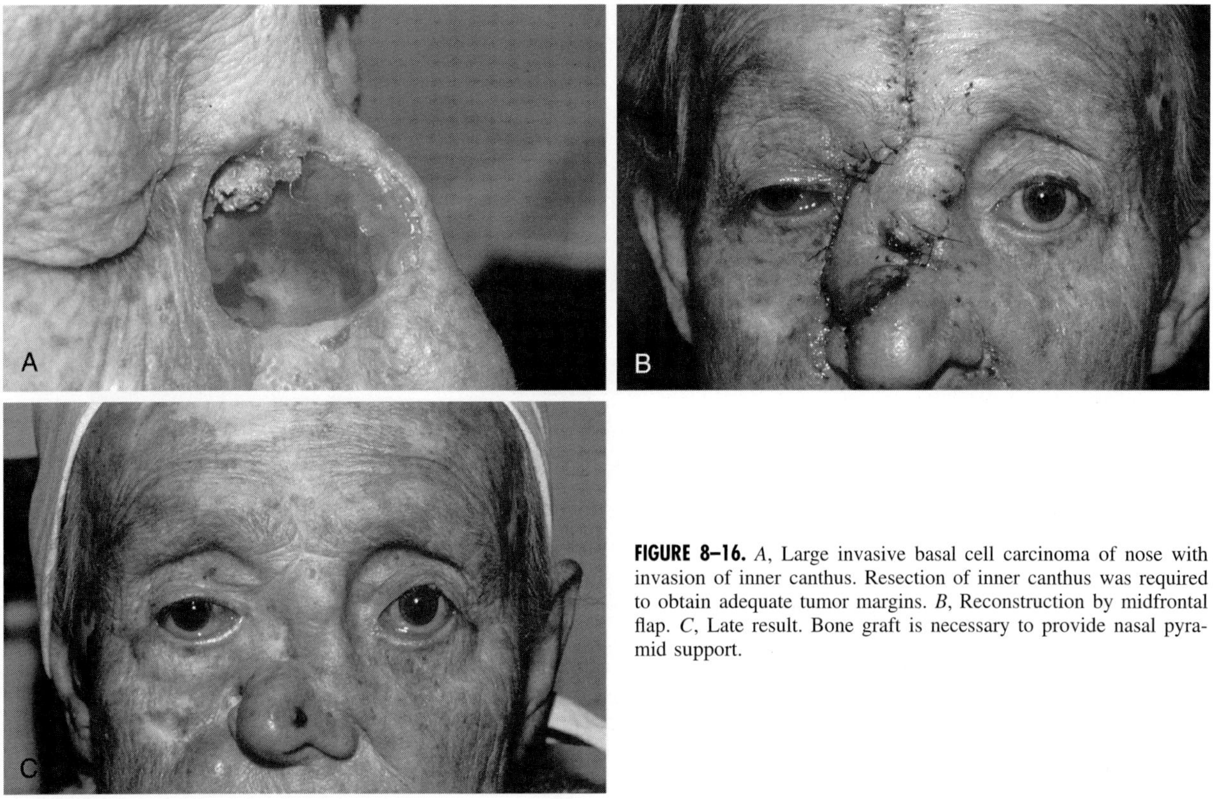

FIGURE 8–16. *A*, Large invasive basal cell carcinoma of nose with invasion of inner canthus. Resection of inner canthus was required to obtain adequate tumor margins. *B*, Reconstruction by midfrontal flap. *C*, Late result. Bone graft is necessary to provide nasal pyramid support.

This flap was covered on the mucosal surface by mobilized conjunctiva, and the other lamella was replaced with a full-thickness retroauricular skin graft. Postoperative views show excellent lid contour, although the skin does not match perfectly with the surrounding tissue (Fig. 8–21).

In another patient with meibomian gland carcinoma of the lower lid with neck metastasis (see Fig. 8–2) a nasolabial flap based medially as originally described by A.J. Maniglia[17] was used. A mucoperichondrial cartilage graft from the nasal septum was also used to reconstruct the tarsal plate. There is need for an epithelial lining of the perichondrium with this procedure because mucosa from the conjunctiva grows in the perichondrium. A conjunctival rhinostomy was done to provide lacrimal drainage (Fig. 8–22). Parotidectomy and radical neck dissection were also performed. Metastasis was present in the neck. Postoperative radiation therapy was given to the parotid and the neck. Figure 8–23 illustrates the postoperative result. The patient died 3 years later from brain metastasis, but there was no evidence of recurrent tumor in the orbit, parotid, or neck.

Upper Lid Reconstruction

Upper lid reconstruction should make use of similar tissues, if at all possible. Small defects (up to 25%) can be corrected by primary suture. For larger defects, a lateral canthotomy is added. If primary repair is not possible, a

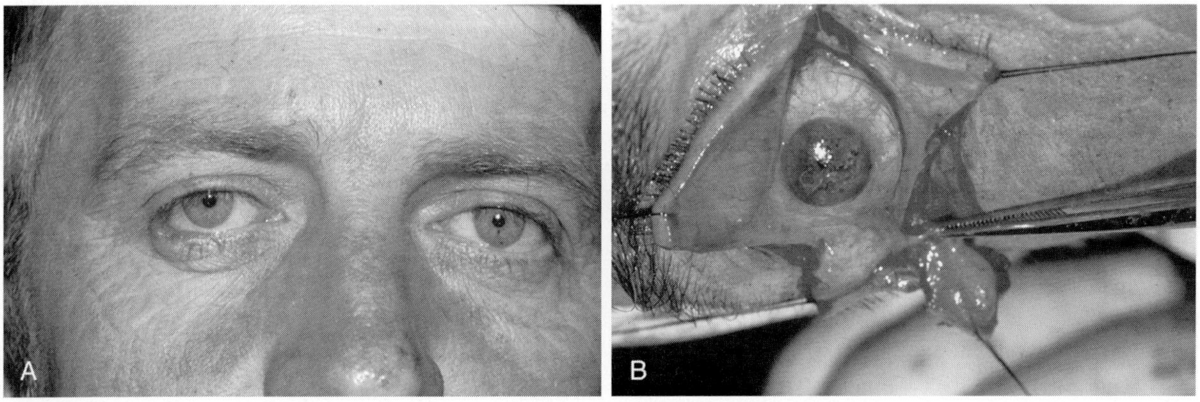

FIGURE 8–17. *A*, Patient with basal cell carcinoma of outer canthus with conjunctival invasion in fornix. *B*, Section of upper and lower lid exposes tumor extension in lateral fornix.

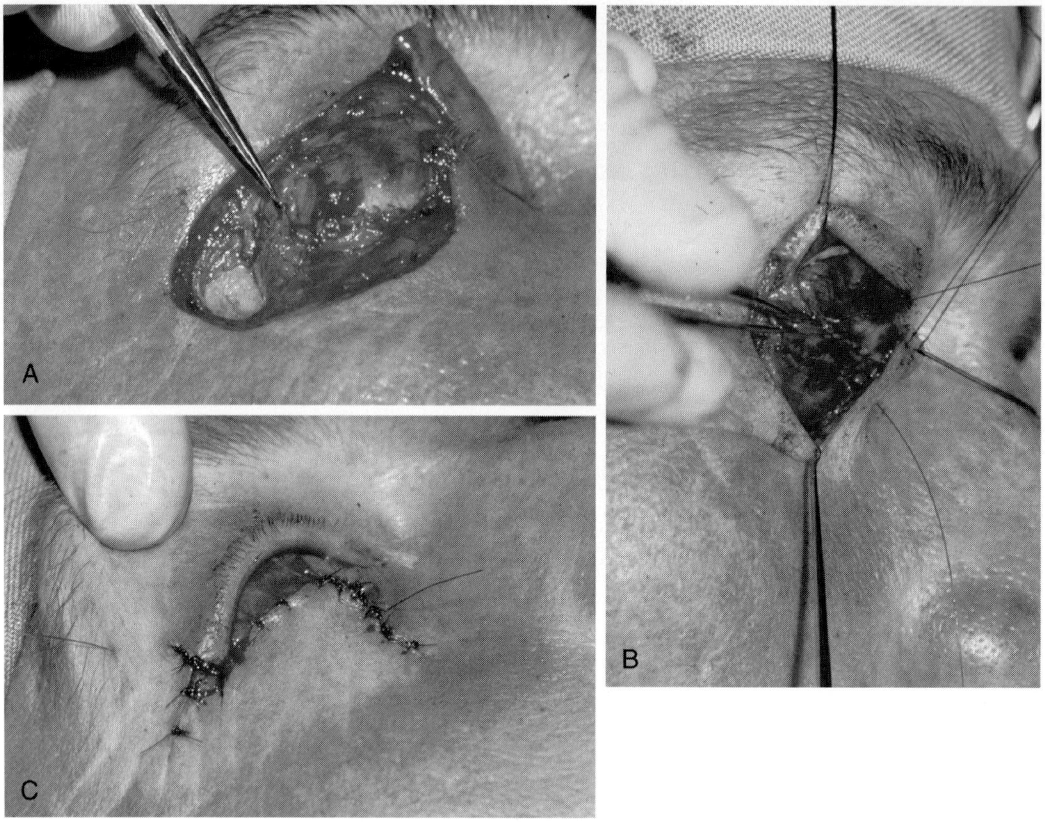

FIGURE 8–18. *A*, A periosteal flap replaces the lateral tendon ligament. Forceps hold flap. *B*, Tarsoconjunctival flap and lids are anchored in the periosteal ligament. *C*, Temporal flap advancement reconstructs the external lamella.

chondromucosal total lid graft from the opposite side may be used. This graft brings eyelashes to the repair. Putterman developed a nice technique in which the skin cover of the graft taken from the opposite upper lid is removed, leaving an intact margin with cilia. A skin flap of the upper lid (with its vascular supply) covers the composite graft, and the donor site of the flap is skin grafted using skin removed from the composite graft. Because of the need to reconstruct the contralateral upper lid (which is the donor site of the composite graft), defects repaired by this technique should not be larger than 30% or 40% to allow for primary suturing of the outer canthotomy and canthoplasty of the contralateral eyelid.

A case of sebaceous carcinoma of the left upper eyelid was diagnosed after a chalazion-like lesion was excised (Fig. 8–23*A* [see Color plate]). The patient was found to have a solitary metastasis to the left parotid gland area. After tumor resection with control of the margins was performed, functional and cosmetic characteristics were considered in the repair of a 45% lid loss including resection of the lacrimal canaliculus and upper crus of the medial canthal tendon (Fig. 8–23*B* [see Color plate]). A Tenzel rotational flap would have left an area laterally without lashes, which would have been quite conspicuous. Instead, taking advantage of an excess amount of lid skin, the tarsus adjacent to the defect was divided horizontally, and the superior portion was transposed medially to attach to the lid margin and medial canthal tendon. Skin and muscle were advanced from above to cover the flap. Postoperatively, the lateral extent of the lash line appears normal (Fig. 8–24*A* and *B* [see Color plate]).

Reconstruction techniques similar to the ones used in the lower lid can be used, but there is a lack of cilia replacement. Mustardé[11] uses whole lower lid for upper lid reconstruction, pedicled on the marginal artery; a second-stage procedure is needed to sever the pedicle and repair the lower lid. Cutler and Beard[16] developed a method for reconstructing the total upper lid by performing a marginal lower lid horizontal blepharotomy and suspending the inferior lid "under the bridge" to the levator aponeurosis and skin. With this method, after severance it is possible to end up with problems in both lids. We prefer to use a tarsoconjunctival flap from the lower lid that can be developed in a similar fashion: "One borrows from Peter to pay Paul only if Peter can afford it."

If a large defect (up to a loss of 100%) is produced by tumor ablation (Fig. 8–25), this tarsoconjunctival flap should be anchored in the levator aponeurosis, and the external lamella should be built by using full-thickness retroauricular skin graft or upper lid skin growth along the flap (Fig. 8–26). If there is a short inner lower lid lamella, a mucoperiosteal graft should correct it very nicely in the second stage (mucosal flap severance).

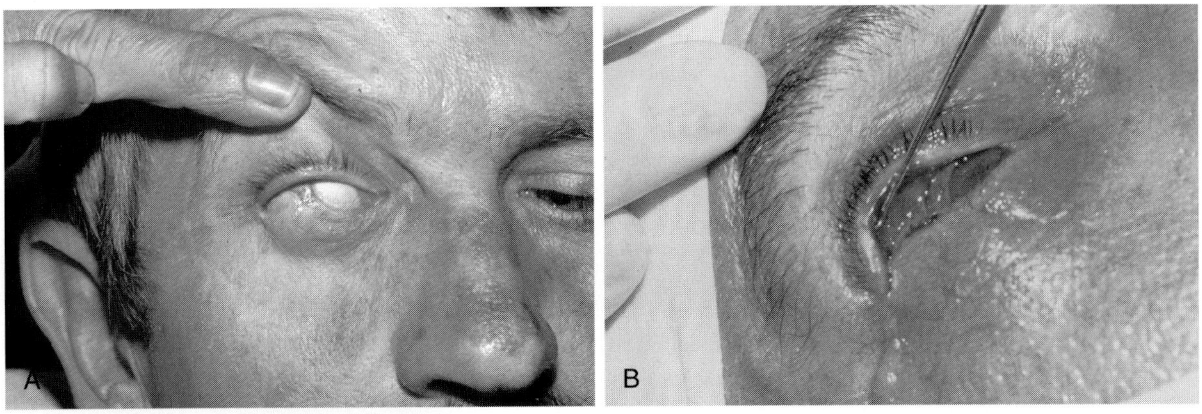

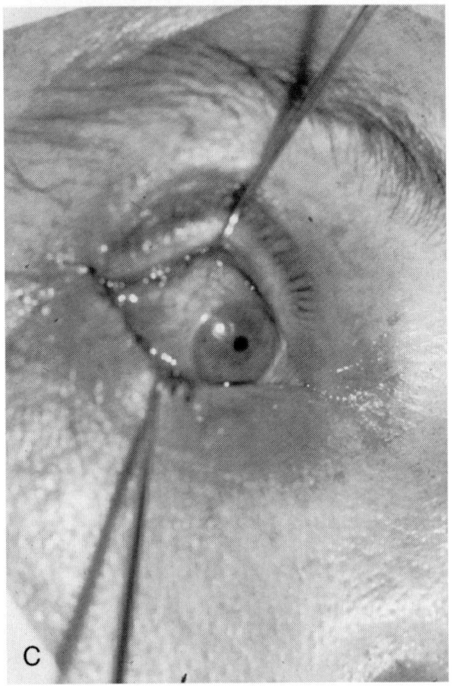

FIGURE 8–19. *A*, Postoperative view of same patient shown in Figure 8–17*A*. Skin growth is evident on the mucosal flap. *B*, View of mucosal flap pedicle. *C*, After severance of the mucosal flap pedicle, the upper lid is detached from the lower lid.

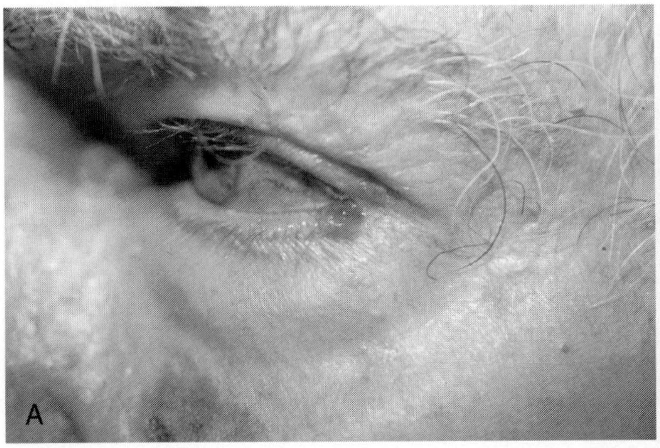

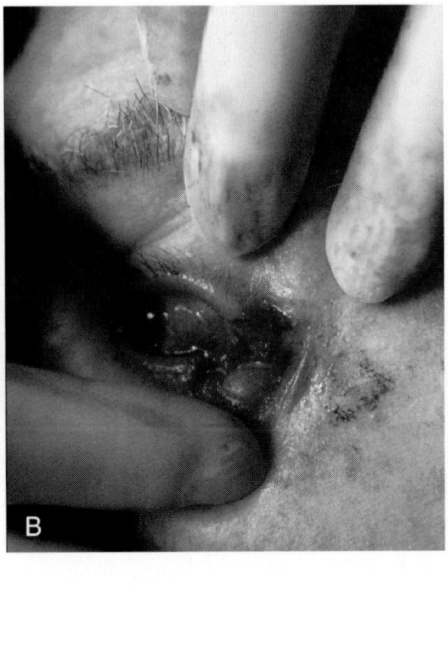

FIGURE 8–20. *A*, Patient with basal cell carcinoma; noduloulcerative lesion of left lower eyelid. *B*, Tissue defect after tumor-free margins were obtained.

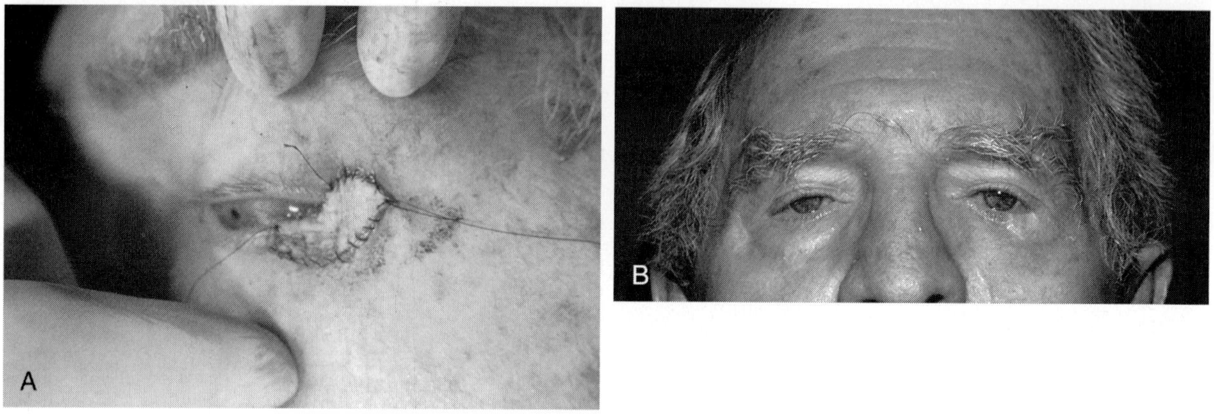

FIGURE 8–21. *A*, Lid after reconstruction using periosteal flap from lateral orbital wall covered internally by mobilized conjunctiva and externally with a full-thickness retroauricular skin graft. *B*, Postoperative result with excellent lid contour. Graft skin is distinguishable from surrounding skin.

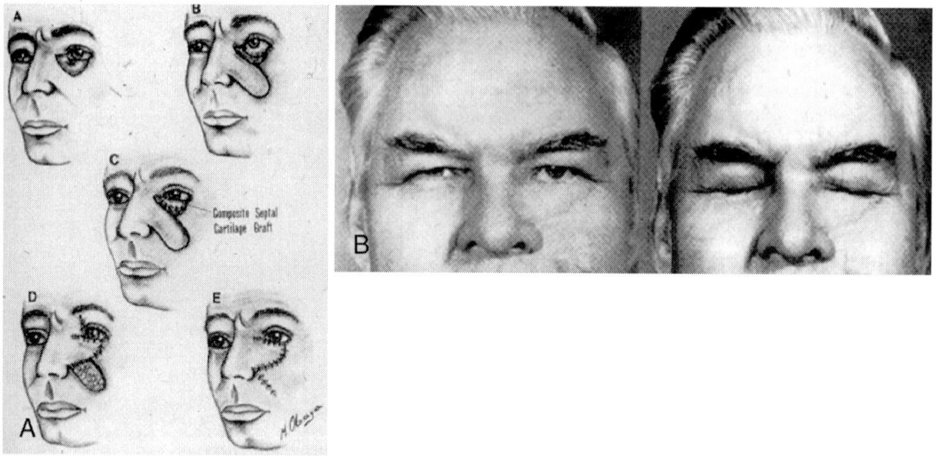

FIGURE 8–22. *A*, Demonstrates the surgical steps required to remove lesion with adequate margins. A medially based rotation nasolabial flap lined with a composite nasal septal graft (cartilage and mucosa) is used for reconstruction of the eyelid, including the conjunctiva and tarsal plate. Step D illustrates a Silastic tube left for 4 weeks as a stent in the reconstruction of the lacrimal drainage system (dacryorhinostomy). *B*, Six-month postoperative photographs of the patient shows the result of the left eyelid reconstruction. The patient was asymptomatic and declined a second-stage cosmetic improvement. (*A* and *B* from Maniglia AJ: Meibomian gland adenocarcinoma of the eyelid with neck metastasis. Laryngoscope 88: 1421–1426, 1978.)

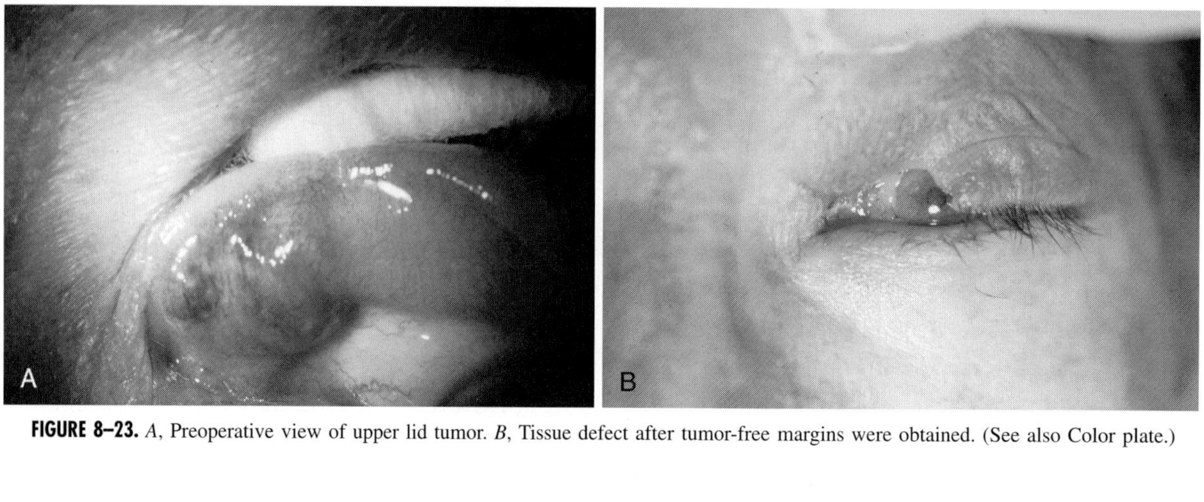

FIGURE 8–23. *A*, Preoperative view of upper lid tumor. *B*, Tissue defect after tumor-free margins were obtained. (See also Color plate.)

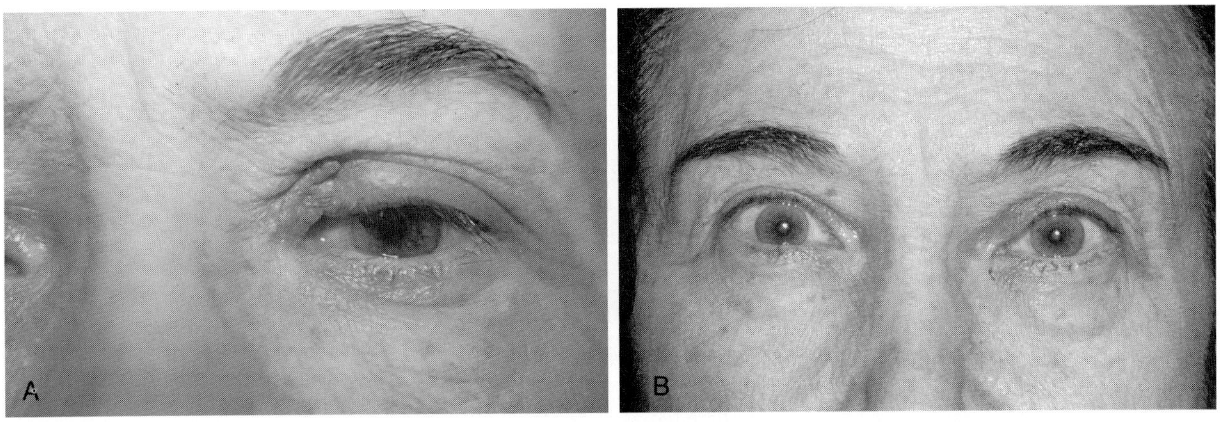

FIGURE 8–24. *A*, After reconstruction, which consisted of the following: Lid was everted, and tarsus was divided horizontally. Flap of tarsus and conjunctiva was mobilized inferomedially to the defect and sutured to the lid margin and the medial canthus. *B*, Reconstructed eyelid showing symmetrical extent of lashes, excellent function, and good contour. (See also Color plate.)

Complex Eyelid Reconstruction

In some situations of tumor extension or multiple skin tumors tumor ablation may extend to neighboring aesthetic units (Fig. 8–27). In these circumstances, each aesthetic unit should be repaired independently (Fig. 8–28).

Highly Malignant Eyelid Tumors

In patients with squamous cell carcinoma, tarsal gland adenocarcinomas, or melanomas, the decision-making process becomes more complicated. The issue of tumor extension must be carefully evaluated because of the need to resect the tumor with a larger margin. Orbital invasion with impairment of ocular motility or loss of vision may contraindicate eyelid reconstruction. Ophthalmological consultation is imperative. High-resolution computerized tomography (CT) is important to determine local extension, and magnetic resonance imaging (MRI) is used to determine soft tissue invasion and the need for orbital exenteration.

Enlargement of the preauricular or submandibular neck nodes indicates regional metastasis, and associated parotidectomy and modified or classic radical neck dissection may be necessary. In the presence of distant metastasis, combined treatment with postoperative radiotherapy is indicated.

On occasion the tumor may not be resectable except with the addition of skull base surgery. This should be performed in a select group of patients. It may very well improve the patient's quality of life, provide control of local disease, or even lead to cure. In the management of eyelid neoplasms, one should never compromise on the margin of resection to save tissue for reconstruction. Sound oncologic principles are imperative.

SUMMARY

Surgical resection with immediate repair if this is also possible remains the gold standard for the treatment of malignant neoplasms involving the upper and lower eyelids, especially in patients with larger lesions. A variety of surgical techniques are available, and selection is based on the type of defect present and the most suitable method of reconstruction. Smaller lesions may be managed by appro-

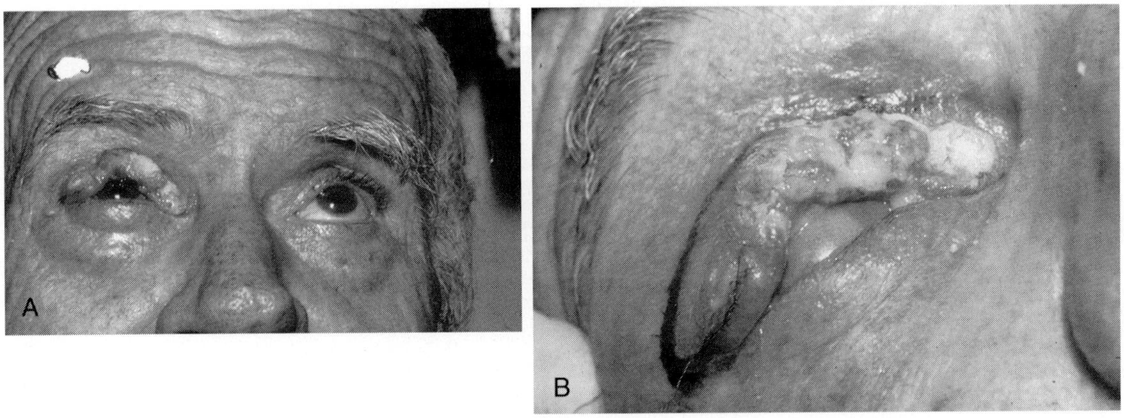

FIGURE 8–25. *A*, Patient with large upper lid basal cell carcinoma. *B*, Close-up of patient shown in *A*.

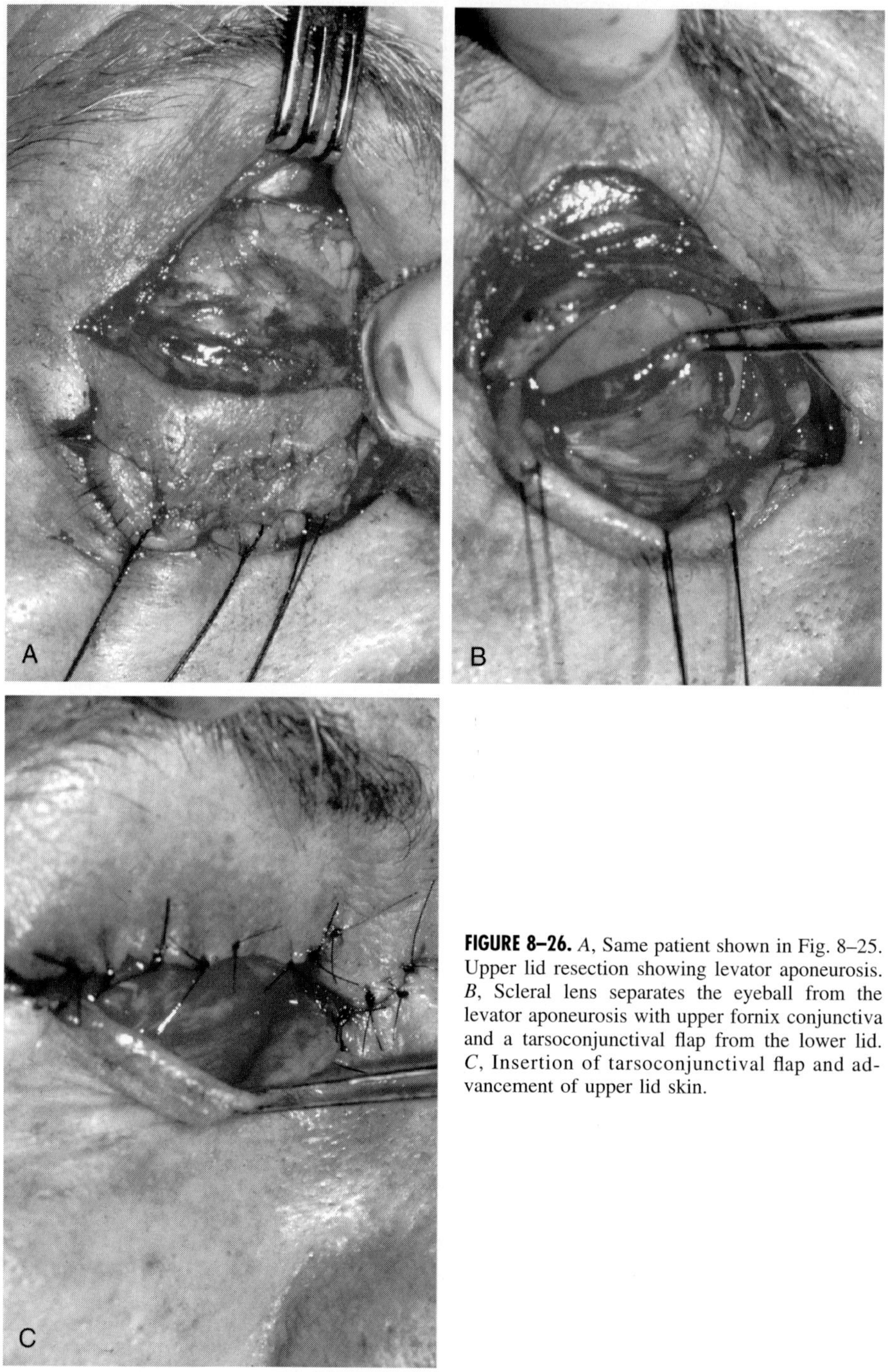

FIGURE 8–26. *A*, Same patient shown in Fig. 8–25. Upper lid resection showing levator aponeurosis. *B*, Scleral lens separates the eyeball from the levator aponeurosis with upper fornix conjunctiva and a tarsoconjunctival flap from the lower lid. *C*, Insertion of tarsoconjunctival flap and advancement of upper lid skin.

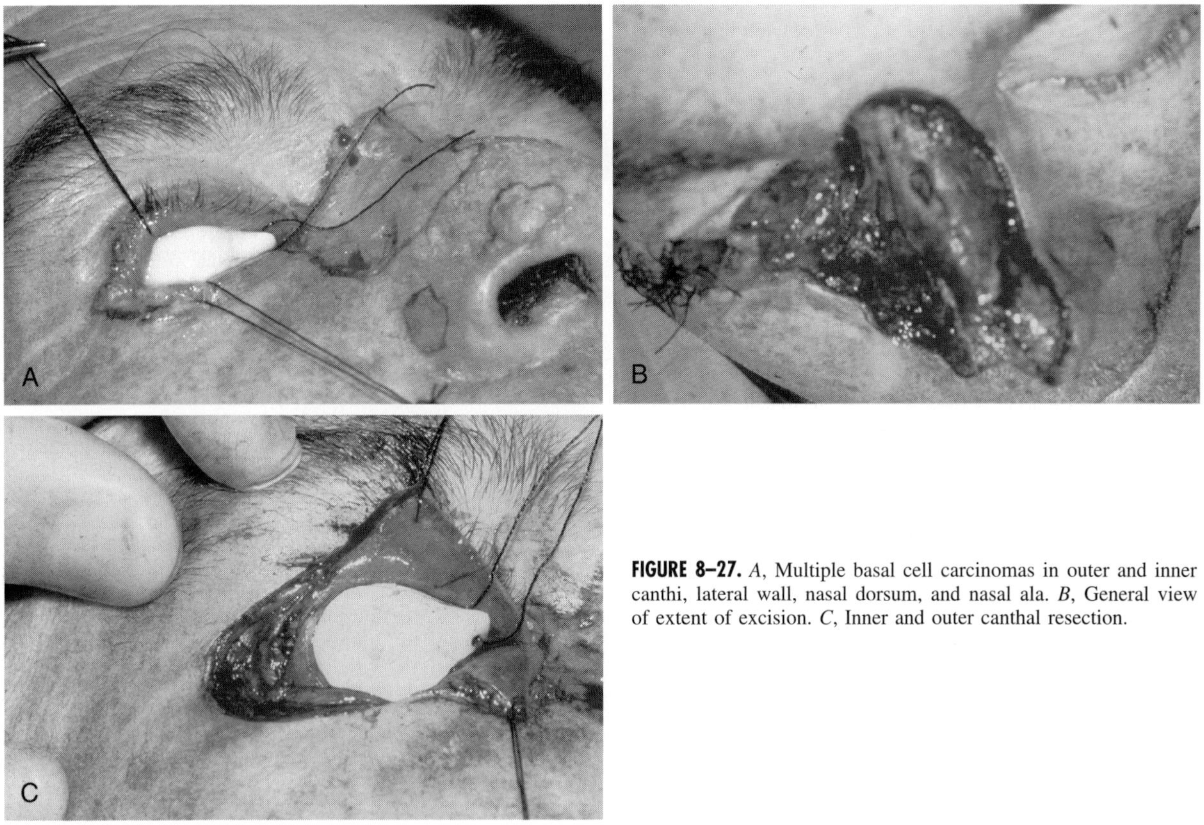

FIGURE 8–27. *A*, Multiple basal cell carcinomas in outer and inner canthi, lateral wall, nasal dorsum, and nasal ala. *B*, General view of extent of excision. *C*, Inner and outer canthal resection.

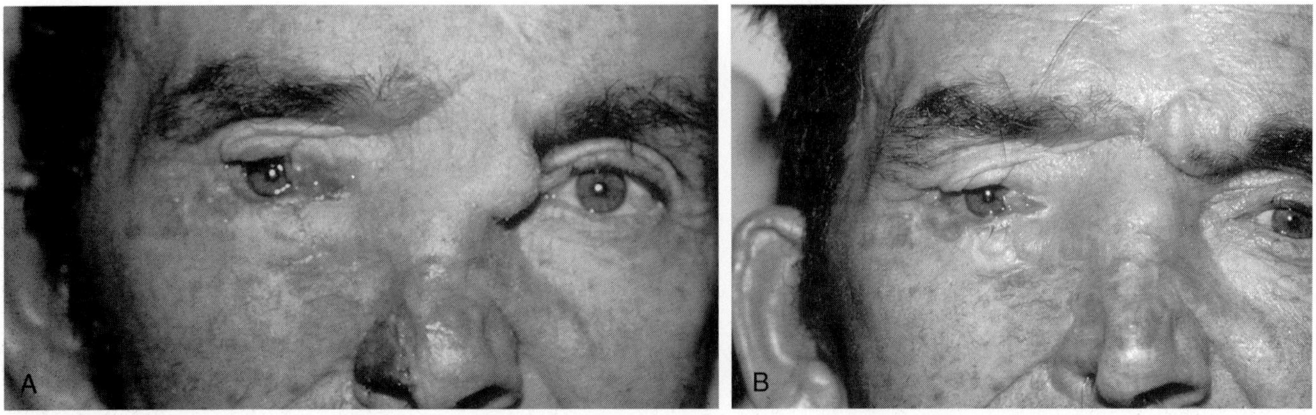

FIGURE 8–28. *A*, Postoperative view of patient shown in Fig. 8–27 with reconstruction of outer canthus (Byron Smith technique) and inner canthus and nose (bivalved forehead flap). *B*, Nasal dorsum is skin grafted (using a full-thickness postauricular graft), and nasal ala is reconstructed with an auricular composite graft.

priate radiation therapy provided that the eyeball is protected to avoid intraocular complications. Nevertheless, cataracts or blindness may occur when radiation is applied to the ocular area regardless of what technique is used. Alternative treatment should be discussed with the patient.

REFERENCES

1. Schlienger P, Brunin F, Des Jardins L, et al: External radiotherapy for carcinoma of eyelid: Report of 850 cases treated. Int J Radio Oncol Biol Phys 34(2): 277–287, 1996.
2. Kumar B, Roden D, Vinciullo C, et al: A review of 24 cases of Mohs surgery and ophthalmic plastic reconstruction. Aust NZ Ophthalmol 25(4): 289–293, 1997.
3. Monheit G, Callahan M, Callahan A: Mohs micrograft surgery for periorbital skin cancer. Dermatol Clin 7(4): 677–697, 1989.
4. Dogru M, Matsuo H, Inoue M, Okubo K: Management of sebaceous eyelid carcinoma. Ophthalmologica 211(1): 40–43, 1997.
5. Aliseda D, Vasquez J, Munuera JM, et al: Medial canthus tumor surgery: A prospective study of microscopically controlled excision. Eur J Ophthalmol 7(3): 216–222, 1997.
6. Tessier P: Eyelid reconstruction or blepharopoiesis. *In* Plastic Surgery of the Orbit and Eyelids. Masson, Paris, 1981, pp. 335–355.
7. Putterman AM: Viable composite grafting in eyelid reconstruction. Am J Ophthalmol 85: 237–241, 1978.
8. Tenzel RR: Eyelid reconstruction by the semicircle flaps technique. Ophthalmol A A O O 85: 1164–1169, 1978.
9. Perry MJ, Langtry J, Martin JC: Lower lid reconstruction using pedicled skin flap and palatal muco-periosteum. Dermatol Surg 23(5): 395–397, 1997.
10. Kollner: Verfahren für den plastischen Ersats des Unterlides. Munchen Med Wchnescher 58: 2166, 1911.
11. Mustardé JC: Repair and Reconstruction in the Orbital Region, 2nd ed. New York, Churchill Livingstone, 1980.
12. Hughes WL: A new method of rebuilding a lower lid: Report of a case. Arch Ophthalmol 17: 1008–1017, 1937.
13. McNab AA: Early division of conjunctival pedicle flap in modified Hughes repair of the lower eyelid. Ophthal Surg Lasers 27(6): 422–424, 1996.
14. Glatt HJ: Tarsoconjunctival flap supplementation; an approach to the reconstruction of large lower lid defects. Ophthal Plast Reconstr Surg 13(2): 90–97, 1997.
15. Smith B: A technique for extirpation and replacement of lateral canthus. *In* Ophthalmic Plastic and Reconstructive Surgery. C.V. Mosby Co., 1987, p. 794. St. Louis.
16. Cutler NL, Beard C: A method for partial and total upper lid reconstruction. Am J Ophthalmol 39: 1–7, 1955.
17. Maniglia AJ: Meibomian gland adenocarcinoma of the eyelid with neck metastasis. Laryngoscope 88 (9 p. 1): 1421–1426, 1978.
18. Maniglia AJ, Megerian CA: The medially based myocutaneous upper eyelid flap for lateral nasal defect reconstruction. Am J Otolaryngol 17(2): 118–121, 1996.
19. Ni C, Searl SS, Kou PK, et al: Sebaceous cell carcinomas of ocular adnexa. Int Ophthalmol Clin 22: 23, 1982.
20. Hewes EH, Sullivan J, Beard C: Lower eyelid reconstruction by tarsal transposition. Am J Ophthalmol 81: 512, 1976.
21. Kersten RC, Anderson RL, Tse DT: Tarsal rotation flap for upper eyelid reconstruction. Arch Ophthalmol 104: 918, 1986.
22. Leone CR Jr, Van Gemert JV: Lower eyelid reconstruction with upper eyelid transpositional grafts. Ophthalmic Surg 11: 315, 1980.
23. Tenzel RR: Reconstruction of the central one half of an eyelid. Arch Ophthalmol 93: 125, 1975.
24. Tenzel RR, Boynton JR, Buffam FV: Technique of combined lid and medial canthal reconstruction. Ophthalmic Surg 7: 25, 1976.
25. Wesley RE, McCord CD: Transplantation of eyebank sclera in the Cutler-Beard method of upper eyelid reconstruction. Ophthalmology 87: 1022, 1980.

CHAPTER 9

Cranial Bone for Midface and Skull Reconstruction

James E. Zins, M.D.
Kimlyn Long, M.D.
Frank A. Papay, M.D.

Major advances in reconstruction of the midface, orbits, and skull were initiated by Paul Tessier over 25 years ago,[1–3] and with these advances the field of craniofacial surgery was born. Tessier made two important observations:

1. Surgeons can operate on craniofacial malformations more safely using a combined intracranial-extracranial approach than an extracranial route alone.
2. The orbit can be completely osteotomized, separated from its blood supply, and moved in any one of three dimensions without any long-term loss of bone volume. Further, these orbital osteotomies and advancements create large bone gaps that need large volumes of bone to fill. A reliable bone graft that can be harvested in large quantities with little morbidity is needed.

During the next 20 years numerous papers investigating the physiology of cranial bone grafting, methods of cranial bone harvest, and the morbidity associated with bone graft harvest were published. Major issues such as the enhanced volume maintenance of membranous bone compared to endochondral bone as a bone graft,[4–6] the importance of rigid fixation to the maintenance of volume in bone grafts,[7–9] and the importance of primary bone grafting in trauma cases, tumor resection, and pediatric craniofacial surgery were hotly debated. These issues have been clarified in recent years, and the use of cranial bone grafting has become increasingly popular in plastic surgery, otolaryngology, neurosurgery, and other surgical specialties.

MEMBRANOUS VERSUS ENDOCHONDRAL BONE: EXPERIMENTAL STUDIES

It is clear that cranial bone and other membranous bone grafts show superior volume maintenance compared to traditional grafts from the iliac crest and rib. This has been demonstrated many times in different animal models and in both mature and immature animals.[4–6] However, the reason for this enhanced volume maintenance is not clear. As suggested by Zins and Whitaker,[4] the superior volume maintenance seen with cranial bone grafting is due either to (1) delayed revascularization and hence delayed resorption, or (2) enhanced vascularization and hence enhanced bone survival and volume maintenance.

Although most surgeons agree that revascularization was integrally related to graft incorporation and volume maintenance, the early revascularization studies were inconsistent. Kusiak and colleagues[10] demonstrated enhanced revascularization in cranial grafts in a rabbit model. Sullivan and Szwajkun[11] demonstrated the opposite in a rat model, and Phillips and Rahn[7] found no correlation. Further, none of these studies correlated long-term vascularization with long-term volume maintenance.

The effect of rigid fixation on bone graft survival was studied by Phillips and Rahn.[8] They demonstrated that fixed membranous grafts maintained 10% greater volume than nonfixed membranous grafts, and fixed endochondral grafts maintained 75% of their volume compared to only 17% for nonfixed endochondral grafts. Vascularization studies by Phillips and Rahn[7] showed enhanced vascularization for fixed membranous grafts at 2 weeks compared with nonfixed grafts, whereas endochondral bone grafts demonstrated just the opposite. They concluded that other factors besides vascularization determined volume maintenance. La Trenta and associates[9] demonstrated in a dog model that rigid fixation led to enhanced volume maintenance in both membranous and endochondral grafts. They concluded that rigid fixation led to enhanced revascularization and hence improved volume maintenance.

Chen and colleagues,[12] in an elegant study, did much to clarify these issues. Whereas the previously mentioned studies concluded that rigid fixation of membranous grafts led to more rapid revascularization and enhanced volume maintenance, the results of the Chen study demand rethinking of this issue. They studied revascularization by microfill injections and osteoclastic activity by tartrate-resistant acid phosphatase (TRAP) staining and, for the first time, correlated these short-term studies with long-term volumetric analysis. In addition, they calculated vascularization indices for cancellous and cortical components of each graft and correlated these indices with an analysis of resorptive activity for each component and with long-term volume maintenance. They found that (1) revascularization rates were similar for the cancellous and cortical components of each graft, and (2) the TRAP activity, a measure of osteoclastic activity, was similar for each component regardless of graft origin. However, if the cancellous and cortical components were combined, the overall rates of revascularization were not statistically different for membranous and endochondral bone. This finding may partially explain the differences seen in the revascularization studies previously mentioned.

From the Chen study it can be concluded that early vascularization leads to graft resorption. Early vascularization and graft resorption occur predominantly in the cancellous portion of the graft, and since the iliac crest graft has a greater percentage of cancellous bone, its long-term volume maintenance is less. Further, as suggested by Glowacki,[13] the terms membranous and endochondral should be de-emphasized, and bone grafts should be referred to by their anatomic location, not their embryonic origin. Finally, the term bone graft survival should be replaced by the term volume maintenance or persistence because it is clear that less than 5% of the osteoblasts from autogenous bone grafts survive transplantation.

CLINICAL ADVANCES

As Tessier and others pushed the clinical envelope with conceptual advances in pediatric craniofacial surgery, technical improvements followed, leading to improved surgical results. This is particularly true for the technical advances of rigid fixation and primary bone grafting techniques.

The Importance of Primary Reconstruction

Primary reconstruction not only saves the patient a second operation, but, more important, it prevents soft tissue contraction. Once soft tissue contraction has occurred, it is extremely difficult to reverse, and secondary reconstruction becomes significantly more difficult, as exemplified by the patient shown in Figures 9–1 and 9–2. This patient was first seen 2 years after he sustained a comminuted LeFort III fracture, which was treated elsewhere. He presented with traumatic telecanthus, orbital dystopia, a saddle nose deformity, and a class III malocclusion. Figure 9–2 shows the same patient after two operations in which an attempt was made to restore the soft tissue and bony skeleton. The patient underwent bilateral medial canthoplasties, bone graft to the floor of the orbit and nasal bone, enophthalmos correction, and scar revisions. The unimpressive surgical result shown

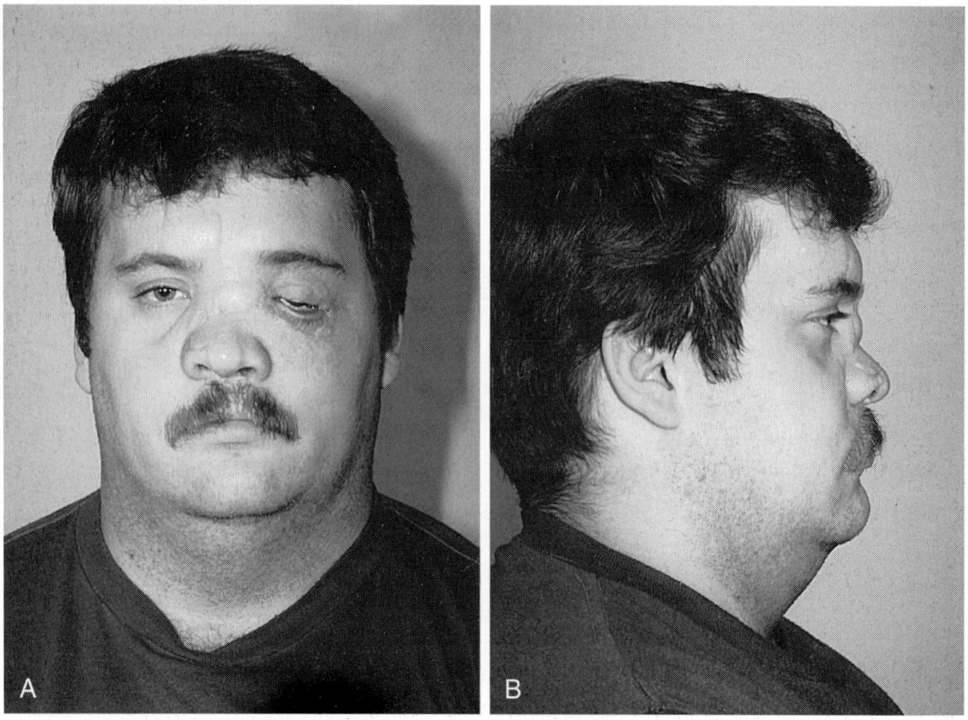

FIGURE 9–1. Two years after repair of a comminuted LeFort III fracture treated at another institution. Note traumatic telecanthus, orbital dystopia, and saddle nose deformity. *A*, Anterior view; *B*, lateral view.

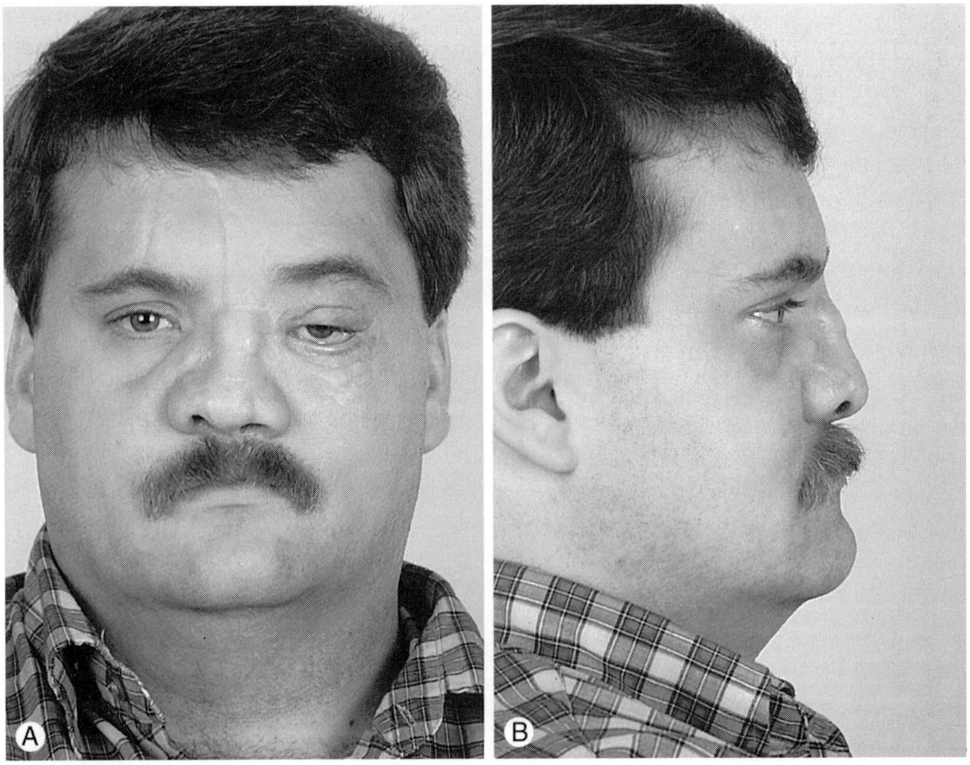

FIGURE 9–2. Same patient as in Figure 9–1 following two further procedures by the author in an attempt to correct the soft tissue deformity and bony skeleton. *A*, Anterior view; *B*, lateral view.

in Figure 9–2 is due, not to lack of surgical expertise, but rather to the difficulty of correcting soft tissue contraction once it has occurred.

In contrast, Figures 9–3 and 9–4 represent preoperative and postoperative photographs of a similar injury (a comminuted LeFort III fracture, traumatic telecanthus, and a complex orbital fracture) treated by the author with open reduction, internal fixation, rigid fixation, and primary bone grafting. Meticulous reconstruction of the bony framework using rigid fixation techniques, primary bone grafting, and careful repair of the soft tissues including reattachment of the detached medial and lateral canthi produced an optimum surgical result. In this case, rigid fixation enhanced the three-dimensional stability of the bony framework reconstruction.

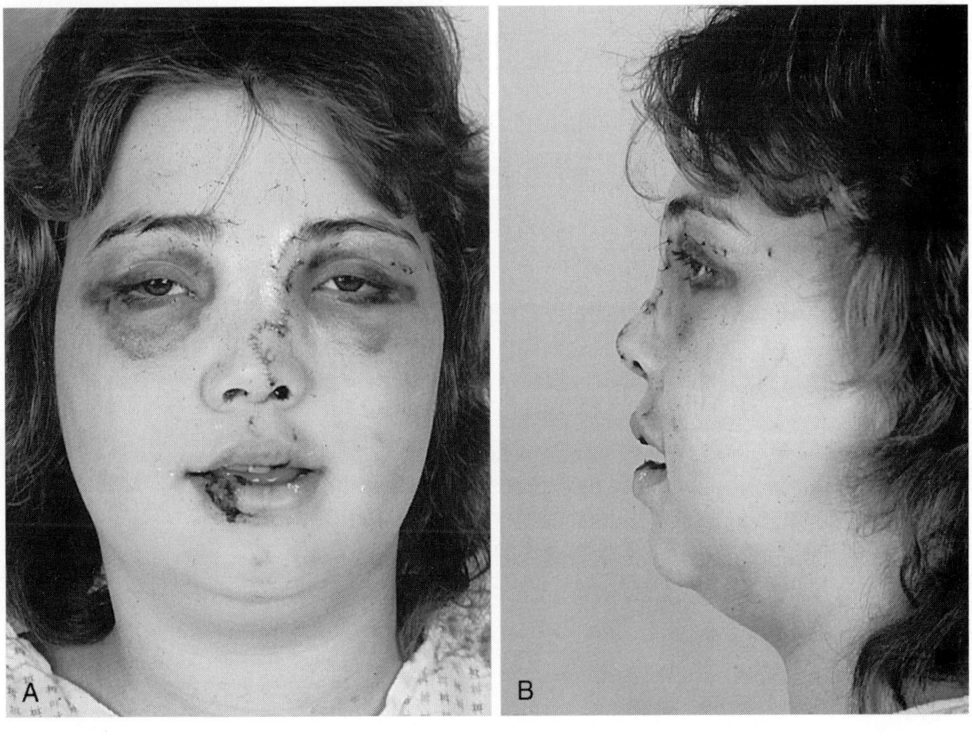

FIGURE 9–3. Preoperative view of patient with a comminuted LeFort III fracture and complex orbital fracture. *A*, Anterior view; *B*, lateral view.

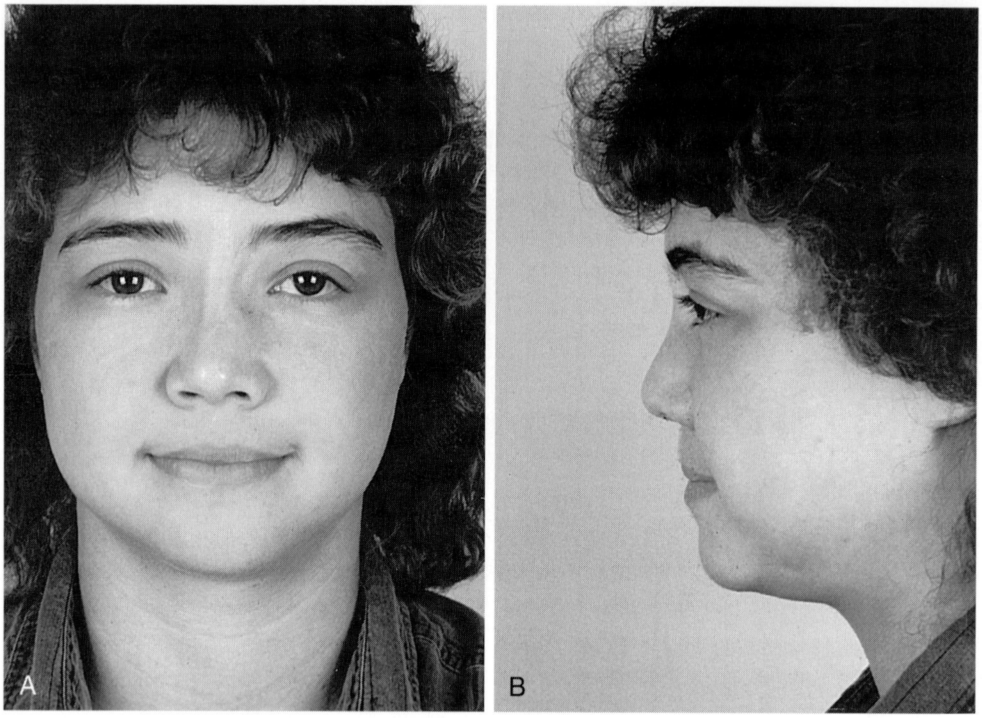

FIGURE 9–4. Postoperative view of same patient as in Figure 9–3 following acute repair of LeFort III fracture with rigid fixation techniques, primary bone grafting, and meticulous soft tissue repair. *A*, Anterior view; *B*, lateral view.

It also significantly reduced the period required for intermaxillary fixation. Finally, rigid fixation made it possible to span the bony gaps and fix the bone grafts to the plates, thus more readily repairing the facial skeleton.

Primary reconstruction of the midface and upper face was first popularized in patients with facial trauma and led to significant improvement in surgical results. These techniques were then naturally extended to primary reconstruction of the upper face, midface, and lower face following tumor resection. Figures 9–5 and 9–6 show the preoperative and postoperative appearance of a patient with proptosis and orbital dystopia with inferior displacement of the globe secondary to a meningioma of the greater wing of the sphenoid. This situation required a combined intracranial and extracranial resection of the meningioma with primary bone grafting of the floor of the orbit and sphenoid wing using cranial bone grafts. As mentioned previously, cranial bone grafting at the time of tumor ablation is straightforward and avoids problems associated with secondary reconstruction such as soft tissue contraction.

Rigid Fixation

Although rigid fixation in the maxillomandibular region is a very unforgiving technique, in the upper face and skull it is less demanding. In the maxillomandibular complex, one must first establish intermaxillary fixation before attempting to apply any fixation in this area. Once intermaxillary fixation has been established, rigid fixation can then proceed. Finally after rigid fixation has been applied, the intermaxillary fixation must be removed in the operating room before the operation is completed. Small discrepancies in the application of the rigid fixation plates will be manifested by occlusal abnormalities.

Rigid fixation in the upper face and skull does not require the absolute precision necessary in the midface and lower

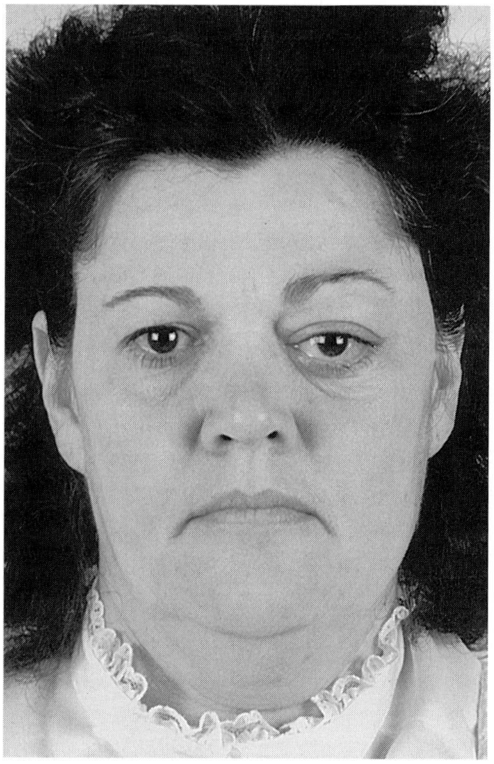

FIGURE 9–5. Preoperative view of a patient with proptosis and orbital dystopia with inferior displacement of the left globe secondary to a meningioma of the greater wing of the sphenoid.

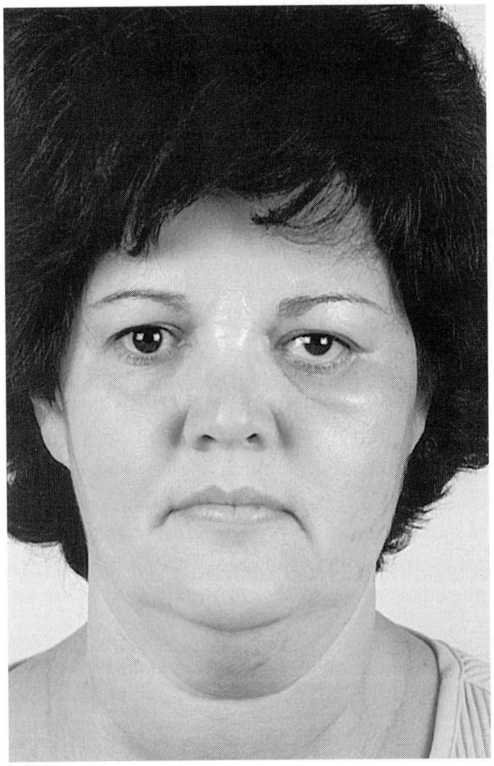

FIGURE 9–6. Same patient as in Figure 9–5 following combined intracranial-extracranial approach for resection and primary reconstruction of the orbit and sphenoid wing using cranial bone grafts to the orbital floor, the lateral orbit, and the anterior cranial base.

face when the occlusion is a concern. Relative rigid fixation will lead to three-dimensional stability, rapid healing, and minimal swelling in the upper face and skull. Masticatory forces require stronger plates in the lower face. In the mid-face, where there are no muscle attachments to bone, mini-plate fixation is adequate. In the orbital and skull regions, microfixation plates are all that is necessary.

Drawbacks of Rigid Fixation. Although the greatest benefit of rigid fixation is the three-dimensional stability it provides, it has several distinct drawbacks. First, rigid fixation can be overutilized, significantly increasing the cost of a given operation. Second, fixation plates may become palpable, especially under the thin skin of the orbital and forehead region. Therefore, it is suggested that the smallest and fewest plates that obtain relatively rigid fixation and accomplish the job be used.

Other theoretical concerns about rigid fixation relate to infant and pediatric surgery. These include (1) the possible adverse effect of rigid fixation on facial growth, and (2) the possibility of "pseudomigration" of fixation plates. Yaremchuk[14] addressed the question of the adverse effect of rigid fixation on facial growth in an experimental monkey model. His data demonstrated that the larger the plate and the more aggressive the dissection, the greater the adverse effect on facial growth. Manson[15] summarized this issue succinctly in a review of this subject, stating that although rigid fixation may have an adverse effect on facial growth in craniofacial surgery in children, this effect is small and is significantly outweighed by the benefit afforded by rigid fixation.

Technique of Cranial Bone Harvesting

Cranial bone may be harvested by either an in-situ or full-thickness technique. Our choice of technique is determined by the size of the cranial bone graft required.[16] When relatively small pieces of bone are required, the in-situ technique is used. Small pieces are arbitrarily limited to grafts in which the smaller dimension of length or width is 3 cm or less.

In-Situ Harvest Technique. This technique is described as follows: The area of the donor site is chosen in the hair-bearing region of the parietal bone, and the skull is exposed. Then, using a bone pencil,[17] an outline of the desired dimensions of the bone graft to be harvested is drawn on the skull. Important landmarks include the sagittal suture and underlying sagittal sinus and the other cranial sutures. In-situ cranial bone is never harvested closer than 2 cm lateral to the sagittal sinus to avoid not only injury to the sinus but also profuse bleeding, which may result from the subarachnoid granulations that are characteristically located in the vicinity of the sagittal sinus. Next, a contouring bur is used to outline the cranial bone graft that is to be harvested and to establish the depth of the outer table cranial bone harvest (Fig. 9–7). The contouring bur is taken down through the outer table into the diploe, exposing the inner table. Our preference at this point is to use a sagittal saw held parallel to the outer table of the skull to enter the diploe separating the outer table from the inner table. If the saw is held parallel to the outer table and the edge of the saw blade is always kept in view by moving the blade from one edge of the cranial bone graft toward the middle (Fig. 9–8), the inner table will not be violated. We find that the sagittal saw used in this way results in very regular pieces of cranial bone with a minimal incidence of inner table violation. Others prefer to use an osteotome to separate the outer table from the inner table at this juncture.

As previously mentioned, the in-situ cranial bone harvest technique is used for small grafts that are arbitrarily limited in size. If the shorter dimension (length or width) of a rectangular piece of bone is limited to 3 cm, it is relatively easy to maintain the sagittal saw blade parallel to the outer table and within the diploe, thus avoiding entrance into the inner table and possible dural tears. If in-situ techniques are used to harvest larger pieces of bone, it is necessary to saw from both edges of the cranial bone to be harvested. This can lead to different levels of entry into the diploe from these different directions and thus to a greater likelihood of violating the inner table. Therefore, when larger pieces of cranial bone are required, the full-thickness cranial bone harvest technique is used.

Full-Thickness Harvest Technique. This technique is accomplished with the aid of a neurosurgeon. Again, the skull is exposed in a hair-bearing area, and the sagittal sinus and other sutures are noted. Care is taken to stay 2 cm lateral to the sagittal sinus and to avoid the other sutures

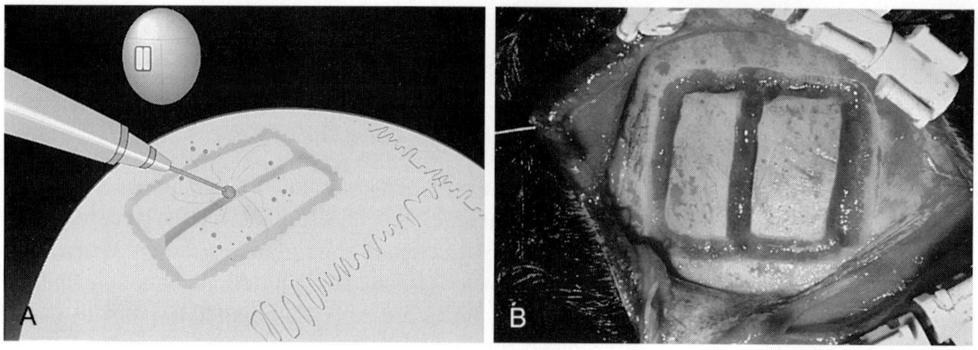

FIGURE 9–7. A contouring bur is used to outline the dimensions of the in-situ split skull graft and bur through the outer table into the diploe, exposing the inner table of the skull. *A*, Schematic drawing. *B*, Graft outlined, diploe exposed. (*A* and *B* from Zins JE, Weinzweig N, Hahn J: A simple fail-safe method for the harvesting of cranial bone. Plast Reconstr Surg 96(6):1444–1447, 1995.)

as well because the dura tends to adhere in the area of the sutures.

The reconstructive surgeon marks out the cranial bone to be harvested using a bone pencil, and then a full-thickness craniectomy is performed by the neurosurgeon. At a separate table the full-thickness piece of cranial bone is then split down the diploe using the sagittal saw, again obtaining a very regular piece of cranial bone for grafting purposes (Fig. 9–9). The outer table is then replaced at the donor site and wired or sutured back in place flush with the rest of the skull to avoid skull depressions and irregularities. The piece taken from the inner table can then be used for the cranial bone reconstruction.

Morbidity of Cranial Bone Graft Harvest. The morbidity of cranial bone graft harvest should be minimal in practiced hands. The largest study reviewing this issue was published by Kline and Wolfe[18]; it consisted of a personal series of 1000 consecutive bone graft harvests using cranial, iliac, costal, tibial, and mandibular bone grafts. No neurologic complications were associated with any of the 586 cranial bone grafts taken in this series. In addition, the authors surveyed members of the International Society for Craniofacial Surgeons about the complications they encountered from bone graft harvest. The survey respondents reported performance of 12,672 cranial bone graft harvests. Temporary neurologic complications were associated with graft harvest in three cases (0.02%). The respondents also identified neurologic complications associated with cranial bone graft harvests performed by other surgeons. In five of these eight cases of neurologic injury, the bone graft harvest was performed by surgeons who had little or no experience in the harvesting of cranial bone. Their conclusion was that cranial bone harvest in proper hands is a very safe procedure. To underscore this point, we cite a report by Cannella and Hopkins.[19] Although they document superior sagittal sinus laceration following attempted cranial bone harvest, we seriously question the reason for harvesting bone from this vicinity.

When cranial bone harvest is compared to harvest of rib and iliac crest bone, the complication rate for cranial bone harvest is found to be quite low. Marx and Morales[20] reported nearly a 20% incidence of wound complications following bone harvest from the anterior iliac crest and significant gait abnormality for several months following iliac crest harvest. Others have corroborated the low incidence of complications with cranial bone harvest. Jackson and colleagues[21] reported 265 cranial bone grafts with no neurologic disturbance, Posnick and colleagues[22] reported 26 in-situ cranial bone graft

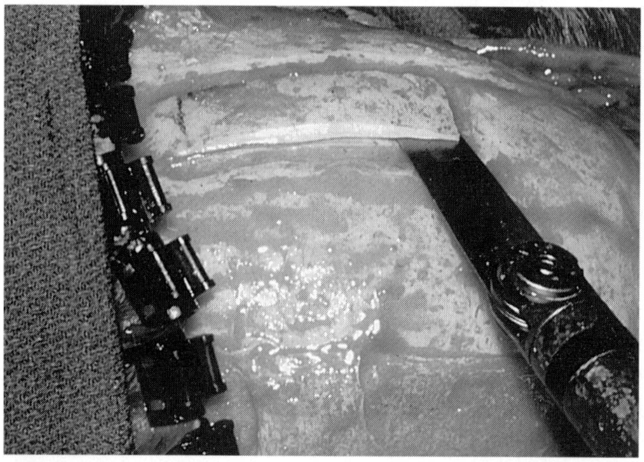

FIGURE 9–8. The sagittal saw is used to separate the outer table from the inner table after contouring has been completed. The sagittal saw blade is kept in view by working the blade from the edge of the graft to the center, thus ensuring the depth of cranial bone harvested. (From Zins JE, Weinzweig N, Hahn J: A simple fail-safe method for the harvesting of cranial bone. Plast Reconstr Surg 96(6):1444–1447, 1995.)

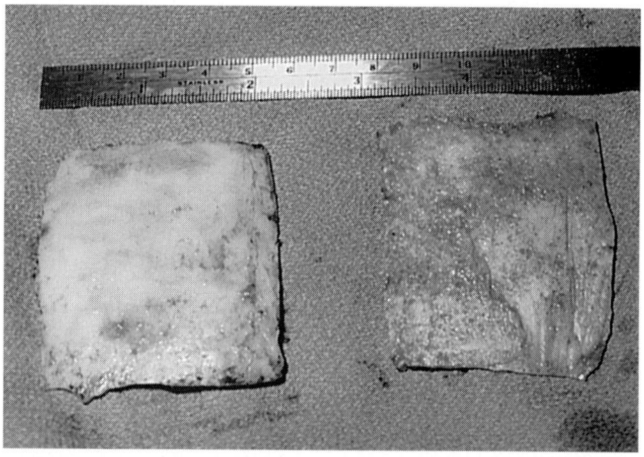

FIGURE 9–9. For large grafts, a formal craniectomy is performed. The full-thickness bone is then split down the diploe. The result is two uniform pieces of bone. One is replaced in the donor site and the second is used for bone grafting. (From Zins JE, Weinzweig N, Hahn J: A simple fail-safe method for the harvesting of cranial bone. Plast Reconstr Surg 96(6):1444–1447, 1995.)

harvests with no morbidity, and Ilankovan and Jackson[23] reported a 4.6% minor complication rate in 279 cranial bone grafts taken for orbital reconstruction.

A potential deleterious effect on the cranial bone graft donor site was suggested by Wilkinson.[24] Our group reported a biomechanical effect of cranial bone harvest on the donor site in a cadaver model.[25] In this study, the entire hemicalvarium was harvested from 16 fresh cadavers. An in-situ defect measuring 4 × 3 cm was then created. A blow to the skull either directly over the harvest site or to the opposite side of the intact skull was simulated using a material testing system cylinder. The force was increased until skull fracture occurred. There was significant variability in skull thickness and hence breaking strength of individual skulls. There was no statistically significant difference in breaking strength of skulls with in-situ defects compared to cadaver skull controls whether the blow occurred directly over the defect or on the opposite side. The greatest variable remained the thickness of the native skull.

Secondary Reconstruction

Although primary reconstruction using cranial bone is favored whenever possible, the need for secondary reconstruction is a frequent occurrence. Cranial bone in these instances is used as either an onlay bone graft, an interposition bone graft, or an en bloc bony movement. Examples of each are described.

Figure 9–10 shows a middle-aged man following an orbital fracture that required enucleation of the left globe followed by prosthetic reconstruction. Preoperatively he had enophthalmos and orbital dystopia of the left prosthetic globe. Figure 9–11 shows 1-year follow-up following orbital reconstruction using an in-situ 2- × 2-cm double stack of

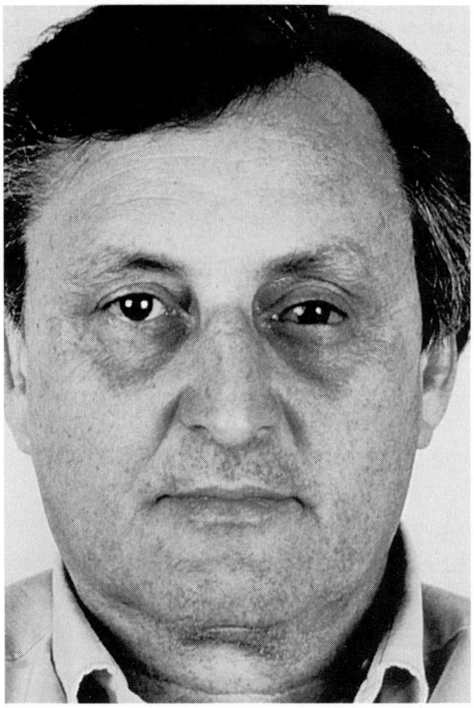

FIGURE 9–11. Same patient as in Figure 9–10 one year following orbital reconstruction using a 2 × 2-cm double stack of in-situ cranial bone onlay graft to the orbital floor, which filled the floor defect and elevated the prosthetic globe.

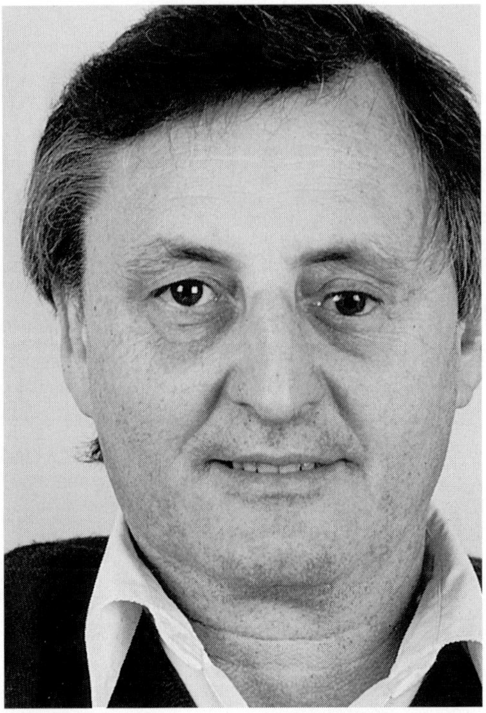

FIGURE 9–10. Preoperative view of a middle-aged man suffering from a previous orbital floor fracture that required enucleation of the left globe followed by prosthetic globe replacement. Note enophthalmos and orbital dystopia of the left prosthetic globe.

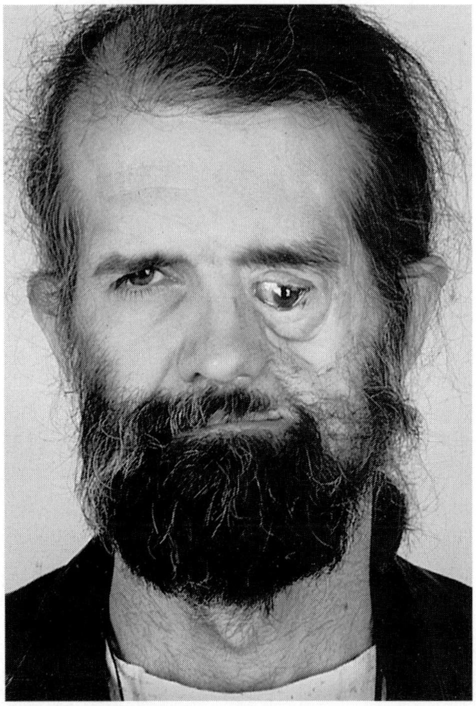

FIGURE 9–12. Preoperative view of a 35-year-old man with a congenital Tessier No. 3 facial cleft who had undergone 20 previous procedures.

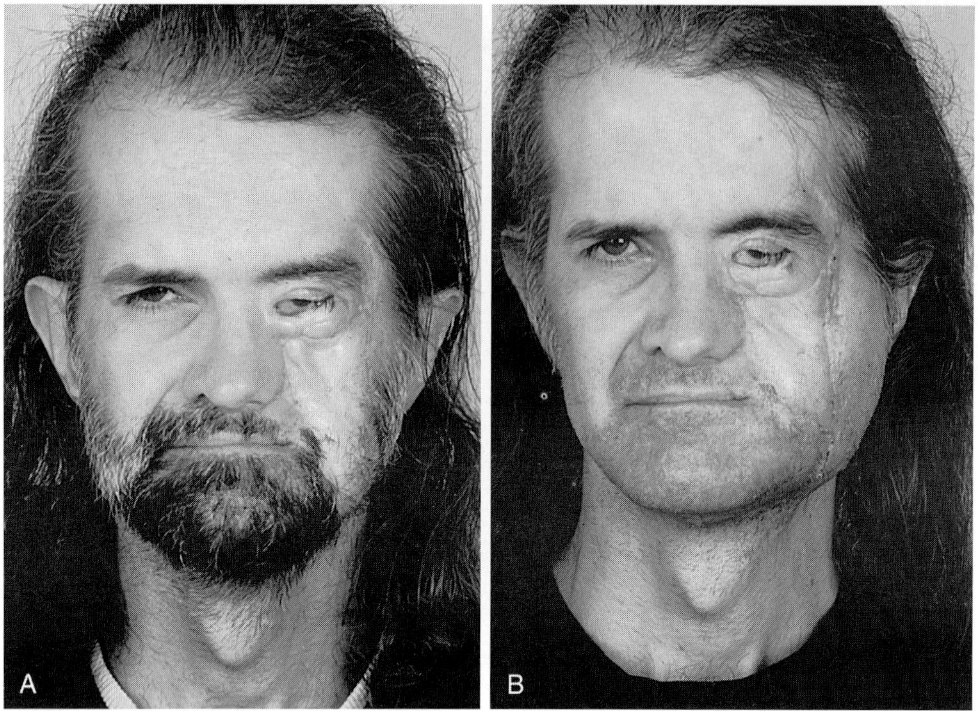

FIGURE 9–13. *A*, Same individual as in Figure 9–12 one year following a left orbital osteotomy using a combined intracranial-extracranial approach, with superior repositioning of the orbit by 8 mm and soft tissue revision. The frontal sinus was entered at the time of frontal craniectomy and obliterated. *B*, Patient is now undergoing multiple additional soft tissue procedures.

onlay cranial bone to the orbital floor to fill in the floor defect and elevate the prosthetic globe.

Figure 9–12 shows a 35-year-old man who had previously undergone multiple operations for correction of a congenital Tessier No. 3 facial cleft. His appearance is shown in Figure 9–13*A* 1 year after left orbital osteotomy using a combined intracranial-extracranial approach in which all four walls of the orbit underwent osteotomy and the orbit was moved superiorly by 8 mm. The resultant inferior bony defect was filled with a cranial bone graft, and the frontal sinus, which was entered at the time of the frontal craniectomy, was obliterated. Six months later (Fig. 9–13*B*) the patient was in the process of undergoing multiple adjunctive soft tissue procedures including tissue expansion and advancement, skin grafting, and lateral canthoplasty.

Figure 9–14 shows the preoperative view of a 40-year-old

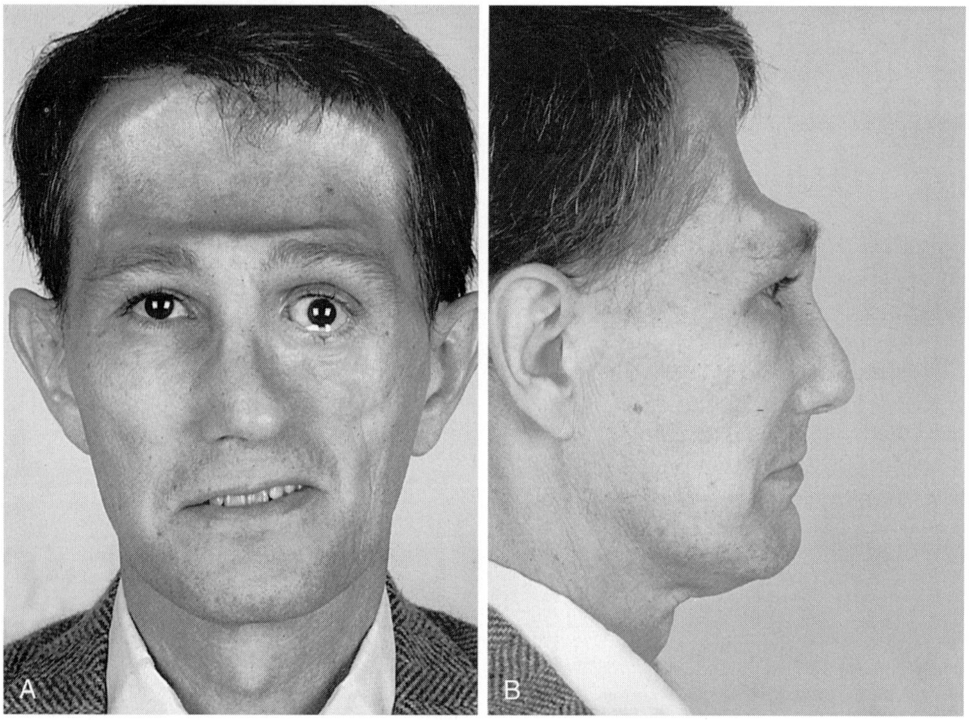

FIGURE 9–14. Middle-aged man who had previously undergone craniofacial resection for an ethmoid sinus tumor followed by radiation and removal of his infected bifrontal craniectomy bone flap. *A*, Anterior view; *B*, lateral view.

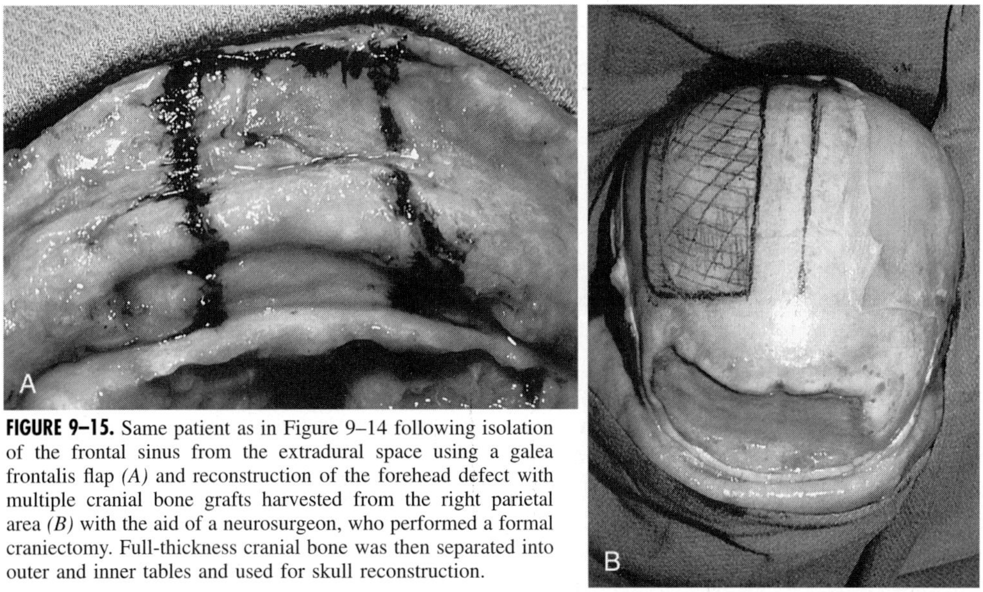

FIGURE 9–15. Same patient as in Figure 9–14 following isolation of the frontal sinus from the extradural space using a galea frontalis flap *(A)* and reconstruction of the forehead defect with multiple cranial bone grafts harvested from the right parietal area *(B)* with the aid of a neurosurgeon, who performed a formal craniectomy. Full-thickness cranial bone was then separated into outer and inner tables and used for skull reconstruction.

man who had previously undergone craniofacial resection for an ethmoid sinus tumor followed by radiation and infection of the bifrontal craniectomy bone flap, which was then removed. Reconstruction included obliteration of the frontal sinus with a galea frontalis flap (Fig. 9–15) and reconstruction of the forehead defect with multiple cranial bone grafts harvested from the right parietal area with the aid of the neurosurgeon, who performed a formal craniectomy. Figure 9–16 demonstrates the postoperative result at 1 year.

Extradural dead space in the forehead reconstruction is not acceptable. Bone graft is applied to dura and skin to bone. Extradural dead space leads to infected seromas and ultimate loss of the forehead reconstruction. Fifty-six such high-risk cranioplasties have been performed by our unit during the past 10 years with no cranial bone graft lost to infection.[26] High-risk cranioplasty patients are those who have had previous cranial bone flap infection, paranasal sinus in continuity with the extradural space, or abnormal soft-tissue forehead cover, secondary to radiation.

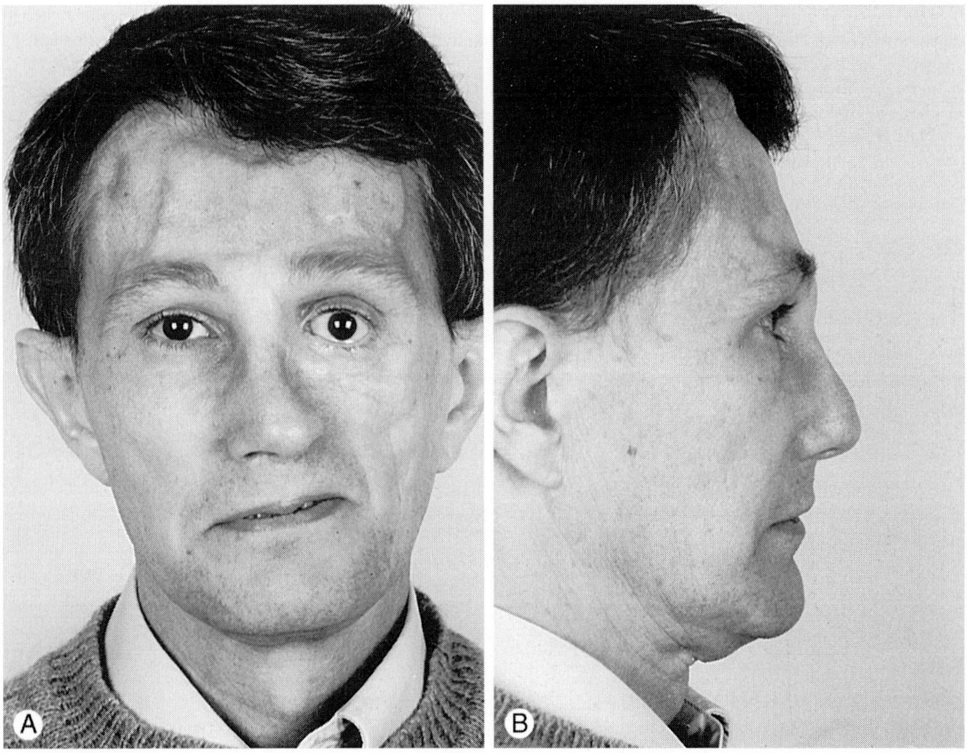

FIGURE 9–16. Postoperative views of this patient. *A*, Anterior view; *B*, lateral view.

SUMMARY

Cranial bone grafting has resulted in significant improvements in surgical outcome in both primary and secondary reconstruction. Primary reconstruction is preferred in patients with trauma and tumor resection because prevention of soft tissue contraction simplifies the surgical correction. However, cranial bone grafting in patients requiring secondary reconstruction is of great assistance, as demonstrated in the foregoing cases. Cranial bone grafts can be safely harvested with minimal morbidity in practiced hands. The technique of cranial bone harvest is described for in-situ and full-thickness cranial bone grafts. It is strongly advised that prior to attempting the harvest of cranial bone, the surgeon become fully familiar with the technique by assisting a surgeon who is well versed in the technique of cranial bone reconstruction.

REFERENCES

1. Tessier P: Relationship of craniostenoses to craniofacial dysostoses, and to faciostenoses. Plast Reconstr Surg 48:224, 1971.
2. Tessier P: The definitive plastic surgical treatment of the severe facial deformities of craniofacial dysostosis: Crouzon's and Apert's diseases. Plast Reconstr Surg 48:419, 1971.
3. Tessier P: Osteotomies totales de la face syndrome de Crouzon, syndrome d'Apert, oxycephalies, scaphocephalies, turricephalies. Ann Chir Plast 12:273, 1967.
4. Zins JE, Whitaker LA: Membranous versus endochondral bone: Implications for craniofacial reconstruction. Plast Reconstr Surg 72(6):778, 1983.
5. Smith ID, Abramson M: Membranous versus endochondral bone autografts. Arch Otolaryngol 99:203, 1974.
6. Hardesty RA, Marsh JL: Craniofacial onlay bone grafting: A prospective evaluation of graft morphology, orientation, and embryonic origin. Plast Reconstr Surg 85:5, 1990.
7. Phillips JH, Rahn BA: Fixation effects on membranous and endochondral onlay bone graft revascularization and bone deposition. Plast Reconstr Surg 85(6):891, 1990.
8. Phillips JH, Rahn BA: Fixation effects on membranous and endochondral onlay bone-graft resorption. Plast Reconstr Surg 82(5):872, 1988.
9. La Trenta GS, McCarthy JG, Breitbart AS, et al: The role of rigid skeletal fixation in bone-graft augmentation of the craniofacial skeleton. Plast Reconstr Surg 84(4):578, 1989.
10. Kusiak JF, Zins JE, Whitaker PA: The early revascularization of membranous bone. Plast Reconstr Surg 76(4):510, 1985.
11. Sullivan WG, Szwajkun PR: Revascularization of cranial versus iliac crest bone grafts in the rat. Plast Reconstr Surg 87(6):1105, 1991.
12. Chen NT, Glowacki J, Bucky LP, et al: The roles of revascularization and resorption on endurance of craniofacial onlay bone grafts in the rabbit. Plast Reconstr Surg 93:714, 1994.
13. Kusiak JF, Zins JE, Whitaker LA: The early revascularization of membranous bone. Discussion by Glowacki J. Plast Reconstr Surg 76(4):517, 1985.
14. Yaremchuk M: Experimental studies addressing rigid fixation in craniofacial surgery. Clin Plast Surg 21:517, 1994.
15. Manson PN: Facial bone healing and bone grafts: A review of clinical physiology. Clin Plast Surg 21:3, 1994.
16. Zins JE, Weinzweig N, Hahn J: A simple fail-safe method for the harvesting of cranial bone. Plast Reconstr Surg 96(6):1444, 1995.
17. Zins JE, Parker M: The bone pencil and the bone surgeon. Plast Reconstr Surg 80(3):453, 1987.
18. Kline R, Wolfe SA: Complications associated with the harvesting of cranial bone grafts. Plast Reconstr Surg 95:5, 1994.
19. Cannella DM, Hopkins LN: Superior sagittal sinus laceration complicating an autogenous calvarial bone graft harvest: Report of a case. J Oral Maxillofac Surg 48:741, 1990.
20. Marx RE, Morales MJ: Morbidity from bone harvest in major jaw reconstruction: A randomized trial comparing the lateral anterior and posterior approaches to the ilium. J Oral Maxillofac Surg 46:196, 1988.
21. Jackson IT, Pellen C, Smith JM: The skull as a bone graft donor site. Ann Plast Surg 11:527, 1983.
22. Posnick JC, Seagle MB, Armstrong D: Nasal reconstruction with full-thickness cranial bone grafts and rigid internal skeletal fixation through a coronal incision. Plast Reconstr Surg 86(5):894, 1990.
23. Ilankovan V, Jackson IT: Experience in the use of calvarial bone grafts in orbital reconstruction. Br J Oral Maxillofac Surg 30:92, 1992.
24. Wilkinson HA: Autogenic skull bone grafts (letter). Neurosurgery 21:760, 1987.
25. Zins JE, Reger SI, Lynch T, Papay FA: Biomechanical analysis of split cranial bone. Presented at the American Cleft Palate–Craniofacial Association Meeting, April 22–27, 1996, San Diego, California, 1996.
26. McNemar T, Zins JE, Hahn J: Autogenous split skull cranioplasty in the high risk patient. Presented at the American Cleft Palate–Craniofacial Association Meeting, April 22–27, 1996, San Diego, California, 1996.

CHAPTER 10

Reconstruction of the Midface and Fronto-orbital Region Following Tumor Resection and Trauma

K. Lädrach, M.D., D.M.D.
J. Raveh, M.D., D.M.D.
T. Iizuka, M.D., D.M.D.

The method of reconstruction of the skeletal facial frame as well as soft tissue and bone following tumor resection and severe high-velocity trauma resulting in defects or disruption of these regions is still subject to controversy. We are well aware of the fact that a meticulously detailed, step-by-step description of the multiple techniques, as well as the state-of-the-art and innovative aspects of these techniques, is most desirable, but the length of such a chapter would have resulted in a book by itself. Thus, this chapter is limited to specific aspects of these techniques, with allusions to the best methods according to our own experience. We assume that the reader is acquainted with the use of the hardware mentioned, the harvesting and application of grafts and flaps, and the basic classic surgical procedures.

RECONSTRUCTION OF THE MIDFACE AND ORBITAL AREA FOLLOWING TUMOR RESECTION

Radical tumor resection does not necessarily imply that the functional and aesthetic reconstruction that follows must be considered as of secondary importance. The choice of the approach for the resection is itself of utmost importance for the outcome, and the correct selection of grafts and flaps is crucial for the achievement of acceptable results and a high quality of life.

Tumors of the Anterior Skull Base Involving the Frontonaso-orbital Region

In this location tumors often involve and extend toward the nasal lumen and the orbital and sphenoethmoidal compartment including the clivus, as well as intracranially. For broad exposure and radical tumor resection, the subcranial-subfrontal approach developed by us (Fig. 10–1) keeps iatrogenic damage to a minimum and allows optimal reconstruction. The anterior to posterior direction of the exposure with direct visualization of the vital structures provided by this approach is a major advantage. Thus, the common lateral rhinotomy or midface degloving procedure or splitting or other osteotomies are unnecessary. Another major advantage is that no intact structures have to be damaged to expose the tumor, thus avoiding any related deformities, and this in turn facilitates the reconstruction. The watertight alignment of the skull base (see Fig. 10–1*D*) and closure of the dural defects are achieved by using several layers of fascia lata. Only in rare cases is it necessary to combine this approach with a pericranium flap or bone grafts to bridge the skull base defect. Further details on the subcranial-subfrontal approach as well as statistical data on results and long-term evaluation would be beyond the scope of this chapter, and we refer the reader to the related literature.[1–4]

As shown in Figure 10–2*B,* following resection and management of the skull base (see Color plate), the osteotomized segment is replaced. The preoperative configuration of the frontonasal segment can be exactly reproduced because the miniplates or microplates (Howmedica-Leibinger GmbH, Freiburg, Germany) have been adapted previous to the osteotomy. Centripetal symmetrical fixation of the canthal ligaments (see Fig. 10–2*A*) is performed with a thread applied to the canthal ligaments guided through the lateral nasal wall fragment beneath the skull base; this is tightened and fixed to the contralateral frontal bone. This moreover achieves not only a symmetrical adaptation toward the midline but also adjusts the traction of the canthal ligament inward and downward, producing optimum symmetry. If a total medial orbital

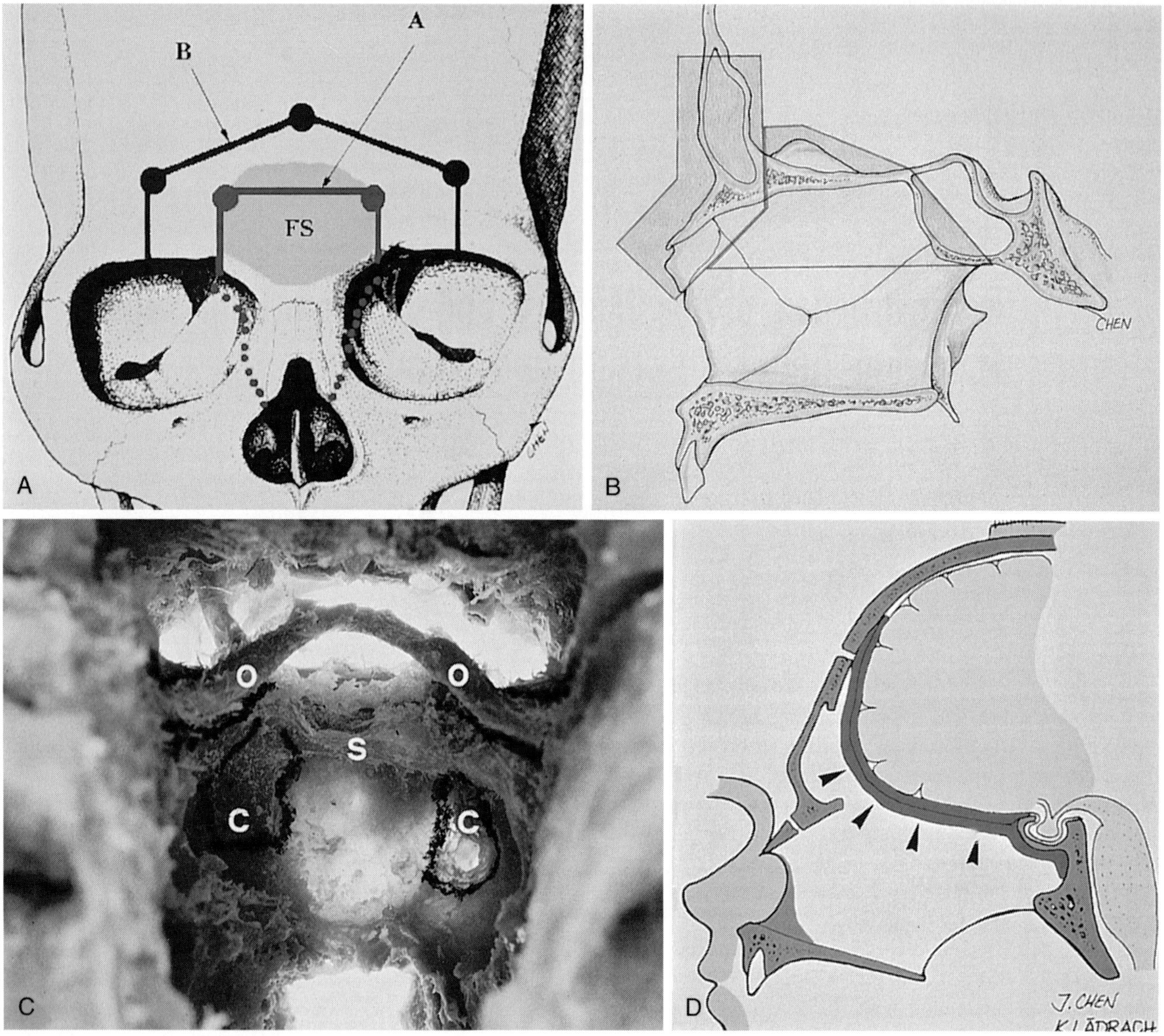

FIGURE 10–1. Anterior approach to the skull base. *A,* The osteotomies are tailored in relation to the tumor extension and can be modified accordingly. (FS = frontal sinus; A = osteotomy within borders of frontal sinus; B = osteotomy outside frontal sinus borders.) *B,* Schematic drawing of the sagittal plane illustrating the exposure following removal of the frontonasal segment. *C,* The exposure of vital structures—optic nerve and chiasm (o), sella (s), and ascending part of the carotid artery (c)—and direct visualization in an anterior to posterior direction allows radical en bloc tumor removal including the sphenoclival extensions. *D,* Reconstruction using fascia lata layers *(arrows)* and replacement of the frontonasal segment.

wall resection including periorbital tissue has been performed, application of a lyophilized or external table graft is indicated. However, in most cases, when the medial wall is only partially removed, the periosteum remains intact, so this step can be omitted.

A different situation common to such extensive tumors is shown in the case illustrated in Figure 10–3. This aesthesioneuroblastoma (see Fig. 10–3*A*) involved the ethmoidal-sphenoidal planes up to the clivus with intracranial and nasal lumen extensions. In this case, the frontonasal frame was partially resorbed by the tumor tissue. Following resection (see Fig. 10–3*B*) the frontonasal frame had to be substituted by external cranial table grafts (the internal table is always left intact). Because the plates are always contoured prior to the osteotomy, fixation of the grafts guarantees that the individual configuration is reproduced exactly (see Fig. 10–3*C–E* [see Color plate]). We prefer to use the Y-shaped Leibinger miniplate developed for this purpose. Further reconstruction of the orbital medial and lateral nasal walls, as well as canthal ligament fixation ensured an excellent aesthetic and functional reconstruction (see Fig. 10–3*F* and *G*). Despite the fact that these bone grafts are free, we have not experienced, apart from two cases out of 153, extensive resorption, any further complications concerning osteolysis, infection, or rejection that obviated secondary corrections.

Tumors Located in the Maxillo-Orbital Region

Depending on the extent of the resection performed at this location, the reconstruction is performed with free bone

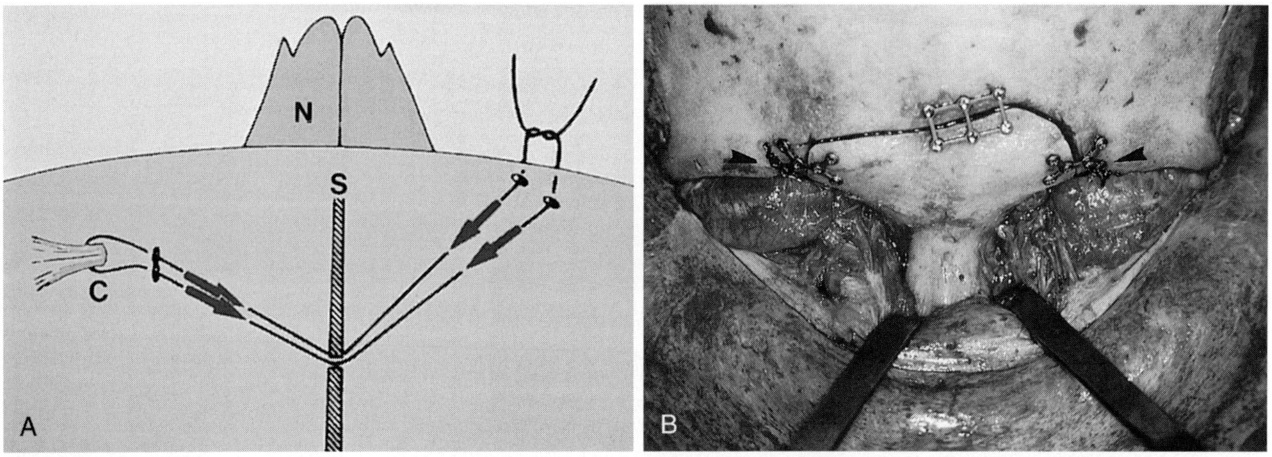

FIGURE 10–2. Replacement of the osteomized segment and canthal ligament fixation. *A,* Centripetal compression and canthal ligament (c) fixation by a thread guided underneath the anterior skull base toward the contralateral frontal bone. (N = nose; s = septum). *B,* Repositioned frontonasal segment fixed with titanium microplates (Leibinger). Arrows show the thread fixed to the contralateral side, which allows not only medial adjustment of the canthal ligaments but also adjustment in an inward posterior direction (see Color plate).

grafts combined with pedicled or local flaps as well as free revascularized soft tissue or osseomyocutaneous flaps. The indications and selection of the method will be described next in representative cases.

Free Bone Graft Application and Local Flaps. The cavernous lymphangioma in the palate and anterior maxillary sinus walls (Fig. 10–4*A–C*) was removed, preserving the major part of the uninvolved mucosa. In such cases, we prefer to use free iliac crest bone grafts with simultaneous application of intraosseous dental implants (see Fig. 10–4*D*). Aware of the high rate of resorption of such grafts, we apply a pedicled buccal fat pad, aligning the graft's inner surface with the maxillary sinus lumen (Fig. 10–4*E–G*). Fixation of the graft is performed with miniplates. In this case, using local soft palate flaps in combination with the partially preserved palatal mucosa, the bone graft was covered on both sides. Further bone grafts were necessary to reconstruct the anterior maxillary sinus walls as well as the medial part of the infraorbital rim. This procedure ensures a sufficient blood supply to keep the anticipated resorption to a minimum. The result is shown in Figure 10–4*H–M* (see Color plate). This procedure can only be recommended in patients who have not been irradiated. A 10% to 15% rate of bone resorption was observed in 12 of 63 cases; it did not affect the stability of the dental implants or require additional secondary surgery.

Combination of Iliac Crest and Temporal Vessel Pedicled Galea Flap. The patient shown in Figure 10–5*A–I* was operated on, alio loco, to remove an osteogenic sarcoma, leaving parts of the tumor along the retromaxillary area and the pterygopalatine fossa. The hemimaxillectomy defect was left unreconstructed (see Fig. 10–5*A*). Following referral of the patient, radical resection of the tumor was performed, and an iliac crest bone graft with dental implants was inserted as a substitute for the palate; grafts for the orbital floor were also performed. Because there was no palatal mucosa left, a temporal vessel pedicled galea-pericranium flap (see Fig. 10–5*B*) was harvested and aligned with the intraoral graft's surface and the pedicled buccal fat pad to cover the exposed inner surface toward the maxillary cavity. Figure 10–5*C–E* depicts the reconstructed palate and the implants. The consolidated soft tissue and bone are shown in Figure 10–5*F–I* as well as the temporary denture and the patient's appearance.

Iliac Crest Graft and Radialis Forearm Flap. In patients undergoing a total maxillectomy, we prefer to use a free osseomyocutaneous flap because of the size of the defect. A compromise is then indicated if the resection is limited to the palate and retromaxillary area. As shown in Figure 10–6*A–N,* a squamous cell carcinoma, the combined procedure includes use of a free iliac crest graft aligned with a radialis forearm flap. The radical resection of the palate is shown in Figure 10–6*B* and *C*. The iliac crest graft, following the simultaneous application of dental implants, was covered on the side facing the oral cavity with a radialis forearm flap that included an anastomosis to the facial vessels (Fig. 10–6*D–F*). The buccal pad was used as previously described. The result is shown in Figure 10–6*G–N*.

Free Revascularized Osseomyocutaneous Flaps for Extensive Resections. In extensive resections of bone and soft tissue, the use of free bone grafts, because of the anticipated osteolysis and resorption rate, is not recommended. Such cases represent an absolute indication for the use of free revascularized flaps. Resection of the squamous cell carcinoma shown in Figure 10–7, which had undergone radiotherapy (65 Gy), required a hemimaxillectomy, including the pterygoid, the anterior and lateral parts of the zygoma, and the orbital floor. An iliac crest osseomyocutaneous flap was harvested. The bone was used to reconstruct the zygomatic-palatinal defect and the orbital floor, the skin flap was used to line the maxillary sinus nasal lumen, and the oblique muscle was used for the closure of the oral cavity (Fig. 10–7*E–H*).

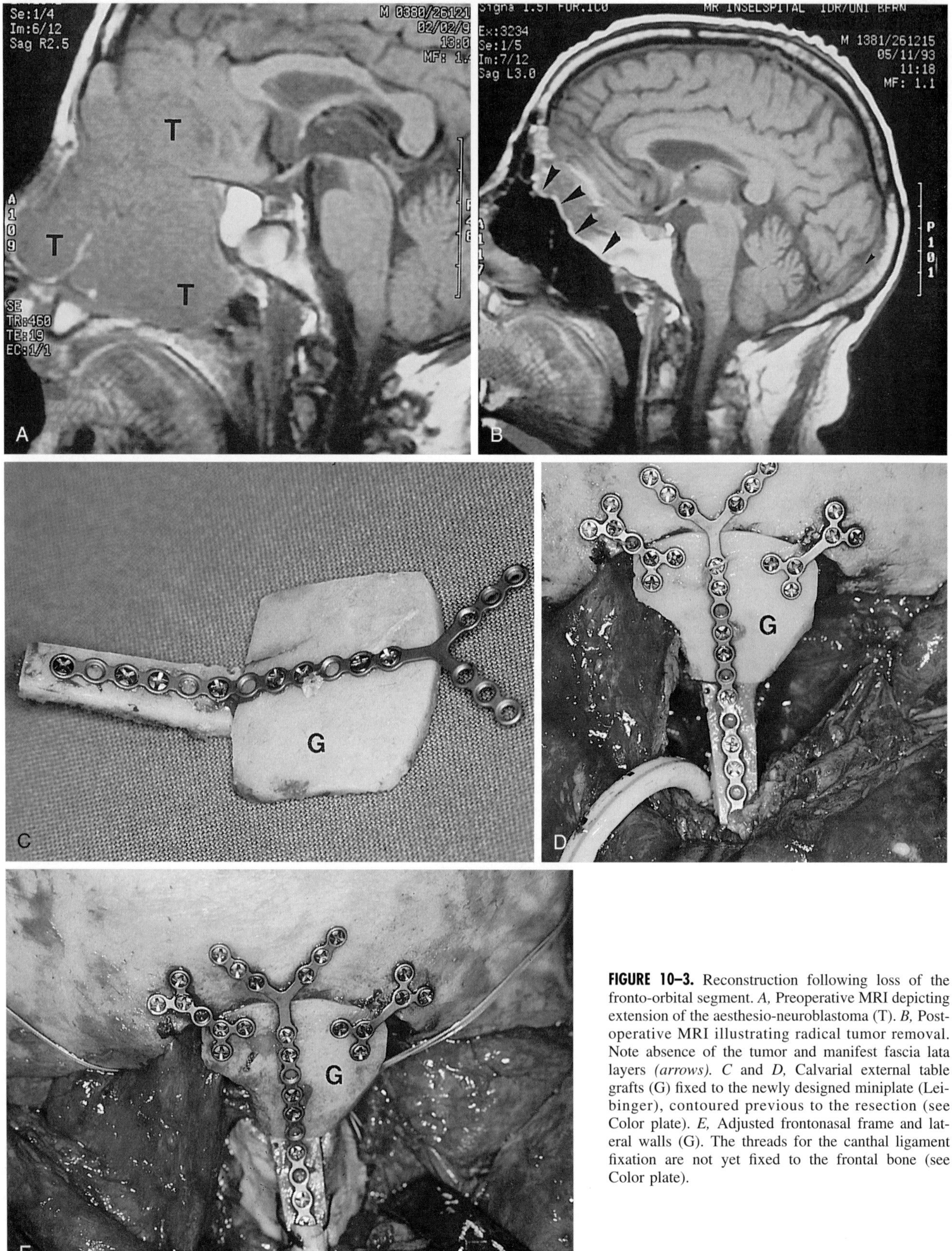

FIGURE 10–3. Reconstruction following loss of the fronto-orbital segment. *A,* Preoperative MRI depicting extension of the aesthesio-neuroblastoma (T). *B,* Postoperative MRI illustrating radical tumor removal. Note absence of the tumor and manifest fascia lata layers *(arrows). C* and *D,* Calvarial external table grafts (G) fixed to the newly designed miniplate (Leibinger), contoured previous to the resection (see Color plate). *E,* Adjusted frontonasal frame and lateral walls (G). The threads for the canthal ligament fixation are not yet fixed to the frontal bone (see Color plate).

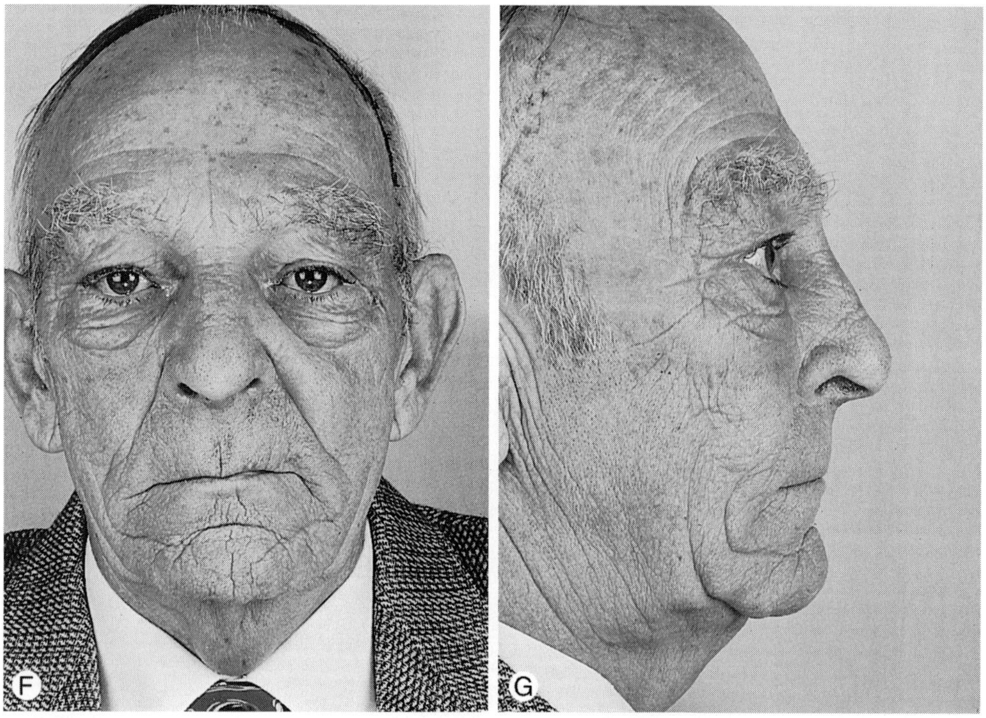

FIGURE 10–3 *Continued. F* and *G,* Postoperative view.

Summary

The choice of methods for reconstruction and for achievement of an acceptable functional and aesthetic result should not be limited to one or two techniques but should take all methods, even "old-fashioned" ones, into consideration. This is particularly important because the temptation, in light of the high success rate of today's microvascular surgery, to consider this method as a standard for all cases is obvious. Despite a success rate of 97% in 158 free revascularized flaps performed in our department in the last 6 years, we do not consider this the method of choice in all the cases. The evaluation of each case in regard to the extent of the defect and the degree of bone and soft tissue loss is of utmost importance. If no radiotherapy has been done and the recipient bed provides a sufficient blood supply, the application of relatively small free bone grafts and local and pedicled flaps or combinations of flaps, if correctly performed, is often sufficient. The advantages of such a wide selection of methods include a reduction in costs and the ability to perform less time-consuming surgical procedures. To avoid repetition here, further aspects of the reconstruction of the orbital cone are described in the next section.

RECONSTRUCTION OF THE ORBITAL COMPLEX AND MIDFACE FOLLOWING TRAUMA

Particularly high-velocity trauma often results in multifragment fractures and a major dislocation and disruption of the internal and external facial skeletal frame. Even relatively minor fractures that have been insufficiently reduced often lead to visible deformities, asymmetry, and functional derangements. The thrust of this section is to emphasize very specific aspects as well as pitfalls.

Reconstruction of the Orbital Cone and the Zygomatic Complex

The selection and choice of the correct hardware is important to avoid late complications. The schematic drawing shown in Figure 10–8 depicts the different indications for miniplates or microplates in our experience. The thicker titanium miniplates should be limited to the load-bearing buttresses. In more peripheral locations, such as the infraorbital rim, anterior maxillary sinus, and lateral nasal walls, wire ligatures, or, even better, microplates should be used. This is particularly important because the bone is often very thin in these locations, and the undersurface of the fragments is covered only by the thin maxillary sinus or the nasal mucosa, which is often lacerated or missing. Thus, multifragment fractures in these locations, if fixed with miniplates, will often, because of the size of the plate, be denuded and separated from the periosteum. In addition, the thin mucosa beneath the fragments often provides an insufficient blood supply. This often results in osteolysis and resorption. A compromise along the nasal frame may be acceptable, particularly if one miniplate is used to fix several fragments, obviating the application of further hardware. But if the fragments are small, and particularly if they are located in the lower part of the lateral nasal walls, microplates are indicated.

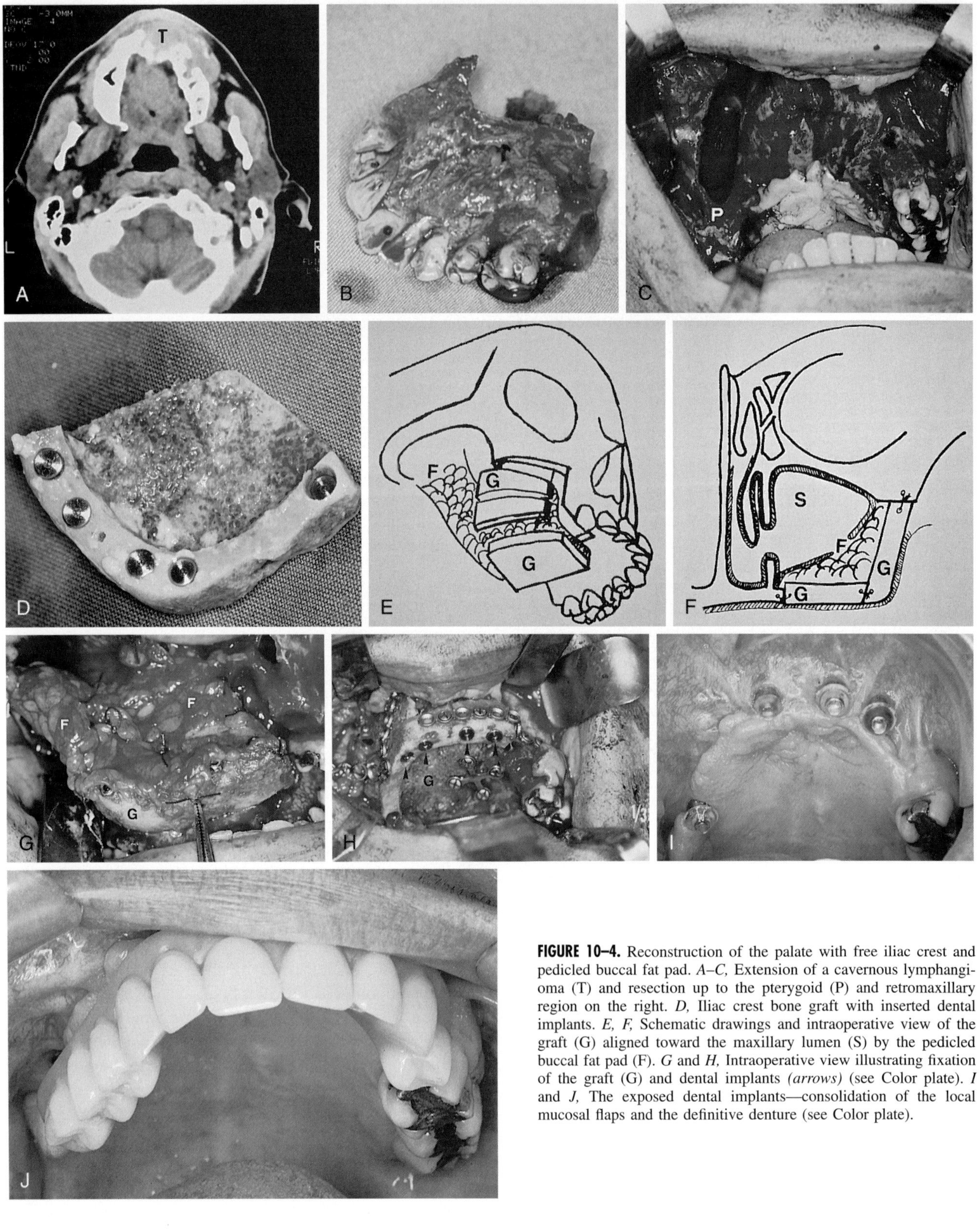

FIGURE 10–4. Reconstruction of the palate with free iliac crest and pedicled buccal fat pad. *A–C,* Extension of a cavernous lymphangioma (T) and resection up to the pterygoid (P) and retromaxillary region on the right. *D,* Iliac crest bone graft with inserted dental implants. *E, F,* Schematic drawings and intraoperative view of the graft (G) aligned toward the maxillary lumen (S) by the pedicled buccal fat pad (F). *G* and *H,* Intraoperative view illustrating fixation of the graft (G) and dental implants *(arrows)* (see Color plate). *I* and *J,* The exposed dental implants—consolidation of the local mucosal flaps and the definitive denture (see Color plate).

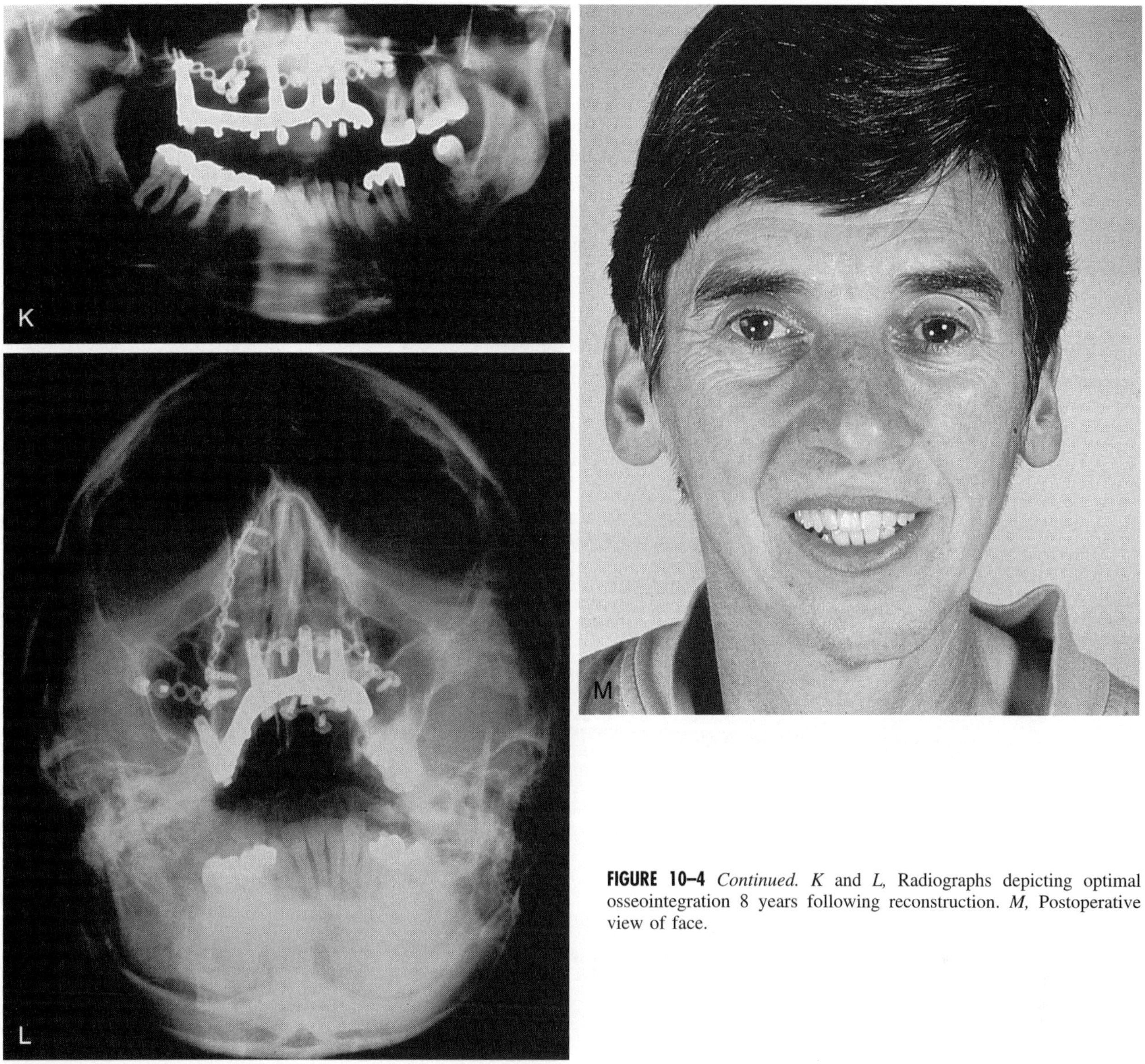

FIGURE 10–4 *Continued. K* and *L,* Radiographs depicting optimal osseointegration 8 years following reconstruction. *M,* Postoperative view of face.

In the case shown in Figure 10–9 of a dislocated zygoma fracture reduced with a miniplate to the frontozygomatic buttress and another one to the zygomatic alveolar arch, the defect along the maxillary sinus walls as a result of the pulverization of the fragments is apparent. Often, if the fracture is a classic simple tetrapod fracture, a closed reduction using a hook is sufficient. In all other cases, open reduction and exposure should include the lateral orbital wall, the infraorbital rim and floor, and the zygomatic alveolar arch. Only this exposure can guarantee the correct three-dimensional configuration. If, unlike the situation in this case, reduction of the further fractures is established and stable, only one miniplate applied to the frontozygomatic buttress is sufficient.

The transconjunctival approach (Fig. 10–10*A*) is exclusively used for all infraorbital and orbital floor fractures, and the intraoral approach is used for the management of the maxillary buttress fractures. Thus, unnecessary skin incisions and scar tissue formation can be avoided. As depicted in Figure 10–10*B–F,* the transconjunctival approach with no additional lateral canthotomy is sufficient to reduce even severely dislocated multifragmented infraorbital and orbital floor fractures. Depending on the size and location of the fracture, this procedure is performed with wire ligatures or microplates. The majority of orbital floor fractures and defects are bridged using lyophilized cartilage. Only in cases in which the entire orbital floor is missing or pulverized and no support is available are bone grafts, mostly external table grafts fixed by lag screws or microplates, indicated (Fig. 10–11). As shown in Figure 10–12*A* and *B,* the results confirm this concept.

In the case shown in Figure 10–12*C* a subciliary-subtarsal approach was used on the left side (alio loco) to treat an orbital floor and isolated infraorbital rim fracture. On the right side the complicated multifragment fracture of the zygoma and orbital floor was reduced using the transcon-

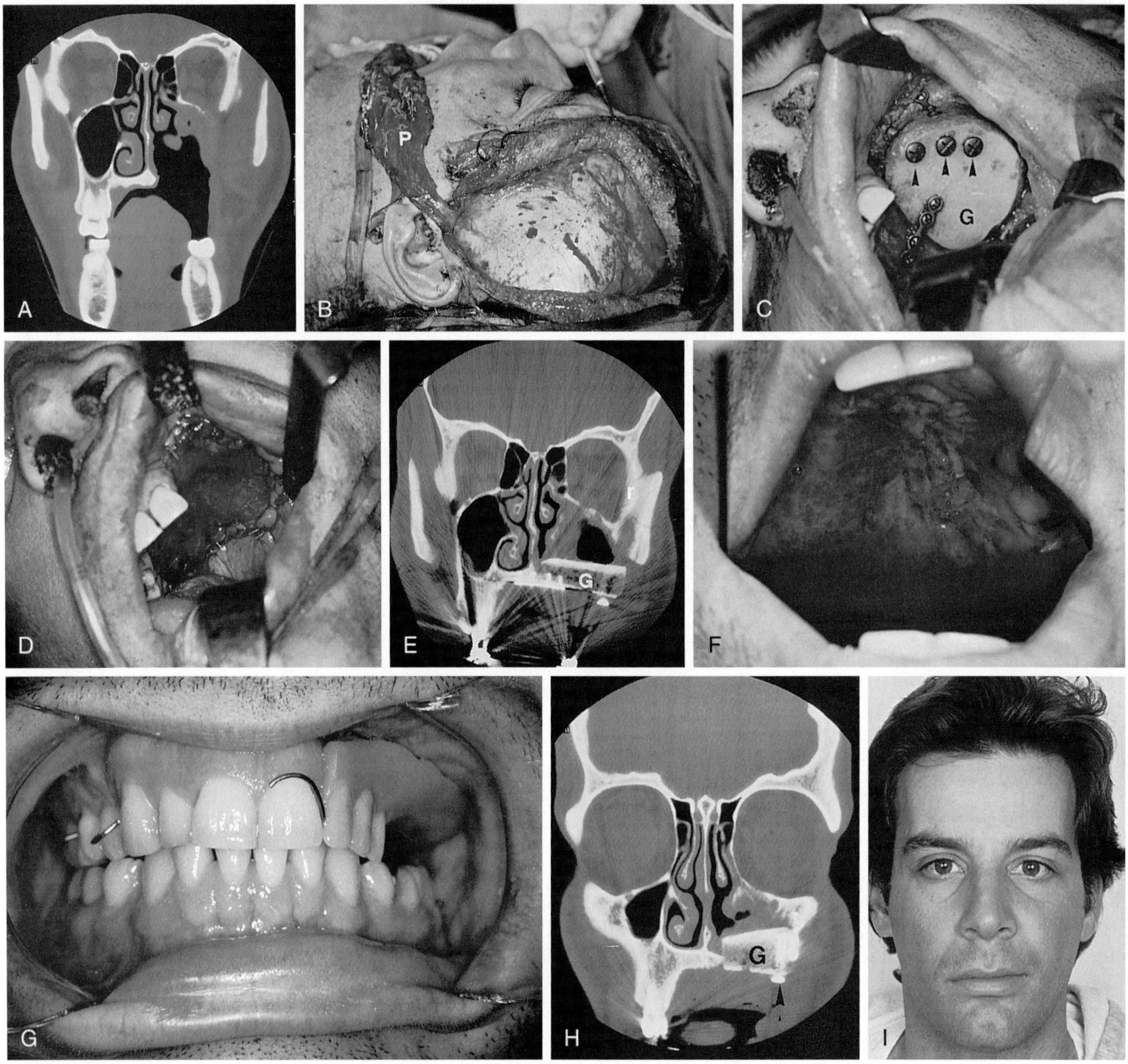

FIGURE 10–5. Combination of an iliac crest graft with a temporalis vessel pedicled pericranium-galea flap and buccal fat pad. *A,* Axial CT scan following partial resection of an osteogenic sarcoma (alio loco), leaving tumor tissue along the orbital floor and retromaxillary area. *B,* Pedicled pericranium flap (P). *C,* Intraoral view showing the iliac crest graft (G) with the dental implants *(arrows)* and miniplate fixation. The inner surface is already aligned by the buccal fat pad. *D,* Intraoperative view showing the intraorally adapted pericranium flap. *E* and *F,* Postoperative radiograph and intraoral view of the consolidated grafts and pericranium flap. *G,* Denture in situ. *H,* Late control radiograph showing the reconstructed orbital floor and palate with the iliac crest grafts. *I,* Postoperative view of face confirming symmetry of the zygoma prominence and eyes.

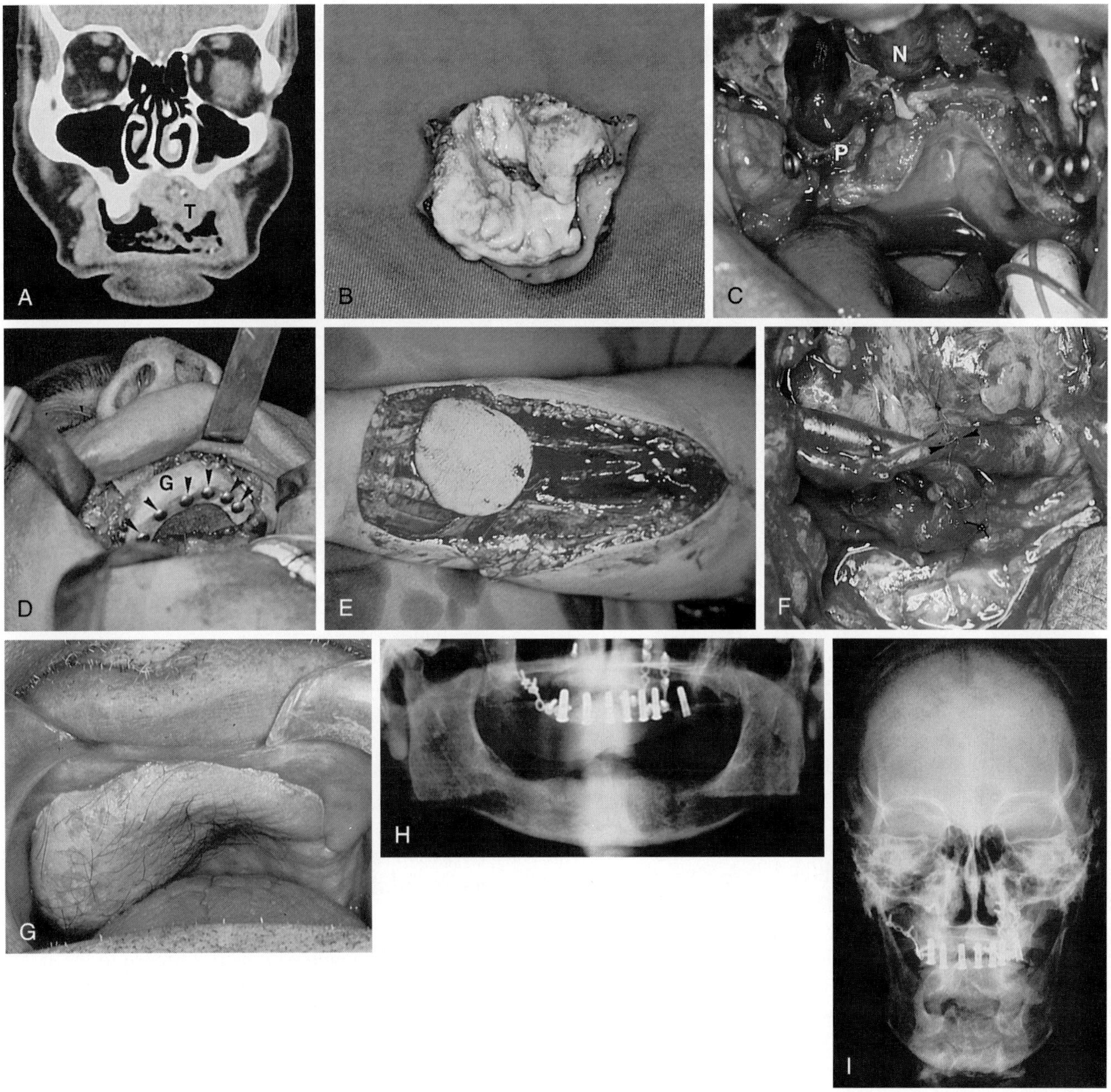

FIGURE 10–6. Combination of a free iliac crest graft and radialis forearm flap. *A* and *B,* Squamous cell carcinoma of the palate (T). *C,* Intraoperative view following resection including the pterygoid (P) and retromaxillary area. The nasal cavity (N) is exposed. *D,* The iliac crest graft (G) including the dental implants; the inner surface was aligned by the fat pad. *E* and *F,* Closure toward the oral cavity with a radialis forearm flap. Arrows show the microanastomosis to the facial vessels. *G,* Intraoral view of the consolidated flap. *H* and *I,* Radiographs depicting osseointegration.

Illustration continued on following page

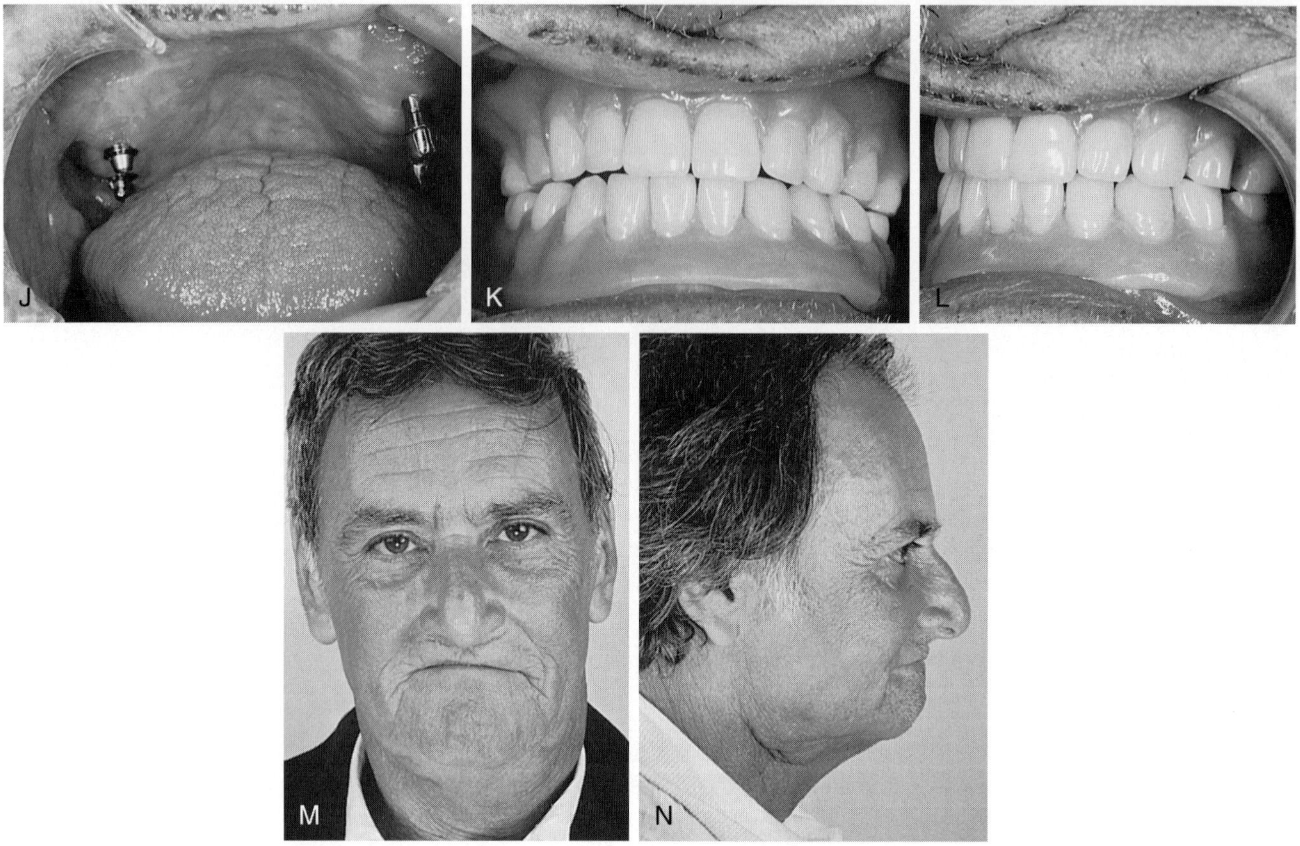

FIGURE 10–6 *Continued. J,* Exposed dental implants and the flap surface following epilation. *K–N,* Denture and view of face.

junctival approach. In contrast to the right side, the scar on the left was visible even several years following surgery. We agree that in many cases scar tissue formation is minimal, but in our experience, this is not predictable, and scar tissue formation, entropion, or ectropion is often manifest. Unlike the situation with the subtarsal-subciliary incision used for blepharoplasties, very different factors must be considered in trauma cases, including the fact that swelling and hematoma are usually manifest and further dissection, exposure, reduction, and fixation of the fractures are necessary, thus leading to further damage of the tissue and interfering with the vascularization and lymphatic drainage at this location. Because of these requirements and the consequent edema and hematoma formation, wound healing is very different than it is in blepharoplasty and explains the higher incidence of complicatons in such cases.

Combined fixation with mini- and microplates is shown in Figure 10–13. An open laceration wound and multifragment and dislocated fractures of the zygomatic complex are demonstrated in Figure 10–14. In such cases the preservation and integration of even small bone fragments instead of removing them and substituting them with bone grafts is crucial to guarantee correct three-dimensional reproduction of the original zygoma-orbital contour.

The case illustrated in Figure 10–15 is representative of the management of large open laceration wounds in combination with extensive bone loss. In such cases, exposure and identification of the intact fracture borders of the zygomatic complex is necessary to allow a symmetrical reconstruction. External table or iliac crest bone grafts are most suitable for the reconstruction. For more detailed information and statistical data we refer to several of our previous publications on this topic.[5–8]

Reconstruction of Comminuted Combined Midface/ Frontonaso-Orbital and Anterior Skull Base Fractures

These fractures can be divided into two major categories as follows: (1) Comminuted fractures limited to the external facial frame (Fig. 10–16*A*), and (2) disruption of the external and internal frame and palisades with intracranial dislocation and skull base involvement (Fig. 10–16*B–D*).

Type 1 represents a challenge in reconstruction in itself. But in type 2 additional vital aspects are involved. The involved anterior skull base along with frequent multiple dural tears, devitalized brain tissue herniation toward the paranasal spaces and orbital cavity, brain contusion, edema, and elevated intracerebral pressure often make it unfeasible to attempt immediate early one-stage definitive management by the conventional transfrontal approach with adequate frontal lobe retraction. Immediate exposure of this area up to the sphenoidal planes is, because of the intracranial pressure, too high a risk and must be postponed 10 days to 2 to 3 weeks. This means not only a prolonged stay in the

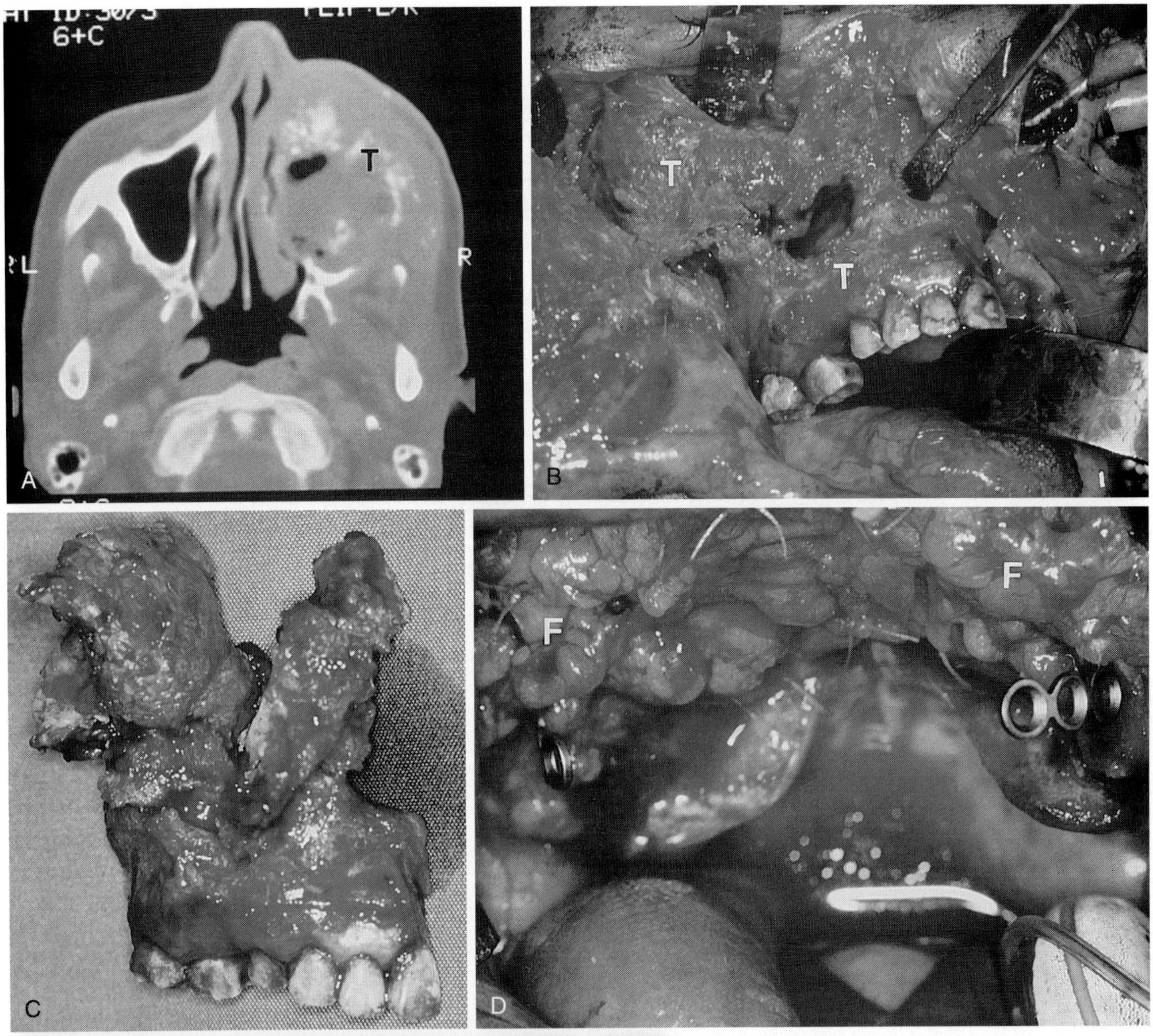

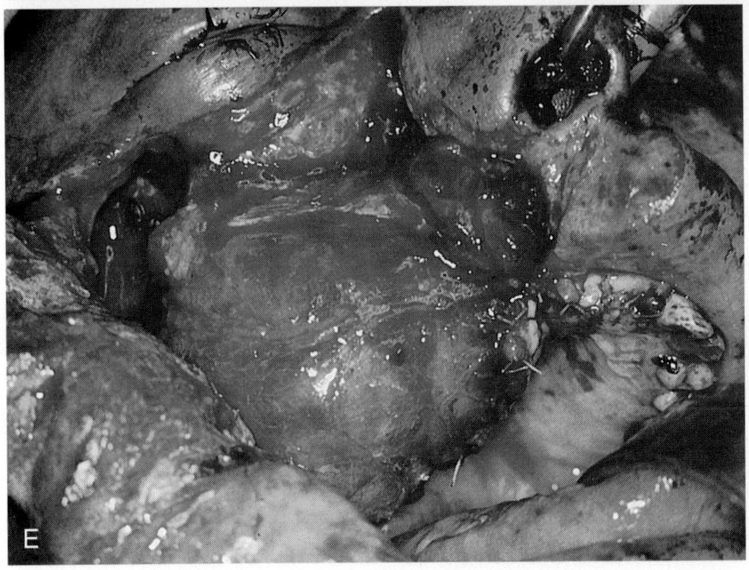

FIGURE 10–7. Reconstruction with a free revascularized iliac crest flap. *A–C,* Extension and resection of a preirradiated squamous cell carcinoma. *D,* Intraoperative view following extensive bone and soft tissue resection (fat pad [F]). *E,* Iliac crest bone was used to substitute for the palate and zygoma including the orbital floor and lateral wall; skin was used for alignment towards the lumen, and the oblique muscle was used for reconstruction of the oral cavity.

Illustration continued on following page

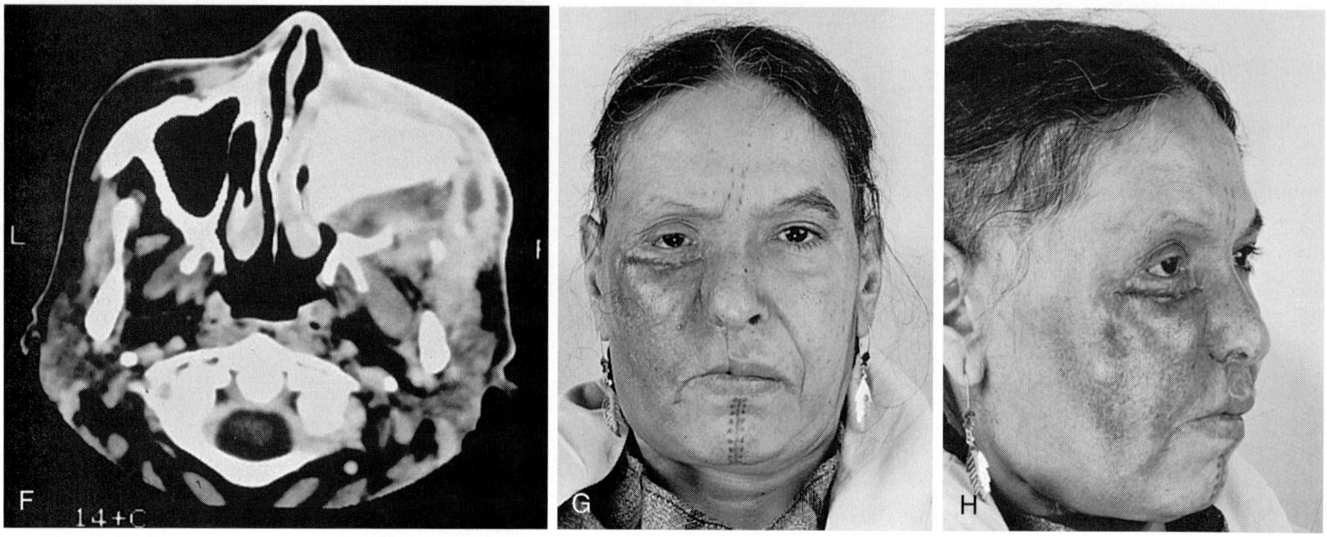

FIGURE 10–7 *Continued. F–H,* Postoperative radiograph and view of face.

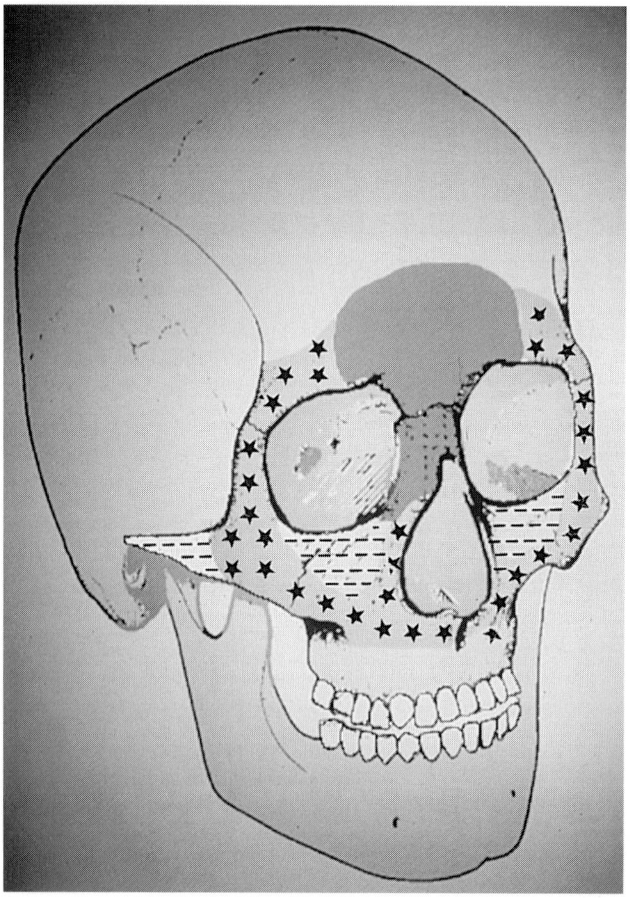

FIGURE 10–8. Preference of plates: (1) miniplates along the buttresses *(stars)*; (2) microplates *(dotted lines)*; and (3) mini- and microplate combinations *(grey area)*.

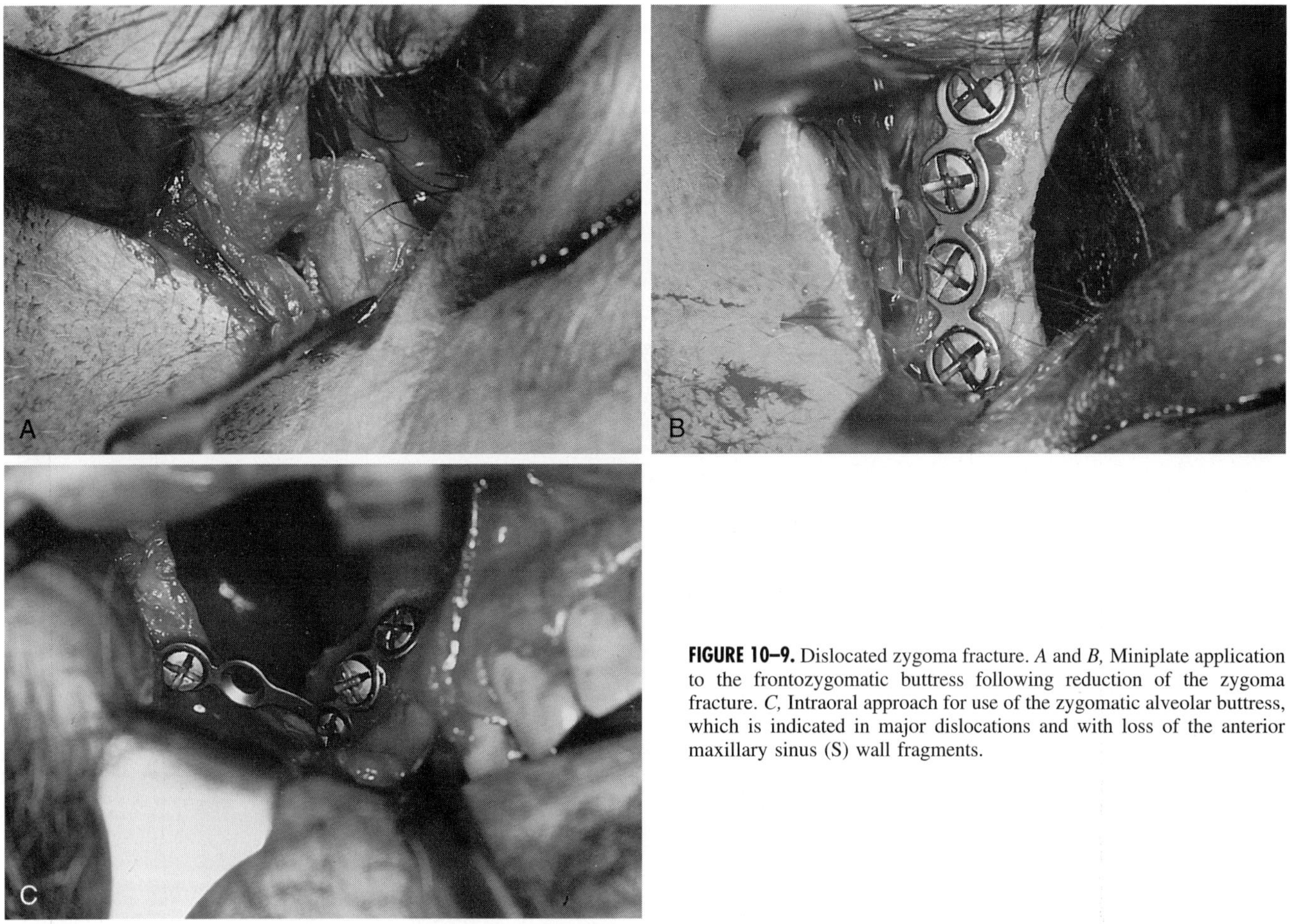

FIGURE 10–9. Dislocated zygoma fracture. *A* and *B*, Miniplate application to the frontozygomatic buttress following reduction of the zygoma fracture. *C*, Intraoral approach for use of the zygomatic alveolar buttress, which is indicated in major dislocations and with loss of the anterior maxillary sinus (S) wall fragments.

intensive care unit and subsequent hospitalization but also further swelling in the first days because of the obstructed lymphatic drainage and insufficient vascularization enhanced by the dislocated bone fragments and hematoma, not to mention further damage to the soft tissues, thus enhancing scar tissue formation. The later the reduction of the fractures and the reconstruction take place, the more laborious and difficult is the achievement of optimal results. In our experience, the term of 24 to 48 hours for the reconstruction should be stressed. Development of the subcranial-subfrontal approach, which obviates the need for frontal lobe retraction, as it does for skull base tumors, enabled us to perform early one-stage definitive management of the skull in concert with the reconstruction of the midface within the first 24 to 48 hours in most of 625 cases. Further, concomitant optic nerve compression often occurs in such complex fractures (Fig. 10–17). Decompression is indicated within the first 8 to 12 hours after trauma. Thus, on the one hand, this approach allows immediate surgical treatment, and on the other it allows simultaneous decompression and removal of the medial optic nerve canal wall.

The major advantage of this method in the reconstruction of the facial frame is that the correct reconstruction of the skull base and the posterior palisades (Fig. 10–18) allows optimal adjustment of the frontal and supraorbital area (Fig. 10–19). Optic nerve decompression is performed using the same approach (Fig. 10–19*D–E*). Once the correct reproduction of the original facial contour at this location is achieved and the osteosynthesis has been performed (Fig. 10–19*F*), the correct relationship for further reduction of naso-orbital and midface fractures is guaranteed. Canthal ligament fixation, as described earlier, is performed, and the nasal fractures are compressed in the correct position (Fig. 10–20*A*), thus reducing the application of plates to an absolute necessary minimum. Also, in such cases even small fragments should be preserved and integrated in the reconstruction to enhance the reproduction of the original contour. In severe cases, a thread can be applied to the intact part of the body of the zygoma to be guided beneath the orbital floor and ethmoidal roof and fixed to the contralateral frontal bone, which has been already reconstructed. Thus, centripetal compression of the replaced and reduced fractures is achieved. Following this, the correct position of each fragment is retained by mini- and microplates.

A combined open laceration wound with a complex craniofacial disruption and bone loss is illustrated in Figure 10–21. Following management of the skull base fractures, reduction and replacement of the inwardly telescoped nasal buttress was achieved, and the bone defects along the frontal bone and supraorbital rim were replaced by external bone

Text continued on page 133

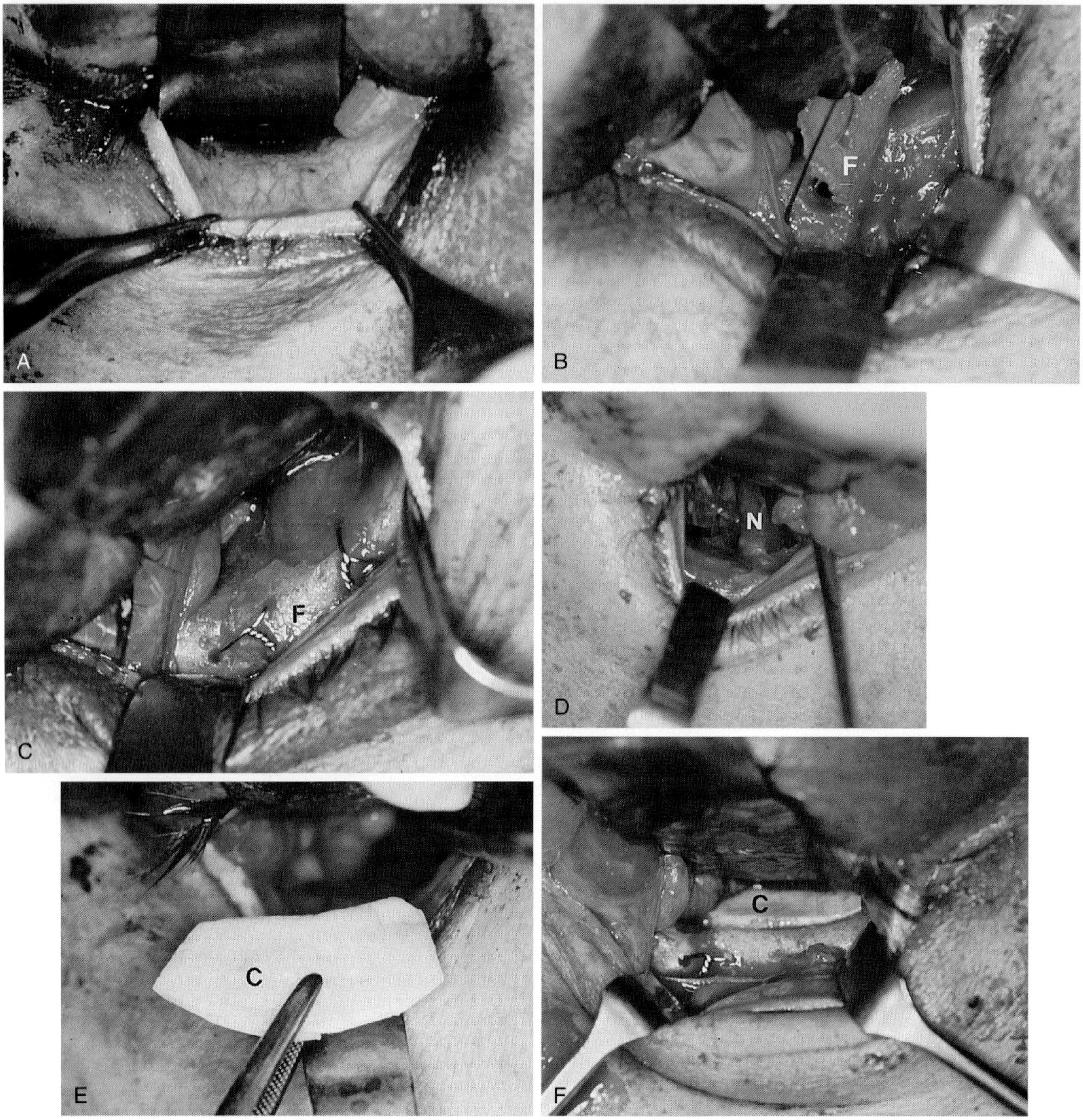

FIGURE 10–10. The transconjunctival approach, avoiding any lateral canthotomy to the infraorbital rim and orbital floor. *A,* This approach allows direct broad exposure of the infraorbital rim and orbital floor. *B* and *C,* Even in patients with multifragmentary fractures (F), this exposure allows optimal reduction with wire ligatures or microplates. *D–F,* Exposed infraorbital nerve (N) following disruption of the orbital floor. Reconstruction of the orbital floor is performed with lyophilized cartilage (C).

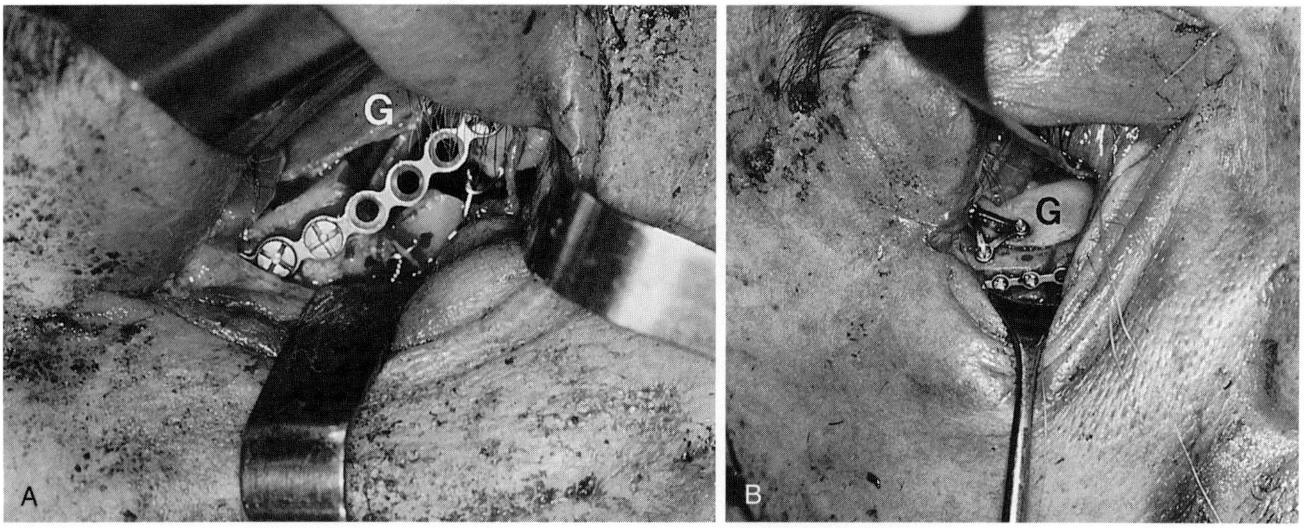

FIGURE 10–11. *A* and *B,* In the presence of a major multifragment disruption of the infraorbital rim, orbital floor, and anterior maxillary wall, combined fixation with microplates and a miniplate for bridging to preserve even small fragments is indicated. The use of external table bone grafts (G) for the orbital floor is indicated only in patients with the most extensive defects (see text). The transconjunctival approach is exclusively used for all cases.

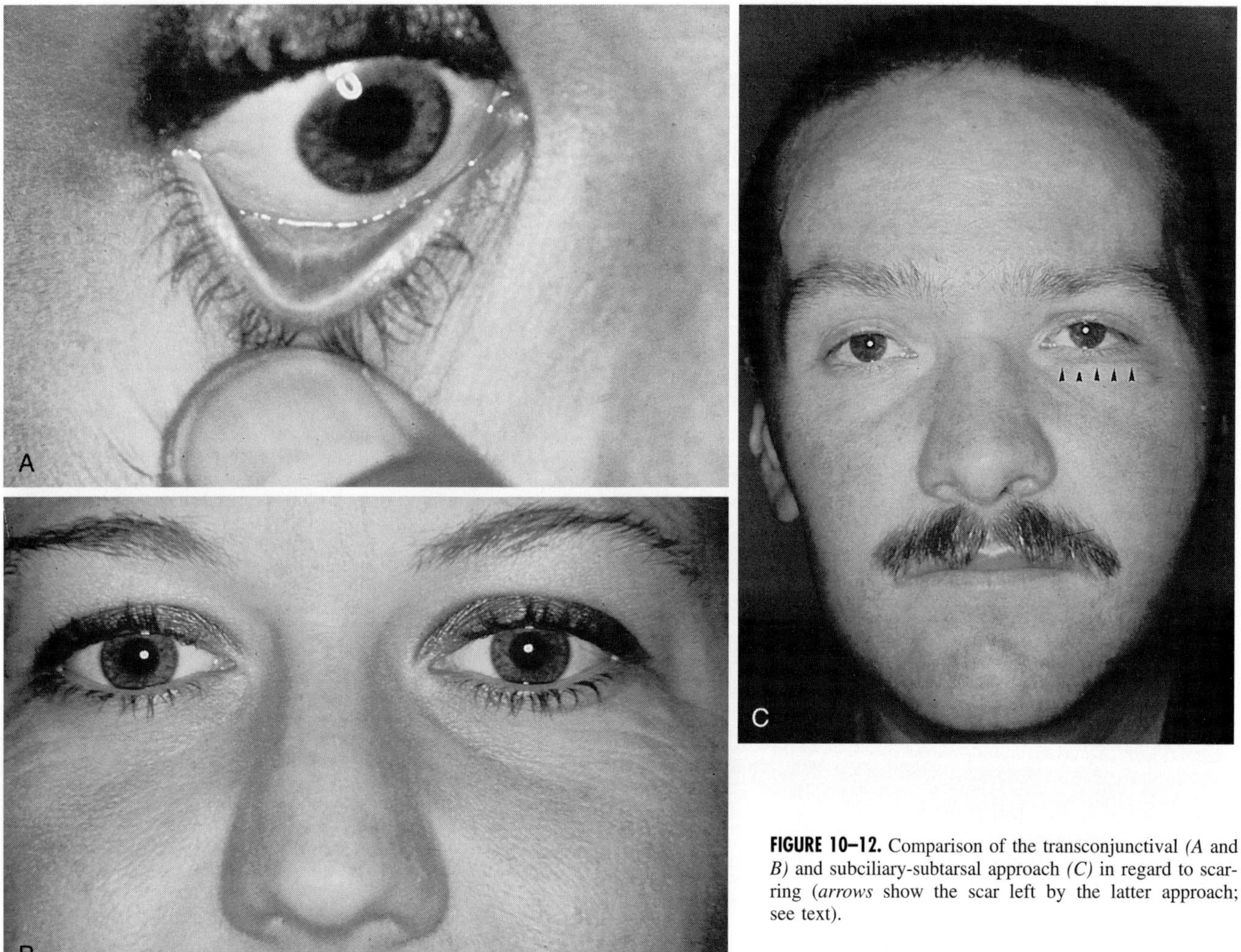

FIGURE 10–12. Comparison of the transconjunctival *(A* and *B)* and subciliary-subtarsal approach *(C)* in regard to scarring (*arrows* show the scar left by the latter approach; see text).

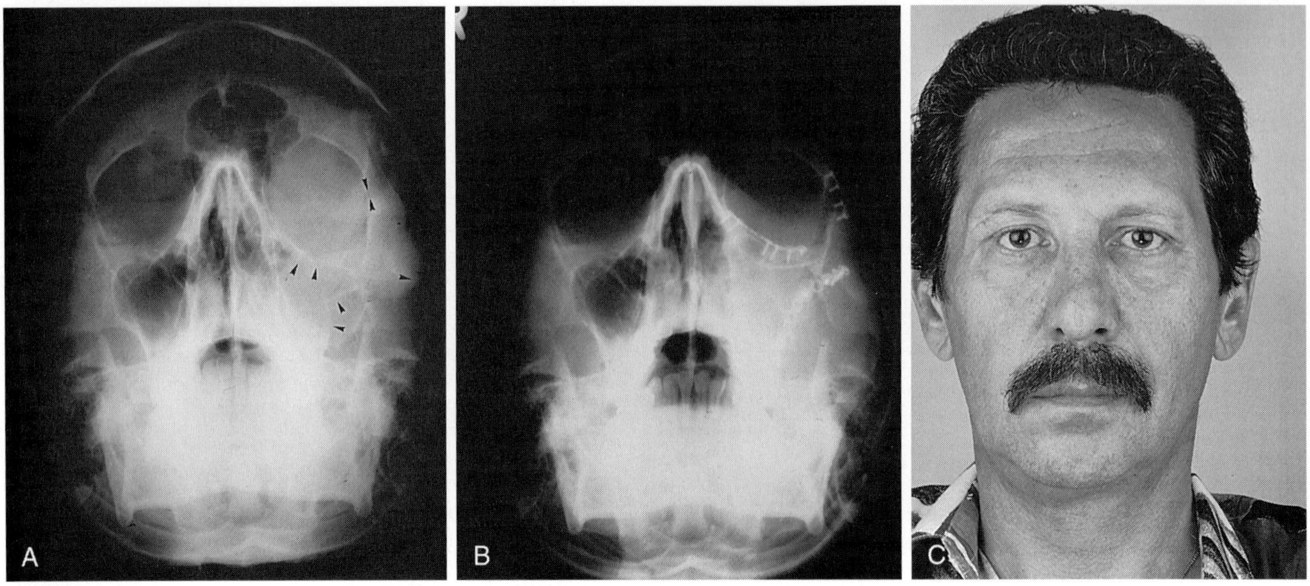

FIGURE 10–13. *A,* Complex multifragment fracture of the orbital rim and orbital floor, including major dislocation of the zygoma as well as a fracture of the zygoma prominence. Reconstruction with mini- and microplates *(B)* and view of face *(C)*.

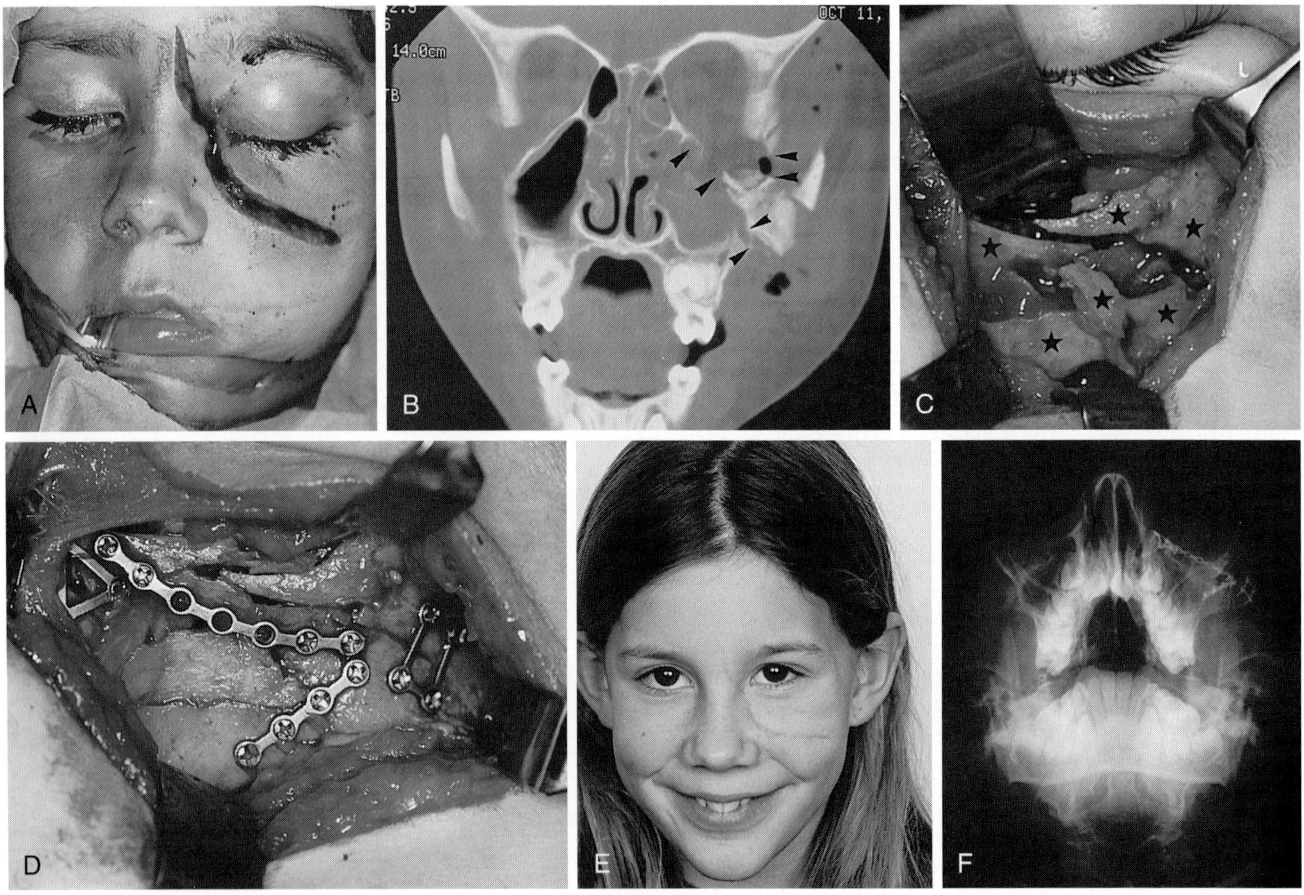

FIGURE 10–14. Open multifragment dislocated zygoma fracture. *A,* Disrupted zygoma fracture combined with an open laceration wound. *B* and *C,* CT and intraoperative view illustrating the extent of this fracture type (*arrows* and *stars*). *D-F,* Combination of microplates. Preservation of all small fragments is crucial for optimal reproduction of the contour.

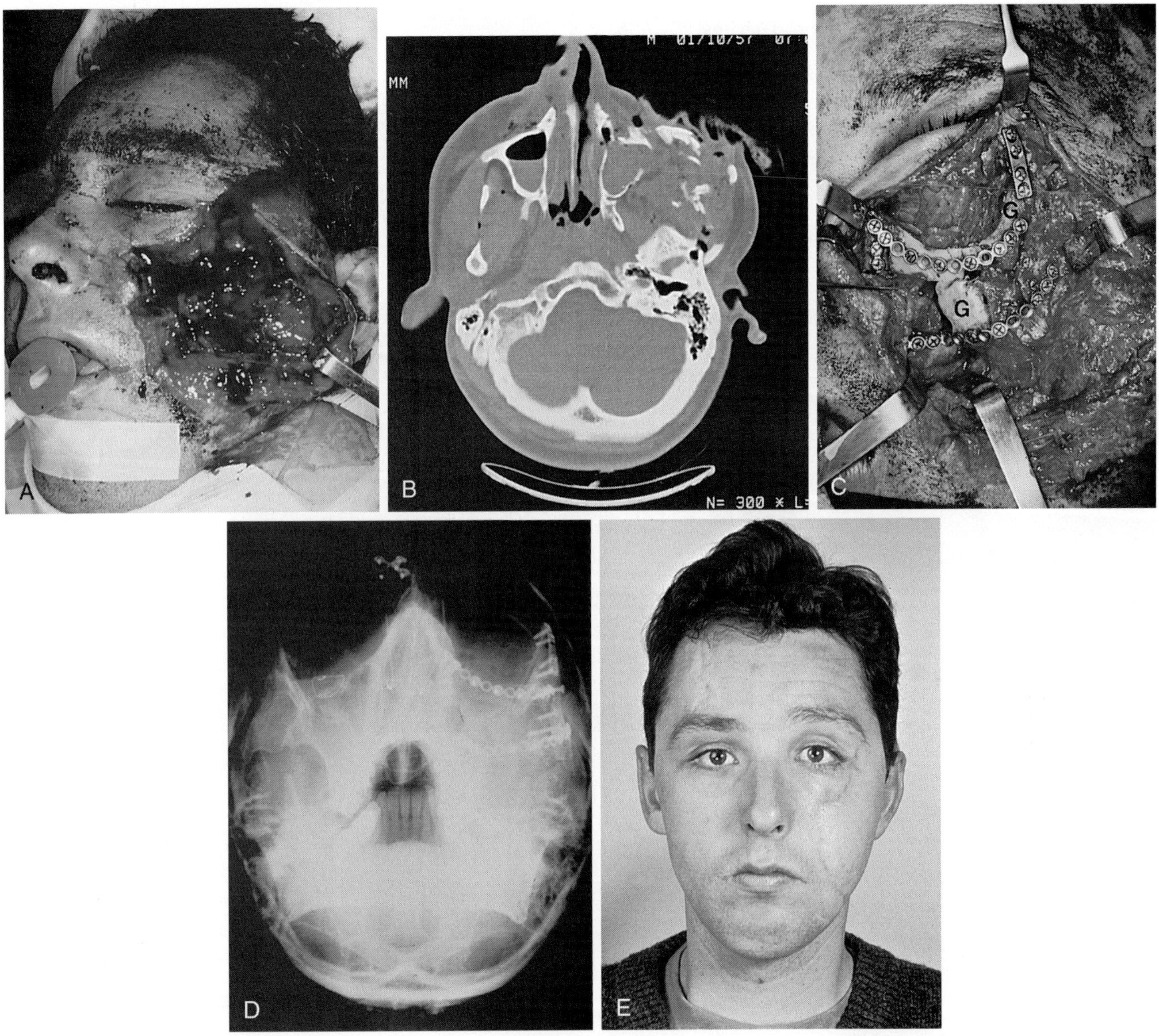

FIGURE 10–15. Zygoma fracture with bone loss. *A* and *B,* Open laceration wound with loss of bone. *C* and *D,* Reconstruction with free iliac crest grafts (G). *E,* View of face.

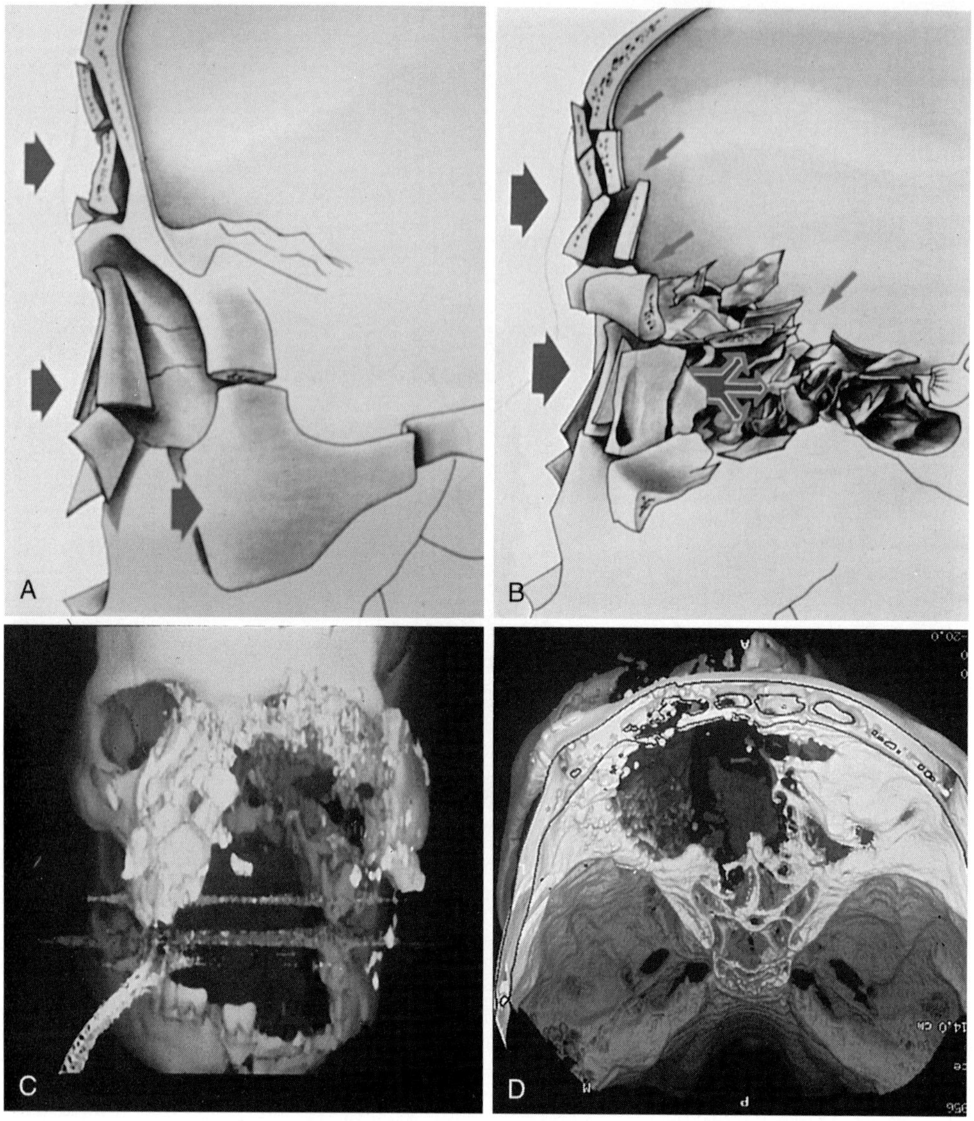

FIGURE 10–16. Combined craniomaxillo-orbital fractures. *A,* Type I: Combined fractures limited to the external craniofacial frame. *B,* Type II: Disruption of anterior and posterior palisades with intracranial and skull base involvement. *C* and *D,* Extensive facial frame and skull base injuries implying a one-stage reconstruction of the frame and the skull base.

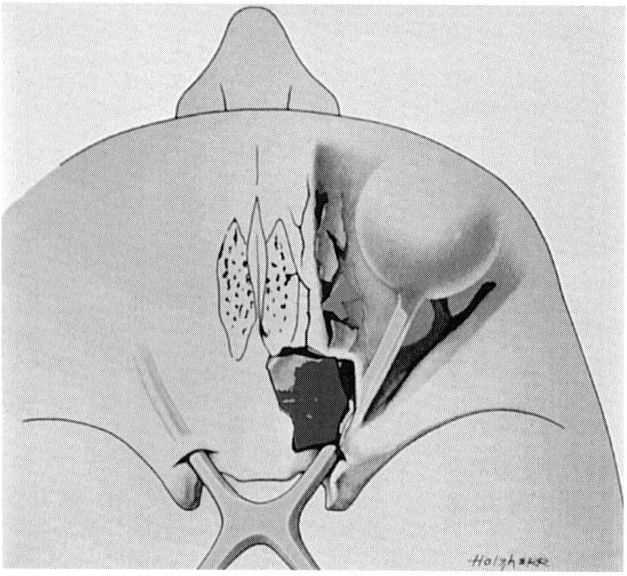

FIGURE 10–17. Direct and indirect involvement of the optic nerve canal (see text).

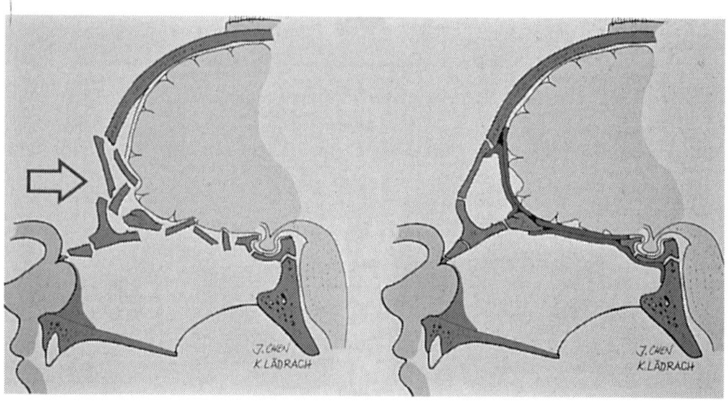

FIGURE 10–18. The subcranial-subfrontal approach allows an early one-stage reconstruction. The watertight skull base alignment is performed with fascia lata.

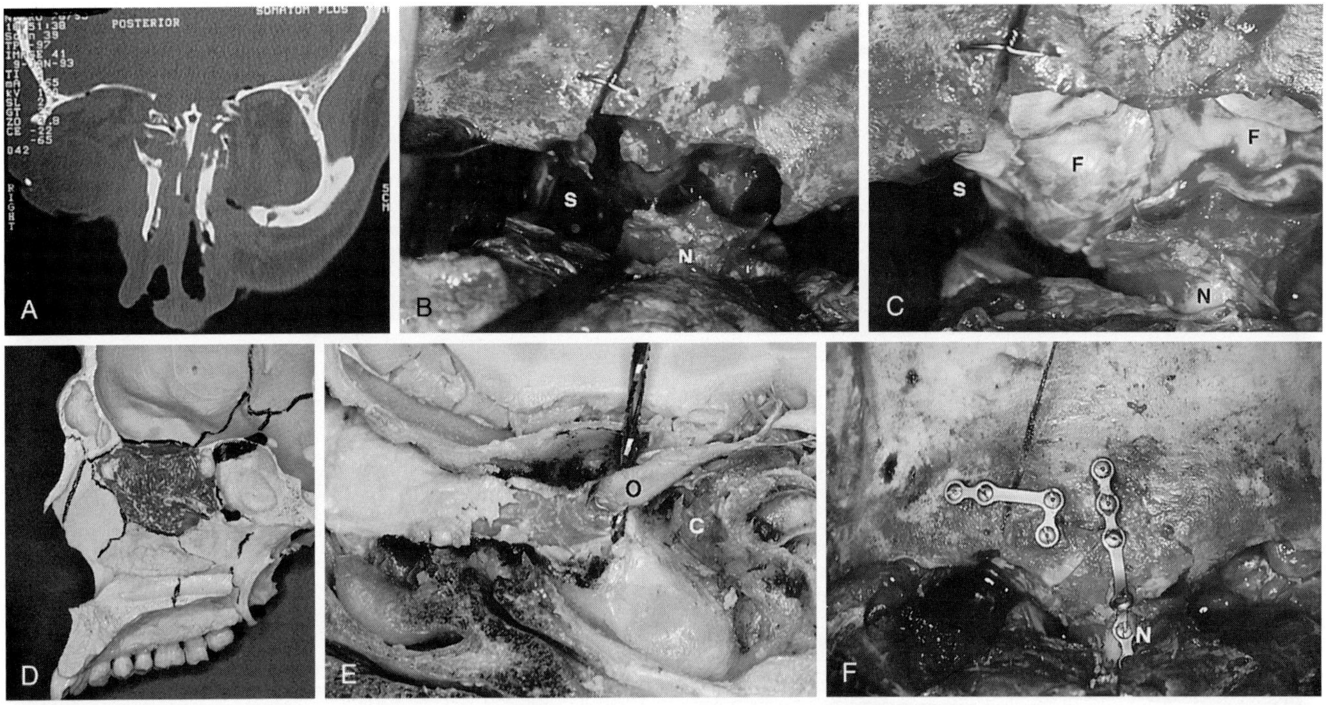

FIGURE 10–19. Complex nasoethmoidal skull base fracture pattern. *A,* Coronal CT scan shows multifragment fractures of the anterior skull base, orbital cone, and nasal frame. *B,* Same patient as in *A.* The dislocated frontal bone fracture is temporarily fixed with a wire ligature. N = disattached nasal buttress; S = the subcranial approach for the management of skull base planes. *C,* Anterior part of fascia lata (F) applied to the sphenoid by the subcranial access (S). The nasal buttress and midface are still disattached. *D* and *E,* Optic nerve is decompressed (O) by this approach, and the medial optic nerve canal is removed. (C = adjacent carotid artery.) *F,* The skeletal frame is reduced and fixed with miniplates. The nasal buttress is also reduced.

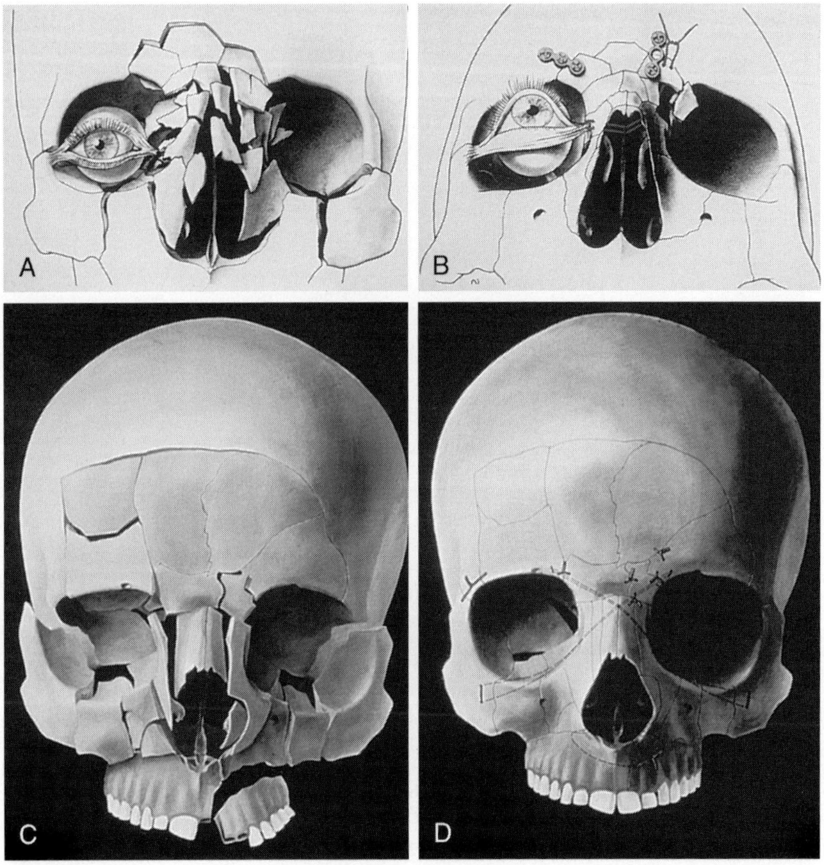

FIGURE 10–20. Centripetal compression and reduction of the telecanthus. *A* and *B,* Subcranial exposure allows fixation of the canthal ligaments by means of a thread guided beneath the exposed skull base that is then tightened and fixed to the contralateral side. This compresses and wedges in even small nasal fragments to achieve an optimal reproduction of the contour with a minimum of plates. *C* and *D,* The same technique can be applied to the adjustment of both zygomas; the thread is guided beneath the orbital floor and the exposed skull base and is then fixed to the contralateral side. Only then are the miniplates and microplates applied.

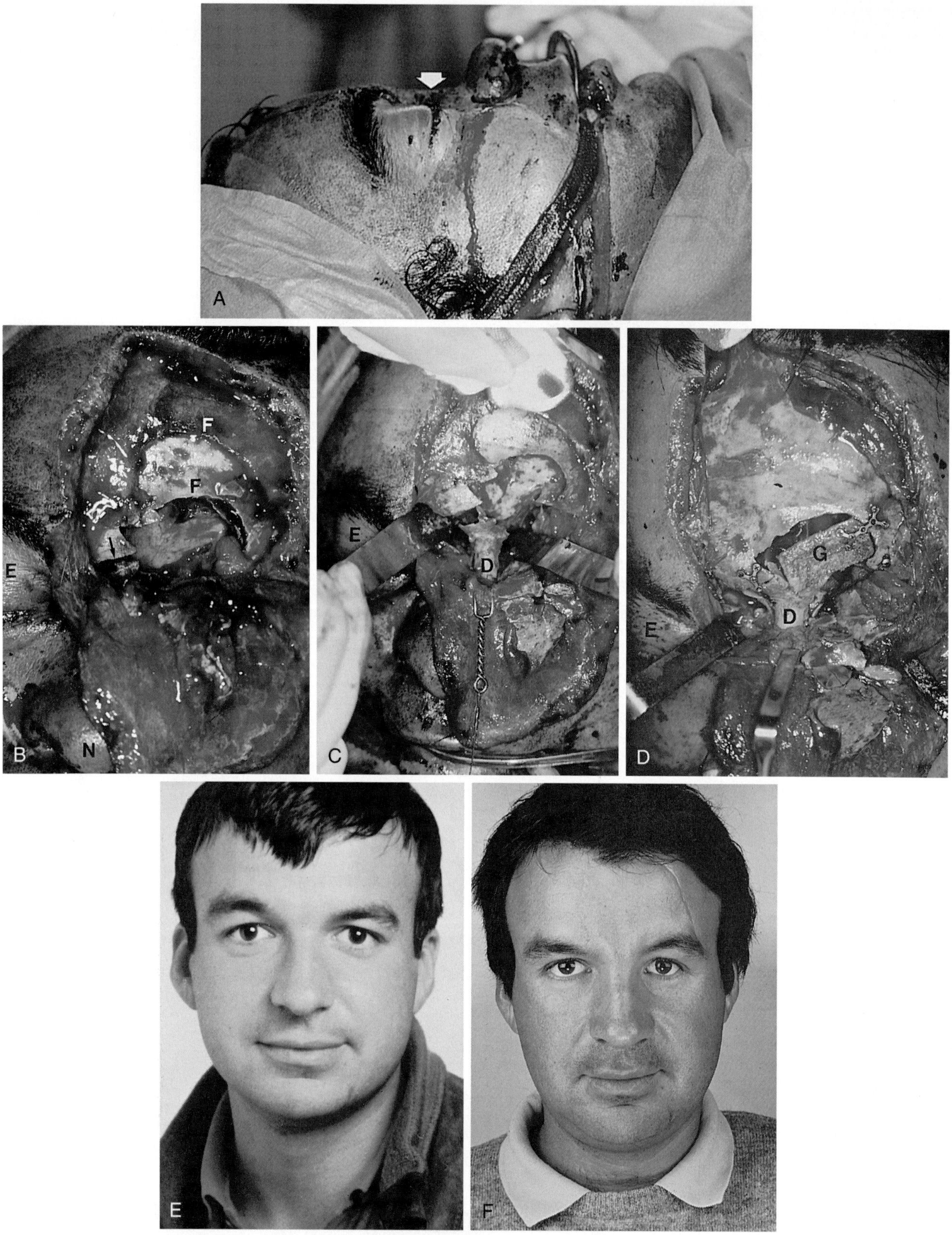

FIGURE 10–21. Complex midface frontonasoethmoidal fractures. *A,* Preoperative view depicting the inwardly telescoped nasal buttress *(arrow)*. *B,* The open laceration wound with loss of the frontal sinus wall (F), disattached nasal buttress *(arrow)*, and midface. (N = tip of nose.) *C,* Intraoperative view following management of the skull base, dural tears, and herniated devitalized brain tissue. The nasal buttress (D) is still disattached. *D,* Reduced midface and nasal buttress fractures and application of external table grafts (G) and microplate fixation (Leibinger). *E* and *F,* Preoperative (8 years before trauma) and postoperative views of the same patient. The laceration wound is still visible.

grafts (Fig. 10–21*B–D*). The optic nerve regained function immediately following decompression. The patient's appearance is shown in Figure 10–21*E* and *F*.

If there are multiple intracranially dislocated frontal and orbital fragments, these are temporarily removed (Fig. 10–22*A* and *B*). However, all the skull base planes including the optic nerve decompression are managed by the subfrontal approach, avoiding any retraction of the exposed frontal lobes or damage to the olfactory structures. Following this, the correct repositioning of the bone fragments is achieved

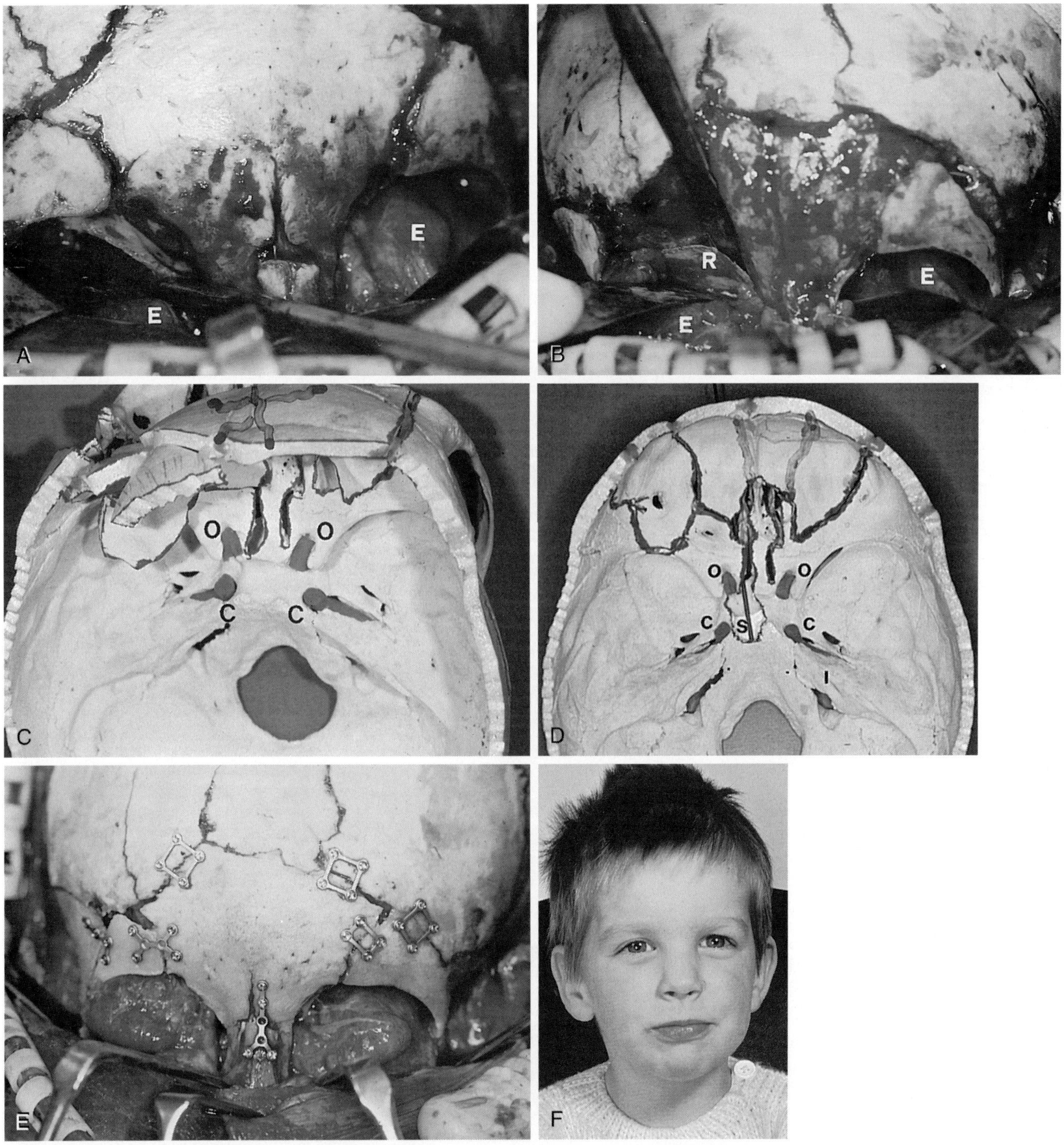

FIGURE 10–22. Intracranially dislocated fronto-orbital fracture pattern. *A*, Intraoperative view of multifragment fracture and intracranial dislocation of the frontal bone. The orbital roof fragments are already partially mobilized on the right, and the nasal buttress and midface are disattached. (E = eyeballs.) *B*, Temporarily removed frontal bone fragments. Further management of the skull base fractures, including fracture of the sphenoid and adjustment of the orbital roof (R) as well as suture and alignment of the dural tears, was performed by the subcranial approach, avoiding any frontal lobe retraction or damage to olfaction. *C* and *D*, Schematic drawing and intraoperative view depicting the intracranial configuration that is accessed by the subcranial approach. Note the adjacent vital structures: optic nerve (O), carotid artery (C), and sphenoid (S). Accurate reduction of the fractures allowed by the anterior (in contrast to the transfrontal) approach is crucial for correct adjustment of the midface fractures. *E* and *F*, Microplate fixation and view of face.

and retained with microplates, and the correct relationships for the adjustment of the nasal and midface fractures are provided (Fig. 10–22*C–F*). In our series deferral of primary definite management, as used with the transfrontal approach, was avoided, and accordingly the morbidity rate was significantly reduced.

Gunshot Injuries and Complex Soft Tissue–Bone Loss

One of the major controversial aspects in the management of gunshot injuries is the timing and extent of the primary reconstruction. Such injuries should be meticulously evaluated in regard to the demarcation zone of the devitalized soft tissue borders and the bone fragments, and the involved soft tissues should be preserved, keeping debridement to an absolute minimum. In our experience, the concept of a simple hemostasis and a limited temporary primary closure of the defects, leaving most of the involved structures to be reconstructed in a later secondary procedure is not to be recommended. The primary treatment should include the reconstruction of osseous tissues as well as soft tissues, even

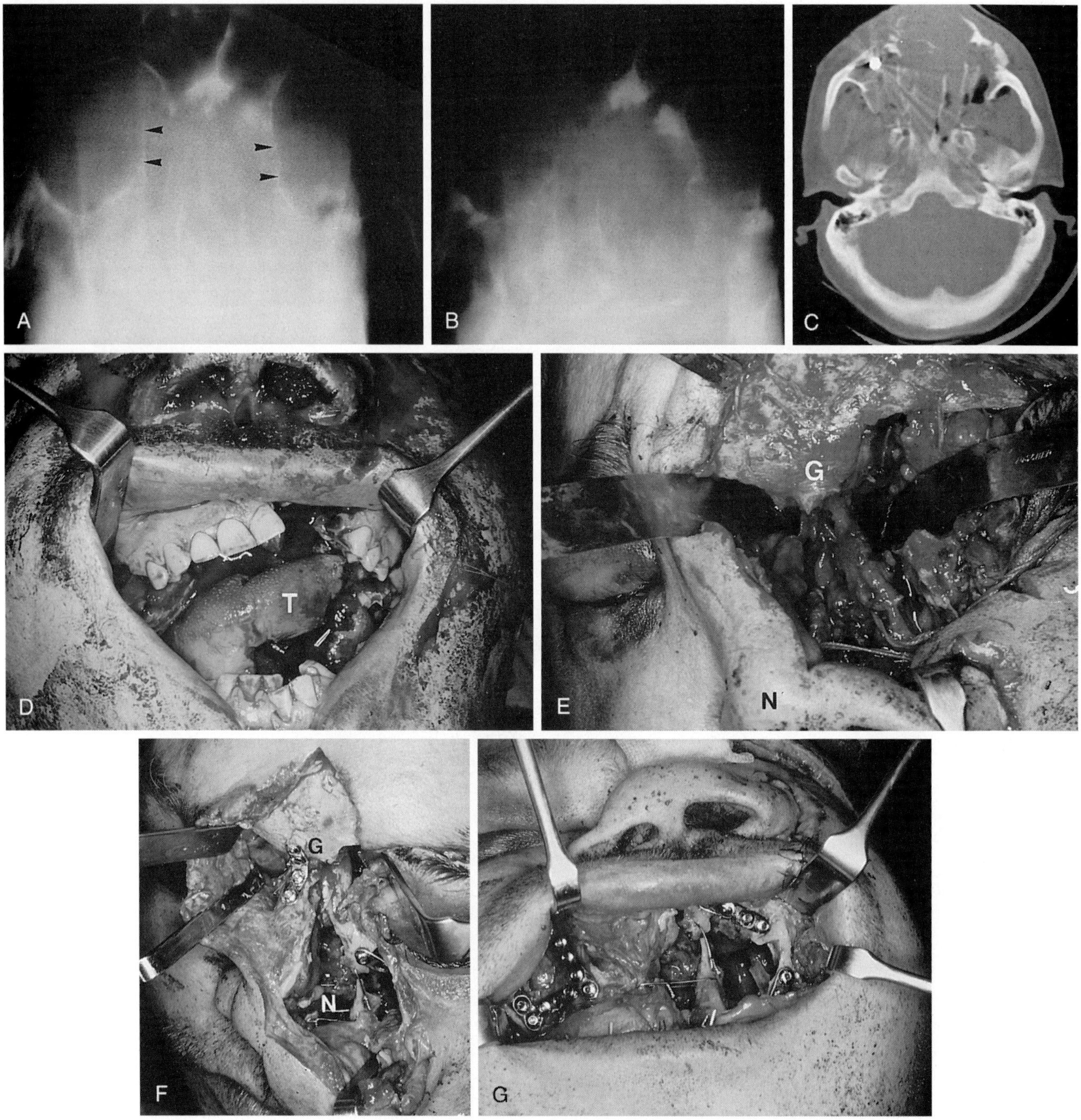

FIGURE 10–23. Gunshot injury and loss of bone. *A–C,* Radiographs illustrating the extent of the dislocation and defects along the midface. *D,* Intraoral view illustrating dislocation of the alveolar fragments of the midface and lower jaw as well as the palatinal defect. (T = tongue.) *E,* The entire midface–nasal frame as well as the orbital floor and medial wall were blown away. Further broad defects along the skull base were manifest. (N = tip of nose; G = glabella.) *F,* Partial stage of the midface and orbital cone reconstruction with bone grafts. *G,* Intraoral view of the partially reconstructed palate and occlusion.

using local flaps to achieve an acceptable primary result or to provide a solid basis for later correction. Only in patients with extensive loss of tissue should free, nonvascularized, and revascularized flaps be deferred to a secondary procedure. Accordingly, the recipient bed must be established in the primary session. Several of these aspects are illustrated in the following cases.

The damaged structures following a gunshot injury to the lower jaw and involving disruption of the palate, midface, naso-orbital area, and skull base region are illustrated in Figure 10–23. The primary surgical procedure included setting and retaining the remaining occlusion and reducing the lower and multiple upper jaw fragments. Preparation of local mucosal flaps allowed closure of the palate. The pieces of bone in the fractured orbital cone and zygoma were reconstructed using lyophilized cartilage and free external table grafts. Because the size of these grafts was relatively small, such a primary procedure was justified. The skull base lesions were managed and the soft tissues were adapted using local flaps. Thus only one secondary procedure involving osseous reconstruction of the nasal frame was necessary, allowing achievement of a satisfactory aesthetic and functional result (Fig. 10–23*H–L*).

A gunshot injury in which the bullet penetrated the oral cavity and disrupted the maxillo-orbital cavity, leading to loss of the right eye and the nasal buttress is depicted in Fig. 10–24. In this case, primary management included reconstruction of the maxilla, enucleation of the eye, and reconstruction of the orbital cone, the skull base lesions, and the nasal buttress. The symmetry achieved and the application of the eye prosthesis made further secondary corrections unnecessary.

A different situation is manifested in patients in whom extensive bone and soft tissue loss occurs (Fig. 10–25*A–C*). In this patient, the loss of the lower jaw bone and the palate, midface, and nasal structures, as well as the two-sided disruption of the zygoma complex and loss of parts of the lower and upper lip had to be treated in secondary sessions. Even so, the primary reconstruction should be performed in a way that minimizes the extent of the secondary corrections needed and guarantees an optimal configuration for any further steps. In this case, the correct relation of the lower jaw stumps was retained with a reconstruction plate, and the palate was closed using soft palate mucosal flaps and replacing multiple bone fragments. The skull base and the multiple dural tears and herniated devitalized brain tissue were managed by the subfrontal approach as already described. The soft tissues were tailored and adapted to allow temporary closure of the defects.

Further secondary procedures were necessary to reconstruct the back of the nose. The collumella and the nasal septum were reconstructed using a labial fold flap combined with a free cartilage graft harvested from the ear concha (Fig. 10–25*D–F*), and the upper lip defect was corrected

Text continued on page 140

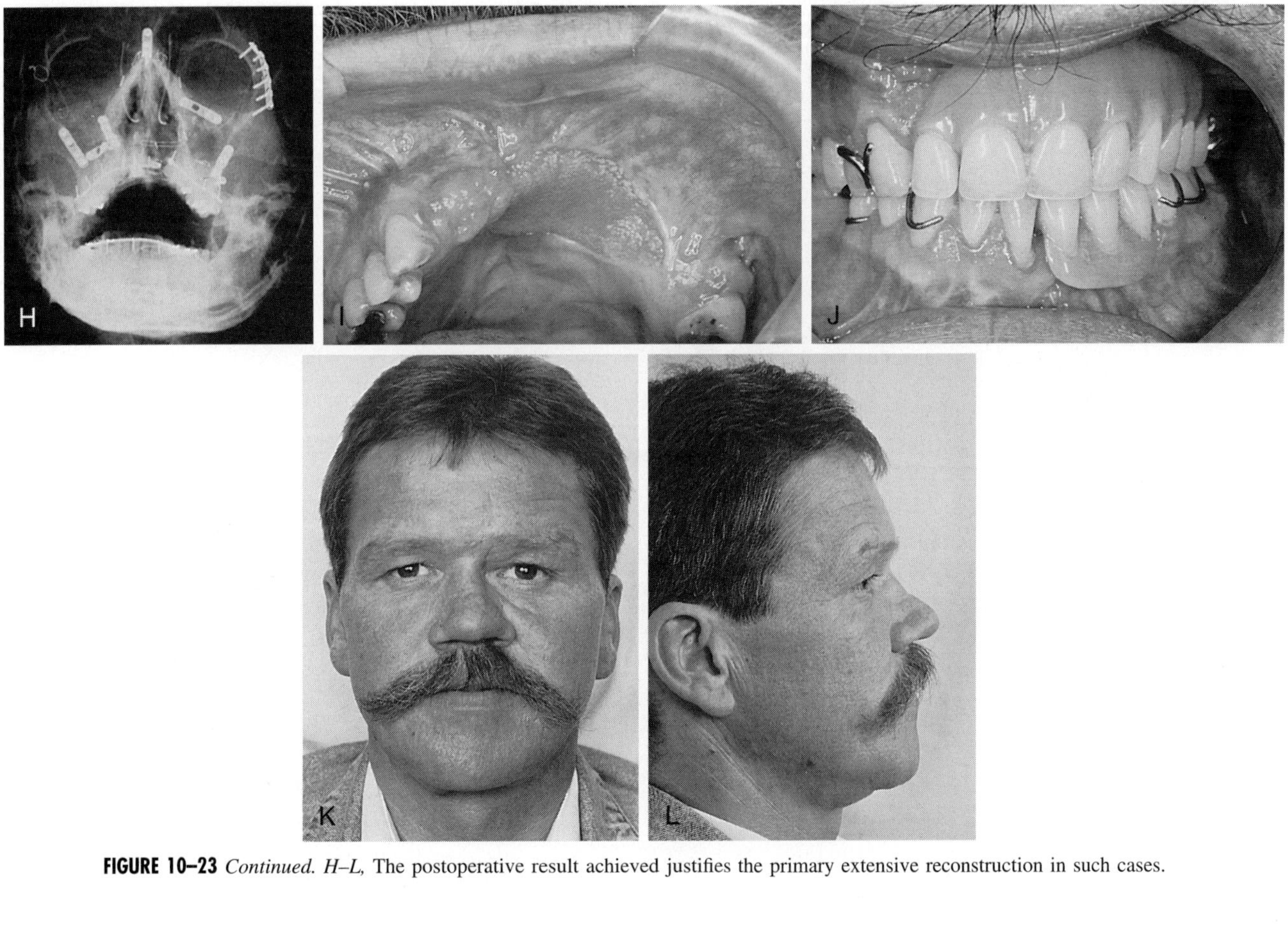

FIGURE 10–23 *Continued. H–L,* The postoperative result achieved justifies the primary extensive reconstruction in such cases.

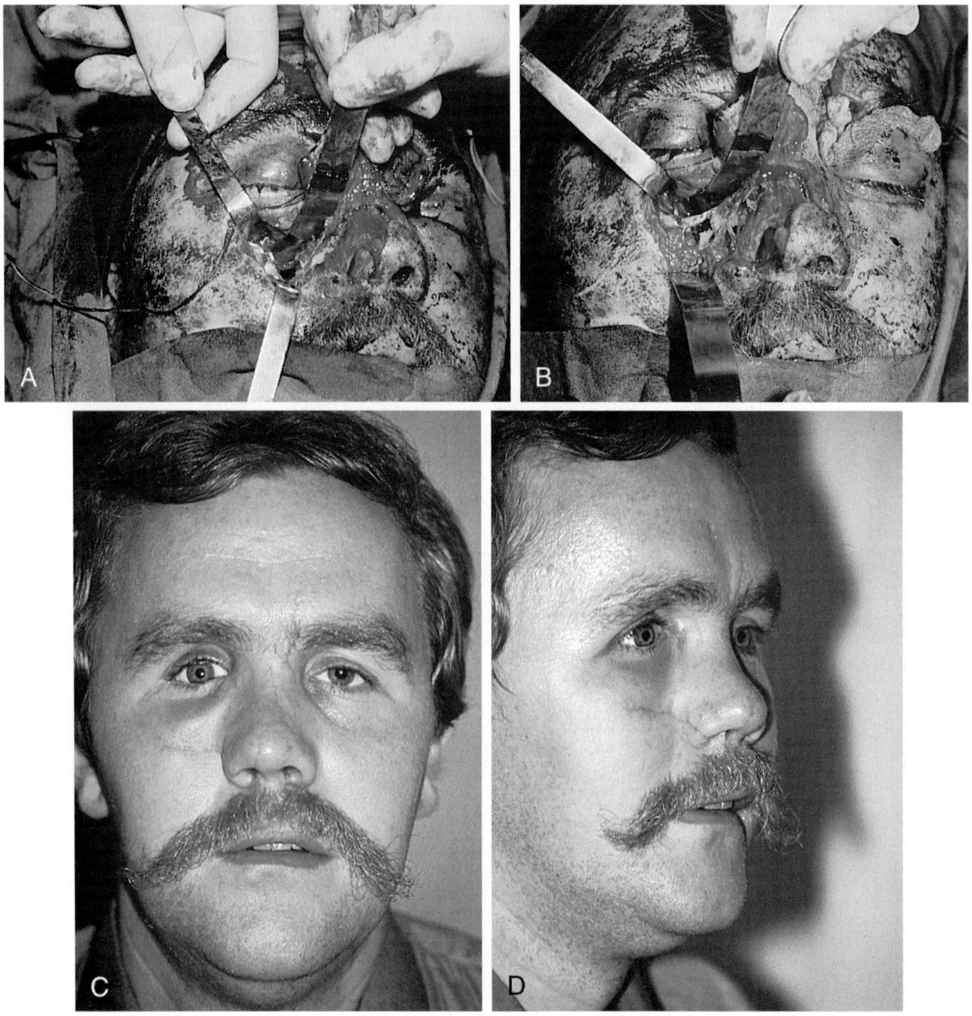

FIGURE 10–24. Gunshot injury—one-stage reconstruction. *A,* Intraoperative view of the gunshot wound, which penetrated the palate and exited from the glabella with loss of the right eye and skull base disruption. *B,* Intraoperative view showing partial reconstruction of the orbital-maxillary sinus and the already redressed skull base. *C* and *D,* Postoperative view of face following application of an eye prosthesis on the right and a reconstructed nasal frame midface and zygoma.

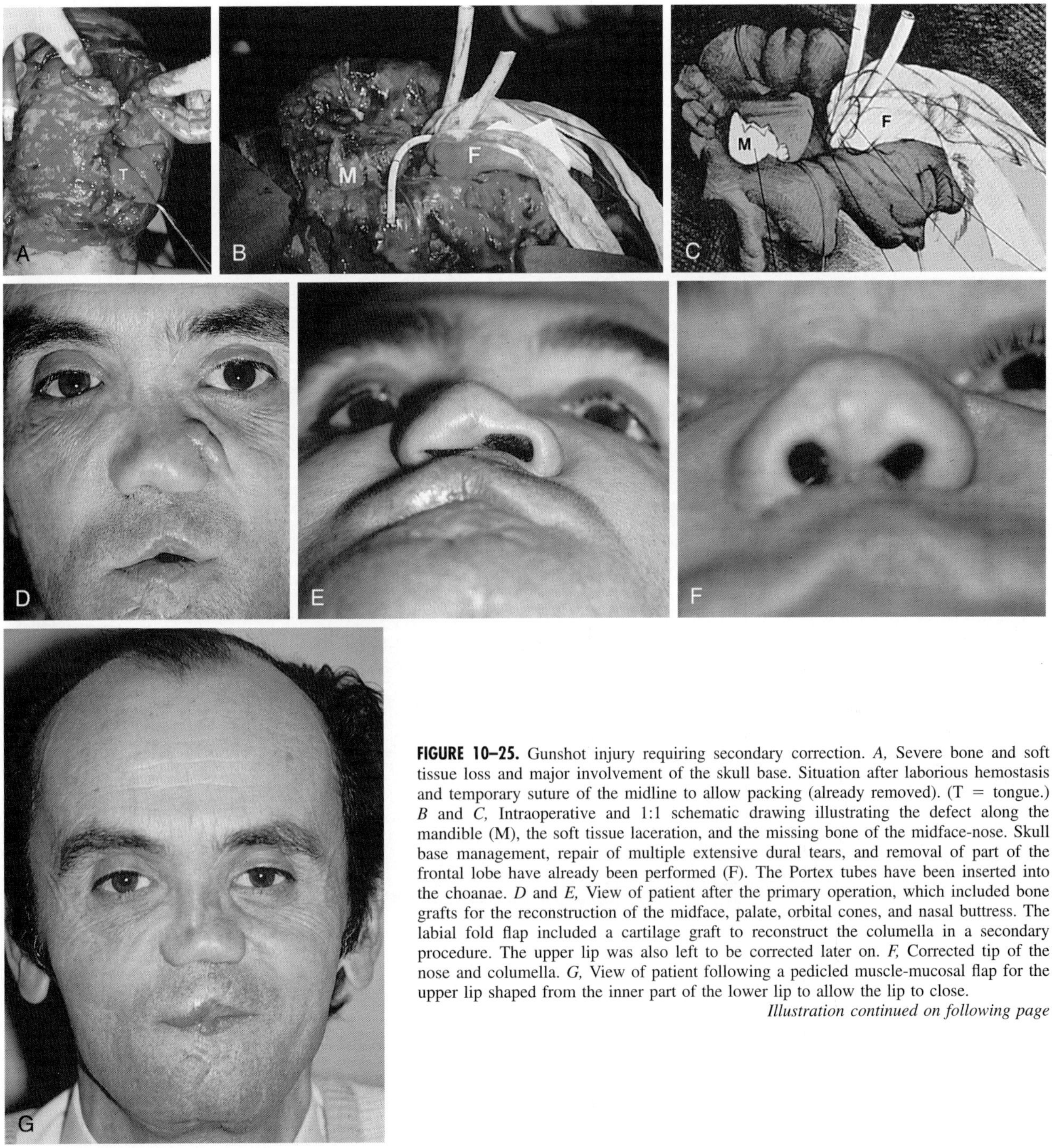

FIGURE 10–25. Gunshot injury requiring secondary correction. *A,* Severe bone and soft tissue loss and major involvement of the skull base. Situation after laborious hemostasis and temporary suture of the midline to allow packing (already removed). (T = tongue.) *B* and *C,* Intraoperative and 1:1 schematic drawing illustrating the defect along the mandible (M), the soft tissue laceration, and the missing bone of the midface-nose. Skull base management, repair of multiple extensive dural tears, and removal of part of the frontal lobe have already been performed (F). The Portex tubes have been inserted into the choanae. *D* and *E,* View of patient after the primary operation, which included bone grafts for the reconstruction of the midface, palate, orbital cones, and nasal buttress. The labial fold flap included a cartilage graft to reconstruct the columella in a secondary procedure. The upper lip was also left to be corrected later on. *F,* Corrected tip of the nose and columella. *G,* View of patient following a pedicled muscle-mucosal flap for the upper lip shaped from the inner part of the lower lip to allow the lip to close.

Illustration continued on following page

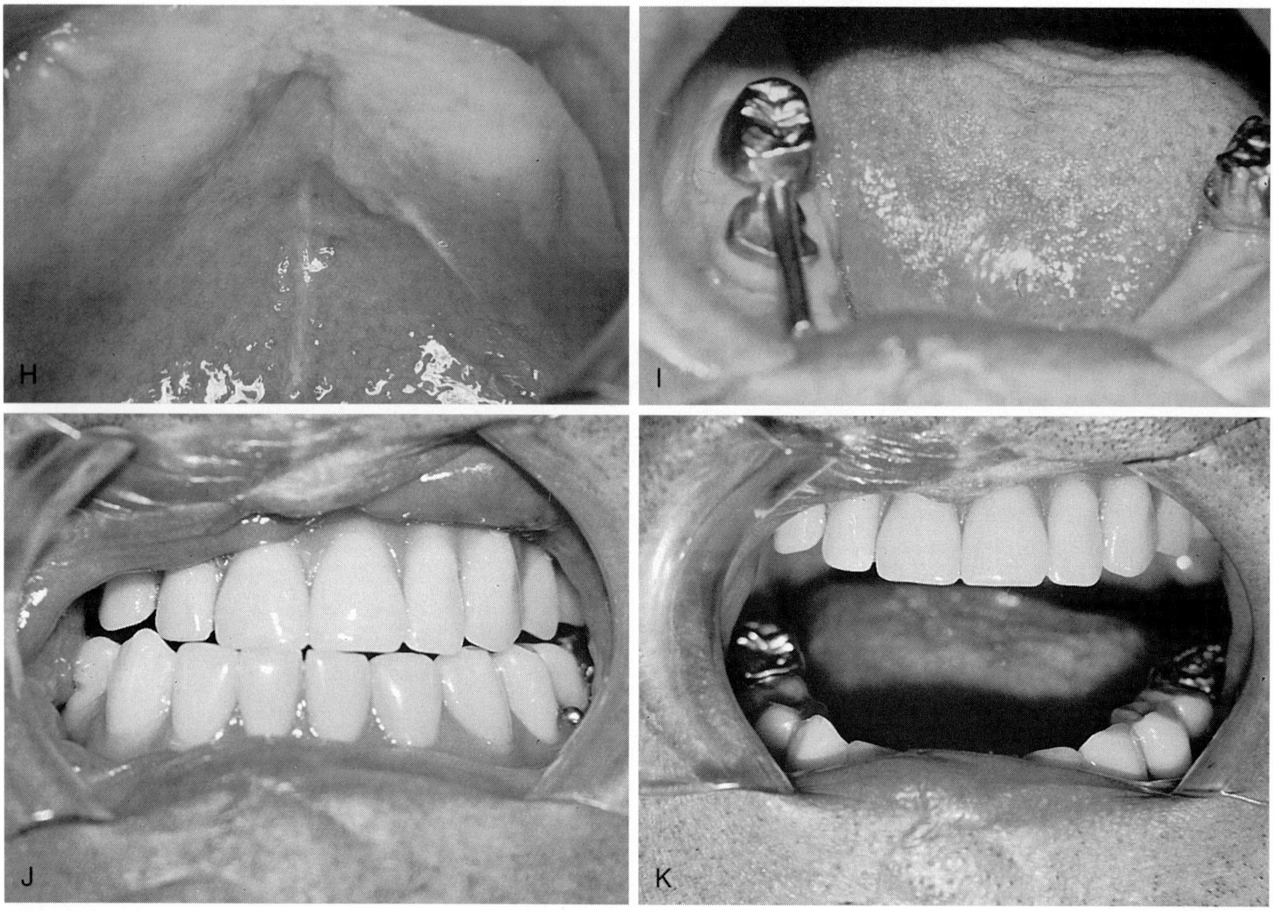

FIGURE 10–25 *Continued. H,* Closed palate and intact consolidated mucosal flaps. *I–K,* Following grafting of the mandibular defect in a secondary procedure, the application of a denture was satisfactory.

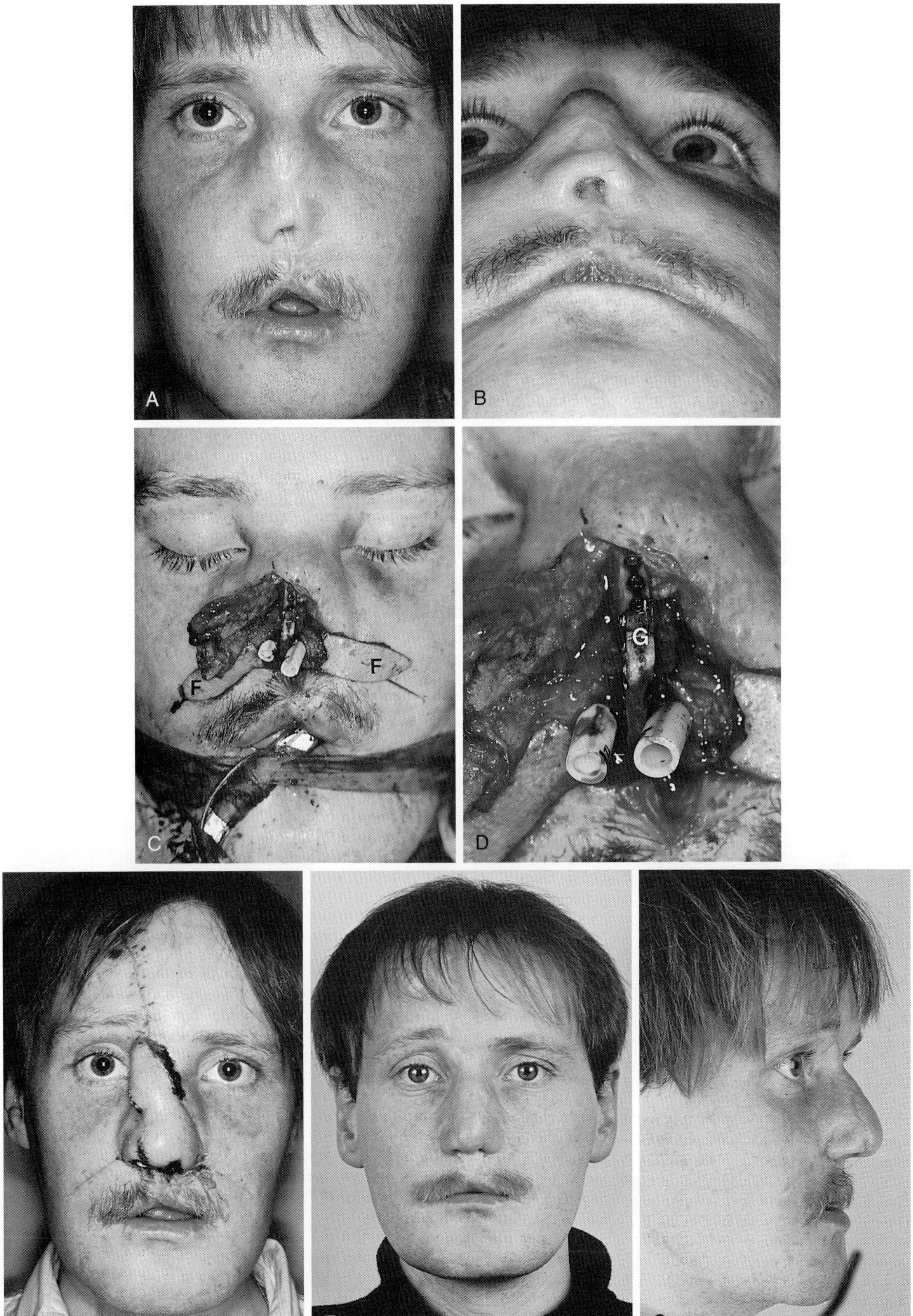

FIGURE 10–26. Gunshot injury requiring secondary correction of the nose. *A* and *B,* View of patient and deformity. *C* and *D,* Bone grafts (G) fixed with microplates for reconstruction of the back of the nose and septum. The Portex tubes have been inserted into the newly formed nasal lumen. (F = nasolabial flaps for the alae.) *E,* Forehead flap following the application of an expander. *F* and *G,* Views of face.

using a muscle-mucosal flap pedicled to the lower lip, thus allowing the lip closure. The lower jaw defect was bridged by an iliac crest graft, and further reconstruction allowing application of a denture was necessary (Fig. 10–25*G–K*).

Extensive loss of nasal tissue also represents an indication for secondary surgery (Fig. 10–26). In this case, a combination of local flaps and a forehead pedicled flap, treated with an expander, achieved an acceptable result.

For more detailed information on trauma we refer the reader to other sources.[9–14]

SUMMARY

In this chapter only very specific aspects of reconstruction have been included; a more detailed and systematic description of these aspects and the variety of methods and techniques used to achieve them would have been beyond the scope of a chapter. We have emphasized the most controversial and actual aspects of reconstruction of the face and orbit, using representative cases to illustrate the various categories. A detailed statistical evaluation and follow-up, as required for scientific papers, was intentionally omitted. Yet by providing the references we tried to compensate for that.

REFERENCES

1. Raveh J, Turk J, Lädrach K, et al: The extended anterior subcranial approach for skull base tumors—long-term results. J Neurosurg 82:1002, 1995.
2. Raveh J, Lädrach K, Speiser M, et al: The subcranial approach for fronto-orbital and anteroposterior skull-base tumors. Arch Otolaryngol Head Neck Surg 119(4):385, 1993.
3. Lädrach K, Raveh J: Advantages of the combined subcranial/transfrontal approach for frontal skull base tumor resection. Fourth International Congress of the International Society of Cranio-Maxillofacial Surgery, Santiago de Compostela, June 1991. Craniofac Surg 4:293, 1992.
4. Raveh J, Vuillemin T: The subcranial-supraorbital and temporal approach for tumor resection. J Craniofac Surg 1(1):53, 1990.
5. Lädrach K, Annino D, Raveh J, et al: Advanced approaches to cranio-orbital injuries. Facial Plast Surg Clin North Am 3(1):107, 1995.
6. Zingg M, Lädrach K, Chen JM, et al: Classification and treatment of zygomatic fractures: A review of 1025 cases. J Oral Maxillofac Surg 50:778, 1992.
7. Chen JM, Zingg M, Lädrach K, et al: Early surgical intervention of orbital floor fractures—a clinical evaluation of lyophilized dura and cartilage reconstruction. J Oral Maxillofac Surg 50:935, 1992.
8. Zingg M, Chowdhury K, Lädrach K, et al: Treatment of 813 zygoma-lateral orbital complex fractures: New aspects. Arch Otolaryngol Head Neck Surg 117:611, 1991.
9. Vuillemin T, Raveh J: The correction of traumatically induced craniofacial skeletal disruption with concomitant hypertelorism and skull base involvement. Fourth International Congress of the International Society of Cranio-Maxillofacial Surgery, Santiago de Compostela, June 1991. Craniofac Surg 4:273, 1992.
10. Raveh J, Lädrach K, Vuillemin T, et al: Management of combined fronto-naso-orbital/skull base fractures and telecanthus in 355 cases. Arch Otolaryngol Head Neck Surg 118(6):605, 1992.
11. Raveh J, Vuillemin T: Advantages of the subcranial approach in craniofacial surgery. *In* Gruss J, Manson P, Yaremchuck M (eds): Rigid Fixation of the Craniofacial Skeleton. Boston, Butterworth-Heinemann, 1992, p. 561.
12. Raveh J, Vuillemin T: Subcranial management of 395 combined frontobasal-midface fractures. Arch Otolaryngol 114:1115, 1989.
13. Raveh J, Vuillemin T: The surgical one-stage management of combined cranio-maxillofacial and frontobasal fractures: Advantage of the subcranial approach in 374 cases. J Craniomaxillofac Surg 16:160, 1988.
14. Raveh J, Redli M, Markwalder T: Operative management of 194 cases of combined maxillofacial-frontobasal fractures: Principles and modifications. J Oral Maxillofac Surg 42:555, 1984.

CHAPTER 11

Free Flap Reconstruction Techniques of the Skull Base

David W. Stepnick, M.D.

Over the past several decades, increasingly more aggressive procedures for resection of neoplasms involving the cranial base have been performed by oncologic surgeons. Now an established field of surgical oncology, skull base oncologic surgery is associated with tumor-free survivals of up to 80% with follow-up periods of as long as 24 months.[3] In one of the earliest analyses of complications following oncologic craniofacial surgery, Ketchum and colleagues[8] in 1966 reported an incidence of 47% for cerebrospinal fluid leaks and 27% for osteomyelitis following resection of cranial base tumors involving the paranasal sinuses. Some 30 years later, these complications still plague the skull base surgeon, although the overall incidence of such complications has plummeted to about 10%.[3] In addition to a more thorough understanding of the surgical principles involved in the procedures themselves, improvements in perioperative imaging and intraoperative monitoring have allowed oncologic surgeons to perform these complicated excisions in a relatively safe manner. Minimizing morbidity depends not only on the techniques used for tumor resection but also on advances made in reconstructive techniques.

Bacterial contamination is usually avoided at all costs in intracranial neurosurgical procedures, whereas otolaryngologists routinely operate in the clean-contaminated environment of the upper aerodigestive tract. These two disciplines are combined in cranial base surgery, as are these two normally separate areas. The dura is routinely opened and often actually resected in the course of these procedures. Successful reconstruction following cranial base surgery necessitates reestablishment of the separation between the intracranial cavity and the upper aerodigestive tract, the creation of a watertight closure following tumor removal, and the elimination of dead space.

Reestablishment of an intact *bony* cranial base remains controversial. Some believe that a three-layered closure consisting of dural repair, bone grafts for skeletal reconstruction, and skin grafts to replace the paranasal sinus mucosa is essential to minimize the risk of complications, whereas others believe that the risk of infection around nonvascularized bone fragments is lower, skin graft take is higher, surgery is easier, and the chances of pseudoencephalocele are minimal when the bony skeleton is *not* reconstructed.[29] Following a retrospective analysis of 16 patients who had undergone cranial base resection without skeletal reconstruction, Spinelli and colleagues[29] concluded that defects involving only the anterior cranial base, regardless of size, do not necessarily require bone replacement, whereas defects involving exposure of both the anterior and middle fossae should be considered for bony reconstruction because problems such as pulsating exophthalmos may result from temporal lobe herniation into the orbit, especially if the periorbita has been opened.

An ideal cranial base reconstructive procedure is one that restores bony and soft tissue defects, thereby obliterating any dead space including the involved paranasal sinuses, while covering exposed vessels and nonvascularized grafts, supporting neural structures, and achieving a watertight dural seal. Additionally, it maintains optimal cosmetic and functional integrity. Reconstruction using local fascial flaps, transposition of locoregional muscle flaps, or microsurgical tissue transfer should be considered when it is desirable to obliterate the paranasal sinuses, cover tenuous dural grafts or repairs, or separate the nasopharynx from the dura of the frontal and temporal lobes and posterior fossa to prevent leakage of cerebrospinal fluid (CSF) and meningitis.[5]

In contrast to similar procedures done for other reasons (e.g., craniofacial trauma or congenital syndromes), a unique aspect of oncologic procedures involving the skull base is the need to deal with the presence of preoperative or postoperative radiotherapy, which is frequently used as part of the cancer therapy. Its inclusion in the treatment regimen appears to increase the probability of complications such as CSF leak. It is widely recognized that the use of vascularized tissue for dural seal and dead space obliteration is associated with a decreased incidence of these complications, especially in irradiated patients.

A variety of vascularized flaps, ranging from local flaps to revascularized free tissue transfers, are available to the reconstructive surgeon. Local tissues that can be advanced into these wounds include pericranial, temporalis or temporalis fascial, temporoparietal fascial, and galeal flaps. When these flaps are impractical because they were sacrificed during tumor resection, are unsuitable owing to radiotherapy, or do not provide sufficient tissue bulk, free flaps or pedicled fasciocutaneous, muscle, or myocutaneous flaps such as the latissimus dorsi, trapezius, pectoralis major, and sternocleidomastoid flaps may be used. Limitations caused by pedicle length or arc of rotation can be circumvented by using free flaps in which distant tissue is transplanted to the cranial base region and revascularized by restoring blood flow through the use of local recipient vessels. Rectus abdominis flaps are most commonly used; less frequently, radial forearm, latissimus dorsi, lateral arm, omentum, and scapular flaps have been used. Analysis of the surgical defect is required to determine which of these flaps is most appropriate for the reconstruction of a particular defect.

LOCAL FLAPS

Anatomy of the Scalp

The outermost layers of the scalp are the skin and subcutaneous tissue, which are essentially inseparable components covering the cranium. Under these layers one finds the galea aponeurotica, a dense, fibrous sheet of tissue formed as a condensation between the frontalis muscle anteriorly and the occipitalis muscle posteriorly. It continues laterally as the temporalis fascia, also called the superficial temporal fascia, galeal extension, and epicranial aponeurosis. As a distinct vascularized entity, the galea aponeurotica can be transposed and used for reconstructive purposes. Laterally, in the temporoparietal region, the subgaleal fascia is quite well developed and richly vascularized from the superficial temporal artery.[34] It overlies the temporalis fascia, which invests the temporalis muscle and directly attaches to the surrounding periosteum. In contrast, it is quite thin at the vertex and consists of loose areolar tissue. Although it is surgically dissectable, it is not particularly useful as a separate layer in cranial base reconstruction. The deepest layer of soft tissue overlying the skull is the periosteum, which, when used alone, can support a graft but is generally of insufficient thickness to be used as a flap. Separately, these layers are of little use, but together, the latter two layers comprise the pericranium, one of the most useful flaps in anterior skull base reconstruction. Snyderman and associates[26] reviewed 30 patients who underwent anterior cranial base reconstruction, mostly for malignant neoplasms, with pericranial, galeopericranial, and galeal scalp flaps without skin grafts. All flaps healed without persistent CSF leaks, meningitis, or brain herniation, and all showed evidence of spontaneous mucosalization of the intranasal surface. Together, these tissues provide an excellent source of tissue for many small anterior skull base defects.

The Pericranium (Pericranial Flap)

The pericranial flap is highly vascularized and can be used alone or in combination with other tissues. It derives its blood supply from both the internal and external carotid systems. Whether its intrinsic blood flow occurs in an axial or random pattern is an element of debate. Its potential use must be considered well before the resection begins because it is developed after the bicoronal incision is made but before tumor resection begins. It is then protected throughout the course of the resection. Once resection is complete, dural tears are repaired and dural defects are covered with fascial grafts. The pericranial flap is then rotated onto the floor of the anterior fossa. Because the primary focus of this chapter is free flap reconstruction of the skull base, further details of the pericranial flap will not be described. However, this important flap must be mentioned because of its significance. Its use is recommended for small to moderate size defects of the anterior fossa or in combination with a laterally based temporalis flap for larger defects that extend laterally from the midline to involve a portion of the orbital roof.[22] Larger defects often require other methods of repair, which are described subsequently.

PEDICLED FLAPS VERSUS FREE FLAPS

Free tissue transfer failure rates in the head and neck are low, in the range of 0 to 6%. Kroll and colleagues[10] compared the use of free rectus abdominis flaps with that of pectoralis major myocutaneous flaps (performed by the same surgeons) and reported a higher failure rate—5% to 14%—in the latter group. Flap reliability, per se, should *not* be cited as a reason not to employ free flaps for skull base reconstruction. Indeed, their reliability with respect to not only flap survival but also their ability to resist infection and to separate the intracranial space from the outside often makes free tissue transfer flaps the option of choice for such defects.

Some have argued against the use of free flaps in patients who require radiation therapy as adjunctive treatment for head and neck cancer. However, studies have demonstrated that radiation does not produce significant untoward effects on the patency of microvascular anastomoses.[9, 14] Even in the presence of comorbid conditions such as diabetes or coronary artery disease in elderly patients, some authors have reported flap success rates of over 90%[23] with acceptable or less postoperative morbidity, flap complication rates, and shorter hospital stays.[7, 24] Neligan and colleagues[15] compared the use of local, pedicled, and free flap reconstruction in 90 skull base procedures and found a higher rate of uncomplicated primary wound healing (95% versus 62.5%) and a lower incidence of flap loss (0%), CSF leak (5%), meningitis, and abscess (0%) for free flaps compared with pedicled myocutaneous flaps.[15] They concluded that microvascular free tissue transfer is the safest and most economical procedure for reconstruction of moderate to large defects of the skull base. In another series the outcomes of free tissue transfers for the reconstruction of extensive defects of the sino-orbital region were reviewed. Cranial base repairs healed without sequelae; the authors concluded that free tissue transfer is the safest and most versatile reconstructive procedure for such defects.[33] Specific reasons for choosing free tissue transfers rather than other techniques include the presence of previous radiation therapy or surgery, distance of the defect from vascular pedicles, making pedicled flaps impossible or impractical owing to a limited arc of rotation, and tissue requirements that can only be met with a free flap.[33]

FREE FLAPS

A number of advantages of free tissue transfers for reconstruction of skull base defects are immediately apparent. First and foremost, they allow placement of richly vascularized tissue that can heal primarily. This tissue facilitates wound healing, resists the deleterious effects of radiation, nourishes poorly vascularized tissues that have been previously irradiated, and helps in the delivery of chemotherapeutic agents to the region. Furthermore, separation of the upper aerodigestive tract from the meninges is easily accomplished, as is the elimination of dead space. With primary wound healing, postoperative radiation can be initiated without delay.

Rectus Abdominis Flap

If any free flap deserves recognition as a "workhorse" flap for cranial base reconstruction, it is the rectus abdominis flap. It is the flap of choice for many cranial base defects, and it has been used to repair anterior, middle, and posterior fossa defects.[6, 36] A variety of features make the flap ideally suited for many reconstructive procedures requiring free tissue transfer to the skull base.

It may be raised either as a vascularized muscle flap or as a true myocutaneous flap. The entire muscle or a small portion thereof can be used according to the anticipated defect. Because of its location, it is readily accessible to a second operating team, allowing concomitant harvest of the tissue while the ablative procedure is underway. Although harvest of the flap requires a thorough knowledge of the anatomy of the abdominal wall, it is relatively easy and can be done fairly quickly. The flap is exceedingly reliable. Its pedicle, the deep inferior epigastric artery (DIEA) and vein (DIEV), is of large caliber (usually 3 to 4 mm) and relatively long. Although there is some variation with respect to the course of the vessels between the external iliac vessels and the medial border of the rectus abdominis muscle, their presence is constant.[13]

The rectus abdominis muscles are paired paramedian muscles of the anterior abdominal wall. The muscles, whose fibers are oriented in a vertical direction, originate from the pubis, span the entire abdomen, and insert into the anterior-inferior thorax. Its function is to flex the trunk; the absence of one of the two muscles is of little functional impact, assuming that closure is adequate and proper healing prevents an abdominal wall hernia or bulge.

According to the Mathes and Nahai classification, the rectus abdominis is a type III muscle[11] that has two dominant blood supplies that anastomose above the umbilicus through small vessels known as choke vessels.[31] The deep superior epigastric artery (DSEA) and vein (DSEV) originate superiorly and course downward, while the DIEA and DIEV originate inferiorly and course upward. The latter vessels may be divided, allowing upward rotation about the superior pedicle and creating a superiorly based pedicled flap that is frequently used for breast reconstruction. However, when used for cranial base reconstruction as a free flap, the superior pedicle is divided, and the flap is carefully dissected along with its larger caliber inferior pedicle vessels. The DIEA originates from the external iliac artery, near the origin of the deep circumflex iliac artery, and courses laterally, entering the muscle medially above its origin. It then passes superiorly on the undersurface of the muscle, arborizes, and connects with the DSEA system.

The muscle with its vascular pedicle can be harvested with or without an overlying cutaneous component. When dissected as a composite flap, fascia, subcutaneous tissue, and skin can be transferred as well as the muscle itself. As a revascularized muscle, it is an excellent source of vascularized tissue that fills dead space, seals the dura from the paranasal sinuses, helps prevent CSF leakage, and resists infection. It can also provide a vascular supply to free bone grafts or areas compromised by prior surgery, infection, or radiation therapy. The anterior sheath can be harvested above the arcuate line without fear of ventral hernia formation and is useful as a thin, tough layer that can be sewn to the margins of a defect to achieve a watertight seal. The muscle readily accepts a skin graft, when necessary.

The cutaneous portion of the flap can be designed with a transverse, vertical, or oblique orientation. As with the muscle, a very small or very large cutaneous paddle can be harvested. Periumbilical perforators send branches from the muscle to the overlying abdominal wall skin, which then course in a radial fashion from an epicenter in the umbilical region. The richest concentration of perforators from the underlying rectus muscles is in this region, and incorporation of skin from this region is essential to ensure skin survival. If an obliquely oriented flap is chosen, an ellipse of skin is designed that has its long axis along a line drawn between the umbilicus and the tip of the scapula. The axial blood

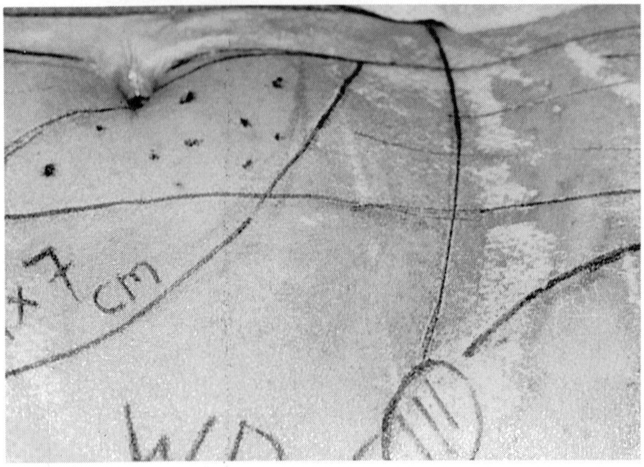

FIGURE 11–1. Rectus abdominis myocutaneous free flap. The obliquely oriented skin paddle of the flap must be designed to include its blood supply from periumbilical perforators, which course through the rectus muscle.

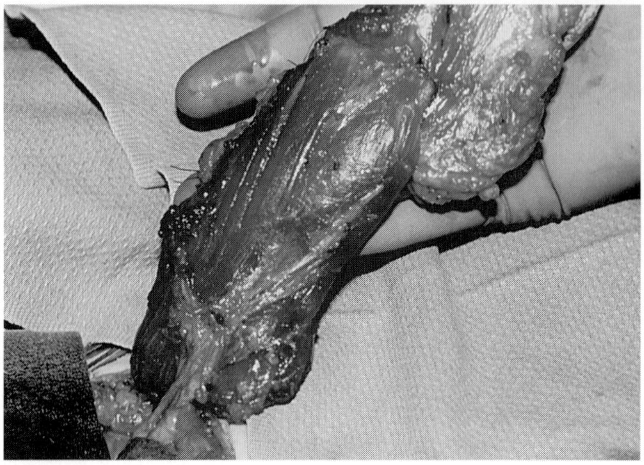

FIGURE 11–3. Rectus abdominis free flap, viewed from its undersurface. Note the deep circumflex iliac artery and vein vascular pedicle, still attached to the femoral vessels.

flow from this critical periumbilical area allows the skin to be harvested well lateral to the lateral border of the rectus muscle. This variation of the flap, also known as a thoracoumbilical flap, allows creation of a flap with varying tissue thicknesses: the skin is thickest in the periumbilical region and thinnest in the lateral region near the costal margin (Figs. 11–1 to 11–3).

Although the technique of flap dissection is beyond the scope of this chapter, it should be emphasized that the surgeon must be familiar with the anatomy of the anterior abdominal wall and must be cognizant of the need for meticulous repair of the fascial layers violated during dissection of the flap; if insufficient fascia is present secondary to its harvest and incorporation into the flap, a material such as Marlex mesh must be used for repair to prevent abdominal wall herniation.

This flap is exceedingly useful for cases in which local or regional tissues are unavailable or insufficient for closure following skull base resection. It has low metabolic requirements and, especially when harvested as a revascularized free muscle flap, readily conforms to the requirements of the surgical defect. It is the technique of choice for the management of problem cases resulting in complications such as local or regional flap failure, persistent CSF leak that does not respond to medical or "simpler" surgical management, and stubborn infections.

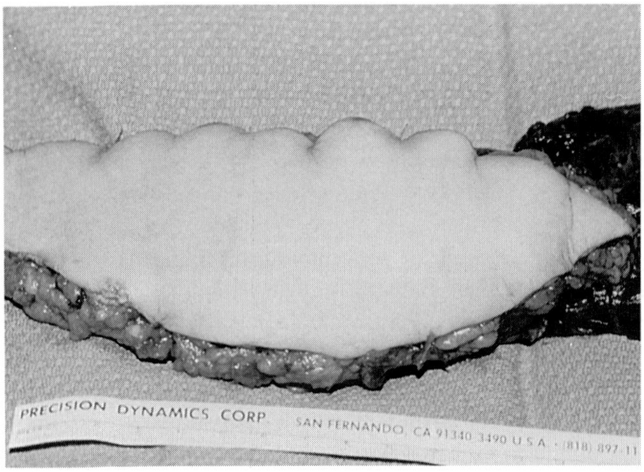

FIGURE 11–2. Large skin paddles are available (17 × 7 cm in this patient) with the rectus abdominis free flap, here viewed from above.

Consideration should be given to selection of this flap for reconstruction of larger defects and those involving the oral, nasal, and intracranial cavities as well as the orbit. We have used this flap to obliterate the entire orbital and maxillary sinus cavity following anterior craniofacial resection with orbital exenteration and maxillectomy. The dead space is easily obliterated, and a flat, skin-covered surface replaces the facial defect where the eye had been. It averts the need for lifetime cleansing of the cavity that would be otherwise needed for such defects.

In summary, this versatile flap is the most commonly used free flap for skull base reconstruction. Because of its reliability and low donor site morbidity, it should be considered as the reconstructive technique of choice for many skull base defects.

Latissimus Dorsi Flap

First described by Tansini in 1896 as a method of reconstructing postmastectomy chest wall defects,[31] and then virtually forgotten for nearly a century before its revival in the 1970s by Olivari,[16, 17] the latissimus dorsi flap has become an important part of the reconstructive surgeon's armamentarium. It has been used to repair a wide variety of defects including chest wall defects, pharyngoesophageal reconstruction, complex midfacial defects, scalp defects, dynamic reconstruction of cheek defects, and cranial base reconstruction. Its exceptionally long pedicle allows it to remain pedicled for many reconstructive applications. Watson and colleagues[35] recognized its potential as a free flap and were the first to report its successful transfer. It has an extremely large surface area and can be reliably transferred with or without overlying skin paddles, which, when used, can be designed as needed as multiple islands overlying the muscle. Donor site morbidity is low. The primary disadvantage is its dorsal location, which usually requires intraoperative repositioning of the patient to allow harvest and transfer. For this reason, it is not usually a first-line choice.

The latissimus dorsi muscle is a broad, flat muscle that arises from the thoracolumbar fascia, the spinous processes of the lower six thoracic vertebrae, and the lower four ribs. Its fibers coalesce and insert on the medial surface of the humerus. Blood supply to the flap is through the dominant thoracodorsal pedicle. According to the Mathes and Nahai classification, it is a type V muscle—one with a single dominant pedicle combined with several smaller segmental pedicles.[11] A large-caliber vessel (the artery is 2 to 3 mm in diameter) provides an excellent blood supply to the free flap. The segmental supply from the paraspinous perforators is divided in the course of the dissection. The thoracodorsal artery and vein arise from the subscapular vessels, themselves branches of the third portion of the axillary artery and vein. Branches to other muscles such as the serratus anterior, the subscapularis, and the teres minor are of clinical importance in composite flaps utilizing the serratus anterior or in scapular or parascapular flaps based on the circumflex scapular artery. They may be harvested with the latissimus dorsi as needed. The pedicle length of the combined thoracodorsal and subscapular arteries can be as much as 14 cm long, thus allowing the flap to reach easily across the midline and often as far as the vertex.

In cases in which pedicle length or the position of the defect limits flap placement at the recipient site, the flap can easily and readily be converted to a free flap. Flap surface area and length of the nutrient pedicle are important considerations in the selection of reconstructive options in the skull base region.

Despite its large size, the latissimus muscle is surprisingly thin. This desirable feature makes it especially useful for reconstruction of the scalp defects that are sometimes associated with skull base defects. Because of its relative pliability, the flap is valuable for various defects of the orbitomaxillary or skull base region in which a complex three-dimensional anatomy must be restored. Transfer of the muscle lined with a skin graft is yet another way of using a very thin flap to cover massive defects while still allowing primary closure of the donor site.

The skin overlying the thoracolumbar aponeurosis is very unreliable as a separate skin island, and its use should be avoided. When this skin is in continuity with skin overlying the more superior portion of the muscle, it must be considered a random extension of the flap. In a rather ingenious application of this (usually) unreliable portion of the flap, Smith and colleagues[25] described a patient with a composite defect of the scalp and skull in which the musculocutaneous portion of the flap was used to replace the scalp and the thoracolumbar fascia was used to patch a dural defect. A variety of other reports have attested to the efficacy of this flap in neurosurgical and cranial base applications.[1, 2, 19, 20, 30]

A wide variety of complications associated with the latissimus dorsi flap have been described in the literature and will not be further chronicled here. Although some of these are significant, they are generally unusual and typically minor in nature. Especially when the flap is designed more caudally near the inferior medial thoracolumbar fascia where perforators are less abundant, marginal necrosis is not uncommon. If this part of the flap is placed in a critical area of the wound, wound dehiscence and resultant problems may occur. Knowledge of the neurovascular anatomy and proper flap design help to minimize the chances of such problems occurring.

Radial Forearm Flap

The radial forearm free flap enjoys enormous popularity among surgeons who perform free tissue transfer. It is suited to a wide variety of reconstructive applications, not only in the head and neck but throughout the body. The radial forearm free flap was once known as the "Chinese flap" because of its introduction by Yang and colleagues[37] and subsequent reports from China.[27] Its use was popularized by Soutar and McGregor in the early 1980s,[28] and it has become perhaps the most frequently used of all free flaps.

As used by most otolaryngologists–head and neck surgeons, it is a fasciocutaneous flap harvested from the palmar aspect of the forearm. It may also be transferred as a composite flap containing vascularized bone, the brachioradialis, and/or the vascularized tendon. Its primary use in the head and neck region is to reconstruct oral cavity defects; it is particularly suited to this purpose because of its extraordinary thinness and pliability. Because of its versatility, it is suitable for a variety of defects. Moderate-sized flaps are readily available, the average size being about 10 × 10 cm. When greater surface area is needed, the flap can be extended up to the antecubital fossa from the flexor crease of the wrist or, although this is not generally recommended, almost circumferentially around the arm, leaving only a few centimeters of intact skin on the contralateral side.

Blood supply to the flap is from the large-caliber radial artery and the venae comitantes or superficial venous system, the former of which can be readily located and mapped before the flap is dissected. Preoperative assessment of adequate blood flow to the hand via the ulnar artery is accomplished using Allen's test, which is imperative before flap harvest is undertaken. There is only one report in the literature of a case in which insufficient blood flow to the hand resulted despite a normal Allen's test,[4] suggesting that this complication is indeed very rare. Donor site morbidity is one of the most frequent complications that may occur. Usually it is the result of skin graft loss due to either shearing of the underlying muscle or failure to preserve paratenon over the flexor tendons. Meticulous attention to details during closure can minimize these complications. Sensory neurologic problems may occur, usually as a result of transection of the antebrachial cutaneous nerve or superficial branches of the radial nerve. Motor function of the hand usually remains normal.

Venous outflow of the flap can occur through either the superficial venous system, the venae comitantes, or both. When the venae comitantes are used, it is usually necessary to follow the pedicle well up the forearm toward the antecubital fossa, where the vessels join and become a larger-caliber vein amenable to microvascular anastomosis. When harvested in this manner, the vascular pedicle is very long and can usually readily reach the neck, if required, to reconstruct a defect located at the base of the skull. A long pedicle can also be created from the superficial venous system.

Other features of this flap include the ability to harvest it as a composite osteocutaneous free flap by harvesting up to a third of the diameter of the radius along with the skin paddle, and its capacity for reinnervation, making it a sensate flap. Most otolaryngologists–head and neck surgeons do not harvest the bone as part of this flap (for skull base or other head and neck reconstruction procedures) because of what is considered an unacceptably high rate of pathologic fractures of the forearm. Furthermore, its sensate potential is of little use in cranial base reconstruction, and thus normally it is not reinnervated for this application.

Other Free and Pedicled Flaps

In the late 1970s and mid-1980s, McCraw and colleagues[12] and Rosen[21] both proposed using the trapezius flap for posterior and middle skull base reconstructions. As with the latissimus dorsi flap, this flap usually requires time-consuming intraoperative position changes. Additionally, its vascular supply is often compromised by ipsilateral radical neck dissection. It can be used, but because of positioning problems, it is difficult. Also, it is somewhat unreliable. Other pedicled flaps have been used as well but extremely infrequently. Free flaps currently provide more and better options.

The lateral arm flap, scapular-parascapular flap, and the omentum have either been used or represent potential sources of tissue for skull base defects. It is important for the reconstructive surgeon to have these flaps at his or her disposal; however, the three flaps previously described in detail should suffice as a source of tissue for skull base defects with rare exceptions.

CASE HISTORY

K.M., a 30-year-old male security guard, had been healthy when he was shot with a small-caliber weapon. The bullet entered the midface, violated the base of the skull, and lodged in the mastoid region of the temporal bone. He presented to the author after undergoing 19 surgical procedures subsequent to the injury over a period of 4½ years. The initial surgery involved an intracranial approach with an intradural repair of the middle fossa CSF leak. Thereafter, recurrent CSF leaks occurred, and the patient underwent multiple intradural and extradural attempts at repair. Complications included chronic or recurrent mastoiditis and cholesteatoma formation. Alloplastic (methyl methacrylate) materials, nonvascularized tissues (abdominal fat, fasica lata), and regional flaps (temporalis muscle) were used in unsuccessful attempts to control the CSF leak and infection.

In February 1990, a contrast cisternogram showed leakage of contrast medium from the area of the petrous roof, the labyrinth, and near the petrous portion of the left internal carotid artery (Fig. 11–4). Debridement of necrotic fat, revision of the mastoidectomy, and drainage of a postauricular abscess were performed. The wound was again packed with fascia lata and fat. Infection and leakage continued, and the patient was referred for revascularized free tissue transfer in July 1990. At that time, all identifiable remaining necrotic tissue was debrided, and a revascularized rectus abdominis flap was placed in the surgical

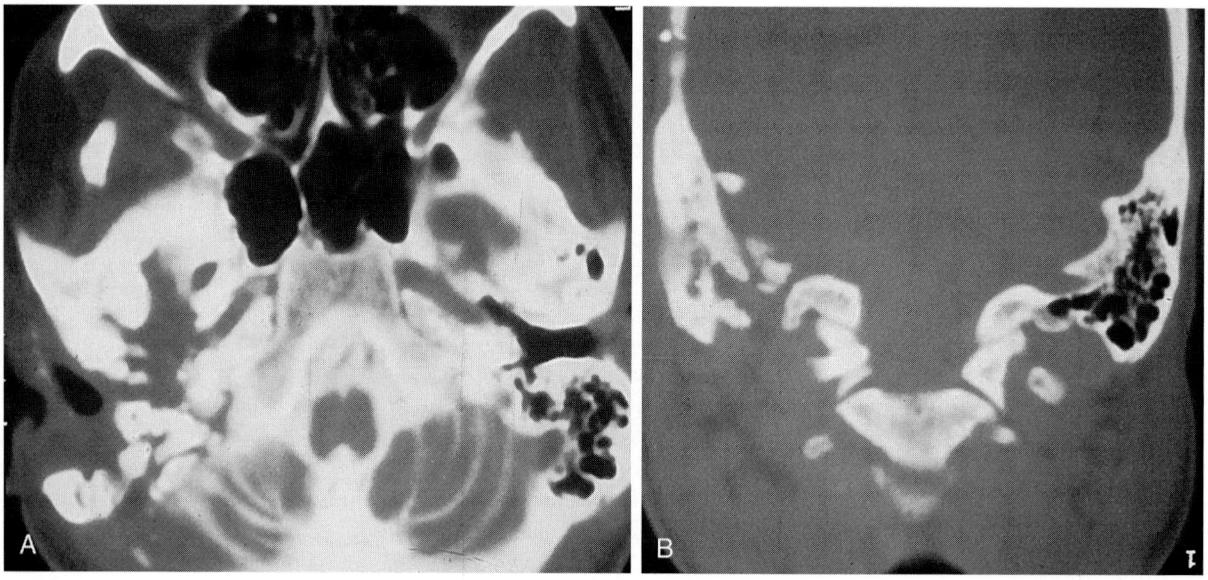

FIGURE 11–4. CT scans (*A*, horizontal cut; *B*, coronal cut) showing a large defect resulting from mastoid-petrous fractures and multiple surgical procedures.

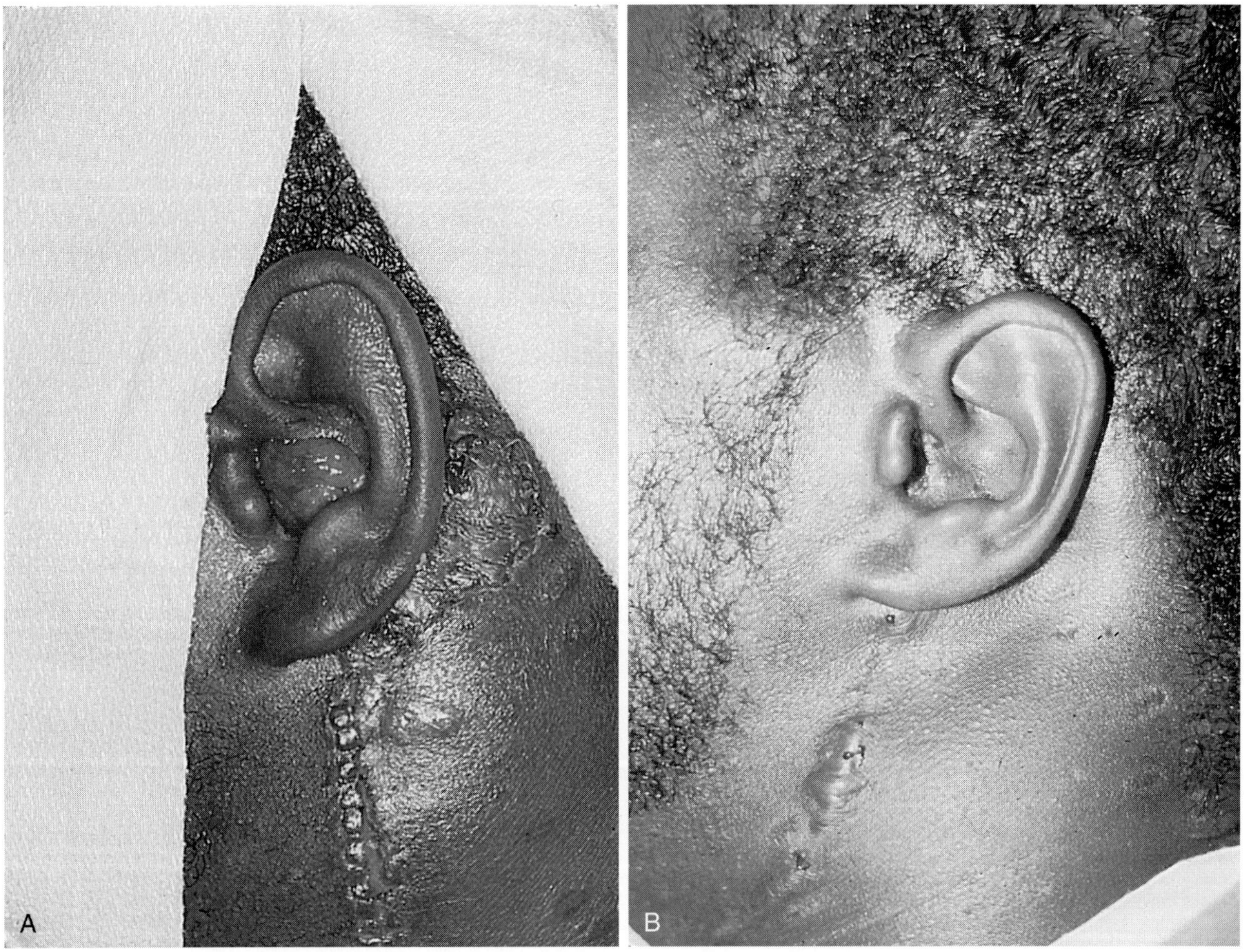

FIGURE 11–5. *A*, Perioperative photograph of patient showing the ear canal defect filled by the rectus abdominis free flap. The visible portion of the flap allows visual inspection and testing of viability. This is the muscle-only variation of the flap depicted in Figure 11–3. *B*, Three months postoperatively, the ear canal defect has healed and is well epithelialized.

defect. The ear canal, which previously had connected with the infected cavity, was amputated about 1 cm medial to the conchal bowl. A small portion of the flap could be seen through this opening, allowing monitoring of its vascularity (Fig. 11–5). During the next several weeks, epithelial migration occurred, and the rectus muscle was covered with skin without subsequent surgery. There has been no evidence of CSF leakage or recurrent infection during the subsequent 8 years.

SUMMARY

Free flaps are the surgical technique of choice for the reconstruction of complex defects of the anterior, middle, and posterior fossae and skull base because they provide a reliable form of reconstruction with a low incidence of complications. Although primary reconstruction of such defects with free flaps is advocated in the majority of cases, these flaps are also useful in patients in whom other more conservative approaches have failed, as exemplified by the patient described in the case report above.

REFERENCES

1. Earley MJ, Green M, Milling M: A critical appraisal of the use of free flaps in primary reconstruction of combined scalp and calvarial cancer defects. Br J Plast Surg 43:283–289, 1990.
2. Hardesty R, Jones N, Swartz N, et al: Microsurgery for macrodefects: Microvascular free-tissue transfer for massive defects of the head and neck. Am J Surg 154:399–405, 1987.
3. Janecka IP, Sekhar LN: Surgical management of cranial base tumors: A report on 91 patients. Oncology 3:69–74, 79–80, 1989.
4. Jones B, O'Brien C: Acute ischemia of the hand resulting from elevation of a radial forearm flap. Br J Plast Surg 38:396, 1985.
5. Jones NF, Schramm VL, Sekhar LN: Reconstruction of the cranial base following tumour resection. Br J Plast Surg 40:155–162, 1987.
6. Jones N, Sekhar L, Schramm V: Free rectus abdominis muscle flap reconstruction of the middle and posterior cranial fossa. Plast Reconstr Surg 78:471–479, 1986.
7. Jones TR, Jones NF: Advances in reconstruction of the upper aerodigestive tract and cranial base with free tissue transfer. Clin Plast Surg 19:819, 1992.

8. Ketchum SD, Hoye RC, Van Buren JM, et al: Complications of intracranial facial resections for tumors of the paranasal sinuses. Am J Surg 112:591, 1966.
9. Kiener JL, Hoffman WY, Mathes SJ: Influence of radiotherapy on microvascular reconstruction in the head and neck region. Am J Surg 162:404, 1991.
10. Kroll SS, Reece GP, Miller MJ, et al: Comparison of the rectus abdominis free flap with the pectoralis major myocutaneous flap for reconstruction of the head and neck. Am J Surg 164:615, 1992.
11. Mathes S, Nahai F: Clinical Applications for Muscle and Musculocutaneous Flaps. St. Louis, Mosby, 1982, pp. 44–45.
12. McCraw JB, Magee WP Jr, Kalwaic H: Uses of the trapezius and sternomastoid myocutaneous flaps in head and neck reconstruction. Plast Reconstr Surg 63:49, 1979.
13. Milloy F, Anson B, McFee D: The rectus abdominis muscle and the epigastirc arteries. Surg Gynecol Obstet 110:293–302, 1960.
14. Mulholland S, Boyd JB, McCabe S, et al: Recipient vessels in head and neck microsurgery: Radiation effects and vessel access. Plast Reconstr Surg 92:628, 1993.
15. Neligan PC, Mulholland S, Irish J, et al: Flap selection in cranial base reconstruction. Plast Reconstr Surg 98:1159–1166, 1996.
16. Olivari N: The latissimus flap. Br J Plast Surg 29:126, 1976.
17. Olivari N: Use of thirty latissimus dorsi flaps. Plast Reconstr Surg 64:654, 1979.
18. Olsen KD, Meland NB, Ebersold MJ, et al: Extensive defects of the sino-orbital region. Results with microvascular reconstruction. Arch Otolaryngol Head Neck Surg 118:828–833, 859–860, 1992.
19. Pennington D, Stern H, Lee K: Free flap reconstruction of large defects of the scalp and calvarium. Plast Reconstr Surg 83:655, 1989.
20. Robson MC, Zachary LS, Schmidt DR, et al: Reconstruction of large cranial defects in the presence of heavy radiation damage and injection utilizing tissue transferred by microvascular anatomoses. Plast Reconstr Surg 83:438–442, 1989.
21. Rosen HM: The extended trapezius musculocutaneous flap for cranio-orbital facial reconstruction. Plast Reconstr Surg 75(3):318–327, 1985.
22. Scher RL, Cantrell RW: Anterior skull base reconstruction with the pericranial flap after craniofacial resection. Ear, Nose, Throat J 71:210–212, 215–217, 1992.
23. Shestak KC, Jones NF: Microsurgical free-tissue transfer in the elderly patient. Plast Reconstr Surg 88:259, 1991.
24. Shusterman MA, Kroll SS, Weber RS, et al: Intraoral soft tissue reconstruction after cancer ablation: A comparison of the pectoralis major flap and the free radial forearm flap. Am J Surg 162:397, 1991.
25. Smith P, Morgan B, Crockard H: Immediate total scalp and skull reconstruction. Microsurgery 4:23, 1983.
26. Snyderman CH, Janecka IP, Sekhar LN, et al: Anterior cranial base reconstruction: Role of galeal and pericranial flaps. Laryngoscope 100:607–614, 1990.
27. Song R, Gao Y, Song Y, et al: The forearm flap. Clin Plast Surg 9:21–26, 1982.
28. Soutar DS, McGregor IA: The radial forearm flap in intraoral reconstruction: The experience of 60 consecutive cases. Plast Reconstr Surg 78:1, 1986.
29. Spinelli HM, Persing JA, Walser B: Reconstruction of the cranial base. Clin Plast Surg 22(3):555–560, 1995.
30. Stueber K, Saloman M, Spence R: The combined use of the latissimus dorsi musculocutaneous free flap and split-rib grafts for cranial vault reconstruction. Ann Plast Surg 15:155, 1985.
31. Tansini I: Spora il mio nuovo processo di amputazione della mammaella per cancre. Riforma Med (Palermo, Napoli) 12:3, 1896.
32. Taylor G, Palmer J: The vascular territories (angiosomes) of the body: Experimental and clinical applications. Br J Plast Surg 40:113–131, 1987.
33. Thomson JG, Restifo RJ: Microsurgery for cranial base tumors. Clin Plast Surg 22:563–572, 1995.
34. Tolhurst DE, Carstens MH, Greco RJ, et al: The surgical anatomy of the scalp. Plast Reconstr Surg 87:603–612, 1991.
35. Watson JS, Craig R, Orton C: The free latissimus dorsi myocutaneous flap. Plast Reconstr Surg 64:299, 1979.
36. Yamada A, Harii K, Ueda K, et al: Free rectus abdominis muscle reconstruction of the anterior skull base. Br J Plast Surg 45:302–306, 1992.
37. Yang G, Chen B, Gao Y, et al: Forearm free skin flap transplantation. Natl Med J China 61:139, 1981.

CHAPTER 12

Management of Carcinoma of the Ethmoids, Craniofacial Resections, and Alternatives for Reconstruction

Valerie J. Lund, M.S., F.R.C.S., F.R.C.S., Ed.
David J. Howard, F.R.C.S., F.R.C.S., Ed.

Sinonasal malignancy, particularly that arising in the ethmoids, has always posed significant management problems because of its late presentation and close proximity to the orbit and intracranial cavity. Although surgery for maxillary cancer has a relatively long history, with the first subtotal maxillectomy being recorded in the English literature in 1829, tumors of the ethmoid were treated by a combination of piecemeal removal through an external approach such as a lateral rhinotomy or maxillectomy, often combined with orbital clearance and radiotherapy, until quite late into this century.[2] This treatment was associated with poor 5-year survival figures of between 23% and 38%[3–8] and led many practitioners to seek alternative surgical approaches that might more satisfactorily address oncologic resection. Thus, a combined intracranial and nasal approach was developed by pioneers such as Smith and colleagues,[9] Ketcham and associates,[10] Clifford,[11] and Terz and colleagues[12] that allowed resection of the skull base and accurate assessment of the dura and orbit. The craniofacial approach has now become the accepted surgical approach in many centers[13–19] for tumors that have breached the anterior cranial fossa, and although some of the technical details may vary from unit to unit, the popularity of the procedure is a tribute to its low morbidity and excellent cosmesis. This chapter is based on our experience with a cohort of over 250 patients who have undergone craniofacial resection during the last 17 years, selected from an experience of more than 600 patients with sinonasal malignant tumors.

CLINICAL PRESENTATION

The late presentation of patients is largely due to the innocuous nature of the initial symptoms. These are often dismissed by patient and doctor alike as representing more common nasal conditions such as allergic or infective rhinosinusitis, although the unilateral nature of the symptoms should alert suspicion. The majority of patients present with nasal obstruction (55%) or epistaxis (38%), while a small number complain of nasal discharge, which may be bloodstained (18%). Twenty-four percent complain of headache, although very few mention anosmia, and nasal deformity is rare. The exact site of origin of ethmoidal tumors is generally difficult to determine at presentation, but those that arise as a consequence of occupational toxins most probably involve the bulla and middle turbinate ab initio, judging by evidence from epidemiologic studies among woodworkers.[20–22] Nevertheless, the ethmoid provides little barrier to tumor spread, and the entire labyrinth is readily involved.

The lamina papyracea, which is frequently dehiscent in the young and old, is rapidly breached, bringing the tumor into contact with the orbit, and although the orbital periosteum may resist penetration for some time, the orbital contents must be regarded as potentially at risk in all cases of ethmoidal malignancy. Thus, orbital symptoms frequently occur in patients with ethmoidal malignancy (62%). The most common symptoms are orbital displacement and periorbital swelling. At least a fifth of patients have evidence of some degree of visual loss, although blindness is uncommon. Tumor involvement can also be relatively silent if the disease spreads posteriorly along the periosteum into the orbital apex and from there into the middle cranial fossa.

The other "silent" area is of course the anterior cranial fossa, which, even when the dura and frontal lobes are extensively involved, produces negligible symptoms. The frontal bone largely constitutes the roof of the ethmoids, so intracranial spread is more often effected through the medial junction between the frontal and ethmoid sinuses, adjacent to the cribriform niche, or through the orbital roof, where the frontal bone is generally thinner.

CLINICAL ASSESSMENT

Tumors occurring in the sinonasal region show the greatest histologic diversity in the body, and it is of considerable importance, given the diverse natural history of these lesions, to determine the extent and type of tumor at the earliest opportunity.[23] Formal biopsy under general anesthesia is greatly facilitated by the use of the rigid endoscope, which allows precise removal of tissue with minimal transgression of normal tissue planes. This tissue must be submitted for expert histologic review because every conceivable tissue can manifest a malignant form in this area, and not infrequently the diagnosis must be revised in patients referred from other institutions, with obvious important implications for management.

The extent of tumor spread can be accurately determined using a combination of high-resolution contrast-enhanced computed comography (CT) scanning (coronal and axial planes[24]) with magnetic resonance imaging (MRI) in the coronal, axial, and sagittal[25] planes, enhanced with gadolinium-DTPA. The coronal CT scan is still essential to show early cribriform plate erosion, and the combination of CT and MRI is 98% accurate in differentiating tumor from normal tissue, inflammation, fluid, and fibrosis.

INDICATIONS

As previously stated, a wide range of malignant tumors may arise in or affect the ethmoid labyrinth. The craniofacial approach offers the possibility of performing a genuine oncologic resection and should be undertaken for tumors of all histologic types that are adjacent to the skull base if the patient's general health permits general anesthesia. Even when gross continuity of tumor with the skull base and anterior cranial fossa is not evident, an understanding of the natural history of the various pathologies of these tumors dictates that tumors such as olfactory neuroblastoma should always be subject to excision of the olfactory bulbs and tracts, in which microembolic disease is frequently found.[26] Table 12–1 shows the distribution by site of the tumors in our own recently analyzed series of 209 cases, which consists largely of malignant tumors (68%), among which adenocarcinoma is the most common type. However, the series also includes a number of benign lesions that, due to their site and extent, necessitated a craniofacial resection.[27] The concept of "benign" is an arbitrary one in this situation because patients rarely survive long enough to manifest metastatic spread, the sine qua non of malignancy, and an inexorable benign tumor such as a meningioma in a young patient may be associated with a high mortality.

Many patients present with extensive intracranial involvement that is beyond the powers of surgery to cure but may be amenable to craniofacial resection if the patients are otherwise fit. The morbidity and mortality of the procedure are sufficiently low to make it a worthwhile exercise in palliation, since it provides a mean of 18 months survival during which the quality of life may be very reasonable.

TABLE 12–1. HISTOPATHOLOGY IN 209 PATIENTS UNDERGOING CRANIOFACIAL RESECTION

TUMOR	NO.
Malignant Histology (n = 167)	
Adenocarcinoma	42
Olfactory neuroblastoma	26
Squamous carcinoma	25
Chondrosarcoma	19
Adenoid cystic carcinoma	15
Anaplastic carcinoma	10
Malignant melanoma	8
Cylindric cell carcinoma	5
Rhabdomyosarcoma	3
Metastasis	3
Malignant fibrous histiocytoma	2
Spindle cell sarcoma	1
Carcinosarcoma	1
Osteogenic sarcoma	1
Angiosarcoma	1
Hemangiopericytoma	1
Alveolar soft part sarcoma	1
Malignant schwannoma	1
Mucoepidermoid carcinoma	1
Ewing's sarcoma	1
Meningioma	7
Fibro-osseous disease	6
Osteoma	5
Phycomycete granuloma	3
Reparative granuloma	2
Osteoblastoma	2
Leiomyoblastoma	2
Meningoencephalocele	2
Osteomyelitis	2
Neurofibroma	2
Angioma	2
Angiofibroma	2
Cholesterol granuloma	1
Pseudotumor	1
Dermoid	1
Pleomorphic adenoma	1
Hemangioma	1

SURGICAL TECHNIQUE

The surgical technique employed in our unit was developed in the late 1970s as an extension of the lateral rhinotomy approach.[19] It has undergone a number of minor changes and is obviously modified in individual cases, but the technique described below is applicable to the great majority of patients.

After bilateral tarsorrhaphies and skin infiltration with adrenalin (1:200,000), a Moore lateral rhinotomy incision on the side of the lesion is extended vertically onto the forehead in the midline or prominent frown crease as far as the hairline (Fig. 12–1) (see Color plate). The soft tissues are dissected off the underlying facial bones with careful preservation of the periosteum. The dissection is carried over the nasal bridge to expose the anterior lamina papyracea on the contralateral side, and the lamina on the side of the lesion is fully dissected as far as the posterior ethmoidal vessels and orbital apex to define the relationship of the tumor to the orbit. Full access to the anterior cranial fossa is effected through a shield-shaped window craniotomy (Fig. 12–2) (see Color plate). The shield is approximately 2.5 × 2.5 cm with an inferior point based over the frontal sinuses. It is outlined using a high-speed 2-mm rosehead drill, and the bone is drilled down almost to the dura. When the bone is sufficiently thin, a small osteotome is used to fracture the last layer, divide the interspinus septum, and fracture the shield outward, resulting in minimal trauma to the underlying dura. The size of this craniotomy has been questioned, but a simple analogy with the view gained through a small hole in the ceiling of a room serves to demonstrate the excellent access that is obtained through this small opening (Fig. 12–3) (see Color plate).

Additional exposure is now gained by removing the posterior walls of the frontal sinuses. Through the craniotomy the

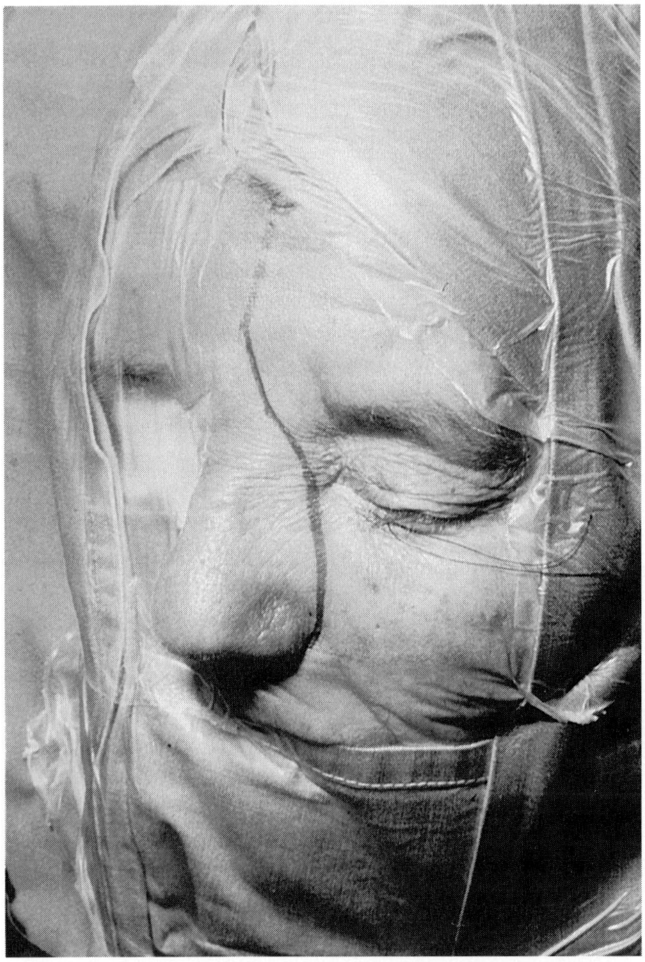

FIGURE 12–1. Intraoperative photograph of extended lateral rhinotomy incision (see Color plate).

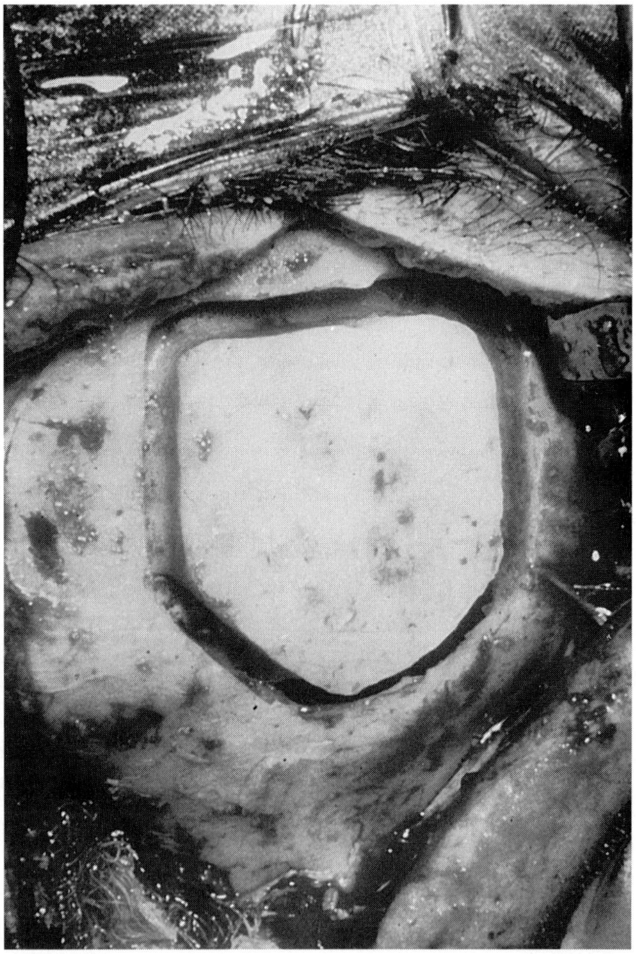

FIGURE 12–2. Intraoperative photograph showing frontal osteotomy (see Color plate).

frontal lobes and overlying dura are retracted as dissection of the dura is carried out on a wide front, progressing onto the smooth bone of the jugum sphenoidale and exposing the crista galli, cribriform plate, and ethmoidal and orbital roofs. The dura is adherent to the cribriform plate owing to the olfactory nerves and their olfactory extensions, and it is often easier and less traumatic to deliberately cut the dura away rather than tear it by blunt dissection. The anterior and posterior ethmoidal vessels are coagulated with bipolar diathermy. The operating microscope is used during the dissection to provide additional illumination and magnification. Shrinkage of the brain is facilitated by deliberate hyperventilation to produce an end-tidal P_{CO_2} of 20 to 25 mm; this is combined with a head-up tilt of 15 to 20 degrees and hypotension of 70 to 90 mmHg systolic pressure. If these measures are not sufficient, intravenous mannitol may be used, but it is rarely necessary. These measures, combined with wide lateral dissection of the dura, allow excellent exposure of the entire anterior cranial fossa, and retractors are rarely required, although they should be available.

En bloc removal of both ethmoidal complexes, the cribriform plate, and the perpendicular plate of the ethmoid forming the posterior part of the nasal septum can now be

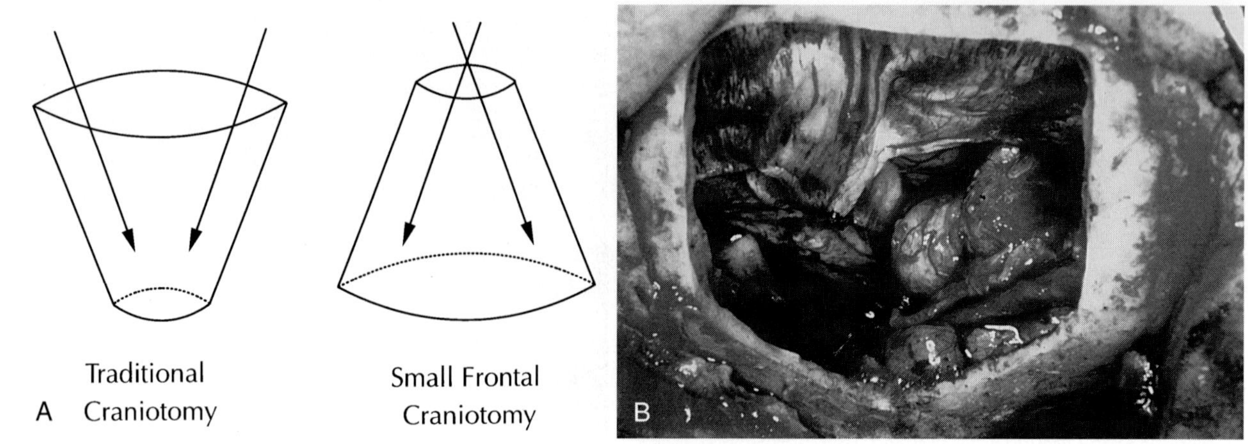

FIGURE 12–3. *A*, Diagram showing view through frontal osteotomy. *B*, Intraoperative photograph showing view through frontal osteotomy (see Color plate).

accomplished using a number of osteotomies. Osteotomy can be performed with a rosehead or fissure bur combined with a curved osteotome. The cranial osteotomy is outlined with a rosehead bur, encompassing both ethmoids and the anterior wall of the sphenoid sinus. Anteriorly the osteotomies are completed with a fissure bur that passes across the midline, and under the nasal bones between both frontal ostia to the orbit on either side, thus uniting intracranial and extracranial cuts (Fig. 12–4). The specimen is freed by dividing the perpendicular plate of the ethmoid from the rest

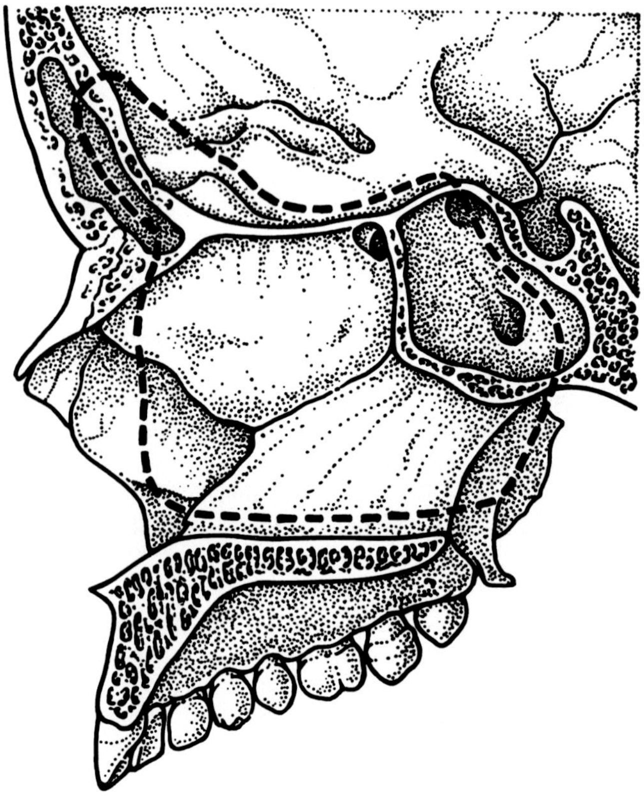

FIGURE 12–4. Diagram showing connection of extracranial and intracranial osteotomies.

of the septum and delivering it through the facial approach. Depending on the extent of disease, additional resection of the overlying skin, nasal bones, orbit, maxilla, pterygopalatine fossa, dura, and brain can now be undertaken under frozen section control.

If tumor is adherent to dura or, in the case of olfactory neuroblastoma when the olfactory bulbs and tracts may be microscopically involved, the area is widely resected, and tumor involvement is be checked by frozen section. Further resection of the olfactory bulbs and adjacent frontal lobes can be performed, but if the frontal lobes are infiltrated with malignant disease, survival for more than 1 year cannot be anticipated. The dural defect is repaired with fascia lata underlaid into the defect and carefully sutured with 4–0 polydianoxylone sulfate (PDS) to form a cerebrospinal fluid (CSF)-proof repair. A thin fenestrated split-thickness skin graft is applied to this inferiorly and "spot-welded" into place with cyanoacrylate glue or autologous fibrin glue.[28] The graft, which provides a biologic dressing while mucosalization takes place, is then also covered with a sheet of absorbable gelatin sponge soaked in Sofradex (framycetin sulfate, gramicidin, and dexamethasone) ear drops and held in place with 2-inch ribbon gauze soaked in Whithead's varnish (compound iodoform paint, composed of iodoform, benzoin, prepared storax, tolu balsam, and solvent ether).

The shield of frontal bone is rewired or fixed in position with miniplates, and the periosteum and skin are closed in three layers with 3–0 Vicryl, 4–0 catgut, and 5–0 Prolene or skin clips. A moderate pressure bandage is applied for 24 hours, and the patient is kept lying flat for 5 days postoperatively. The Whithead's pack is removed under general anesthesia 10 days later. If a gross CSF leak is seen at that time, a further pack may be reinserted, but this is rarely required.

Patients are given prophylactic antibiotics (cefuroxime axetil 750 mg every 8 hours and metronidazole 500 mg every 8 hours) throughout the treatment period until the pack is removed and they are are also given phenytoin (100 mg twice a day) beginning 48 hours prior to the operation and continuing for 2 months.

MANAGEMENT OF THE ORBIT

In cases of obvious intraperiosteal orbital involvement by malignant disease, the orbit can be cleared (Fig. 12–5). The eyelids do not need to be sacrificed on oncologic grounds because they are infrequently compromised by direct tumor spread, so they may be preserved to line the socket. The lashes and tarsal plates are removed, but the orbicularis muscle is preserved to reinforce the flaps. The orbital periosteum is completely dissected circumferentially, detachment of the lateral palpebral ligament allowing removal of the orbital contents as far into the apex as possible (the medial ligament having been previously detached). The mobilized orbital contents are released in a lateral to medial direction, and the ophthalmic vessels are subsequently clipped or tied in the apex. The eyelids are stitched together in two layers with fine plain catgut, which avoids the need for difficult suture removal. If medial canthal skin is involved, the area may be resected and repaired with a variety of flaps, among which the glabellar flap has been used most often.

When the tumor is found to be adherent to the periosteum, the periosteum is opened well away from the tumor margin.[29] Obvious involvement of the inner periosteal surface makes orbital clearance mandatory. In the absence of macroscopic intraperiosteal disease, the periosteum is widely excised with a small amount of adjacent orbital fat and submitted to frozen section analysis. Clearance of the orbital contents must be performed if there is any evidence of tumor penetration. In its absence, adequate periosteal excision is then undertaken. This can include almost the entire medial aspect from the level of the ethmoidal vessels superiorly to the attachment of the inferior oblique muscle inferiorly without significant compromising orbital function. A thin fenestrated split-thickness skin graft is then applied directly to the denuded medial orbital fat and held in place with autologous fibrin glue or cyanoacrylate glue. The graft is then covered with a sheet of absorbable gelatin sponge soaked in Sofradex ear drops. Although mucosalization of the exposed fat would occur quickly without grafting, as shown by orbital decompression performed for thyroid eye disease, subsequent contracture of the skin graft may help minimize the occurrence of postoperative diplopia. This is certainly a prominent feature in the immediate postoperative period following decompression in thyroid disease when no graft is used.

Decompression of the orbital apex may be required primarily in patients with benign disease or when tumor recurrence has affected the contralateral eye following previous orbital clearance. The medial two thirds of the optic canal can be removed throughout its entire length under direct vision. It is inadvisable to incise the meninges, although this has sometimes been advocated in cases of trauma,[30] because hematoma is not a factor and the chances of a CSF leak and damage to the nerve are increased. It is particularly important to assess the optic apices bilaterally, especially in patients with sphenoidal involvement, and to decompress the chiasma anteriorly as much as possible without compromising safety.

In patients in whom orbital clearance is necessary it is now possible to enhance prosthetic rehabilitation considerably by inserting primarily an osseointegrated implant in the orbital margin prior to skin closure. There is no doubt, however, that osseointegration of implants in the orbital rim is slower and less predictable than in other areas of the head such as the mandible, and it is preferably performed as a secondary procedure. A 1-year interval is allowed before proceeding to the second stage exposure and attachment of abutments is undertaken. An orbital prosthesis attached with adhesive or to a spectacle frame is used during the intervening period.

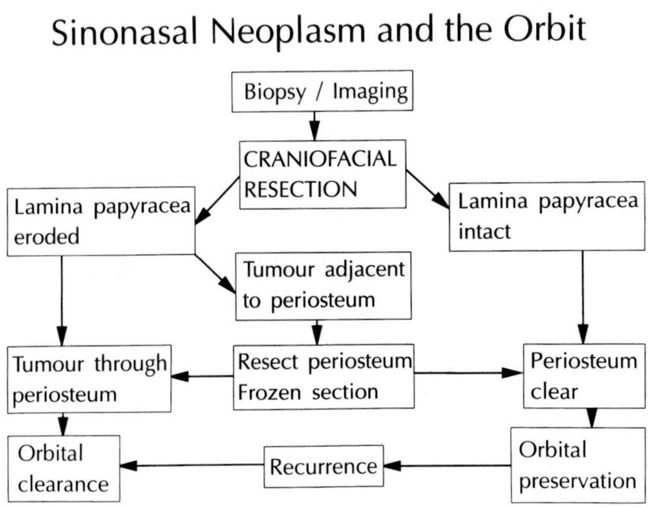

FIGURE 12–5. Algorithm of orbital management during craniofacial resection.

MODIFICATIONS OF CRANIOFACIAL RESECTIONS

Patients occasionally require some modifications in the incision and the closure. The extended lateral rhinotomy can be replaced by a combination of a midfacial degloving procedure and a bicoronal flap (see Chap. 6) when it is desirable to produce no facial scar. It should be stressed that the extended lateral rhinotomy incision heals extremely well and is virtually undetectable in most middle-aged or elderly patients (Fig. 12–6) (see Color plate). However, in children the incision is more obvious, and because most children are undergoing the procedure for benign lesions, a facial scar of any sort is generally undesirable.

The extent of the tumor may necessitate more extensive resection, including removal of overlying skin, which may be reconstructed with a median forehead or glabellar flap. Adenocarcinoma frequently spreads anteriorly through the nasal bones. The nasal bones themselves may be resected and repaired with iliac bone or rib.

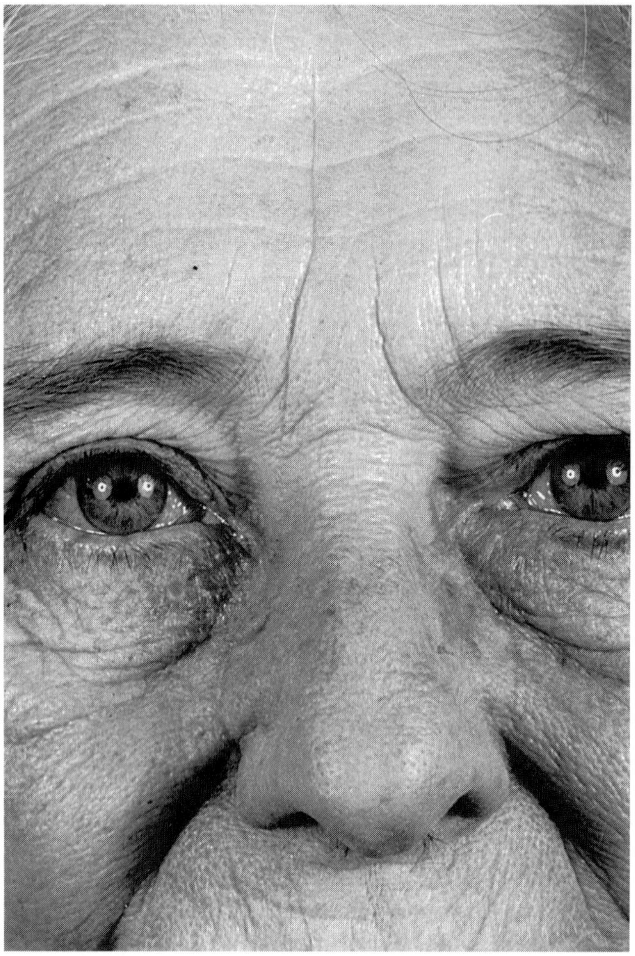

FIGURE 12–6. Clinical photograph of patient 5 years after craniofacial resection (see Color plate).

POSTOPERATIVE FOLLOW-UP

It is important to keep patients undergoing such procedures under close review over the long term because a 5-year follow-up period is irrelevant with many of the tumors occurring in this region. Patients regularly undergo formal examination under anesthesia, initially every 6 months, as well as MRI at similar intervals to assess in particular the orbit and adjacent cranial cavity.[31] Recurrence can thus be determined at the earliest opportunity and salvage surgery performed. Revision craniofacial resection has been performed up to five times in certain individuals without difficulty.

A number of tumors are best managed using a combination of surgery and radiotherapy. Although the sequence is a subject of some discussion, the literature does not show any marked difference in survival regardless of which is given first. Our preference has been to administer full-course radiotherapy followed by craniofacial resection 6 weeks later regardless of the apparent response of the tumor to the radiotherapy. It is not possible to determine the presence of residual microscopic disease with imaging, no matter how detailed, and only an oncologic resection can accurately determine response. Thirty-five percent of our patients with craniofacial resection received preoperative radiotherapy, and 16% received it postoperatively, usually in the earlier part of the series. It should also be noted (see the later section on complications) that a longer time interval must be left between the two therapies if radiotherapy is given after our method of skull base repair.

RESULTS

The purpose of this chapter is primarily to describe the details of a particular technique, but it would be inappropriate not to discuss the results of such a procedure. A recent analysis has been performed of a group of 209 patients[27] whose ages ranged from 7 to 77 years; the male-to-female ratio of the group was 2:1. The actuarial survival at 5 and 10 years is shown in Table 12–2 for the group as a whole, for benign versus malignant lesions, and for some of the individual histologic types. Further analyses have shown that in those tumors requiring combined surgery and radiotherapy, there is no difference in survival regardless of which modality is given first. Multivariant regression analysis shows that, not surprisingly, brain involvement and orbital involvement are the most important prognostic factors for malignant tumors. A Kaplan-Meier graph for adenocarcinoma shows the effect on survival of frontal lobe infiltration compared with dural involvement or no intracranial involvement (Fig. 12–7).

In this series of 209 patients, 41 (20%) underwent primary orbital clearance at the time of craniofacial resection. Since the introduction of the osseointegrated technique in 1990, 19 patients also received implants at the time of resection. Twenty-three patients underwent periosteal resection, five of whom then underwent secondary clearance 5 months to 4 years later. Two patients had massive recurrence of the tumor in the preserved eye, and they succumbed to this disease. Two other patients, who had had no periosteal resection, required a secondary orbital clearance 2 and 6 years after the initial surgery.

TABLE 12–2. ACTUARIAL SURVIVAL FOR WHOLE GROUP OF 209 PATIENTS AND INDIVIDUAL HISTOLOGIES

	ACTUARIAL SURVIVAL		
	5 yr	**10 yr**	***n***
Overall	51	41	209
Benign	75	75	44
Malignant	44	32	155
Adenocarcinoma	43	38	42
Olfactory neuroblastoma	2	47	26
Squamous cell carcinoma	32	32	25
Chondrosarcoma	79	47	19
Adenoid cystic carcinoma	51	36	15

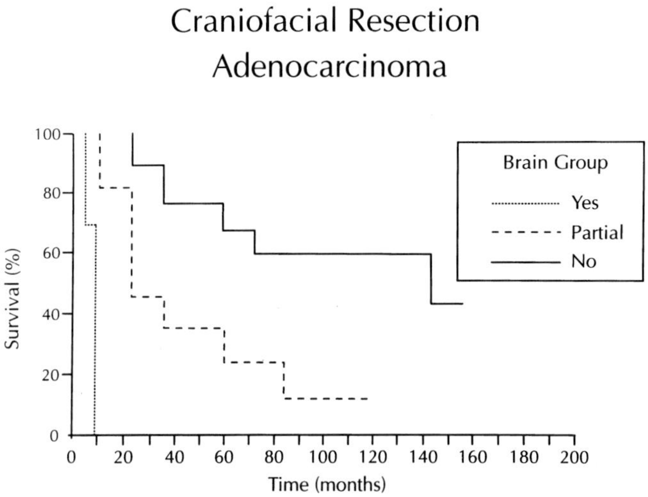

FIGURE 12–7. Kaplan-Meier graph showing survival for patients with adenocarcinoma with involvement of the frontal lobes and dura but no intracranial involvement.

Involvement of the orbit confers a worse 5- and 10-year prognosis (29% and 22%, respectively) compared to no involvement (69% and 62%, respectively), but resection of the orbital periosteum does not compromise survival in that it is no worse than if the eye is removed. Thus, in selected cases when patients are available for close long-term follow-up, an eye that would previously have been sacrificed may be preserved.

Decompressions were performed in seven patients; in three of these it was part of the primary craniofacial resection, and in three others, two of whom had already lost one eye, it was a secondary procedure. Decompression can be repeated, as it was on five occasions in one individual with chondrosarcoma. Although in four cases disease ultimately rendered the patients blind, decompression preserved or improved failing vision in two individuals until close to their deaths and was successful in two long-term survivors with chondrosarcoma. Following craniofacial resection, three patients with fibro-osseous disease, adenocarcinoma, and adenoid cystic carcinoma lost vision in both eyes at 2½ years, 18 months, and 1 year, respectively. The extent of disease precluded any useful intervention.

COMPLICATIONS

Complications resulting from this surgery are few (Table 12–3). The operation is performed in a mean of 3.6 hours (range 1 to 6 hours), and the inpatient stay averages 16 days. Serious problems such as massive hemorrhage from the internal carotid artery may occur occasionally either during the surgery or in the immediate postoperative period. The general well-being of patients led us initially to encourage vigorous early mobilization, which may have contributed to cerebrovascular accidents in two older patients. Consequently, we now keep patients relatively supine for the first 5 postoperative days.

Cerebrospinal fluid leaks may occasionally persist after removal of the pack on the tenth postoperative day, but these heal in the majority of cases with conservative management and rarely require further reinforcement to obtain closure. Meningitis and convulsions in the immediate postoperative period are prevented by prophylactic antibiotics and phenytoin, although fits may occur during longer term follow-up if tumor or radiation fibrosis affects the frontal lobes.

Orbital complications can occasionally result from craniofacial surgery. The nasolacrimal duct is usually transected obliquely during removal of the lateral nasal wall. This rarely produces problems, but eight of our patients required formal dacrocystorhinostomy for persistent epiphora. In selected cases a nasolacrimal duct stent can be placed at the time of resection. All patients who present with orbital symptoms should receive a formal preoperative (and when appropriate, postoperative) ophthalmic assessment. Despite considerable manipulation, diplopia is rarely severe enough to require subsequent surgical correction, even in patients undergoing orbital periosteal resection.

Other long-term complications have been few. The more serious ones were associated with radiotherapy that was begun within 6 weeks of surgery; such therapy can result in frontal lobe abscesses and brain herniation. Occasionally, problems can also occur with the frontal shield, which may undergo radiation necrosis.

Craniofacial resection as described here has been performed in patients of all ages, including 19 children and adolescents who were under 16 years old at the time of surgery. Although the pathologies have been predominantly benign, our cases have included some malignancies, and it has been reassuring to find that on follow-up with sequential standardized photographs, there is no significant distortion of facial growth[32] when these measurements are compared with those found in a standardized maxillofacial database. Although large amounts of tissue are removed from the midfacial region, the anterior (cartilaginous) septum, hard palate, and upper lateral cartilages are not disturbed by this approach.

TABLE 12–3. COMPLICATIONS FOLLOWING CRANIOFACIAL RESECTION

LONG-TERM COMPLICATIONS	NO.	RESULTS
Hemorrhage	1	Death
Frontal abscess or encephalitis	2	Death
Bone necrosis	4	Recovery after debridement
CSF leak	8	Surgical repair (4) Spontaneous recovery (4)
Convulsions	1	Control with phenytoin
Epiphora	6	Dacrocystorhinostomy
Diplopia	6	Spontaneous recovery
Serous otitis media	10	Grommets
Sinusitis	3	Surgery
Cellulitis	5	Antibiotics
Pituitary deficiency	1	Steroid replacement

REHABILITATION

The oncologic surgeon must balance the task of achieving complete excision of disease with that of maximal preservation of appearance and function. This is particularly true in the sinonasal region, where any disfigurement is difficult to hide. Physical and psychological rehabilitation is of considerable importance when the principal criterion of cure has been satisfied, and it must be the primary consideration when only therapeutic palliation can be offered. In a study designed to assess the perception of the relative severity of 11 common facially disfiguring operations, orbital exenteration and radical maxillectomy scored equally with total rhinectomy, outweighed only by mandibulectomy.[33] In an assessment of quality of life in patients with head and neck cancer, the anosmia that inevitably accompanies craniofacial resection was considered a significant disability.[34]

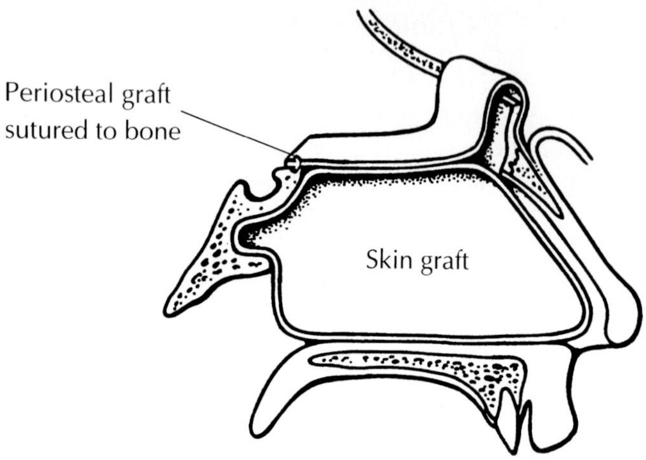

FIGURE 12–8. Repair of surgical defect in skull base with pedicled periosteal flap and skin graft. (Redrawn from Shah JP, Galicich JH. Craniofacial resection for malignant tumors of ethmoid and anterior skull base. Arch Otolaryngol 103:514, 1977. Copyright 1977. American Medical Association.)

ALTERNATIVES FOR RECONSTRUCTION

Craniofacial resection, by definition, implies an approach from above and below to the skull base. The incisions and osteotomies by which this approach can be achieved are numerous, and because most heal well with minimal scarring, the choice is largely determined by personal preference. However, it should be noted that some approaches take longer to perform than others. Similarly, reconstruction of the skull base after resection of bone and dura can be achieved with a variety of tissues. Fascia lata is one of the strongest soft tissues in the body and offers a repair that is both quick to perform and rapidly "waterproof." It is used in a number of centers,[35, 36] although a host of flaps and other tissues have been advocated to provide additional reinforcement to the area (Figs. 12–8 and 12–9). These include temporalis muscle and/or fascia,[37] galeal-pericranial flaps,[38] and latissimus dorsi myocutaneous free flaps.[39] Some of these techniques add considerably to the length of the procedure and may make interpretation of postoperative imaging more difficult. Occasionally resection of the nasal or frontal bones is necessary, and these may be reconstructed with iliac bone, rib, or split calvarial bone, while the overlying skin can usually be replaced with a local pedicled flap such as a median forehead or glabellar flap.

SUMMARY

Craniofacial resection has been one of the major surgical contributions to the management of head and neck cancer in this century and must be regarded as the gold standard in the management of sinonasal malignancy affecting the skull base. It has significantly affected survival of patients with a small but important group of tumors by allowing surgical oncologists to approach the anterior skull base and assess and excise tissues at the intracranial and orbital interface.[27, 35–42] It is particularly appropriate in the management of adenocarcinoma and olfactory neuroblastoma, as evidenced by the published series.[43–45] When cure cannot be achieved, the low morbidity and excellent cosmesis associated with the procedure offer genuine palliation; patients survive a mean of 18 months under these circumstances and enjoy a reasonable quality of life during much of this time. Many sinonasal malignancies have natural histories that must

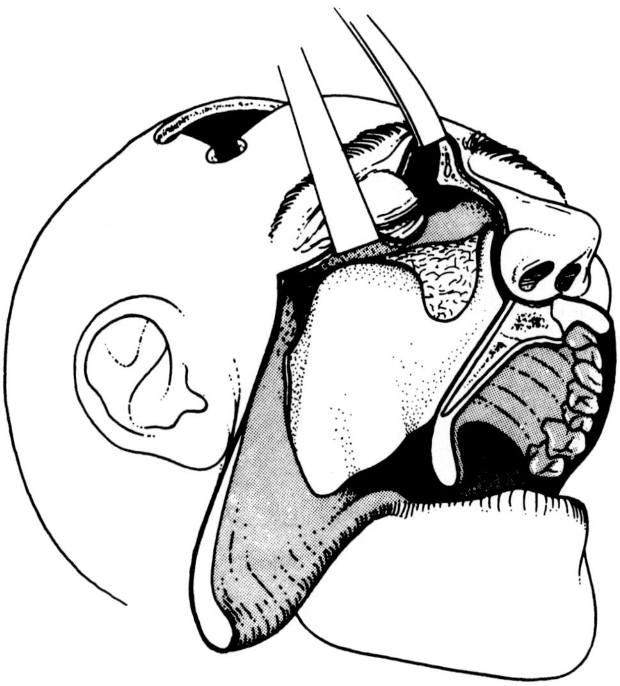

FIGURE 12–9. Diagram showing skin graft applied against periosteal flap. (Redrawn from Shah JP, Galicich JH. Craniofacial resection for malignant tumors of ethmoid and anterior skull base. Arch Otolaryngol 103:514, 1977. Copyright 1977. American Medical Association.)

be measured in decades rather than in the customary 5-year interval, and it is only lately that the actuarial survival at 10 years or longer has been assessable in sufficiently large numbers of individual tumor types. It may be that the evolution of these tumors may be altered by our intervention, and a higher incidence of metastatic disease may be manifest in the survivors some years after treatment, but prior to craniofacial resection it is likely that the patients died of local disease before secondary deposits became apparent. There can be no doubting the intrinsic benefit of this procedure in providing local control at minimal cost to the patient.

ACKNOWLEDGMENT

We would like to recognize the enormous influence of A.D. Cheesman, who is largely responsible for the introduction and evolution of craniofacial resection in the United Kingdom and whose patients are included in the series discussed in this chapter.

REFERENCES

1. Syme J: Excision of the superior maxillary bone. Edin Med Surg J. 32:238, 1829.
2. Stell PM: The history of surgery of the upper jaw. *In* Harrison D, Lund VJ: Tumours of the Upper Jaw. London, Churchill Livingstone, 1993, pl.
3. Harrison DFN: The management of malignant tumours affecting the maxillary and ethmoidal sinuses. J Laryngol Otolaryngol 90:69, 1976.
4. Weymuller EA, Reardon EJ, Nash D: Comparison of treatment modalities in carcinoma of the maxillary sinus. Arch Otolaryngol 106:625, 1980.
5. Lee F, Ogura JH: Maxillary sinus carcinoma. Laryngoscope 91:133, 1981.
6. St Pierre SB Sr: Squamous cell carcinoma of the maxillary sinus: Analysis of 66 cases. Head Neck Surg 5:508, 1983.
7. McNicoll W, Hopkin N, Dalley VM, et al: Cancer of the paranasal sinuses and nasal cavities, Part II. Results of treatment. J Laryngol Otolaryngol 98:707, 1984.
8. Linderman P, Eklund V, Petruson B: Survival after surgical treatment for maxillary neoplasms of epithelial origin. J Laryngol Otolaryngol 101:564, 1987.
9. Smith RR, Kloop CT, Williams JM: Surgical treatment of cancer of the frontal sinus and adjacent areas. Cancer 7:991, 1954.
10. Ketcham AS, Chretien PB, Van Buren JM, et al: The ethmoid sinuses: A reevaluation of surgical resection. Am J Surg 126:469, 1973.
11. Clifford P: Transcranial approach to cancer of the antroethmoidal area. Clin Otolaryngol 2:115, 1977.
12. Terz JJ, Young HF, Lawrence W Jr: Combined craniofacial resection for locally advanced carcinoma of the head and neck. Am J Surg 140:613, 1980.
13. Shah JP, Galicich JH: Craniofacial resection for malignant tumors of ethmoid and anterior skull base. Arch Otolaryngol 103:514, 1977.
14. Schramm VL, Myers EN, Maroon JC: Anterior skull base surgery for 1benign and malignant disease. Laryngoscope 89:1077, 1979.
15. Sisson GA, Bytell DE, Becker SP, et al: Carcinoma of the paranasal sinuses and craniofacial resection. J Laryngol Otolaryngol 90:59, 1976.
6. Jackson IT, Marsh WR, Hide TAH: Treatment of tumors involving the anterior cranial fossa. Head Neck Surg 6:901, 1984.
17. Biller HF, Slotnick DB, Lawson W, et al: Superior rhinotomy for en bloc resection of bilateral ethmoid tumors. Arch Otolaryngol Head Neck Surg 115:1463, 1989.
18. Nuss DW, Janecka IP, Sekhar LN: Craniofacial disassembly in the management of skull base tumours. Otolaryngol Clin North Am 24:1465, 1991.
19. Cheesman AD, Lund VJ, Howard DJ: Craniofacial resection for tumours of the nose and paranasal sinuses. Head Neck Surg 8:429, 1986.
20. Black A, Evans JC, Hadfield E, et al: Impairment of nasal mucociliary clearance in woodworkers in the furniture industry. Br J Ind Med 31:10, 1974.
21. Drettner B, Wilhelmsson B, Lundh B: Experimental studies on carcinogenesis in the nasal mucosa. Acta Otolaryngol 99:205, 1985.
22. Wilhelmsson B, Hellquist H, Olofsson J, et al: Nasal cuboidal metaplasia with dysplasia. Acta Otolaryngol 99:641, 1985.
23. Lund VJ, Howard DJ: Tumors of the paranasal sinuses. *In* Gershwin ME, Incaudo GA (eds): Diseases of the Sinuses. Ottowa, Humana Press, 1996, p. 291.
24. Lund VJ, Howard DJ, Lloyd G: CT evaluation of paranasal sinus tumours for craniofacial resection. Br J Radiol 56:439, 1983.
25. Lund VJ, Howard DJ, Lloyd GAS, et al: Magnetic resonance imaging of paranasal sinus tumours for craniofacial resection. Head Neck Surg 11:279, 1989.
26. Harrison BFN: Surgical pathology of olfactory neuroblastoma. Head Neck Surg 7:60, 1984.
27. Lund VJ, Howard DJ, Wei WI, et al: Craniofacial resection for tumors of the nasal cavity and paranasal sinuses—a seventeen year experience. Head Neck Surg 20:97–105, 1998.
28. Toma AG, Fisher EW, Cheesman AD: Autologous fibrin glue in the repair of dural defects in craniofacial resections. J Laryngol Otolaryngol 106:356, 1992.
29. Lund VJ, Howard DJ, Cheesman AD: The orbit: Evaluation and intraoperative management. Proceedings of the Fourth International Conference on Head and Neck Cancer. Head Neck Cancer Proce. 4:1020, 1996.
30. Uemura T, Isaka Y, Kazuno T, et al: Optic canal decompression: The significance of simultaneous optic canal sheath incision. Neurol Med Chir (Tokyo) 18:151, 1978.
31. Lund VJ, Lloyd GAS, Howard DJ, et al: Enhanced magnetic resonance imaging and subtraction techniques in the postoperative evaluation of craniofacial resection for sinonasal malignancy. Laryngoscope 106:553, 1996.
32. Lund VJ, Neijens H, Clement P, et al: The treatment of chronic sinusitis: A controversial issue. Int J Pediatr Otorhinolaryngol 32:21, 1995.
33. Dropkin MJ, Malgady RG, Scott DW, et al: Scaling of disfigurement and dysfunction in postoperative head and neck patients. Head Neck Surg 6:559, 1983.
34. Jones E, Lund VJ, Howard DJ: Quality of life of patients treated surgically for head and neck cancer. J Laryngol Otolaryngol 106:238, 1992.
35. Richtsmeier WJ, Briggs RJS, Koch WM, et al: Complications and early outcome of anterior craniofacial resection. Arch Otolaryngol Head Neck Surg 118:913–917, 1992.
36. Shah JP, Kraus H, Arbit E, et al: Craniofacial resection for tumors involving the anterior skull base. Otolaryngol Head Neck Surg 106(4):387, 1991.
37. Sundaresan N, Shah JP: Craniofacial resection for anterior skull base tumors. Head Neck Surg 10:219, 1988.
38. Kraus DH, Shah JP, Arbit E, et al: Complications of craniofacial resection for tumors involving the anterior skull base. Head Neck Surg 16:307, 1994.
39. Ketcham AS, Van Buren JM: Tumors of the paranasal sinuses: A therapeutic challenge. Am J Surg 150:406, 1985.
40. Bridger GP, Mendelsohn MS, Baldwin M, et al: Paranasal sinus cancer. Aust NZ J Surg 61(4):290, 1991.
41. Levine PA, Debo RF, Meredith SD, et al: Craniofacial resection at the University of Virginia (1976–1992): Survival analysis. Head Neck Surg 16:574, 1994.
42. McCaffrey TV, Olsen KD, Yohanan JM, et al: Factors affecting survival of patients with tumors of the anterior skull base. Laryngoscope 104:940, 1994.
43. Dulguerov P, Calcaterra T: Esthesioneuroblastoma: The UCLA experience 1970–1990. Laryngoscope 102:843, 1992.
44. Morita A, Ebersold MJ, Olsen KD, et al: Esthesioneuroblastoma: Prognosis and management: Neurosurgery 32(5):706, 1993.
45. Eden BV, Debo RF, Lamer JM, et al: Esthesioneuroblastoma. Long term outcome and patterns of failure—the University of Virginia experience. Cancer 73(10):2556, 1994.

CHAPTER 13

Reconstructive Surgery of the Midface for Large and Massive Defects: Cancer, Fungal Infections, Gunshot Wounds

Anthony J. Maniglia, M.D.
Lawrence J. Marentette, M.D.
David W. Stepnick, M.D.

Malignant neoplasms involving bone and soft tissue of the orbit, cheek, maxilla, and zygoma are often treated surgically. To have tumor-free oncologically sound margins, massive excision may be necessary. Infectious diseases including those caused by fungal organisms such as mucormycosis may cause extensive damage and infiltration, especially in compromised hosts such as patients suffering from diabetes mellitus, leukemia, lymphomas, and so on. Severe trauma, especially gunshot wounds, may cause anatomic defects of great magnitude that produce functional and cosmetic disabilities. Gunshot wounds of the face, especially those caused by shotguns, cause the most massive and serious traumatic injuries. Firearms in the United States account for 65% of all homicides and 57% of all suicides. They also cause more than half as many fatalities (33,000) each year as are caused by motor vehicle accidents (50,000).[1–5]

In cases of cancer, trauma, or necrotic fungal infections, extensive surgical excision or debridement can be the treatment of last resort to save patients' lives. If reconstruction in such cases cannot be done primarily after a period of healing, large and rather difficult surgical defects represent an even greater challenge to surgeons. Many centers prefer to use anaplastology to deal with such defects. Artistically crafted prostheses are sculpted and fixed with cements, glues, or osseointegrated implants. Often, radiation therapy is used in combination with surgery to manage malignant neoplasms. Previous surgical procedures combined with the effects of radiation therapy cause severe scarring accompanied by a poor blood supply in the remaining adjacent tissues. Osseointegrated titanium implants used to retain prostheses may fail, especially if hyperbaric oxygenation is not used.

Closing these extensive surgical defects is a true challenge for the reconstructive surgeon. Ideally, the reconstruction should be functional, reliable, and long-lasting and should provide acceptable aesthetic results that include good skin color matching and minimal scarring. Donor sites used to correct such defects include those classified as local, regional, or distant. Pedicled or free flaps appear to offer the best results for reliable transfer of the large amounts of tissue used in these reconstructions. Adequate color matching and bulk and factors involved in the long-term atrophy of tissues, especially fat and muscle, must be taken into account when planning these reconstructions and during their actual reconstruction. Composite flaps, composed of the maxillofacial bones, calvarium, muscle, and fat, should be carefully studied for proper selection in relation to the defect to be reconstructed. Several donor areas have been reported in the literature.[6–17] Deltopectoral and latissimus dorsi flaps with or without rib have also been used. A new method using a scapular free flap has been reported by Holle and colleagues.[15] Osseointegrated titanium implants are applied to the scapula in the donor site prior to transplantation. Three months later, the free flap is harvested, transplanted, and anastomosed to the maxillary surgical defect.

MATERIALS AND METHODS

The following four cases illustrate the management of these patients and the use of distant pedicle and free flaps for reconstruction of large and massive defects.

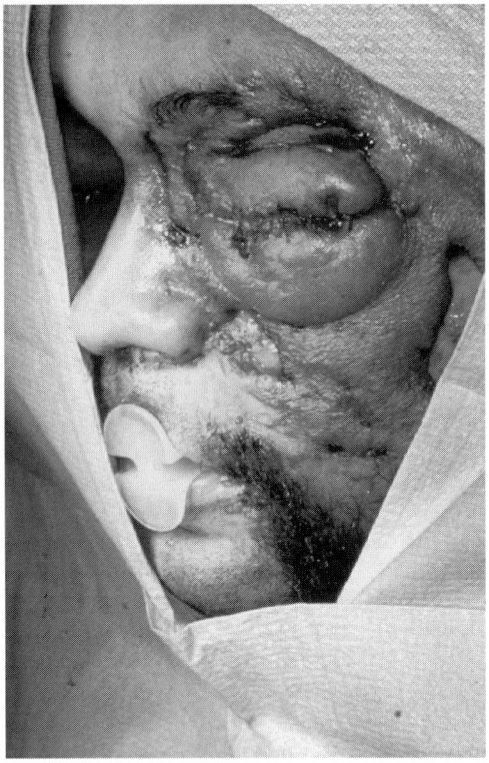

FIGURE 13–1. Necrotic tissues involving the orbit, midface, sinuses, and mandibular area due to mucormycosis.

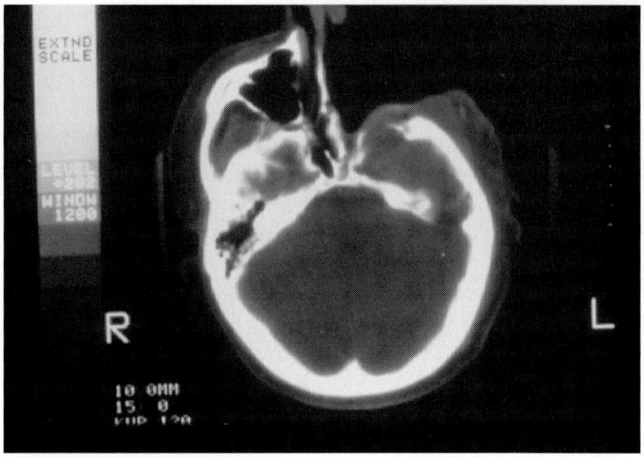

FIGURE 13–3. CT scan showing a horizontal cut of the skull and face shows a large bony defect involving the middle cranial fossa.

▼ CASE 1

A 26-year-old male was involved in a car accident in a foreign country, sustaining severe right midface and orbital trauma. The lacerations were sutured 12 hours after the injury. He developed orbital cellulitis and was treated with cephalosporin and dexamethasone. Severe mucormycosis occurred with vascular occlusion and massive necrosis of facial tissues and paranasal sinuses. The patient also developed secondary infection due to *Pseudomonas aeruginosa* (Fig. 13–1). He was then transferred to the United States. He survived after several surgical procedures including orbital exenteration, maxillectomy, pansinusectomy, and extensive debridement, as well as therapy with amphotericin B and other antibiotics (Figs. 13–2 to 13–5). (See Color plate for Fig. 13–5.) Two parietal lobe brain abscesses were treated conservatively without craniectomy. After about 1 year, with the patient completely free of any infection, options for reconstruction of the defect were reviewed. A trapezius flap was considered as well as a latissimus dorsi flap and pectoralis major myocutaneous flap. At that time (during the late 1970s), a composite free flap with bone (scapula, tibia) was not considered an option because of the lack of adequate experience in the field and, more important, because of the need for tissue volume to reconstruct the maxillary area and provide cheek bulk for facial symmetry. Finally, a pectoralis major myocutaneous flap was selected, and this procedure was carried out in two stages (Figs. 13–6 to 13–11). (See Color plates.) Postoperative photographs taken 1 year following the reconstruction showed very good results. The patient considered wearing an orbital prosthesis retained with adhesive, but he actually preferred to use an orbital patch and dark eyeglasses for camouflage (Figs. 3–12 to 13–14). (See Color plates.) Currently, a good alternative for this patient would be an osseointegrated titanium implant for retention of an artistically made orbital prosthesis and eyeglass camouflage. Because the patient had not been irradiated, a good long-term result would be very likely.

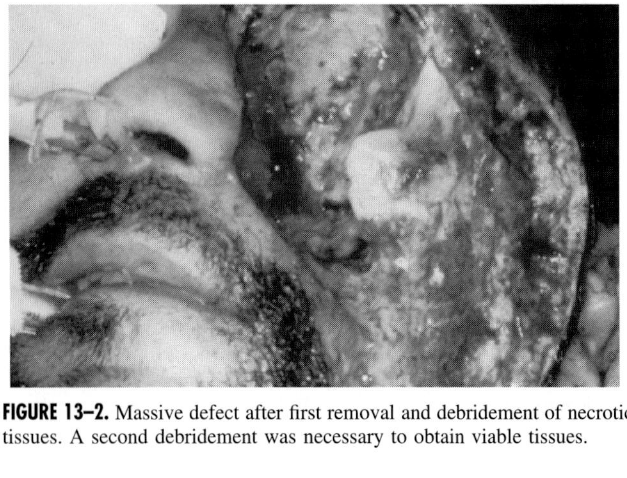

FIGURE 13–2. Massive defect after first removal and debridement of necrotic tissues. A second debridement was necessary to obtain viable tissues.

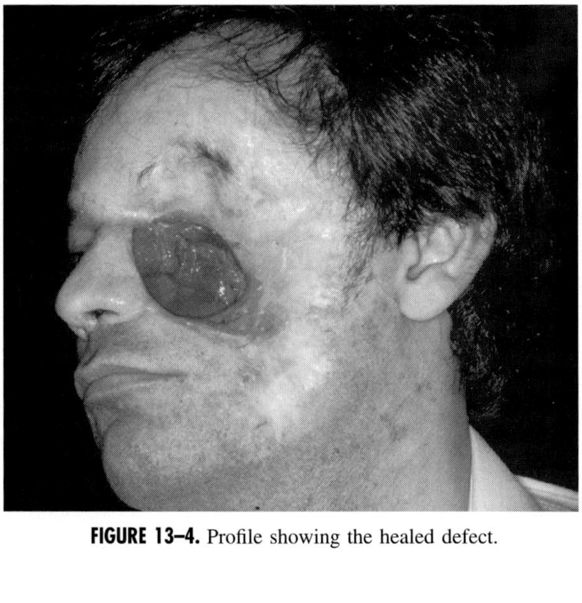

FIGURE 13–4. Profile showing the healed defect.

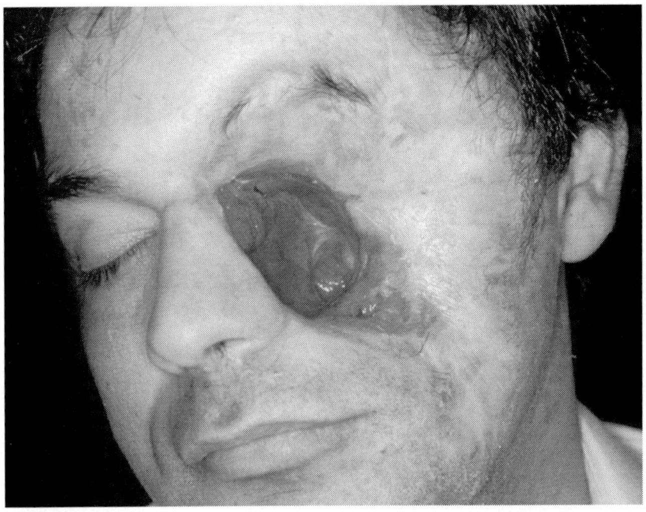

FIGURE 13–5. Close-up view of healed defect after 1 year. The sphenoid sinus cavity is also visible. (See also Color plate.)

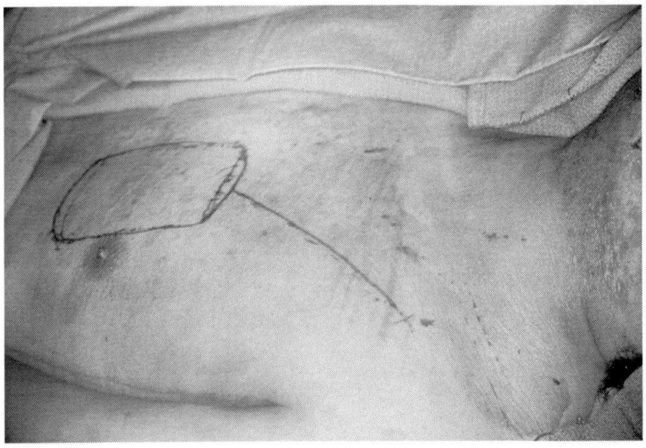

FIGURE 13–6. Views of the chest wall showing an outline of the pectoralis major flap (PMF). (See also Color plate.)

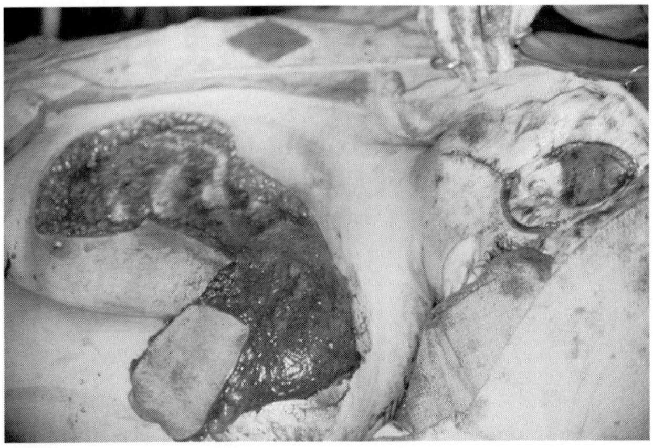

FIGURE 13–7. The PMF is dissected and elevated, ready for trimming and transfer. (See also Color plate.)

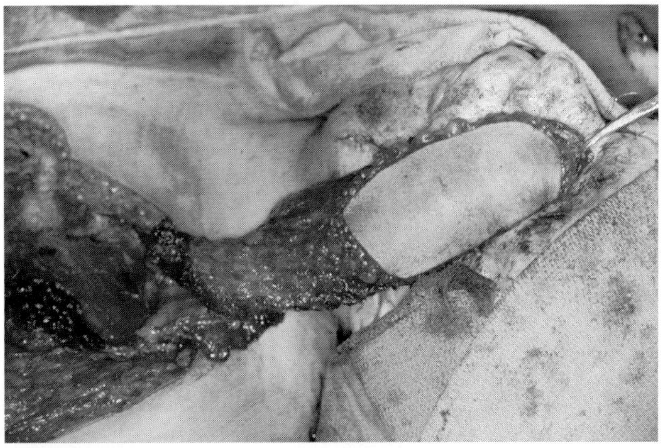

FIGURE 13–8. The PMF is trimmed and tried for size on the defect. (See also Color plate.)

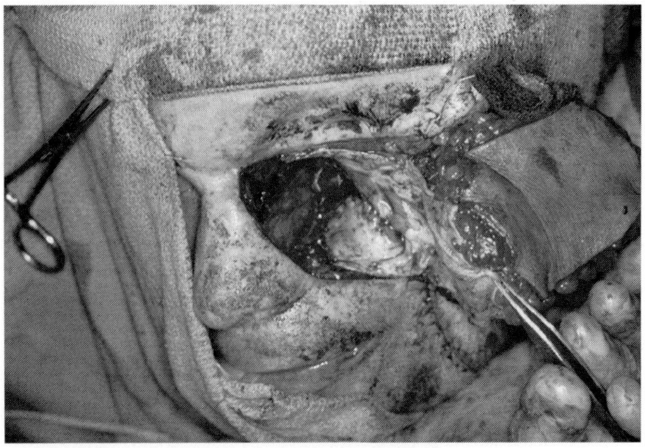

FIGURE 13–9. Local flaps are developed and used for lining the defect.

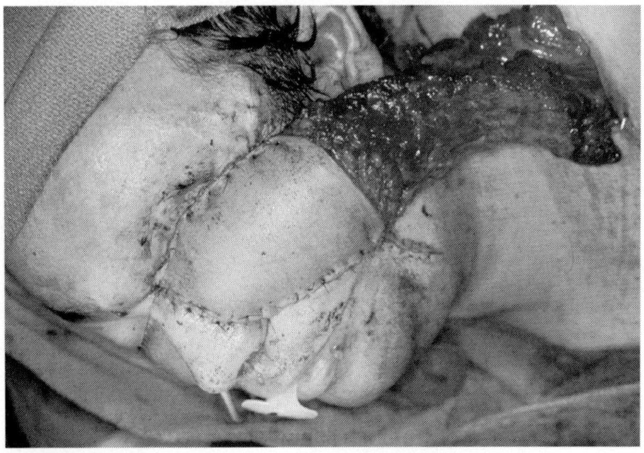

FIGURE 13–10. The PMF sutured in place to reconstruct the defect. The pedicle is externally placed. (See also Color plate.)

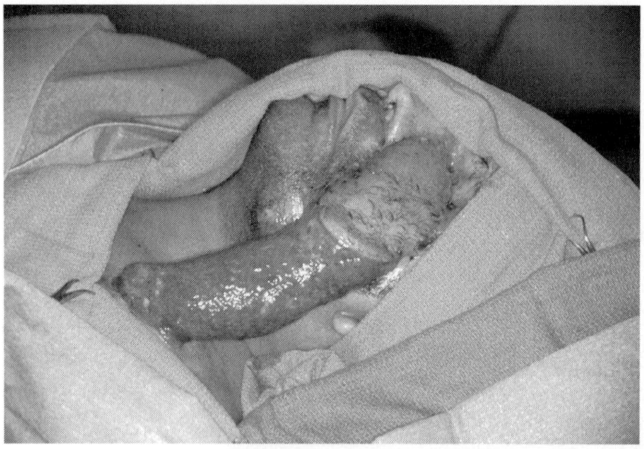

FIGURE 13–11. Three weeks after transfer of the PMF, the pedicle is constricted with a large Penrose drain. There is a good autonomic blood supply on the face derived from blood vessels from local tissues. (See also Color plate.)

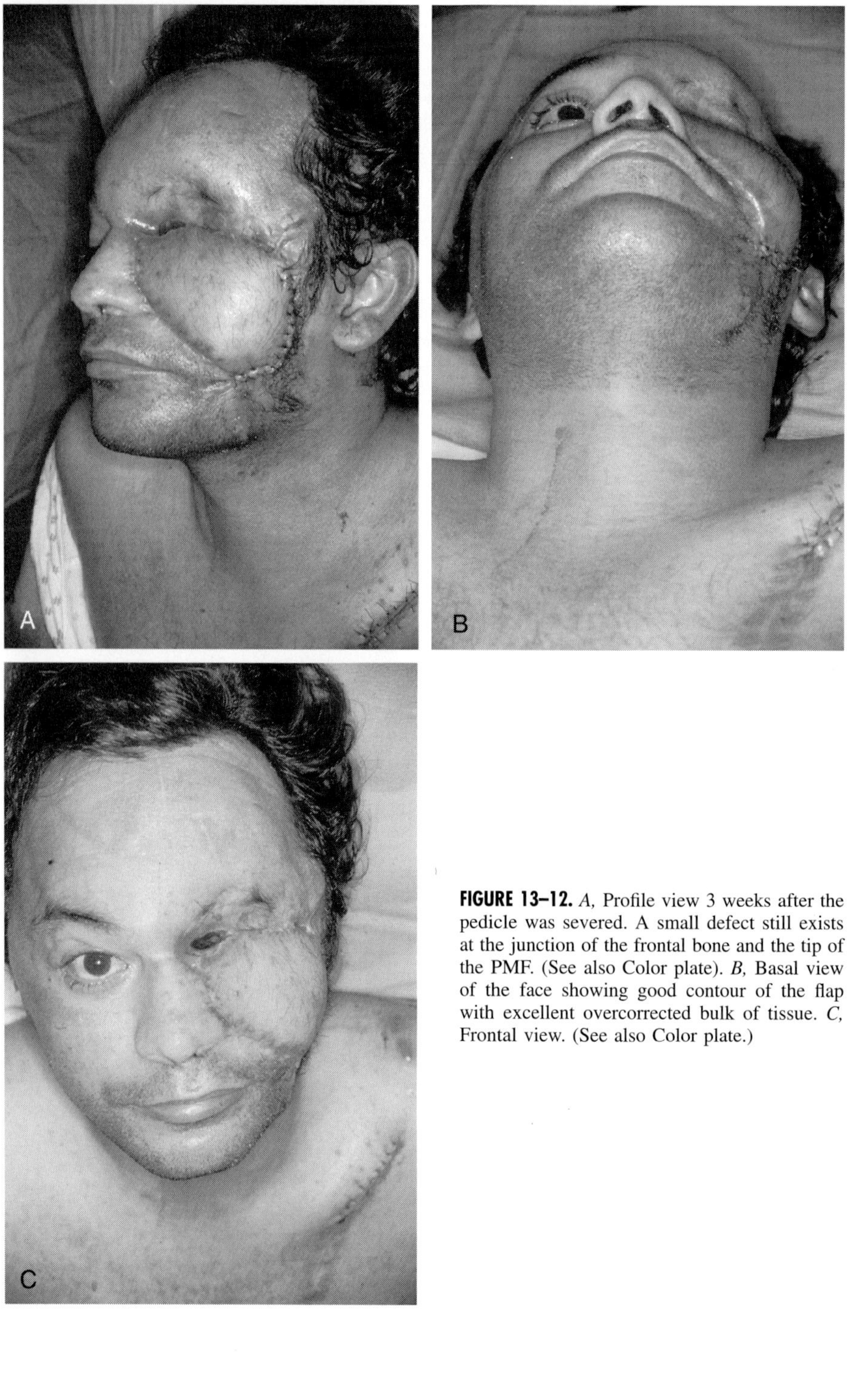

FIGURE 13–12. *A,* Profile view 3 weeks after the pedicle was severed. A small defect still exists at the junction of the frontal bone and the tip of the PMF. (See also Color plate). *B,* Basal view of the face showing good contour of the flap with excellent overcorrected bulk of tissue. *C,* Frontal view. (See also Color plate.)

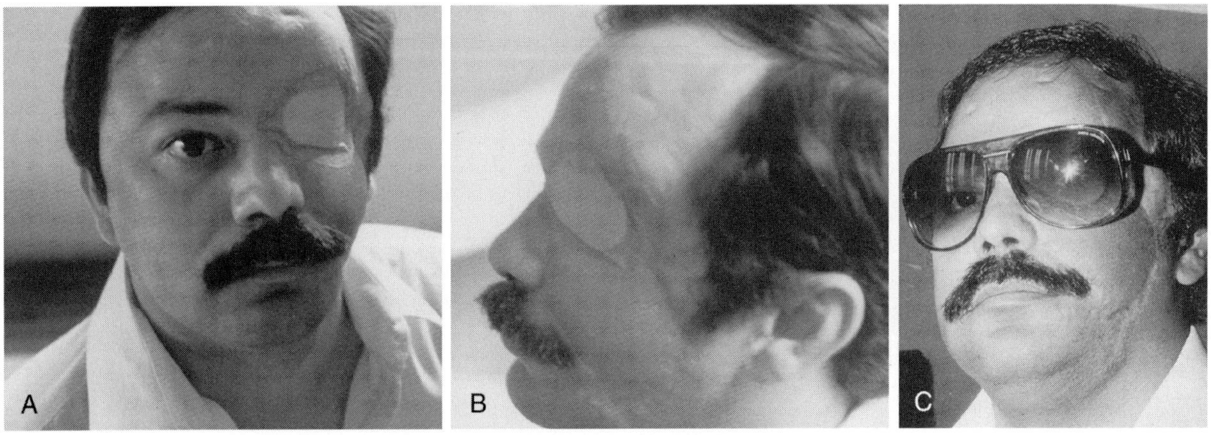

FIGURE 13–13. *A,* Frontal view 1 year postoperatively showing good bulk and color matching of the flap. *B,* Lateral view. (*A* and *B,* see also Color plate.) *C,* Three-quarter view 2 years after reconstruction. The eyepatch and glasses camouflage the defect.

CASE 2

W. B. is a 48-year-old pig farmer who previously had undergone maxillectomy and orbital exenteration with limited anterior craniofacial resection for a mucosal melanoma, the origin of which was believed to be in the maxillary sinus. Although several years had gone by with no evidence of recurrence, a great deal of time was needed during each office visit to clean purulent secretions and remove crusts from this large and very malodorous cavity. The patient was not willing (or able) to care properly for the cavity and later developed a brain abscess, which was treated on two occasions by neurosurgical drainage and long-term antibiotics, and, at the second surgery, by removal of a piece of infected calvarium.

Because the likelihood of additional serious complications was high, it was decided that obliteration of the cavity with a free flap would provide a more sanitary area that would be relatively care free. Computed Tomography (CT) scans show the large bony defect (Fig. 13–15). The patient underwent surgery, which included cleansing of the cavity, wound debridement, and a rectus abdominis myocutaneous free flap. This satisfactorily obliterated the cavity.

Twenty-two days after what initially appeared to be successful surgery, the flap was noted to exhibit compromised perfusion, and the patient was returned to the operating room for exploration of the vascular pedicle. An infected hematoma was found that had not been identified by other clinical indicators (e.g., unexplained swelling, redness, fever, or elevated white cell count). Adequate perfusion could not be reestablished, and the flap failed. It was subsequently debrided, and the wound was cared for over several weeks with dressing changes and allowed to mature as the infection was controlled (Fig. 13–16).

Instead of another (contralateral) rectus flap, it was decided to obliterate the defect with a latissimus dorsi myocutaneous flap (Fig. 13–17). Again, surgery was uneventful, and this time the patient did well and was discharged without evidence of flap compromise (Fig. 13–18). Follow-up visits revealed dehiscence of the wound at the superior medial margin and development of a nasal cutaneous fistula. This fistula apparently developed because the weight of the flap pulling downward on the heavily radiated skin caused the wound to separate before healing took place (Fig. 13–19).

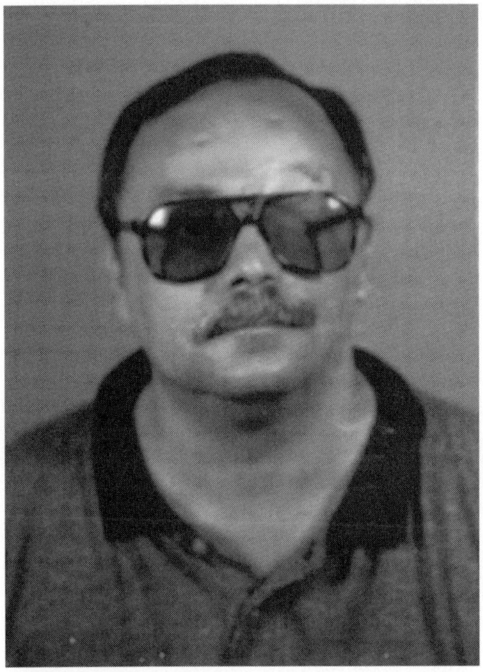

FIGURE 13–14. Twenty-year, full-face follow-up view.

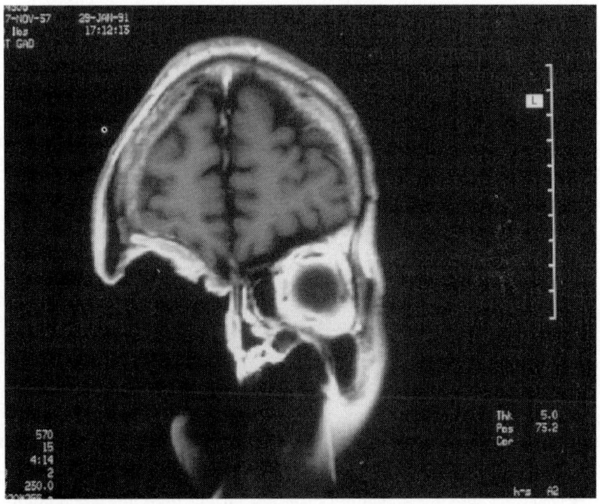

FIGURE 13–15. Coronal CT scan showing status of a large orbitomaxillary defect after excision of a tumor.

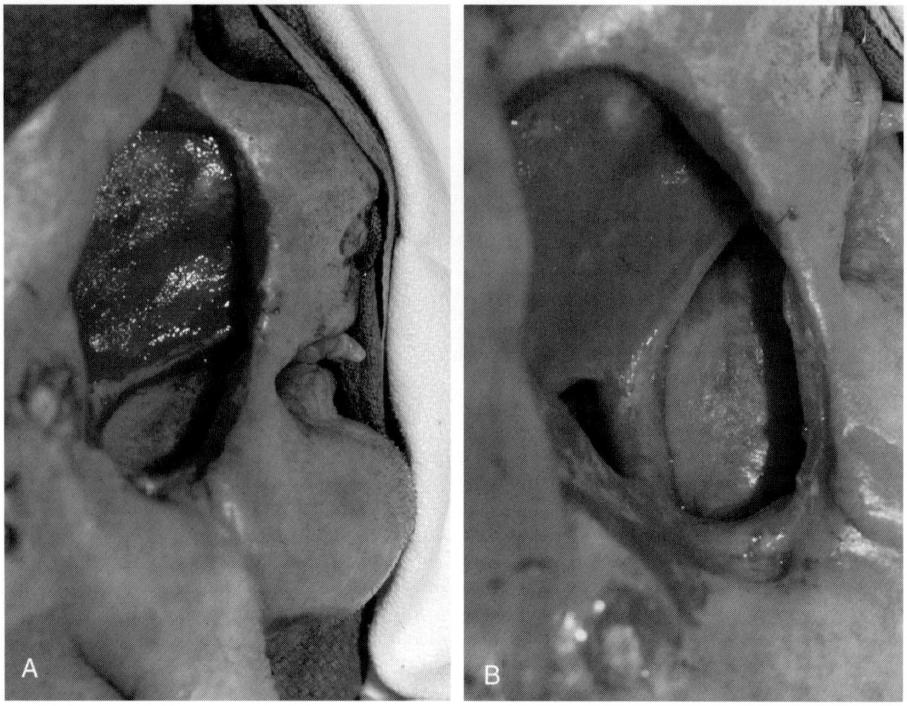

FIGURE 13–16. Orbitomaxillary defect following removal of failed rectus free flap. The nasal septum is visible in the superior two thirds of the cavity. Beneath it is the patient's tongue. *A,* Panoramic view. *B,* Close-up view.

A midline forehead flap fashioned some weeks later was successful in closing the relatively small remaining defect (Fig. 13–20). No further flap problems have occurred to date. The orbital cavity has been nicely obliterated, and the patient wears a prosthetic eye over the flap for cosmetic purposes. Six years later he is back at work on the farm, free of tumor, and has had no further infections, intracranial or otherwise.

CASE 3

W. S. is an otherwise healthy 72-year-old white male who had had a history of a parotid mass for approximately 20 years. The mass had been growing very slowly and did not produce symptoms of facial nerve paralysis or pain. Then it began to grow rapidly several months before evaluation and became increasingly painful owing to facial nerve palsy. A diagnosis of carcinoma ex pleomorphic adenoma was suspected (and was confirmed on final pathologic examination). The patient underwent radical parotidectomy with facial nerve sacrifice and resection of an extensive area of facial skin and muscle to secure tumor-free margins.

Reconstruction was accomplished using a pedicled latissimus dorsi flap, which

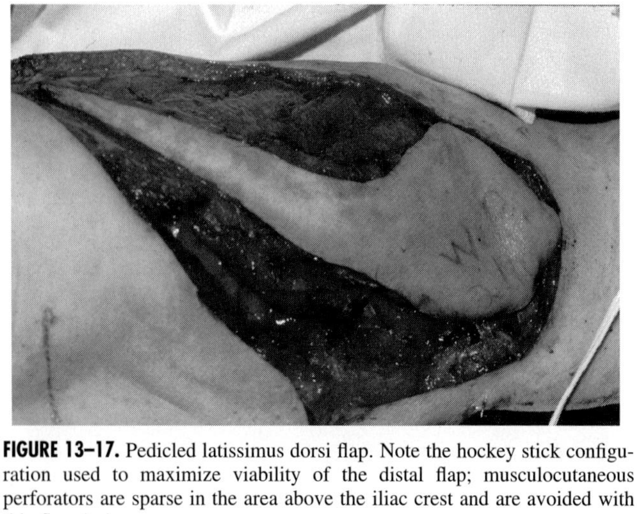

FIGURE 13–17. Pedicled latissimus dorsi flap. Note the hockey stick configuration used to maximize viability of the distal flap; musculocutaneous perforators are sparse in the area above the iliac crest and are avoided with this flap design.

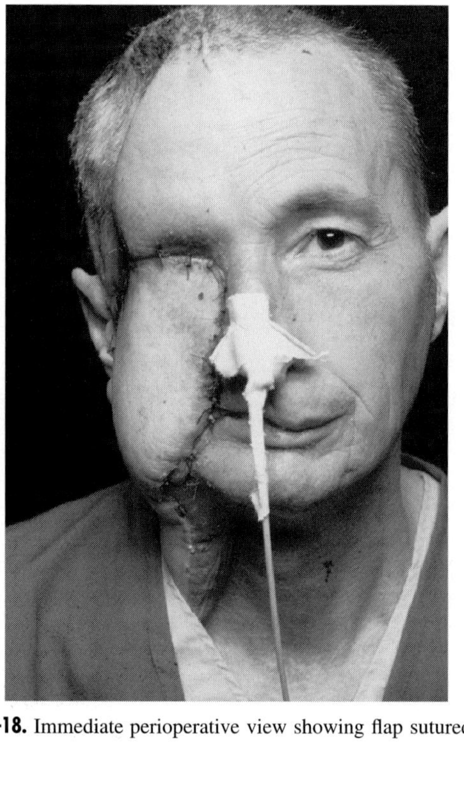

FIGURE 13–18. Immediate perioperative view showing flap sutured in place.

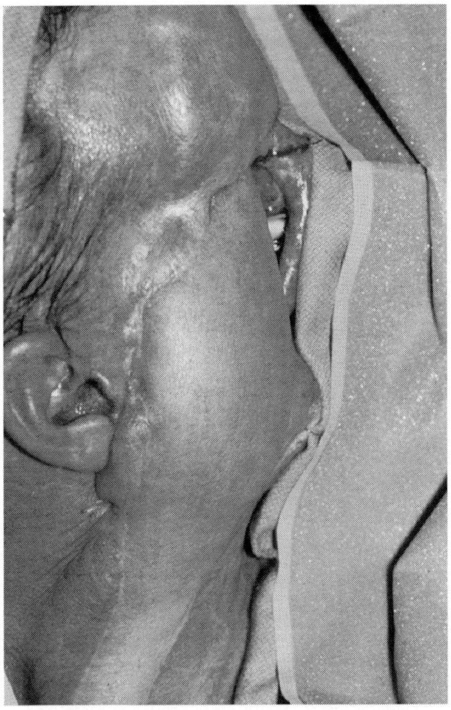

FIGURE 13–19. Latissimus dorsi flap healing in position, with interval development of nasal cutaneous fistula in the superior-medial aspect of the flap. This complication is not infrequently seen if the heavy latissimus dorsi flap is not secured to tissue capable of supporting its weight.

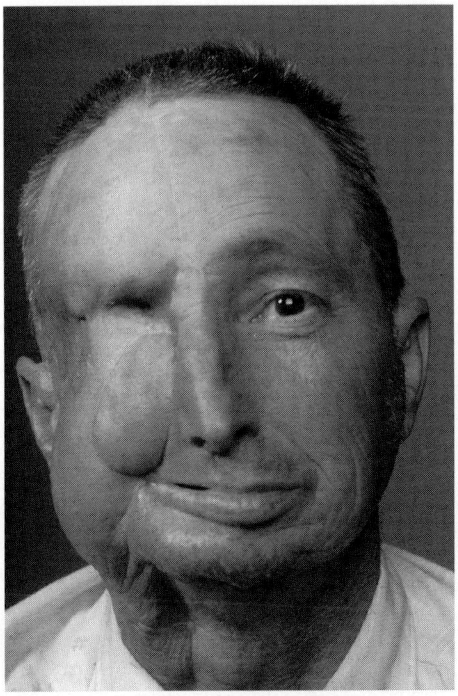

FIGURE 13–20. Same patient 1 year later, with the latissimus dorsi flap completely healed and the fistula closed with a midline forehead flap. No further flap complications occurred, and the patient did not want additional surgical procedures to revise the flap.

readily filled the defect and reached its uppermost margin without difficulty (Fig. 13–21). Postoperative radiation therapy resulted in additional swelling in the infraorbital area, but the procedure nevertheless produced good cosmetic results. Unfortunately, the patient developed spinal metastases and ultimately died from the disease.

CASE 4

The patient was a 31-year-old male who attempted suicide by using a 12-gauge shotgun. At the initial presentation, he had experienced significant destructive loss with total disruption of the midfacial and lower facial architecture and a portion of the mandible. There was no clinical evidence of intracranial injury. The patient was neurologically intact and had normal vision in both eyes (Fig. 13–22).

A careful inspection of the skull base was performed to ensure that there was no fracture or evidence of spinal fluid leak. Traumatic telecanthus was noted (Fig. 13–23). The patient was intubated to secure an adequate airway, intravenous fluids were started, and blood loss was assessed. Once he was stabilized, CT scans of the head, face, and neck were performed to ascertain the extent of the injuries. Extensive damage to the bony structures of the midface were documented. After the patient had been properly evaluated by the neurosurgical service, initial treatment was instituted under general anesthesia. Nonviable facial bony and soft tissues were debrided conservatively. Tissues were placed in their normal position and retained there. Care was taken not to transfer other normal tissues to an abnormal position (Fig. 13–24). A tracheostomy was performed. The telecanthus, orbital, and zygomatic fractures were repaired with appropriate sutures and plating. The mandibular defect was reconstructed with titanium plating.

After several weeks, the facial tissues had healed. The amount of loss of the bony structures was then assessed using a three-dimensional CT scan (Fig. 13–25). The maxilla and palate were reconstructed using a scapular free flap (Fig. 13–26). The excess amount of skin gained from the composite scapular free flap was used to line the nasal area in preparation for reconstructive rhinoplasty (Fig. 13–27).

A nasal airway was obtained by resection of the excess skin and scar tissue. Tissue expanders were used to provide more soft tissue surface area in the forehead to be used for future nasal reconstruction (Fig. 13–28). Then reconstructive rhinoplasty was performed by forming a proper lining with local tissues. Support was obtained by using a titanium plate framework anchored to a cranial bone graft secured to the frontal bone. The midline forehead flap provided the covering. The nasal tip was tailored accordingly (Fig. 13–29).

Unfortunately, the patient was lost to follow-up and did not undergo return of the glabellar area of the midline forehead flap. Later, he was involved in an altercation and was hit hard on the nose, exposing the titanium framework. This area became infected, and the titanium implant had to be removed. No further reconstruction was done in this patient, and no other photographs could be obtained. (The free flaps and reconstructive rhinoplasty were performed by Drs. Ramon M. Esclamado and Shan R. Baker, at the University of Michigan, Ann Arbor, Michigan.)

Comments

Reconstructive surgery is especially challenging when the skin, soft tissues, and bones of the face are missing or have

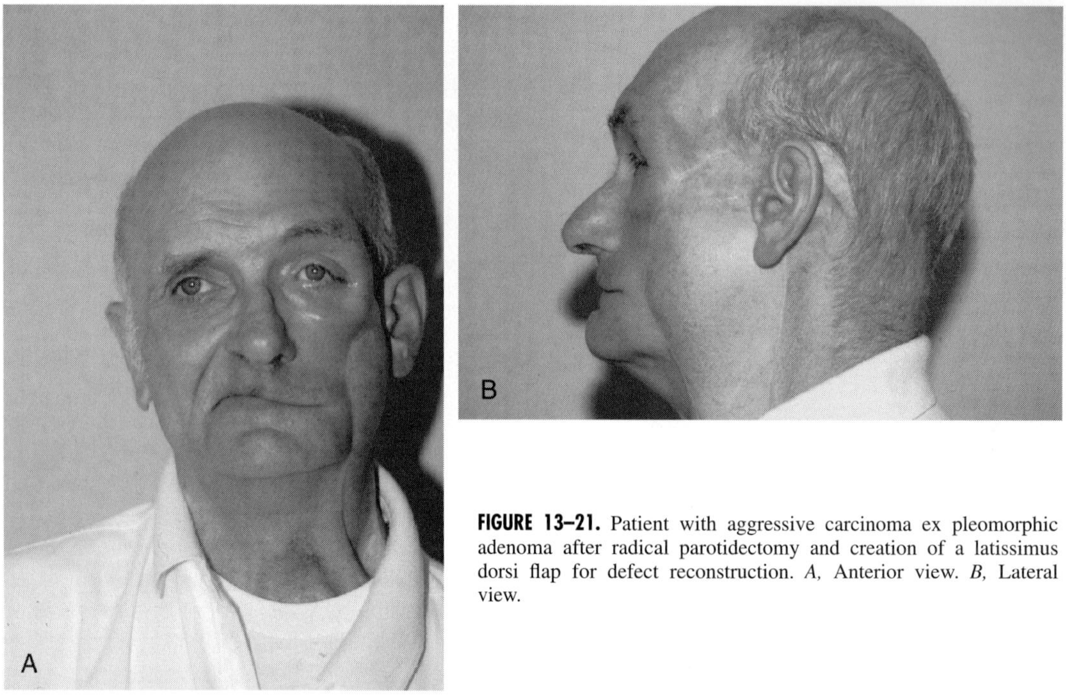

FIGURE 13–21. Patient with aggressive carcinoma ex pleomorphic adenoma after radical parotidectomy and creation of a latissimus dorsi flap for defect reconstruction. *A*, Anterior view. *B*, Lateral view.

been markedly distorted by scar tissue as a result of healing by second intention. When the premaxillary skin and cheek flap are present, reconstruction is easier because the covering provided by these structures is an important factor in the overall success of the transfer of tissues, either pedicled or revascularized. The combination of tissue transfer and anaplastology is advantageous, especially when a prosthesis is accepted by the patient for camouflage, particularly when the eyelids and eyeball are absent. In Case 1, the patient preferred to conceal the orbital defect with large dark glasses rather than using an orbital prosthesis. This patient was treated in the late 1970s, and osseointegrated titanium implants for fixation of the prosthesis were not available at that time. Nevertheless, even more recently, this patient has not seen the need for orbital camouflage with a prosthesis. Once the transferred tissue heals, the results are permanent, and the prosthesis is for the most part trouble-free. Osseointegrated implants may with time result in some failures, especially in patients who have undergone radiation therapy. Again, hyperbaric oxygen therapy may be necessary in such patients prior to implantation to improve local tissue blood supply and the success of the implant.

Cases 2 and 3 illustrate the use of the latissimus dorsi flap, which is a very good alternative for filling large defects. It may be combined with other free or pedicle flaps as needed. It has a rich blood supply and tolerates postoperative radiation therapy very well.

GUNSHOT WOUNDS OF THE FACE

Initial Assessment

On initial examination of the patient, the clinician's impression is usually that of massive soft tissue and bone loss

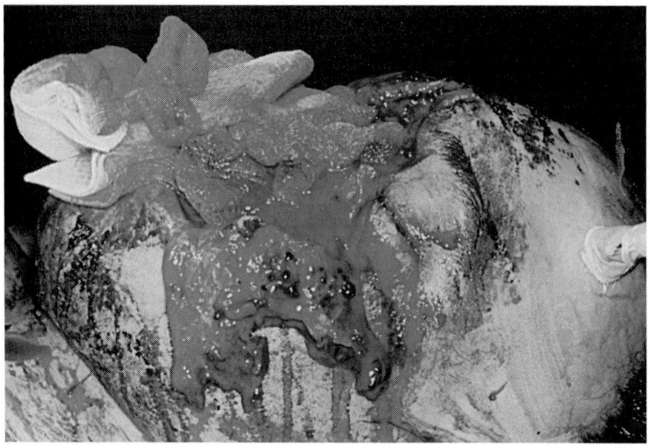

FIGURE 13–22. Initial presentation to the emergency room of a patient with a self-inflicted gunshot wound.

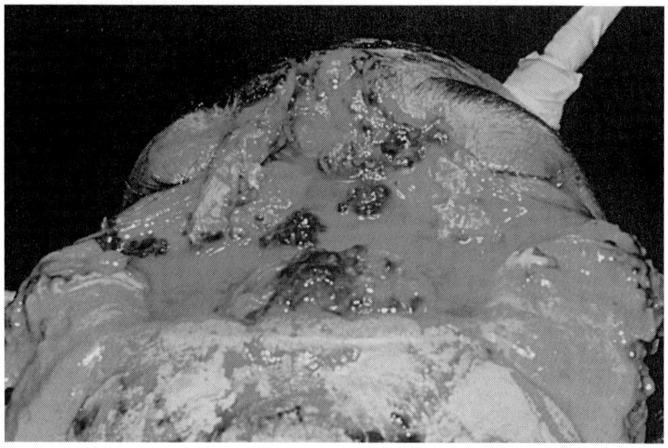

FIGURE 13–23. Submental vertex view exhibiting significant facial disruption and severe traumatic telecanthus.

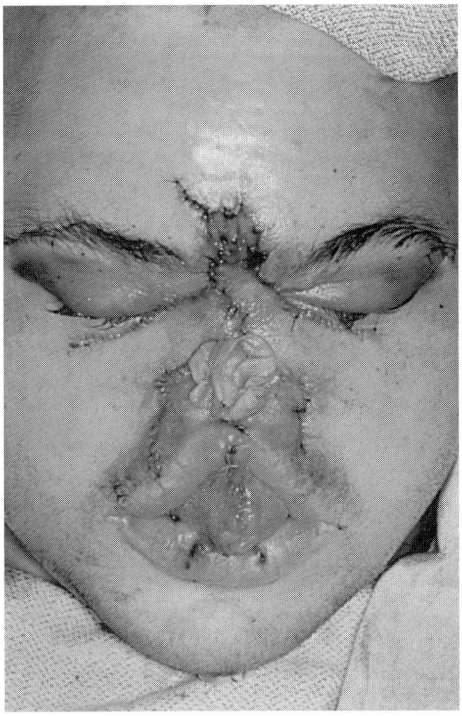

FIGURE 13–24. View of completed initial repair. Note the distortion of the normal structures and soft tissue architecture.

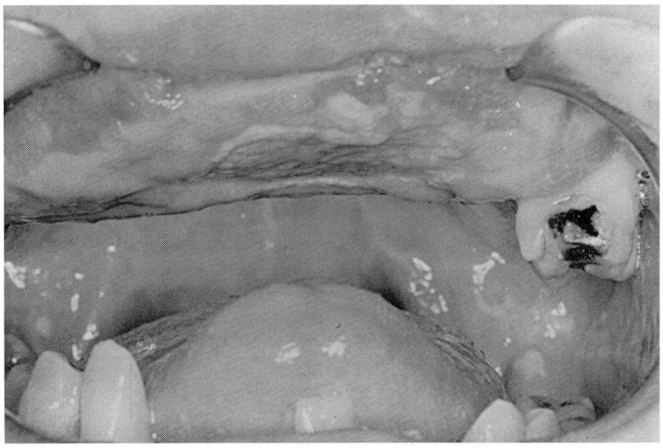

FIGURE 13–26. Reconstruction of the maxilla and palate through use of a scapular free flap.

as a result of a large gaping wound that has splayed the face open. If possible, it is important to determine the type and caliber of weapon that caused the injury because these facts may play an important role in the initial management of the patient. Although the extent of injury depends on the trajectory of the bullet, handgun injuries usually involve a relatively low velocity bullet and, generally speaking, cause greater bone injury than soft tissue destruction. Rifles, on the other hand, produce significantly more injury because of a higher missile velocity. As a rifle bullet passes through the soft tissue, it produces a shock wave that results in a cavitation effect along the path of the bullet. Similarly, a high-velocity projectile striking bone causes bone fragments to become secondary projectiles that produce even further bone and soft tissue injury. Shotguns usually produce the worst types of injury consisting of significant bone and soft tissue losses that depend on the trajectories of the multiple pellets.[4]

At the time of presentation, patients with gunshot injuries of the midface are usually intubated, and intravenous lines are placed for initial resuscitation. Once the patient has been stabilized, a CT scan should be obtained before surgical

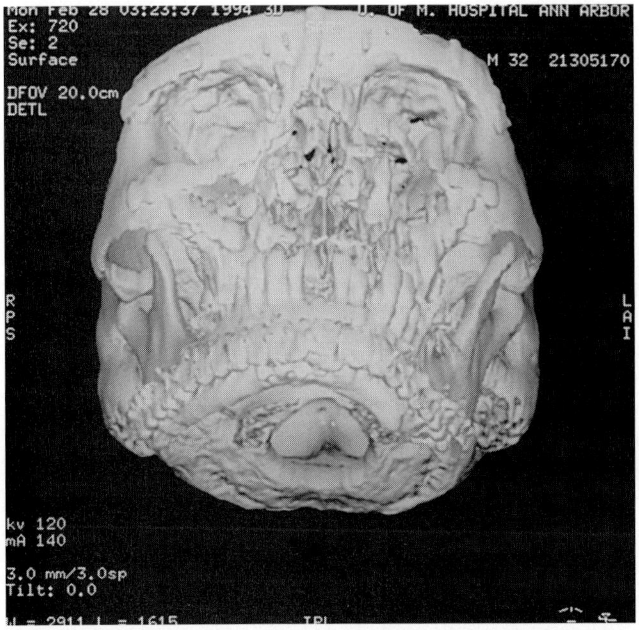

FIGURE 13–25. Three-dimensional CT scan demonstrating the deficient bone of the midface. Mandibular continuity has been achieved by stabilizing the fragments with a reconstruction plate.

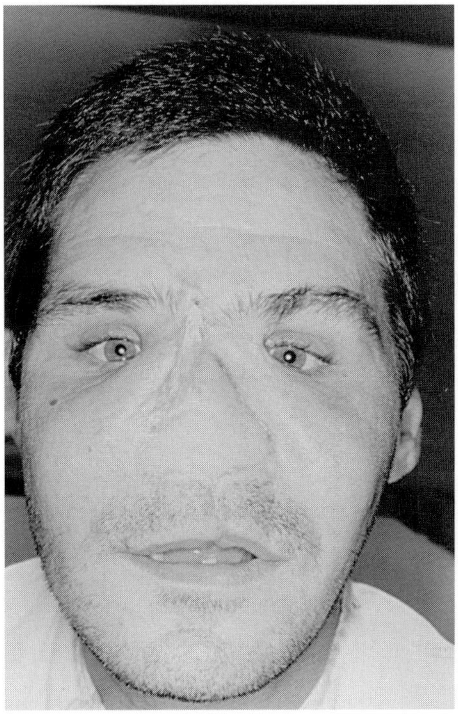

FIGURE 13–27. Excess skin from the scapular free flap has been used to provide bulk to the midface.

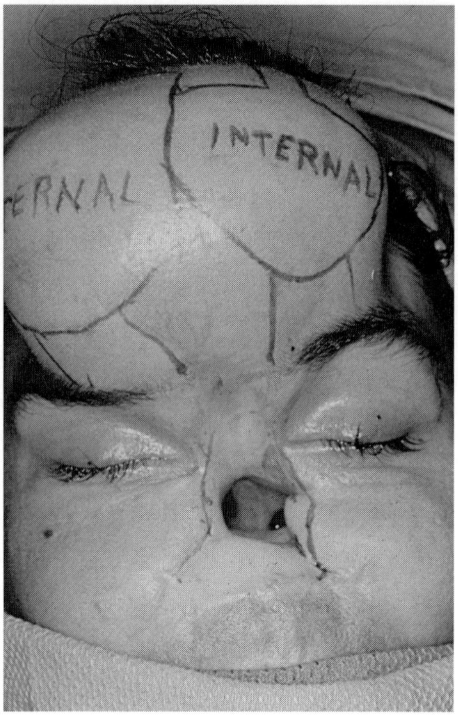

FIGURE 13–28. Tissue expanders are used to provide sufficient skin for nasal reconstruction. The nasal airway has been established by excising skin and scar tissue.

repair is performed. The CT scan is helpful in evaluating the amount of remaining bone and in locating bone fragments that have been driven into soft tissues removed from the immediate area of injury. The surgeon should examine the scan carefully for the presence of pneumocephalus because this finding indicates violation of the anterior cranial fossa, disruption of the dura, and subsequent cerebrospinal fluid (CSF) leak. The presence of a small CSF leak may be difficult to detect during evaluation of a patient with a self-inflicted shotgun wound to the face in whom there has been significant tissue destruction and bleeding. CSF leaks should be repaired at the time of the initial repair of facial injuries. Neurosurgical evaluation is of utmost importance, and neurosurgical treatment as necessary should precede any maxillofacial trauma treatment.

Initial psychiatric evaluation is imperative in patients with self-inflicted gunshot injuries. Few patients who sustain gunshot wounds may try this form of suicide a second time.

After patient evaluation and review of the CT scan, separate areas of the face should be considered for reconstruction in an orderly fashion. Following well-established principles of facial trauma repair, that is, working from the more stable to the unstable areas, reconstruction should begin with the skull base and extend inferiorly to the naso-orbital-ethmoid complex, zygoma, maxilla, and mandible, and, finally, to the overlying soft tissue. The basic principles of craniomaxillofacial surgery should apply, the most important of which is to repair the underlying bony injury first and the overlying soft tissue next.

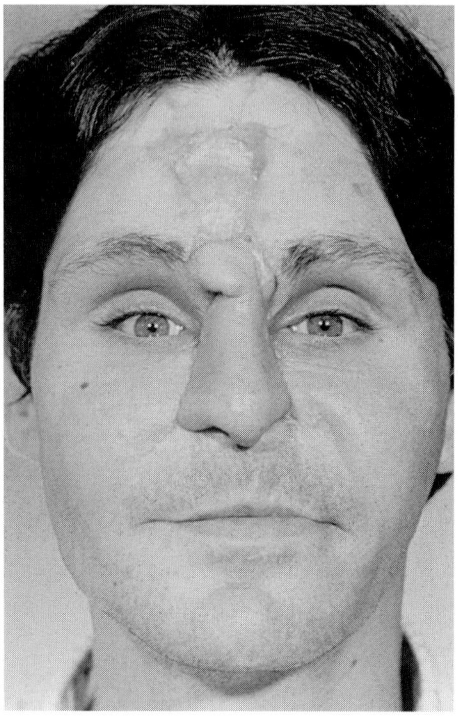

FIGURE 13–29. Forehead flaps have been used for the nasal reconstruction. Pedicle division and scar revisions have yet to be done.

Initial Treatment

The intent at the time of the initial repair should be to save all attached bone and soft tissue fragments. Nonviable tissues should be debrided conservatively, particularly the soft tissues of the face. Tissue that may appear dusky at the time of initial presentation usually regains its blood supply and heals quite well; tissue that becomes necrotic in the postoperative period may be replaced in the subsequent bone and soft tissue reconstruction phase.

Gilles developed many principles as a result of his experience with gunshot injuries to the face during World War I.[18] Of these, the first was to place tissue in its normal position and retain it there. Second, normal tissue should not be transferred into an abnormal position. Gilles' experience established that it was advisable to leave gaps in the wound field where tissue was missing. Tissue transferred to an abnormal position results in scar contracture that can be extremely difficult if not impossible to correct postoperatively several months later.

From a surgical standpoint, the naso-orbital-ethmoid complex fracture with traumatic telecanthus is probably the most important and the most difficult problem to correct secondarily. Proper anatomic reduction of the medial canthal region is essential because traumatic telecanthus is almost impossible to correct fully if revision is delayed. The medial canthal ligaments should be identified and tagged with sutures to allow proper positioning. In the absence of medial orbital walls, calvarial bone grafts should be placed to secure the ligaments to the grafts. If bone grafts are not used, contracture of the scar tissue will bring about lateralization of the medial canthi, causing telecanthus during the postoperative period. In securing the medial canthi, it is essential that the sutures placed through the nasal cavity are aimed in a posterior direction because this will ensure that the lacrimal puncti come into contact with the globes. If the nasal septum is absent, bone grafts should be used to replace it as well. The transcanthal-transnasal sutures should be passed through this bone graft to ensure a posterior pull by these sutures. In this situation, bone grafts may have to be plated directly to the skull base because the entire nasoethmoid complex is often missing. Generally speaking, the adult interorbital distance as measured from each anterior lacrimal crest should be 25 mm. This measurement should be considered when reconstructing a traumatic telecanthus. If possible, traumatic telecanthus should be overcorrected so that the medial canthal ligaments are secured 20 to 25 mm apart.

Typically, in patients with a self-inflicted gunshot wound, the zygomas are fractured and displaced laterally. It is important to expose these bones fully through a coronal approach so that anatomic reduction can begin from the root of the zygoma and proceed anteriorly. As the reduction and fixation phase of surgery proceeds, the surgeon should keep in mind the relationship of the zygomas to the naso-orbital-ethmoid complex and take care to reduce the zygomas medially to avoid excessive bizygomatic facial width. As a general rule, the zygomas should be positioned medially on a line tangent properly to the most anterior portion of the cornea lying 5 mm anterior to the inferior orbital rim in a vertical plane. The farther the zygomas are positioned medially, the greater the globe projection obtained. If orbital floor fractures that also require reduction are present, this procedure should be done at the same time as anatomic reduction of the zygomas to avoid entrapment, particularly of the inferior rectus muscle. Any defects in the orbital floor should be repaired by an implant of whatever type is preferred by the surgeon. It should be noted that the implant also aids in establishing the proper vertical position of the globes.

Anterior maxillary defects are extremely common in self-inflicted gunshot wounds. These may range from small defects of the premaxilla to total absence of the premaxilla, hard palate, and right and left posterior maxillae. However, careful inspection often reveals that fragments of the posterior maxilla are in place, and, although fractured, these fragments usually contain the first and second molars, which may be sufficient to establish the posterior facial height. Because the anterior maxilla has been lost, only the lateral (zygomaticomaxillary) buttresses can be used to reduce these posterior maxillary fragments anatomically. In cases of severe comminution, bone grafts may be used to add stability to the segments. Rigid fixation of the lateral buttress is imperative, and additional fixation may be required to stabilize these fragments to the existing zygoma or, in some instances, to the pterygoid plates or the skull base itself.

Following fixation of the buttress, consideration is given to the mandibular injury. The remaining mandibular bone fragments are carefully assessed again. Typically, the anterior mandible is fragmented or lost, but the rami and angles are usually intact. Often, however, there is a concomitant condylar injury resulting from the force of the blast being transmitted through the weight-bearing portion of the mandible to the condylar heads. If the condyles are fractured and displaced, open reduction and internal fixation of these fracture sites is useful to help restore the posterior facial height. A reconstruction plate is attached to the existing mandible, paying attention to the overlying soft tissues so that the position of the plate neither overcorrects nor undercorrects the defect. The plate is securely fastened to the mandibular rami bilaterally, and then the bone fragments are secured to the plate. These may be further supported by miniplates placed across each fracture line to further stabilize the segments. However, the remaining mandible is supported by the heavier reconstruction plate.

Once skeletal repair has been achieved, repair of the soft tissues is undertaken. It should be kept in mind that questionably viable tissue often regains its blood supply and heals satisfactorily. Therefore, only conservative debridement, if any, should be performed. Lacerations in these patients tend to have a starburst pattern because of the sudden expansion of the oral cavity from the trajectory of the gunshot pellets. The soft tissue should be cleansed meticulously to remove as much gunpowder residue as possible along with any lead pellets that remain embedded in the wound. Lacerations are closed in multiple layers, paying particular attention to eversion of the skin edges to minimize the degree of widening of the scars. Because the lacerations result from a tearing or ripping action rather than a clean incision, they are more prone to scarring, and follow-up assessment of the scar on a long-term basis is advisable. Whenever soft tissue is found to be deficient, it is prudent to leave the gaps open to avoid significant distortion of the normal facial architecture, which can be extremely difficult to correct secondarily. If it is deemed necessary to use normal tissue to close gaps, the next phase of reconstruction should be undertaken early before any definitive healing of the overlying soft tissues has occurred.[19]

Initial Bone and Soft Tissue Reconstruction

Following the initial repair, it is essential to (1) thoroughly assess the position of the bone and soft tissues still present, and (2) determine the areas of bone and soft tissue that are missing. Bone replacement may require free bone grafts or free tissue transfer, but the choice depends on the amount of adjacent soft tissue that remains. As is true in any maxillofacial fracture, it is best to start from the stable areas and proceed to the unstable areas—i.e., to begin with areas that have the least amount of tissue loss and work toward areas with greater amounts of tissue loss. Typically, this type of repair begins at the medial orbital walls and orbital floors if this area has not been repaired at the time of the initial surgery. Free calvarial bone grafts are most often used in this region to reconstruct the orbital walls, and these are fixed directly to the anterior skull base as would be the case with medial orbital wall grafts. The medial canthal tendons are secured to the bone grafts to prevent delayed drift and post-traumatic telecanthus.

The maxilla should be the next area analyzed by the surgeon. Small defects may be reconstructed with either calvarial bone grafts or multiple-layered decorticated split-rib grafts. In either case, it is important to place the grafts, if at all possible, in such a position that dental implants may be placed at a later date to ensure complete prosthetic rehabilitation. If a large segment of the maxilla has been lost, strong consideration should be given to free tissue transfer.

The three flaps most commonly used in maxillary reconstruction are the radial forearm free flap, the scapular free flap, and the fibular free flap, each of which has unique advantages and disadvantages. The radial forearm free flap can transfer skin with an extremely small amount of subcutaneous tissue and bone that requires little debridement to fit the patient with a maxillary prosthesis. The flap has a long pedicle, and the artery and veins are of sufficient caliber to allow relative ease of anastomosis and thus an increased rate of success. The disadvantage of this flap, however, is that the bone that is transferred encompasses only 40% of the diameter of the radius, and typically this is not sufficient to allow successful implantation of osseointegrated dental implants and requires additional bone grafting at a later stage.

The scapular free flap is a highly versatile flap that may be harvested with skin and bone and transferred with multiple skin paddles to reconstruct the surface of the maxilla as well as the nasal surface and any defects that may occur in the skin of the midface. Although the bone is sufficiently long to allow total maxillary reconstruction, in some cases it may not be thick enough to allow adequate anchorage for dental implants.

The fibular free flap is a reliable flap that allows transfer of both bone and skin. The bone is of sufficient quantity to provide solid anchorage for osseointegrated implants, but the skin transferred in this flap is less versatile and has a smaller surface area than that provided by the scapular free flap.

Mandibular reconstruction is a significant consideration in these patients, and the reconstruction of choice is free tissue transfer. The two best choices for mandibular reconstruction are the iliac crest and the fibular free flap. The iliac crest not only provides a significant amount of cancellous bone, it also readily accepts dental implants. Unfortunately, it has the disadvantage of carrying with it a significant amount of soft tissue that will require postoperative debulking several months later. More recently, fibular free flaps have become the gold standard for mandibular replacement because they provide a significant amount of strong bone that more than tolerates the axial loading imposed by dental implants as well as skin coverage for intraoral or extraoral soft tissue deficiencies. At this stage of reconstruction, it is important to obtain a lateral cephalogram for accurate determination of the position of the maxilla and mandible. Although the goal in post-trauma reconstruction is to restore pre-injury occlusion in patients with self-inflicted gunshot wounds, it is not difficult to reestablish a class I dental occlusion and class I skeletal relationship even when a significant amount of tissue has been lost. The position of the maxilla can be determined best by using cephalometric radiography preoperatively and then analyzing the radiographs during the reconstruction. Reconstruction may require many steps, including (1) initial positioning of the bone and/or soft tissue, and (2) revision surgery in which the bone of the maxilla is placed in the proper position to accept dental implants to secure a prosthesis in a skeletal class I relationship. Also, when reconstructing the maxilla or the mandible in these patients, it is best to transfer more tissue than that initially required. Because soft tissues atrophy and contract around the transferred bone, what appears to be an excess amount of tissue at the time of initial surgery may actually result in a merely adequate amount of tissue over an extended period of time. Therefore, it is recommended that excess tissue be provided initially and debrided during subsequent stages of reconstruction rather than bringing in additional soft tissue at a later stage.[18]

Secondary Reconstruction

Following mandibular and maxillary reconstruction, the surgeon should assess what is required for any remaining soft tissue reconstruction and dental rehabilitation. Hypertrophic scar tissue excision is done prior to nasal reconstruction to correct the midface properly. This may be done at the time of nasal reconstruction or at a separate stage preceding definitive repair. In patients with less extensive injuries, only soft tissue revisions such as scar revision or nasal alar reconstruction may be required. These procedures may be performed with local flaps; conchal cartilage grafts may be used to reconstruct the nose. In more severe cases, total nasal reconstruction may be required to provide an adequate nasal airway and cosmesis. If total nasal reconstruction is necessary, paramedian or horizontal forehead flap reconstruction is the treatment of choice. Alternatively, the radial forearm free flap provides another excellent method of reconstructing total nasal defects, but subsequent revision and thinning of the flap are required. If subtotal or total nasal reconstruction is required, both internal and external lining tissues are needed in addition to bone support for the nasal dorsum. The paramedian forehead flap provides an adequate amount of soft tissue covering for the nasal framework, but it may require tissue expanders to provide adequate soft tissue. Nevertheless, tissue expanders should be avoided unless one is dealing with a very large defect. If lip incompetence is apparent when oral competence is assessed, additional soft tissue should be transferred to the oral area to achieve improvement in swallowing, speech, and cosmesis.

Tertiary Reconstruction

By the time of tertiary reconstruction, patients have undergone both maxillary and mandibular reconstruction as well as soft tissue reconstruction. Scar revision may involve excision of excessive scar tissue as well as redirection of scar tissue contracture into normal skin tension lines. If dental implants have been placed, this is the phase in reconstruction when they are uncovered. Although dental rehabilitation is the goal in reconstruction of patients with gunshot injuries to the face, this is not always completely possible. At this point in the reconstructive process, the maxilla and mandible should ideally be in a class I skeletal relationship or as close to that relationship as possible. If sufficient bone is present, dental implants may be placed in the mandible and maxilla that will allow dentures to be used at a later date. If dental implants cannot be used, it may be possible to place simple dentures over the existing bone. This usually requires some degree of soft tissue or intraoral reconstruction to provide a good stable base for the dentures with adequate retention. In patients requiring mandibular dentures, attention must be paid to the lingual and buccal aspects of the mandibular alveolar ridge because often the floor of the mouth is elevated and the buccal sulcus is obliterated. In these situations, a procedure to lower the floor of the mouth may be combined with simultaneous vestibuloplasty. The use of buccal inlay skin grafts allows successful reconstruction of the mandibular vestibule and also prevents instability of the denture during swallowing and speech. Maxillary vestibuloplasty may be necessary also using buccal inlay skin graft techniques to allow adequate retention of the maxillary dentures and prevent upper lip retraction caused by the labial flange of the denture or an excessive anterior maxillary show of teeth from the denture. Reconstructive rhinoplasty, preferably using a forehead flap with titanium and cranial bone support, completes the rehabilitation of the patient's maxillofacial injuries.

SUMMARY

Massive midfacial defects involving the orbit, maxilla, cheek, and lower face can be successfully reconstructed with good functional and aesthetic results by applying sound principles of osteosynthesis and plating, repair of soft tissue injuries, and local regional and distant pedicled flaps. More recently, free flaps (skin, soft tissue, or composite flaps with bone) have allowed great advances in reconstructive techniques. The alternatives to reconstruction and the options should be discussed with the patient. Anaplastology, surgery, or a combination of both may offer the best or most proper solution to each patient.

REFERENCES

1. Baker SP, O'Neill B, Korpf RS: The Injury Fact Book. Lexington, MA, Lexington Books, 1984.
2. Khalil AF: Civilian gunshot wounds to the face and jaws. Br J Oral Surg 18:205, 1980.
3. Osborne TE, Bays RA: Pathophysiology and management of gunshot wounds to the face. *In* Fonseca RJ, Walker RV (eds): Oral and Maxillofacial Trauma, Vol 2. Philadelphia, W.B. Saunders, 1991.
4. Banks P, Mellor S, Haywood IR, Wilson JSP, Sanders R: Gunshot wounds. *In* Williams JLL (ed): Rowe and William's Maxillofacial Injuries, Vol 2. London, Churchill Livingstone, 1994.
5. Igawa HH, Minakawa HM, Sugihara T, Homma K: Cheek reconstruction with an expanded prefabricated musculocutaneous free flap: Case report. Br J Plast Surg 48:569, 1995.
6. Schliephake H, Schmelzeisen R, Neukam FW: The free revascularized rectus abdominis myocutaneous flap for the repair of tumour related defects in the head and neck area. Br J Oral Maxillofac Surg 34:18, 1996.
7. Niranjan NS, Watson DP: Reconstruction of the cheek using a "suspended" radial forearm free flap. Br J Plast Surg 43:365, 1990.
8. Hunter D, Baker S, Sobol S: Split calvarial grafts in maxillofacial reconstruction. Otolaryngol Head Neck Surg 102:345, 1990.
9. Ewers R: Reconstruction of the maxilla with a double musculoperiosteal flap in connection with a composite calvarial bone graft. Plast Reconstr Surg 81:431, 1988.
10. Granick MS, Ramasastry SS, Newton ED, et al: Reconstruction of complex maxillectomy defects with the scapular-free flap. Head Neck 12:377, 1990.
11. Guillamondegui OM, Campbell BH: The folded trapezius flap for through-and-through cheek defects. Otolaryngol Head Neck Surg 97:24, 1987.
12. Brown JS: Deep circumflex iliac artery free flap with internal oblique muscle as a new method of immediate reconstruction of maxillectomy defect. Head Neck 18:412, 1996.
13. Endo T, Nakayama Y, Soeda S: Reconstruction of the cheek and palate using a three-paddle tensor fasciae latae free. Br J Plast Surg 44:234, 1991.
14. Papachristou DN, Valinos P, Skandalakis P, Sechas M: Reconstruction of full-thickness defects of the cheek in cancer surgery. Am Surg 53:592, 1987.
15. Holle J, Vinzenz K, Wuringer E, et al: The prefabricated combined scapula flap for bony and soft-tissue reconstruction in maxillofacial defects—a new method. Plast Reconstr Surg 98:542, 1996.
16. Cheung LK: An animal model for maxillary reconstruction using a temporalis muscle flap. J Oral Maxillofac Surg 54:1439, 1996.
17. Williams RW, Speculand B, Robin PE, Simms M: Second reconstruction of the posterior maxilla with a free latissimus dorsi muscle flap. Int J Oral Maxillofac Surg 21:284, 1992.
18. Gilles HD: Plastic Surgery of the Face: War Injuries of the Face. London, Oxford University Press, 1920.
19. Kellman RM, Marentette LJ (eds): Atlas of Craniomaxillofacial Fixation. New York, Raven Press, 1995.

CHAPTER 14

Skeletal Reconstruction Following Extended Maxillectomy

Richard E. Davis, M.D.
Francisco J. Civantos, M.D.
Barry Shipman, D.M.D.

The human midface defines facial appearance more than any other anatomic subunit. In addition to cosmesis, the midface is also of critical importance in numerous vital functions such as speech, mastication, deglutition, breathing, vision, and facial expression. Not surprisingly, large surgical defects of the midface, such as those arising from total maxillectomy, are associated with severe functional and cosmetic morbidity. Owing to the intricate three-dimensional shape and complex functional role of the midface, bilateral maxillectomy defects remain a formidable challenge for the reconstructive surgeon.

With the advent of microvascular tissue transfer technology and improved bone reconstruction techniques, effective approaches are slowly emerging for the functional and aesthetic reconstruction of patients with extensive maxillectomy defects. Although these techniques remain preliminary, they hold promise for long-term surgical rehabilitation of patients following bilateral maxillectomy. This chapter reviews the structural anatomy of the midface and the morbidity of composite midfacial resection. Our approach to reconstruction and rehabilitation of complex midfacial defects is also presented.

SKELETAL ANATOMY OF THE MIDFACE

The facial skeleton is composed of dense membranous bone organized into a series of integrated vertical and horizontal load-bearing struts (Fig. 14–1). The framework created by these skeletal struts maintains the normal facial dimensions by providing rigid support for the overlying soft tissues. Facial height is provided by three pairs of vertically oriented maxillary struts, known as the *nasomaxillary, zygomaticomaxillary,* and *pterygomaxillary* buttresses.[1] In addition to maintaining facial height, the vertical maxillary buttress system also provides a stable resistance platform for the powerful forces of mastication by uniting the upper jaw with the orbit, frontal bar, malar eminence, and pterygoid bone, which in turn are united with the overlying skull base. Similarly, facial projection and width are provided by the paired zygomatic arches, which form a horizontal buttress between the lateral skull base and the malar eminence, orbital rim, and upper jaw. Although small bony defects of the anterior maxilla or lateral nasal wall are usually asymptomatic, significant disruption of the maxillary buttress system predisposes the overlying soft tissue envelope to unopposed scar contracture and progressive soft tissue collapse.

MAXILLECTOMY DEFECTS

Tumors arising in the premaxilla, septum, alveolus, hard palate, paranasal sinuses, or orbit frequently require maxillectomy for surgical control of neoplastic disease. Spiro and co-workers formally classified surgical defects of the maxilla into limited, subtotal, or total according to the extent of tissue removed.[2] *Limited* maxillectomy defects result from removal of a single antral wall, usually the anterior or medial antral wall. Often these defects are asymptomatic and require no reconstructive management. *Subtotal* maxillectomy defects result from resection of the ipsilateral palate and at least two adjacent antral walls. As with limited maxillectomy defects, some or all of the midfacial buttress framework is

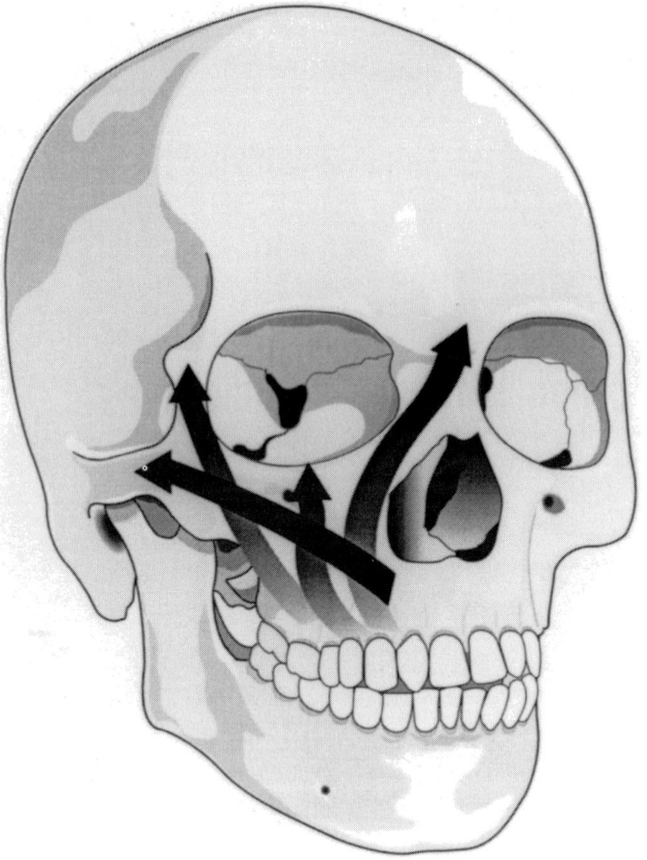

FIGURE 14–1. Schematic illustration of the horizontal and vertical buttress framework of the midfacial skeleton.

preserved, and collapse of the facial soft tissues is seldom observed. However, the palatal defect produced by subtotal maxillectomy results in nasal regurgitation as well as speech, chewing, and swallowing dysfunction. Not surprisingly, rehabilitation efforts have been directed at functional separation of the oral and sinonasal cavities. Although various local or regional flaps have been used for this purpose,[3] direct inspection of the surgical cavity for tumor recurrence is restricted. As a consequence, palatal defects arising from subtotal maxillectomy have typically been managed with an obturator-prosthesis anchored by the remaining teeth and supported by the surrounding palatal and dental structures. The obturator-prosthesis, which may be either tooth-borne or tissue-borne, has become the workhorse of partial maxillectomy rehabilitation because it provides adequate functional capacity and good patient satisfaction without the need for additional surgery.[4, 5] The obturator-prosthesis can also be removed to allow convenient hygiene of the cavity and direct inspection of the surgical site.

According to the classification system established by Spiro and co-workers, *total* maxillectomy is defined as complete surgical resection of the maxilla, usually including orbital exenteration.[2] However, because total maxillectomy *without* orbital exenteration often results in severe deformity of the orbital adnexa owing to disruption of the bony orbit (and thus requires special consideration of reconstructive procedures), we prefer to classify this defect separately as total maxillectomy *with globe preservation.* In either case, total maxillectomy and total maxillectomy with globe preservation are both defined by severe loss of the midfacial skeletal support, which creates profound functional and cosmetic morbidity. In addition to hypernasal speech, nasal regurgitation, and masticatory dysfunction produced by the pathologic union of the oral and nasal cavities, the total maxillectomy defect is also associated with the loss of all bony support to the midface. If support is not promptly reestablished, the lack of skeletal support will quickly yield to unopposed soft tissue scar contracture, producing progressive midface retrusion, nasal airway collapse, and upper lip retraction (Fig. 14–2). Moreover, total maxillectomy with globe preservation is predisposed to additional morbidity from ectropion, vertical lid shortening, globe displacement, gaze restriction, diplopia, or epiphora (see Fig. 14–2).[6] When bilateral, the total maxillectomy defect leads to a devastating surgical deformity that is associated with severe functional disabilities.

Prior to the advent of microvascular free tissue transfers, the intricate nature of bilateral maxillectomy defects posed a virtually insurmountable challenge for the reconstructive surgeon. Early attempts at reconstruction using local or regional tissues were largely disappointing and usually required multiple stages.[7–14] Moreover, complete bony restoration was rarely achieved, and soft tissue collapse was usually severe. Although pedicled temporalis flaps have proved effective for orbital or palatal reconstruction, the temporalis flap has seldom proved adequate for reconstruction of the multifaceted total maxillectomy defect.[14, 15] Other regional flaps have also been tried but with unsatisfactory results.

In addition to the complex anatomic demands of advanced reconstruction of the midface, oncologic management considerations such as the traditional preference for delayed reconstruction and the frequent use of adjuvant radiotherapy further complicate reconstructive efforts. Although primary reconstruction avoids the severe tissue distortion produced by progressive scar contracture, secondary reconstruction has traditionally been advocated following midfacial cancer surgery to facilitate visual detection of recurrent tumor.[16] Moreover, midface surgical defects often arise from high-grade malignancies, and adjuvant radiotherapy is commonly used to enhance local tumor control. In addition to further delaying definitive reconstruction and exacerbating the soft tissue deformity, external beam radiotherapy produces a fibrotic hypovascular wound bed that has characteristically poor healing properties. Although some of the radiotherapeutic tissue effects diminish after 12 to 24 months, chronic soft tissue deformities of the midface following radiotherapy have proved highly resistant to secondary surgical correction.

Because traditional management approaches have failed to fully eliminate the sequelae of bilateral maxillectomy, patients have historically been confronted with harsh long-term morbidity. Adverse alterations in facial appearance combined with deficits in speech, eating, and vision typically lead to depression, social isolation, and reduced quality of

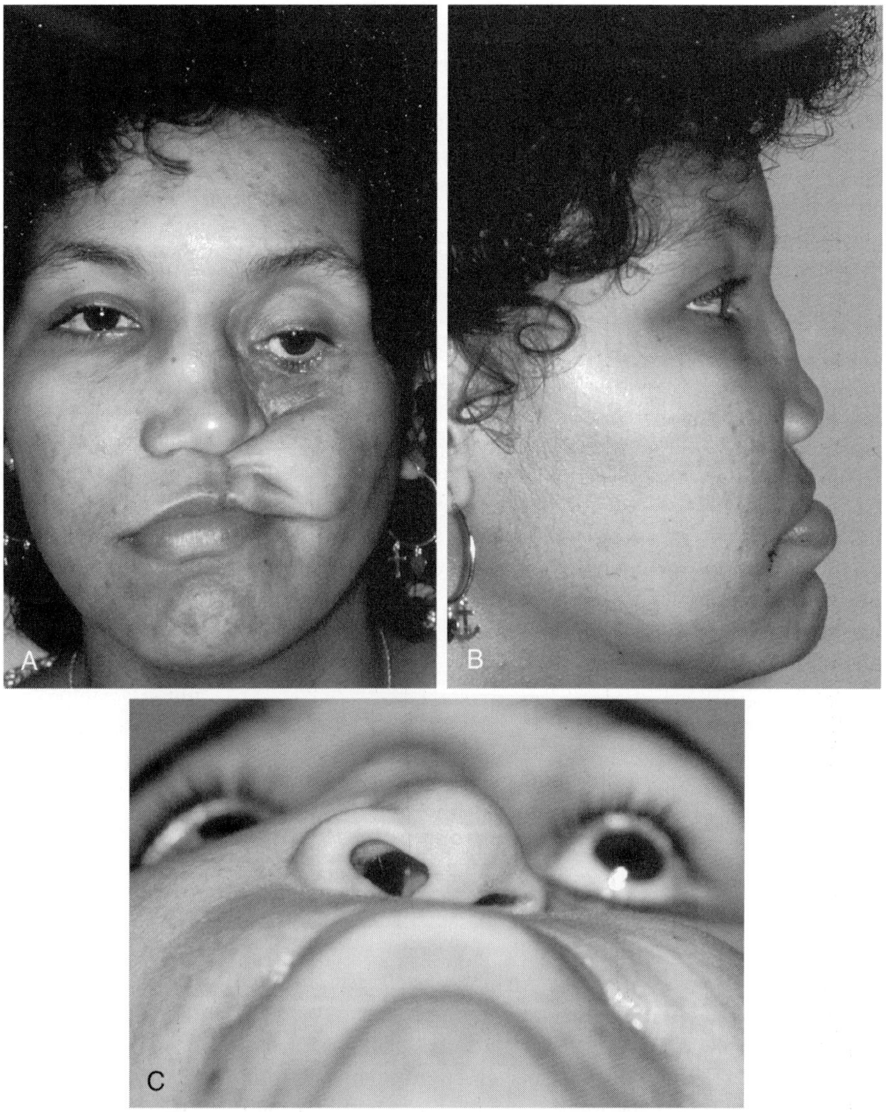

FIGURE 14–2. Severe soft tissue collapse following total maxillectomy with globe preservation and postoperative radiotherapy despite multiple attempts at secondary reconstruction elsewhere. *A,* Frontal view demonstrating orbital dystopia and vertical contracture of the upper lip. *B,* Lateral view demonstrating midface retrusion. *C,* Basal view demonstrating nasal airway collapse.

life.[4] Although patients are often cured of local disease and spared the hardship of uncontrolled primary neoplasia, the impact of tumor treatment in this patient population is considerable.

PROSTHETIC REHABILITATION

In an attempt to reduce the morbidity of bilateral maxillectomy, some practitioners have begun to explore the use of implant-borne prosthetic rehabilitation, particularly in light of the historic limitations of traditional reconstructive surgery. As with surgical reconstruction, significant treatment challenges exist with this type of rehabilitation. Unlike the limited or subtotal maxillectomy defect, in which the surface anatomy and dental structures provide excellent retention, stabilization, and support for a tissue-borne denture-obturator-prosthesis, bilateral maxillectomy defects are characterized by a highly unfavorable anatomy. The challenges of maintaining even simple cosmetic retention of a large tissue-borne midfacial prosthesis are formidable in this patient population and have been well described.[17]

Recently, reports of successful rehabilitation of patients with bilateral maxillectomy defects using implant-borne midfacial prostheses have begun to appear in the medical literature.[18, 19] In 1992, Sjovall and co-workers published a case report describing successful functional rehabilitation with an implant-borne prosthesis following bilateral maxillectomy.[18] Their technique involved bridging the midface with a titanium hollow-screw reconstruction plate (THORP) held in position with paired interlocking titanium screw implants placed in the remaining malar bones. After successful implantation, rehabilitation was accomplished using an implant-borne prosthesis, and clinical follow-up at 18 months revealed good functional and cosmetic results. Similarly, Panje and colleagues reported successful prosthetic rehabilitation of eight patients with bilateral maxillectomy defects using a Steinmann pin to secure the midfacial prosthesis to the skull base.[19] The authors reported good long-term oral function with the implant-borne prosthesis in all patients studied. Unfortunately, bone thickness requirements, angulation limitations, and length restrictions currently limit the use of implant-borne prostheses to a small subset of bilateral maxillectomy patients.[17] Moreover, rehabilitation with a large denture-obturator-prosthesis is also associated with numerous chronic problems including compromised retention and stability, mucosal irritation from the changing fit of the prosthesis, poor hygiene of the cavity, fluid leakage, and persistent speech abnormalities.[17, 20] The long-term success of this approach and the impact of perioperative radiotherapy on implant longevity also remain undetermined.[18] Although many bilateral maxillectomy patients have inadequate bone remaining for optimal implant-borne prosthetic rehabilitation, patients who are poor surgical candidates for microvascular free tissue transfers may still derive partial benefit from this developing technology. Ultimately, improvements in implant-borne prosthetics may supplant the use of microvascular tissue transfers in all but a few selected bilateral maxillectomy patients.

RECONSTRUCTION WITH MICROVASCULAR FREE TISSUE TRANSFER

The success of functional mandibular reconstruction using vascularized free tissue transfers is now well established. Numerous studies have documented the high success rate of free tissue transfers in reconstruction of the upper aerodigestive tract despite their frequent use in elderly patients who are often burdened with multiple medical comorbid problems.[21] The ability to provide large amounts of independently vascularized tissue also minimizes the problems of poor recipient blood supply secondary to radiotherapy, surgical scarring, or chronic infection.

As a consequence of successes in reconstruction elsewhere in the upper aerodigestive tract, reconstructive surgeons have gradually begun to explore the use of free flap technology in the reconstruction of large maxillectomy defects. Baker published the first report of midfacial reconstruction using a microvascular free tissue transfer in 1984.[22] He reported three patients with large orbitoantral exenteration cavities who all underwent successful cavity obliteration using latissimus dorsi soft tissue free flaps. In 1988, Shestak and coworkers reported the use of the same flap for eight patients with similar midface defects.[23] Similarly, in 1989, Coleman published a landmark series of 43 patients with large orbitomaxillary defects who underwent reconstruction with a variety of free flaps including omentum, rectus abdominis, and latissimus dorsi flaps.[15] Coleman concluded that staged local flaps were only useful for limited midface defects and that nonvascularized bone grafts could be used successfully if they were draped with a microvascular free flap. Several patients also received vascularized bone grafts contained within composite free flaps, and most reconstructed patients were able to speak and eat with good to excellent results.

As the experience with free flap midfacial reconstruction has grown, several other reports have appeared advocating functional reconstruction of large maxillectomy defects with free vascularized bone flaps.[17, 24–27] Numerous advantages of such flaps for maxillary reconstruction are now evident. Clearly, the biggest advantage is the availability of abundant robust, durable bone stock for skeletal reconstruction. Unlike nonvascularized endochondral bone grafts, vascularized bone enjoys relative resistance to infection, rapid healing, high osteogenetic regenerative capacity, and a diminished dependence on recipient bed vascularity.[24] Because of their osteogenetic regenerative capacity, free vascularized bone flaps also provide viable bone stock that is suitable for successful implantation with osseointegrated implant-borne prostheses. The prosthesis is mounted on the osseointegrated implants. By combining free vascularized bone flaps, osseointegrated implant technology, and rigid internal fixation (to immobilize the recipient-donor interface and produce a solid bony union), complete functional and aesthetic maxillofacial rehabilitation of the patient with bilateral maxillectomy defects may now be possible.[17, 20, 24–26] Although experimental evidence in humans is lacking, both initial clinical studies and animal experiments indicate that successfully placed vascularized bone grafts enjoy consistent long-term viability and stability despite postoperative radiotherapy.[24] The diminished risk of long-term bone resorption following radiotherapy makes free vascularized bone flaps the method of choice for maxillary reconstruction when functional dental restoration is desired or when recipient bed vascularity is compromised.

Unfortunately, as the experience with maxillary reconstruction has expanded, several disadvantages of vascularized bone reconstruction have also become apparent. Vascularized bone is typically quite bulky and may not readily conform to the precise three-dimensional contour of the human maxilla. Although vascularized bone can be osteotomized for improved three-dimensional adaptation to the surgical defect, extensive changes in bony contour may disrupt vital periosteal attachments, reducing the blood supply and thus jeopardizing bone viability.[28] Moreover, the attached skin paddle, which is vital for palatal reconstruction, antral ablation, or internal epithelial lining, may also be inadvertently jeopardized with aggressive manipulation of the bony contour. As a consequence, overcorrection of facial contour, malposition of bone grafts, or incomplete bone reconstruction is often unavoidable, and revision surgeries are frequently indicated.[15, 29] Other technical limitations, such as inadequate pedicle length, inadequate size of recipient vessels, conflicting juxtaposition of the soft tissue and bony insets, excessive skin paddle thickness, and inadequate skin paddle dimensions, also limit the application of free vascularized bone flaps.[27, 28] To date, numerous donor tissues have been used for composite free flap reconstruction of the maxilla including scapular, iliac crest, fibular, and radial vascularized bone flaps.[17, 20, 24–28] Despite the wide variety of available donor tissues, the uniformly ideal tissue composite for maxillary reconstruction has yet to be reported.

Another contemporary approach to midfacial reconstruction combines the use of autologous split calvarial bone grafts with an envelope of vascularized soft tissue from thin pliable free flaps such as the radial forearm flap.[15] Using this approach, skeletal contour can be restored with greater precision owing to the diminished bulk and greater adaptability of split calvarial bone (Fig. 14–3). Since calvarium is membranous bone, there is little difference in survival in the adult population between it and vascularized bone grafts.[24] Furthermore, the morbidity of calvarial bone harvest is comparatively low, and up to 50 cm^2 of outer cortical bone can be easily harvested from a single donor. Unfortunately, split calvarial bone is generally only 2 to 4 mm thick and cannot satisfactorily accommodate functional osseointegrated implants. Despite its embryologic origin, calvarial bone grafts are also susceptible to gradual resorption when subjected to postoperative radiotherapy or poor recipient blood supply. Although postoperative radiotherapy does not appear to jeopardize the viability of free vascularized bone flaps, in some patients free calvarial bone grafts may demonstrate resorption, infection, or extrusion following postoperative radiotherapy, and their use in planned radiotherapy is best avoided in patients with a poor local blood supply. However, in our experience, the three-dimensional contour that can be achieved with calvarial bone is unparalleled. If complete dental restoration is desired, cancellous iliac bone grafts can be placed to augment existing bone thickness and provide the osteogenic activity necessary to allow the integration of functional dental implants.[30] As with vascularized bone flaps, fasciocutaneous free flaps offer multiple skin paddles that may be used to reconstruct the palate, augment the soft tissues of the cheek, or obliterate the maxillary antrum.

Given the wide range of contemporary management options and the heterogeneity of surgical maxillectomy defects, surgical patient management must be carefully individualized, since no single management approach is appropriate for all patients. The minimum objectives for patient management should include functional restoration of the palate, preservation of orbital support, and maintenance of facial contour. Numerous factors such as the characteristics of individual defects, the status of the recipient bed, donor site morbidity, the risk of tumor recurrence, cost, anesthetic risk, need for radiotherapy, and patient preference must all be considered when devising the surgical treatment plan. Furthermore, patients with a bilateral maxillectomy should also

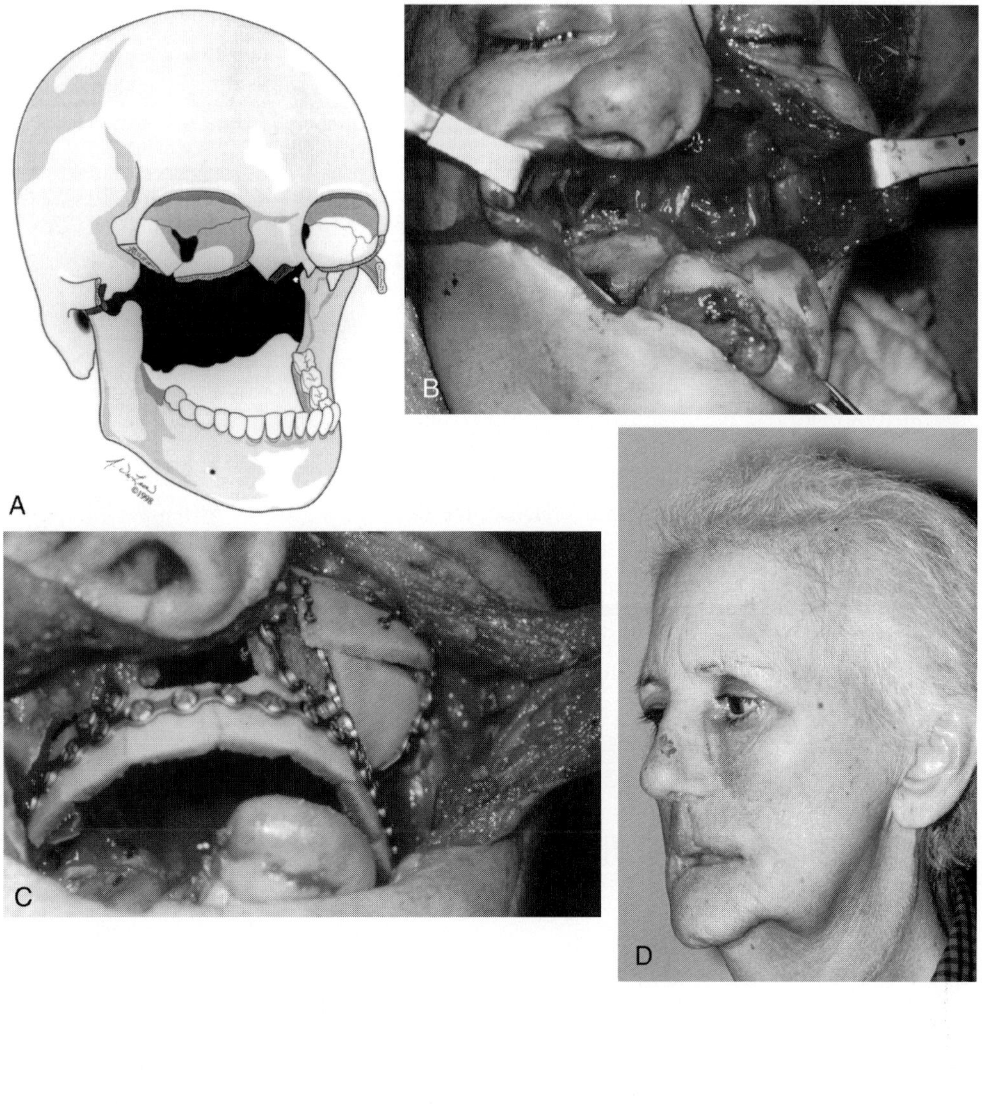

FIGURE 14–3. *A,* Schematic illustration of bilateral total maxillectomy defect with preservation of the globe. *B,* Intraoperative view of this defect. *C,* Defect following reconstruction with calvarial bone grafts prior to placement of lateral arm free flap. *D,* Facial contour 1 month postoperatively.

be advised that virtually any treatment approach will probably require one or more surgical revision procedures, particularly if complete maxillofacial prosthetic restoration is desired.

TIMING OF RECONSTRUCTION

Without prompt restoration of midfacial anatomy following bilateral maxillectomy, a harsh decline in the patient's quality of life is inevitable. Fortunately, with the advent of microvascular free flap reconstruction, the quality of life following bilateral maxillectomy has dramatically improved. Moreover, because of the availability of immediate microvascular reconstruction, extirpative surgeons are now free to enlarge the surgical margin of resection without causing a disproportionate increase in surgical morbidity. When combined with frozen section clearance, the use of aggressive surgical margins is likely to have a favorable impact on local tumor control. Although primary reconstruction remains controversial because it impedes direct inspection of the surgical cavity for recurrence, it has become increasingly popular among oncologic surgeons and has now been adopted by numerous authors.[15, 17, 20, 23, 27, 28, 31] Initial clinical reports of primary reconstruction confirm its significant functional and cosmetic advantages relative to traditional management approaches even when postoperative radiotherapy has been administered.[20] Although the risk of local recurrence is not eliminated with aggressive surgical margins, local recurrences are confined to contiguous anatomic sites (since the midface is removed en bloc), and detection of tumor recurrence in anatomic sites such as the orbital apex, cavernous sinus, nasal cavum, or anterior skull base is often best accomplished using contemporary radiographic surveillance techniques such as computed tomography (CT) or magnetic resonance imaging (MRI) scanning combined with close clinical follow-up and nasoendoscopy.[20, 31] Moreover, recurrences of this type are often incurable, calling into question the benefit of prolonged oncologic surveillance and postponement of definitive reconstruction.[17] Hence, the decision to perform primary reconstruction should be individualized and should take into account such factors as the anticipated morbidity of the surgical defect, recurrence risk, contraindications to free flap surgery, and patient preference. On this basis, immediate reconstruction of the bilateral maxillectomy defect is often justified.

RECONSTRUCTIVE SURGICAL TECHNIQUE

When definitive primary reconstruction of extensive midfacial defects is desired, contemporary surgical management is best provided using a coordinated surgical team approach. This approach not only takes advantage of subspecialty surgical skills, it also leads to a significant reduction in operating time and thus anesthetic morbidity. The extirpative team begins by performing complete tumor resection as directed by frozen section clearance of the surgical margin. Unless tumor invasion of the facial skin is suspected, surgical exposure of the midface is preferentially achieved using the midfacial degloving approach. The midfacial degloving approach avoids visible external incisions, affords excellent surgical exposure, and preserves the facial tissues to provide vascular support to free bone grafts. Concurrent with the tumor resection, the microvascular team isolates the free flap on its vascular pedicle in anticipation of free tissue transfer. Synchronous flap harvest is easily accomplished with most free flaps including the lateral arm, radial forearm, iliac crest, and fibular free flaps. Following removal of the tumor, a third surgical team then prepares the recipient bed, harvests and places membranous bone grafts, or isolates the recipient vessels while awaiting frozen section results.

For large midfacial skeletal defects in which partial maxillary dentition is preserved, free membranous bone grafts are often preferred for skeletal reconstruction of the midface. Although the technique for harvesting outer split-calvarial bone grafts has been described elsewhere, several points are worth emphasizing here. Undercutting the bone grafts with an oscillating saw will minimize graft fracture, provide maximum thickness of the outer cortex, and diminish the risk of intracranial penetration (Fig. 14–4) (see also Color plate).

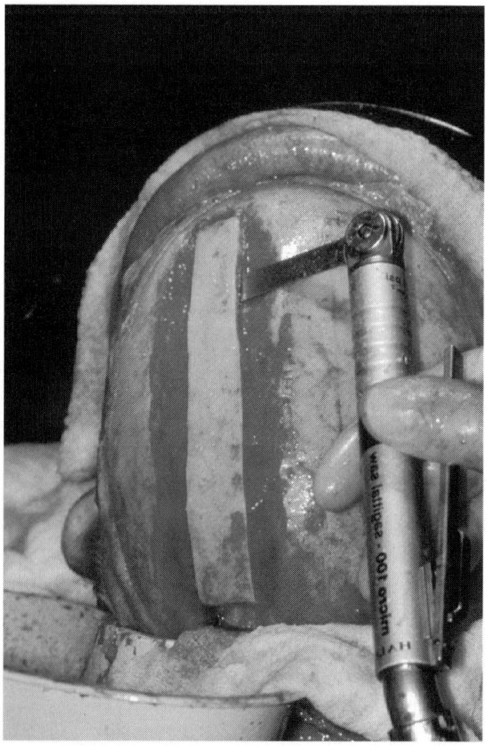

FIGURE 14–4. Use of the oscillating saw to harvest calvarial bone from the outer table. Note how the peripheral saucerization of the donor site facilitates blade angulation. (See also Color plate.)

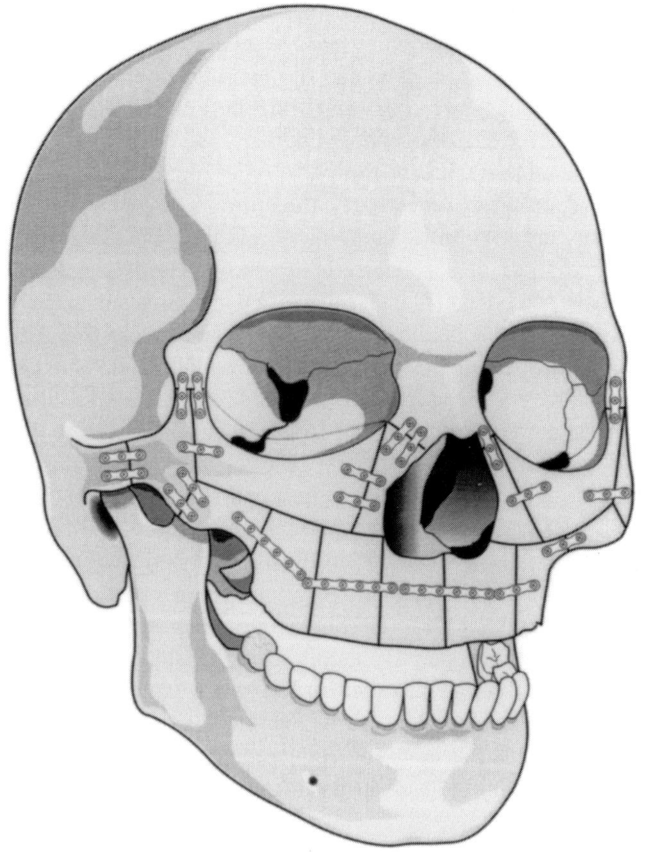

FIGURE 14–5. Schematic illustration of placement of calvarial bone graft following bilateral total maxillectomy.

Heavy saucerization of the donor defect is necessary to facilitate proper angulation of the saw blade and to camouflage the donor site deformity. While performing saw cuts, generous saline irrigation is used to reduce thermal bone injury.

Once harvested, membranous calvarial bone is used carefully to reconstitute the facial skeletal framework. Particular attention is paid to reconstructing the orbital rim, pyriform aperture, posterior maxillary buttresses, and alveolar ridge (Fig. 14–5). Bone segments are carefully sculpted and positioned to approximate the external surface contour of the native maxillary bone as closely as possible. The bone segments are then stabilized using rigid fixation systems (miniplates or microplates) to unify the reconstructed skeletal subunit. In addition to providing proper projection of the soft tissue envelope, skeletal reconstruction restores the vertical and horizontal buttress system and stabilizes the midface against unwanted soft tissue collapse. Although plated calvarial bone grafts do not adequately withstand the full forces of mastication, the rigidity provided by internal fixation easily withstands the load-bearing forces produced during speech, swallowing, and mastication of soft foods.

Once the free calvarial grafts have been secured with rigid fixation, a diamond polishing bur is used to remove all sharp protruding edges in preparation for soft tissue reconstruction. A microvascular free flap, usually a lateral arm flap or a radial forearm flap (with or without bone), is then used to envelop the antral surface of the reconstructed bony framework and reconstruct the palatal defect. Typically, the proximal skin paddle is retained for palatal lining while the remaining pedicle is de-epithelialized for placement within the antral cavity (Fig. 14–6). In this manner, the skeletal framework receives vascular support from both the outer facial soft tissues and the inner revascularized free tissue transfer. The peripheral skin or muscle paddle is then inset to the lip, cheek, and palate, and the vascular pedicle is tunneled through the cheek into the neck, where the microvascular anastomosis is performed (see Fig. 14–6). Typically, the nasal cavity is obliterated, and nasal patency is restored secondarily. With radial forearm free flaps, a small segment of radial bone may also be included to provide vascularized support for the skeletal reconstruction, particularly when adjuvant radiotherapy is planned.

For patients with total maxillectomy defects in which no serviceable maxillary dentition has been preserved, reconstruction is performed using free vascularized bone flaps with or without calvarial bone. For full dental implant rehabilitation, we prefer to use free vascularized fibular bone to

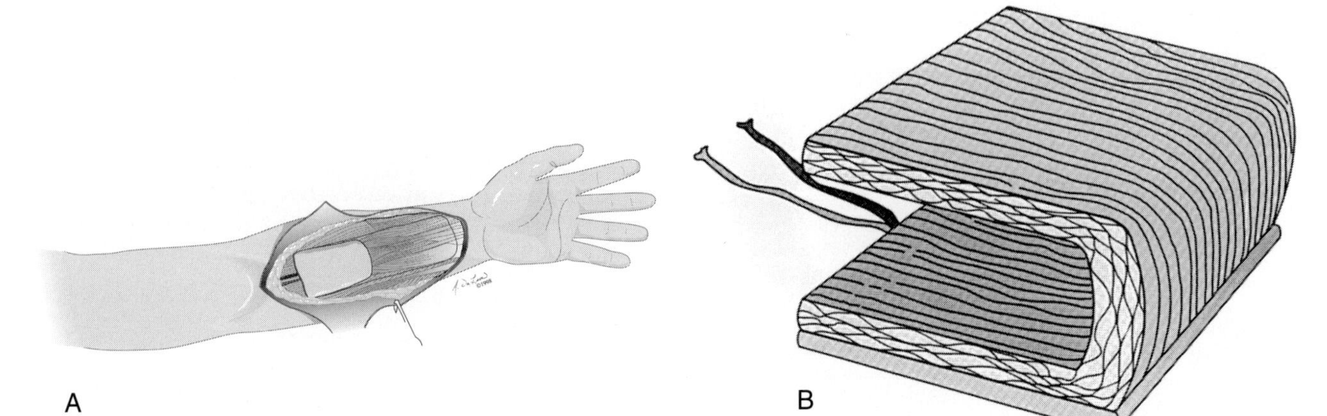

A B

FIGURE 14–6. Schematic illustration of radial forearm fasciocutaneous free flap. *A,* Flap in situ prior to harvest (note the retained skin paddle for palatal lining). *B,* Three-dimensional flap configuration following inset.

reconstitute the alveolar arch and permit placement of dental implants in the future. Calvarial bone grafts may be used to reconstruct the vertical buttress system and stabilize the reconstituted alveolar arch for load bearing when direct contact with the malar bone is not possible. Up to 25 cm of fibular bone, with or without attached soft tissue, may be safely harvested from patients who have no peripheral vascular impairment. Unfortunately, the vascular pedicle, which measures only 6 cm, is excessively short and often requires vein grafting to extend its length. Although fibular bone flaps generally tolerate multiple osteotomies and accept primary dental implants,[24] limitations in the availability and positioning of the soft tissue paddle may necessitate a second free flap for soft tissue coverage. Nevertheless, fibular bone can be expected to tolerate reasonable forces of mastication, and, owing to its three-dimensional adaptability, it may represent the best available scaffold for implant-borne dental rehabilitation.[25, 26] As with calvarial bone grafts, the fibular bone is first stabilized to the retained facial skeleton using rigid fixation. If desired, dental implants may then be placed within the neo-alveolus once the soft tissue inset and vascular anastomosis are complete.

COMPLICATIONS

Owing to the magnitude and complexity of reconstruction following total maxillectomy, the potential for perioperative surgical complications cannot be ignored. However, in our experience, life-threatening perioperative complications following microvascular free flap surgery are seldom observed, and our findings are consistent with the low operative morbidity of free flap surgery reported by other authors.[21] Perhaps the most significant complication of microvascular midface reconstruction is early thrombosis of the vascular pedicle, resulting in ischemic flap necrosis. We estimate that the initial rate of flap failure is approximately 5%, although a small percentage of these flaps can be salvaged through aggressive resuscitation measures. With the fibular free flap, isolated ischemic necrosis of the skin paddle is observed in up to 20% of cases. Extreme care is advised when handling the flap to avoid unnecessary traction and ischemic injury. Due to the short vascular pedicle of the fibular flap, a saphenous (vein) interposition graft is often required to eliminate tension on the microvascular anastomosis. Although this necessitates two anastomoses, the elimination of tension reduces the incidence of flap thrombosis in our hands. Finally, patients undergoing fibular free flap reconstruction must undergo preoperative angiographic evaluation to ensure that vascular collateralization to the lower extremity is adequate prior to sacrifice of the peroneal artery. Following fibular free flap harvest, all patients must also undergo postoperative splinting to avoid foot drop from progressive scar contracture.

In contrast to the fibular free flap, the lateral arm, radial forearm, and rectus abdominis free flaps are seldom associ-

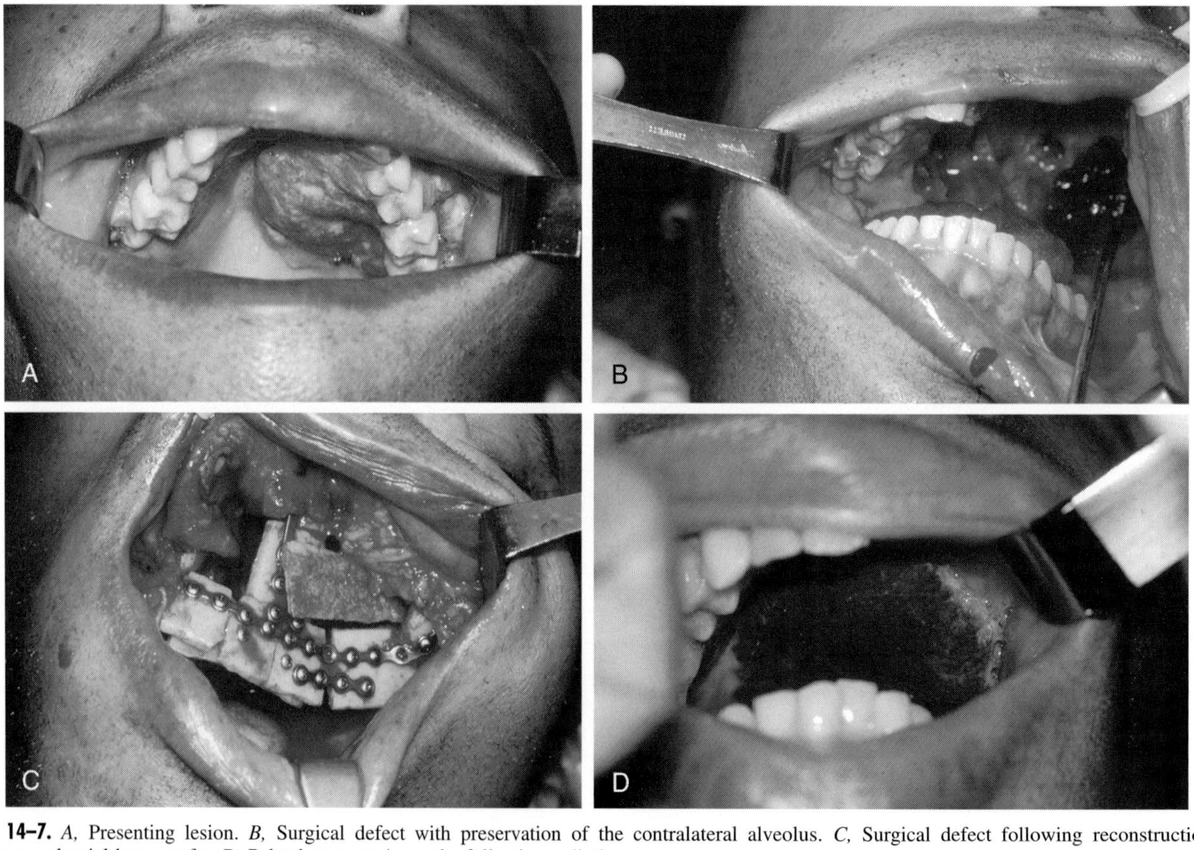

FIGURE 14–7. *A*, Presenting lesion. *B*, Surgical defect with preservation of the contralateral alveolus. *C*, Surgical defect following reconstruction with autologous calvarial bone grafts. *D*, Palatal contour 4 months following radiotherapy.

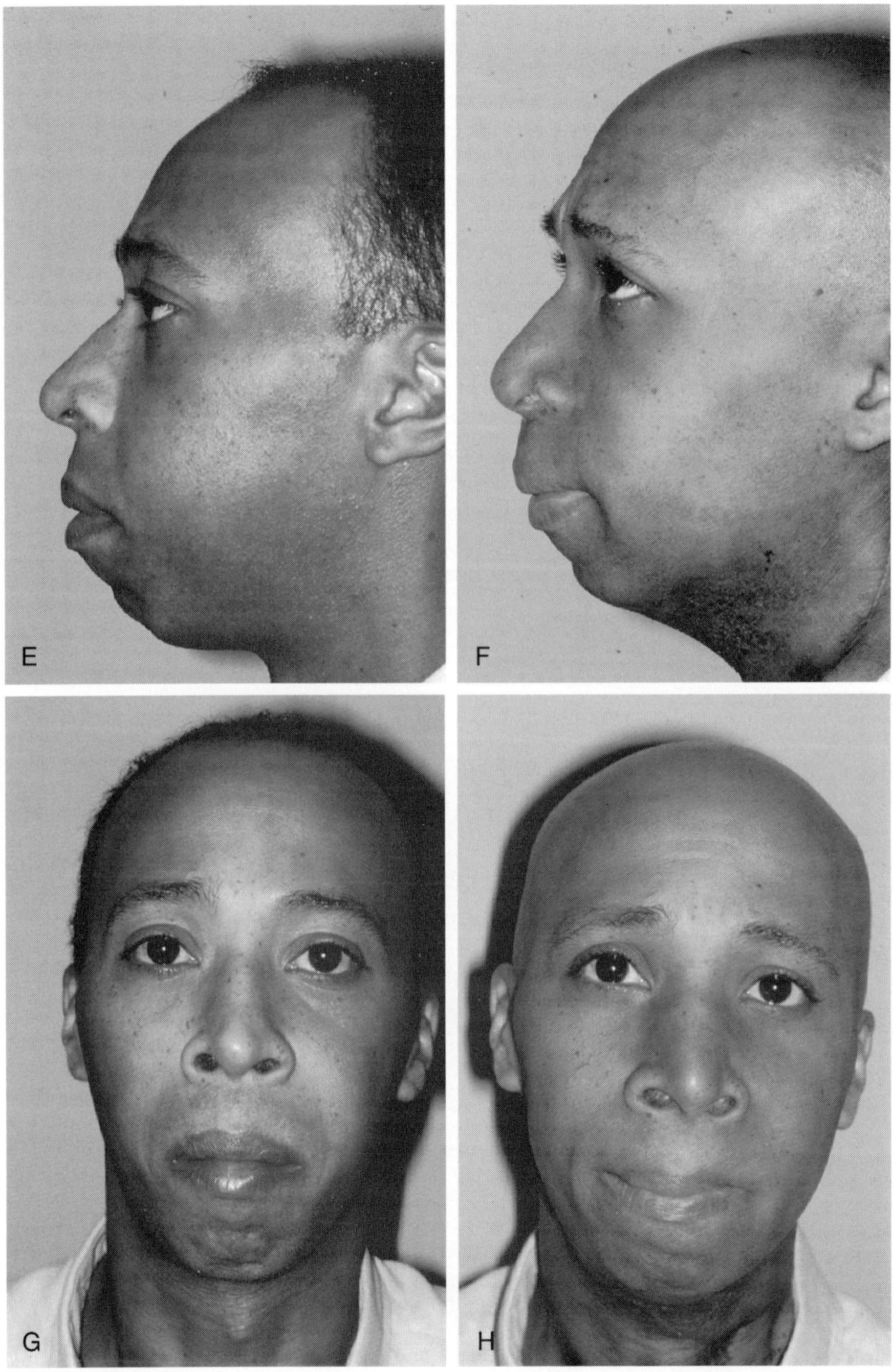

FIGURE 14–7 *Continued. E–H,* Cosmetic results at 7 months. (See also Color plate.)

ated with soft tissue ischemic loss. However, secondary soft tissue modifications are usually necessary, since appropriate flap selection can only approximate the volume requirements of the defect. In addition, the radial forearm donor site requires placement of a split-thickness skin graft directly over the exposed flexor tendon sheaths, and postoperative physical therapy must be instituted to avoid permanent scar contracture. Tendon exposure is a rare complication, but when it occurs it often requires secondary reconstructive procedures to cover the exposed tendon.

In addition to complications resulting from free flap reconstruction, various problems are also observed following midfacial skeletal reconstruction with autologous calvarial bone grafts. Although various injuries have been reported secondary to inadvertent intracranial penetration during calvarial bone harvest, we have yet to experience these complications using the technique described earlier. However, delayed calvarial bone graft infection and/or exposure, with or without plating hardware extrusion, have been observed in approximately 50% to 60% of patients undergoing postoperative radiotherapy. Prompt surgical debridement of nonviable bone, removal of exposed hardware, and aggressive hyperbaric oxygenation have provided satisfactory improvement in nearly all cases to date. In two cases, extensive bone debridement prompted a second free flap reconstruction to provide support and contour for the midface.

CASE HISTORIES

Case 1

A 40-year-old black male presented with a $T_4N_0M_0$ squamous cell carcinoma of the right hard palate (Fig. 14–7*A*). Surgical management included right globe-sparing total maxillectomy through a midfacial degloving approach (Fig. 14–7*B*) and primary reconstruction using autologous split calvarium and a lateral arm osseofasciocutaneous free flap (Fig. 14–7*C* and *D*) (see also Color plate 14–7*A–D*). Two years following postoperative adjuvant radiotherapy the patient can speak and swallow normally and has an excellent facial contour (Fig. 14–7*E–H*).

Case 2

A 28-year-old white female presented with a recurrent juvenile ossifying fibroma of the right hard palate extending to the adjacent orbital floor. Surgical management included a right total maxillectomy with globe preservation through midfacial degloving and transconjunctival approaches. Preservation of the incisor teeth allowed placement of a temporary surgical obturator-prosthesis prior to reconstruction (Fig. 14–8*A*). Following pathologic clearance of the bone margin (2 weeks after tumor removal), delayed reconstruction was performed using autologous split calvarium and a radial forearm fasciocutaneous free flap (Fig. 14–8*B* and *C*) (see also Color plate 14–8 *A–C*). Three weeks postoperatively the patient can speak, eat, and swallow normally and has an excellent facial contour (Fig. 14–8*D–G*).

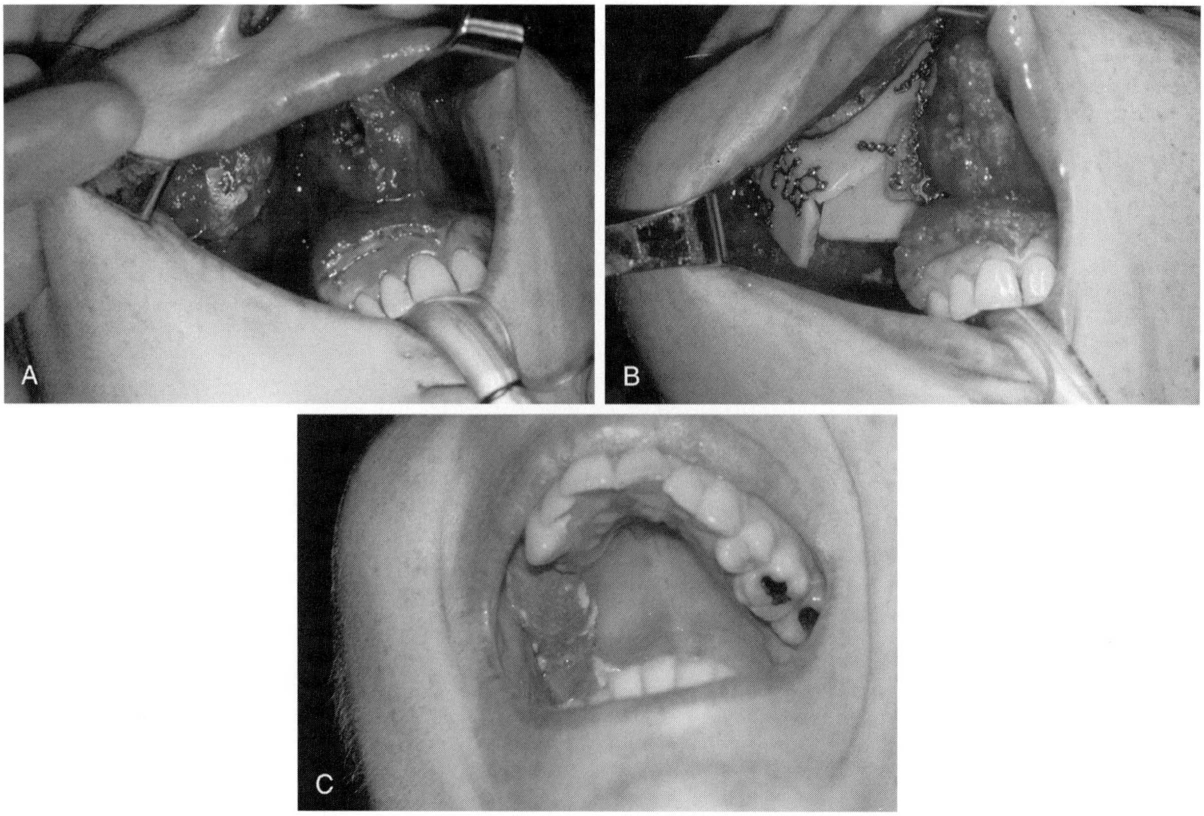

FIGURE 14–8. *A,* Surgical defect. *B,* Surgical defect following reconstruction with autologous calvarial bone grafts. *C,* Palatal contour at 3 weeks.

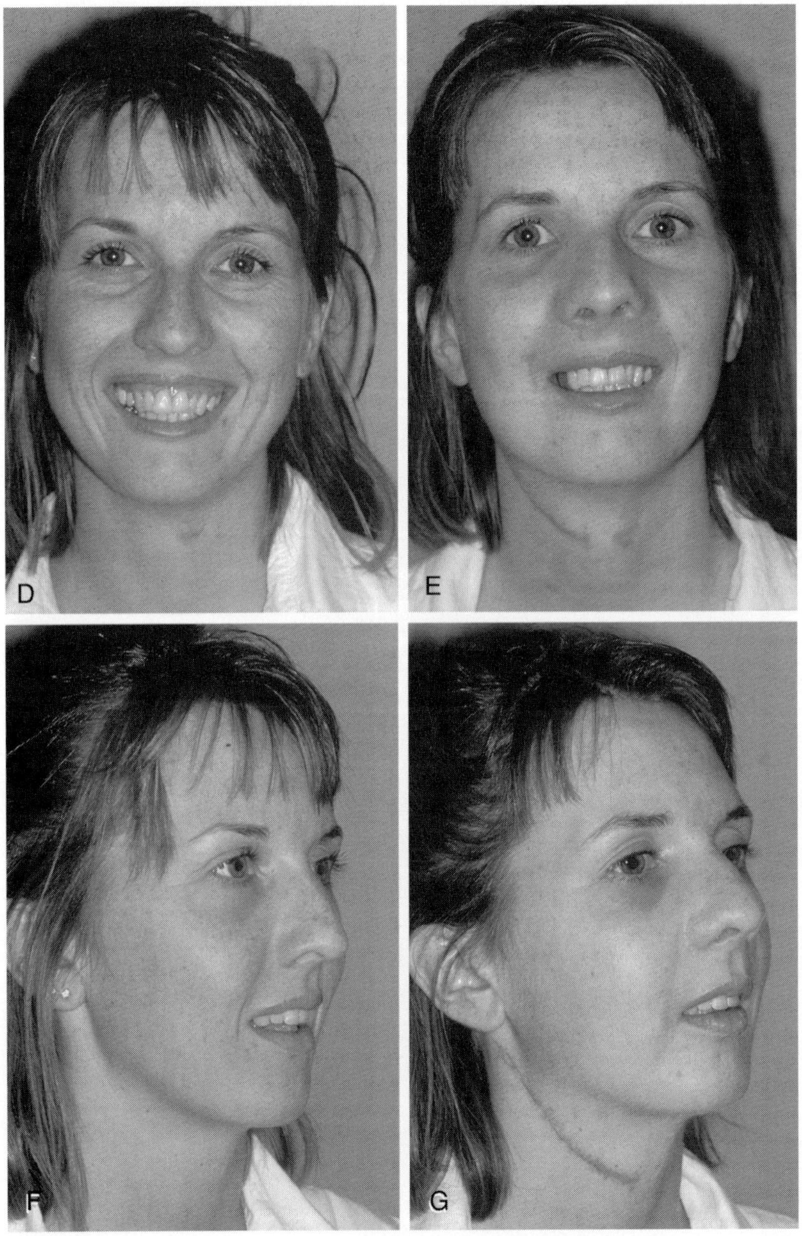

FIGURE 14–8 *Continued. D–G,* Cosmetic results at 3 weeks. (See also Color plate.)

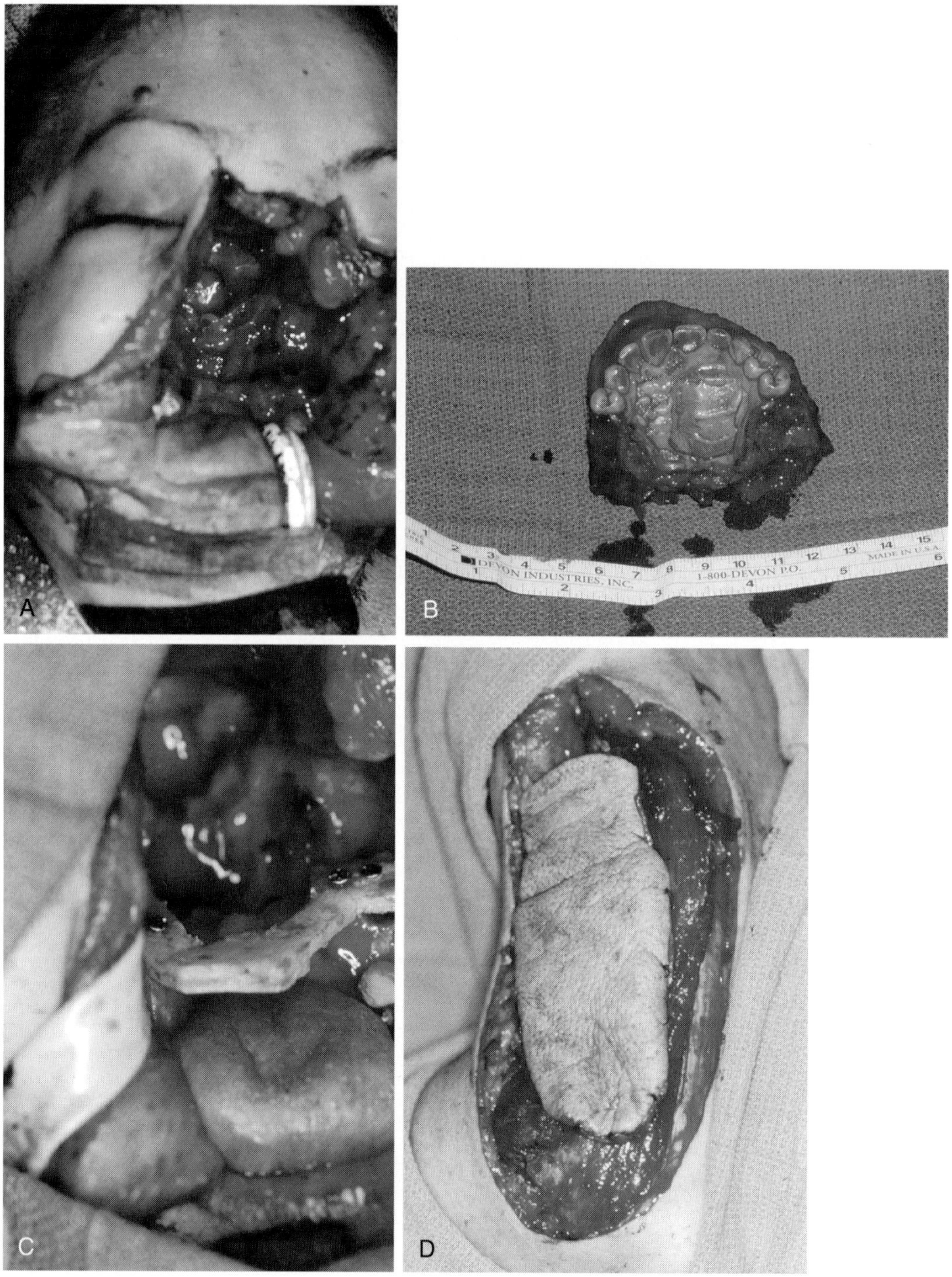

FIGURE 14–9. *A,* Surgical defect. *B,* Surgical specimen. *C,* Placement of calvarial bone graft. *D,* Lateral arm free flap prior to final harvest.

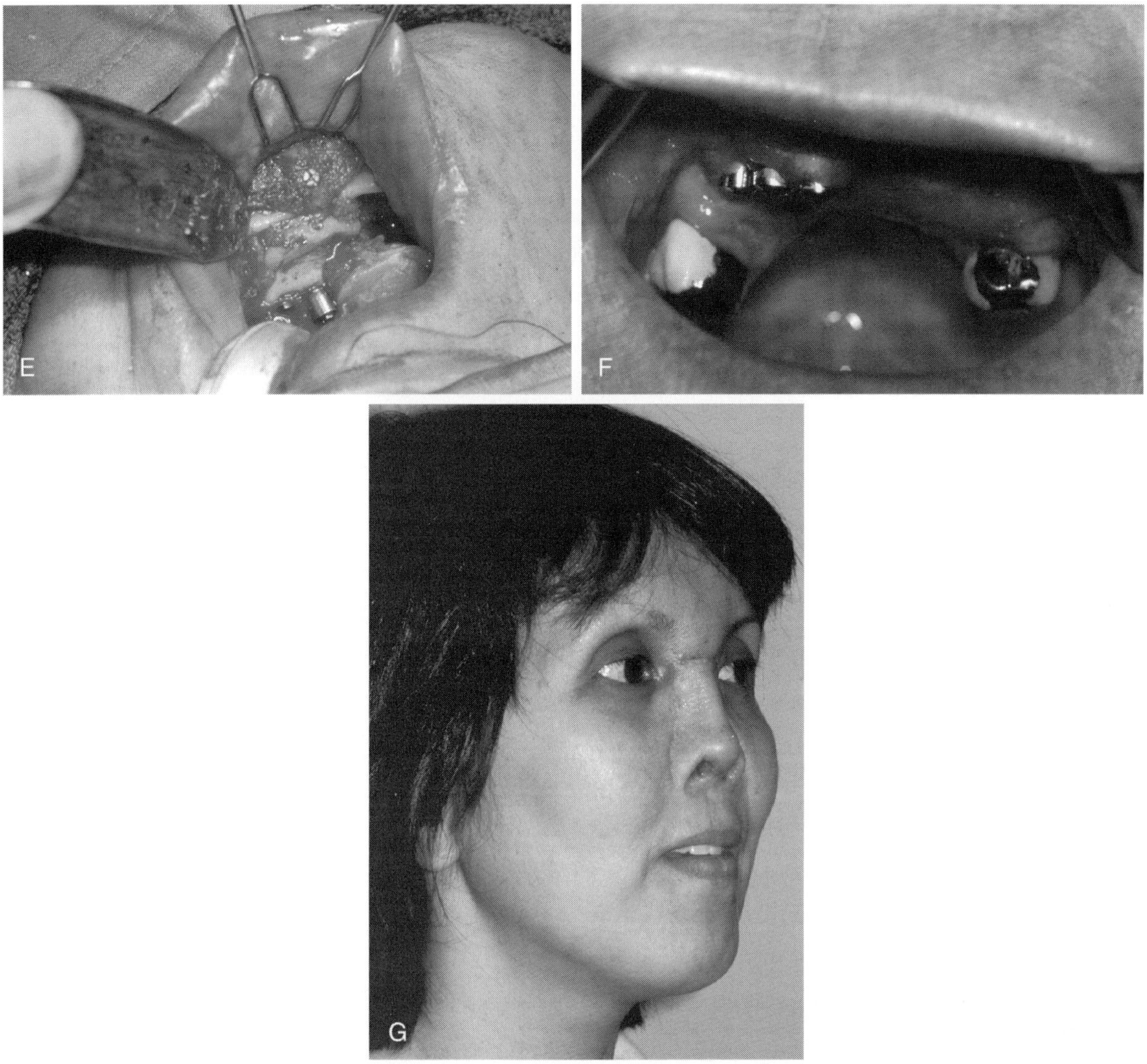

FIGURE 14–9 *Continued. E,* Placement of cancellous bone augmentation grafts. *F,* Osseointegrated implants. *G,* Cosmetic result at 2 years.

Case 3

A 39-year-old white female presented with a large chondrosarcoma of the anterior nasal septum. Surgical management included total septectomy and bilateral total maxillectomy (globe-sparing) with resection of the nasal bones via lateral rhinotomy (Fig. 14–9*A* and *B*): Primary reconstruction was performed using horizontally oriented split calvarium enveloped in a lateral arm fasciocutaneous free flap (Fig. 14–9*C* and *D*). Subsequent operations were performed to place additional calvarial bone, after which the patient was referred to the oral and maxillofacial surgery service for iliac cancellous bone graft placement and osseointegrated dental implants (Fig. 14–9*E* and *F*). Five years after tumor resection, the patient has normal speech and a normal facial contour (Fig. 14–9*G*). With the use of an implant-borne dental prosthesis, she is also able to chew all foods of moderate consistency.

REFERENCES

1. Mathog RH: Classification and pathophysiology of maxillary fractures. *In* Atlas of Craniofacial Trauma. Philadelphia, W.B. Saunders, 1992, pp. 145–148.
2. Spiro RH, Strong EW, Shah JP: Maxillectomy and its classification. Head Neck 19(4):309–314, 1997.
3. Cheung LK, Samman N, Tideman H: Reconstructive options for maxillary defects. Ann R Aust Coll Dent Surg 12:244–251, 1994.
4. Kornblith AB, Zlotolow IM, Gooen J, Huryn JM, Lerner T, Strong EW, Shah JP, Spiro RH, Holland JC: Quality of life of maxillectomy patients using an obturator prosthesis. Head Neck 18:323–334, 1996.
5. Davison SP, Sherris DA, Meland NB: An algorithm for maxillectomy defect reconstruction. Laryngoscope 108:215–219, 1988.
6. Schusterman MA, Reece GP, Miller MJ: Osseous free flaps for orbit and midface reconstruction. Am J Surg 166:341–345, 1993.
7. Owens N: Compound neck pedicle designed for the repair of massive facial defects: development and application. Plast Reconstr Surg 15:369–389, 1995.
8. Bakamjian V: A technique for primary reconstruction of the palate after radical maxillectomy for cancer. Plast Reconstr Surg 31:103–117, 1963.
9. Bakamjian VY, Poole M: Maxillofacial and palate reconstruction with the deltopectoral flap. Br J Plast Surg 30:17–33, 1977.
10. Thomson HG: Reconstruction of the orbit after radical exenteration. Plast Reconstr Surg 45:119–123, 1970.
11. Naquin H: Orbital reconstruction using temporalis muscle. Am J Ophthalmol 41:519–521, 1956.
12. Landra AP: One-stage reconstruction of a massive gunshot wound of the lower face with a local compound osteomusculocutaneous flap. Br J Plast Surg 34:395–397, 1981.
13. Obwegeser HG: Late reconstruction of large maxillary defects after tumor resection. Maxillofac Surg 1:19–29, 1973.

14. Colmenero C, Martorell V, Colmenero B, Sierra I: Temporalis myofascial flap for maxillofacial reconstruction. J Oral Maxillofac Surg 49:1067–1073, 1991.
15. Coleman JJ: Microvascular approach to function and appearance of large orbital maxillary defects. Am J Surg 158:337–340, 1989.
16. Schuller DE: Extensive defects of the sino-orbital region (discussion). Arch Otolaryngol Head Neck Surg 118:859–860, 1992.
17. Funk GF, Arcuri MR, Frodel JL: Functional dental rehabilitation of massive palatomaxillary defects: Cases requiring free tissue transfer and osseointegrated implants. Head Neck 20(1):38–51, 1998.
18. Sjovall L, Lindqvist C, Hallikainen D: A new method of reconstruction in a patient undergoing bilateral total maxillectomy. Int J Oral Maxillofac Surg 21(6):342–345, 1992.
19. Panje WR, Hetherington HE, Toljanic J, LaVelle WE, Fyler A: Bilateral maxillectomy and midfacial reconstruction. Ann Otol Rhinol Laryngol 104:845–849, 1995.
20. Brown JS: Deep circumflex iliac artery free flap with internal oblique muscle as a new method of immediate reconstruction of maxillectomy defect. Head Neck 18:412–421, 1996.
21. Jones TR, Jones NF: Advances in reconstruction of the upper aerodigestive tract and cranial base with free tissue transfer. Clin Plast Surg 19(4):819–831, 1992.
22. Baker SR: Closure of large orbital-maxillary defects with free latissimus dorsi myocutaneous flaps. Head Neck 6:828–835, 1984.
23. Shestak KC, Schusterman MA, Jones NF, Johnson JT: Immediate microvascular reconstruction of combined palatal and midfacial defects using soft tissue only. Microsurgery 9:128–131, 1988.
24. Turk JB, Vuillemin T, Raveh J: Revascularized bone grafts for craniofacial reconstruction. Otolaryngol Clin North Am 27(5):955–982, 1994.
25. Nakayama B, Matuura H, Ishihara O, Hasegawa H, Mataga I, Torii S: Functional reconstruction of a bilateral maxillectomy defect using a fibula osteocutaneous flap with osseointegrated implants. Plast Reconstr Surg 96(5):1201–1204, 1995.
26. Nakayama B, Matsuura H, Hasegawa Y, Ishihara O, Hasegawa H, Torii S: New reconstruction for total maxillectomy defect with a fibula osteocutaneous free flap. Br J Plast Surg 47:247–249, 1944.
27. Cordeiro PG, Bacillous N, Schantz S, Spiro R: The radial forearm osteocutaneous "sandwich" free flap for reconstruction of the bilateral subtotal maxillectomy defect. Ann Plast Surg 40(4):397–402, 1998.
28. Granick MS, Ramasastry SS, Newton DE, Solomon MP, Hanna DC, Kaltman S: Reconstruction of complex maxillectomy defects with the scapular-free flap. Head Neck 12:377–385, 1990.
29. Schmelziesen R, Schliephake H: Interdisciplinary microvascular reconstruction of maxillary, midfacial, and skull base defects. J Craniomaxillofac Surg 26:1–10, 1998.
30. Carlson ER, Marx RE: Mandibular reconstruction using cancellous cellular bone grafts. J Oral Maxillofac Surg 54:889–897, 1996.
31. Olsen KD, Meland NB, Ebersold MJ, Bartley GB, Garrity JA: Extensive defects of the sino-orbital region—results with microvascular reconstruction. Arch Otolaryngol Head Neck Surg 118:828–833, 1992.

CHAPTER 15

Complex Midface Fractures

Gregory A. Antoine, M.D.

LeFort's studies of the fracture patterns of the midface have remained the cornerstone of the basic description of fractures of the midface.[1, 2] This basic description allows surgeons involved in the management of these patients to communicate on a level where everyone has a clear and basic knowledge of the severity and complexity of the injury. The LeFort fracture patterns also serve as an invaluable building block in the advancement of craniofacial surgical techniques and the management of traumatic complex midface injuries in ways that were inconceivable in LeFort's time. LeFort fractures may be associated with other maxillofacial injuries. This chapter addresses the complex midfacial injuries that often occur with the LeFort pattern of injury.

ANATOMY

Two pyramidal-shaped components form the maxillae. The maxillae form a large portion of the facial part of the skull. They form portions of the orbit, the nasal cavity, the palate and the oral cavity. The body of the maxillae contains the maxillary sinuses and bears 16 teeth. The maxilla consists of four processes: the zygomatic, frontal, palatine, and alveolar processes (Fig. 15–1). Three structural pillars, or buttresses, absorb the load of vertically directed forces in the maxilla. The anterior or canine (nasofrontal) buttress forms the lateral boundary of the anterior nasal aperture and continues as the frontal process of the maxilla to the frontal bone.[3] The middle or zygomatic buttress starts just superior to the first molar, bends upward and outward as the zygomaticoalveolar crest and the zygomatic process of the maxilla, and continues into and ends at the zygomaticofrontal junction. The posterior or pterygoid buttress is the pterygoid process of the sphenoid bone (Fig. 15–2). In addition to these three vertical pillars there are two horizontal pillars between them, the inferior and superior orbital rims.[4]

CLASSIFICATION OF LEFORT MIDFACE FRACTURES

LeFort identified three great lines of weakness through the maxillae. The common denominator is that the pterygoid process of the sphenoid bone is always fractured in all three types of LeFort fractures. Fractures that occur above the apices of the teeth include the entire palate and the pterygoid process en block and are classified as LeFort I (horizontal) fractures (Fig. 15–3). The LeFort II fracture (pyramidal, because of its general architecture) begins laterally above the level of the apices of the teeth, extends through the pterygoid plates, and travels medially through the orbital rim into the floor of the orbit and across the nose. The level at which the fracture crosses the nose varies. This fracture may produce lacrimal sac injuries. The LeFort III (craniofacial dysjunction) fracture is a complete bony separation of the midface from the skull base. This fracture extends through the zygomaticofrontal sutures, the nasofrontal suture, and the floor of the orbits to effect a complete bony separation. The maxilla is not necessarily separated from the zygoma or the nasal bones. With today's high-velocity injuries, these classic LeFort patterns hold true in most instances, but associated injuries commonly occur that do not fit this pattern in a straightforward manner.

OTHER MIDFACE FRACTURES

Fractures of the alveolar process of the maxilla may occur. The fracture segment may contain teeth, and in most instances it is attached by soft tissue. Fractures may split the maxilla vertically in the sagittal plane. This type of fracture may lead to an increase in the width of the dental arch if it

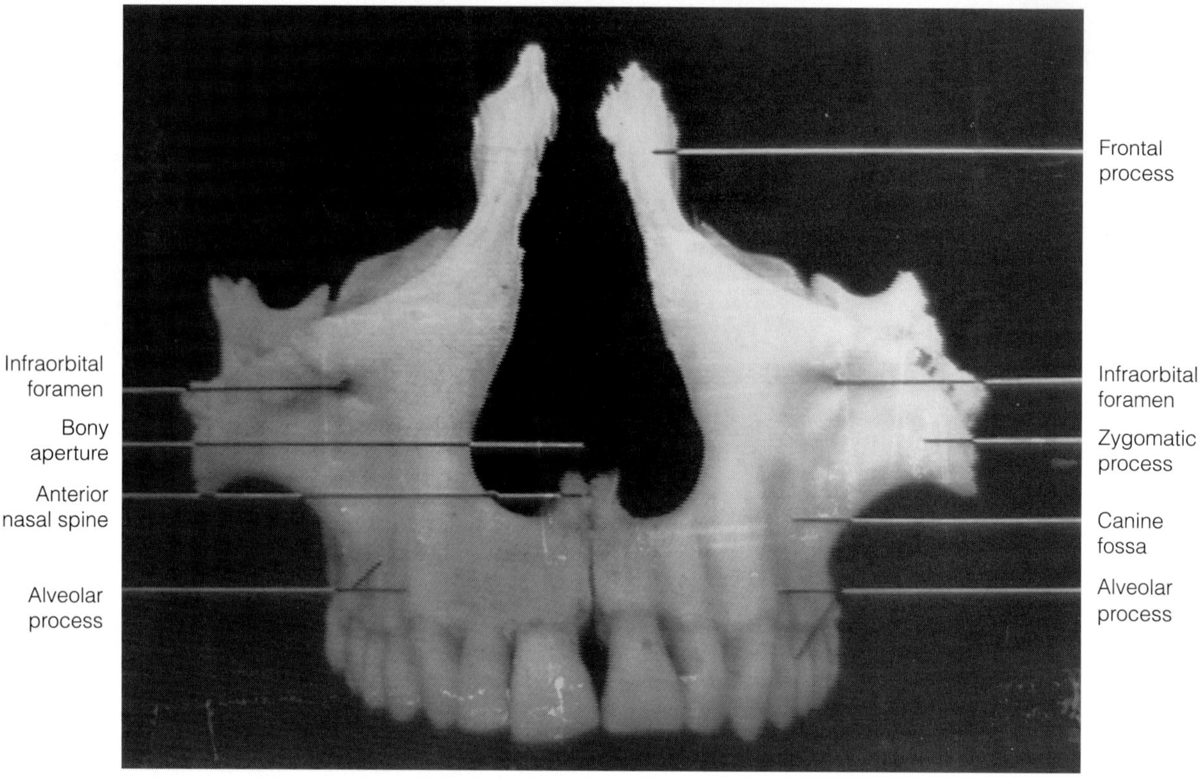

FIGURE 15–1. Paired components and processes of the maxilla.

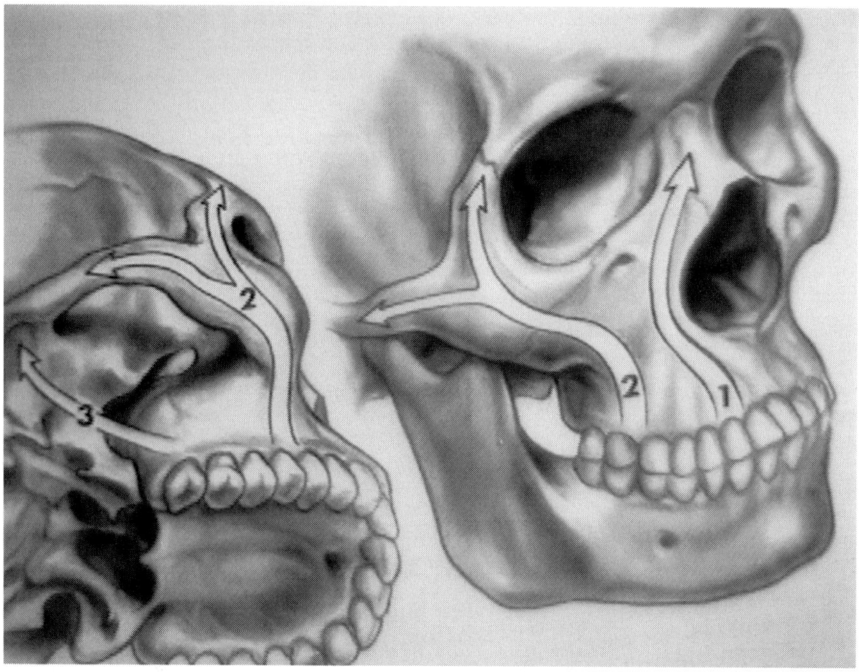

FIGURE 15–2. Structural buttress of the maxilla.

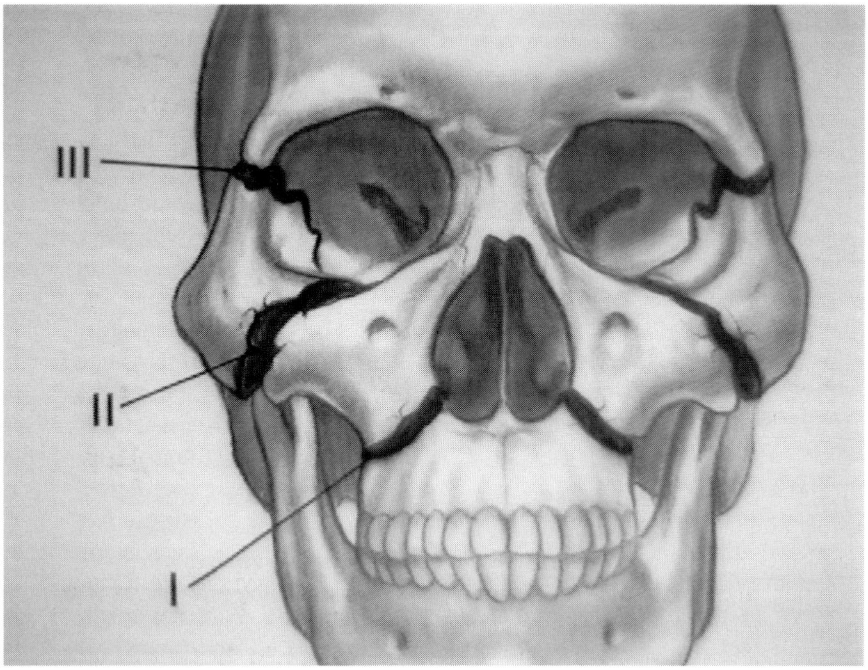

FIGURE 15–3. LeFort classification.

is unrecognized and can lead to difficulty in correcting the occlusal relationships (Fig. 15–4).

MECHANISMS AND DYNAMICS OF MIDFACIAL FRACTURES

The type of injury that occurs depends on the amount of force, the direction of the force, and the anatomic location of the force. Since the force of impact is usually not anatomically centered on the face, the fracture pattern that results is unpredictable. The patterns of injury are asymmetrical, with the level of injury higher on one side than the other.[5] The maxilla is most commonly fractured by frontal and laterally directed forces. An impact directed low on the maxilla is likely to cause a vertical (sagittal) or alveolar fracture. Force directed at the nasofrontal region creates central fractures that involve the frontal sinus and the medial orbital wall. A severe impact on the lateral zygomaticofrontal buttress results in a fracture of the LeFort III pattern. Malalignment of the buttresses can result in any combination of maxillary retrusion, rotation, malocclusion, increase in midface width, and flattening with or without elongation.

DIAGNOSIS

Patients may present with periorbital ecchymosis, epistaxis, cerebrospinal rhinorrhea, and malocclusion with an anterior open bite. Intraoral examination may reveal a torn palate mucosa signifying the presence of a sagittal fracture of the maxilla. Generally, marked instability of the midface, loss of nasal projection, and telecanthus may be present.

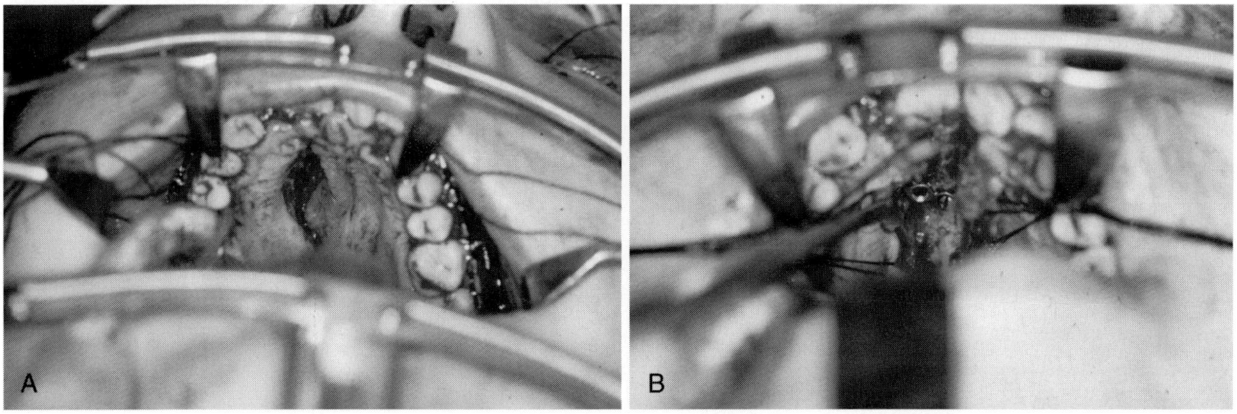

FIGURE 15–4. *A,* Sagittal fracture of the maxilla. *B,* Rigid fixation of sagittal fracture.

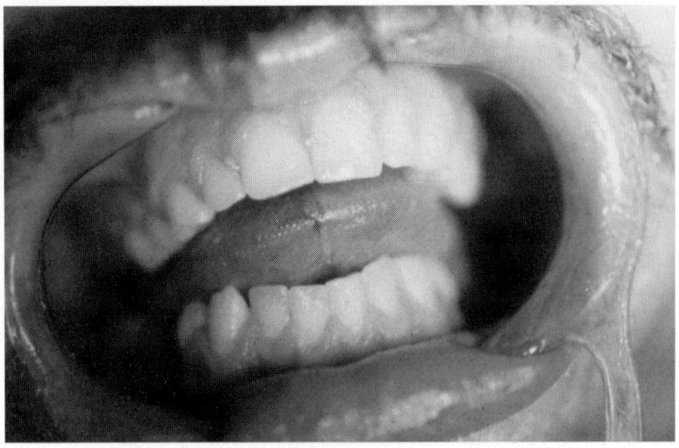

FIGURE 15–5. Patient demonstrates anterior open bite.

Manual examination reveals mobility of the midfacial structures. There are exceptions when the midface is impacted or greenstick fractures occur. The maxillary segments usually are displaced downward and posteriorly. Elongation and retrusion of the midface is evident. The downward displacement of the maxilla causes an anterior open bite, which can occur on one or both sides (Fig. 15–5).

RADIOLOGIC EXAMINATION

Computed Tomographic (CT) scans allow a better understanding of complex fracture patterns and the other fractures that occur in association with these injuries. High-resolution CT scanners are an invaluable tool in assessing the types and extent of injury (Fig. 15–6). Plain film examination is of historic interest only and has been largely discarded in the evaluation of these injuries. CT scans provide precise anatomic details that aid in planning the repairs needed. Three-dimensional scans are an excellent teaching tool but are not necessary for planning the management of these injuries.

MANAGEMENT

The key principles in the management of the patient with midfacial trauma begin with establishing an airway, controlling hemorrhage, and clearing all potential cervical spine injuries. High-resolution CT scanning is the key to planning the surgical approach to treatment (Fig. 15–7). The goal of repair of LeFort fractures is to establish the correct midfacial height, projection, and pretrauma occlusion as a three-dimensional unit. Ideally, fracture repair should be started as soon as the patient is cleared for general anesthesia. I try to repair all complex midface fractures within the first 24 to 48 hours of injury if the patient is cleared for anesthesia. This allows minimal soft tissue retraction. Wide exposure and early repair with primary bone grafting have been championed by many and currently constitute the standard treatment for complex midface fractures.[6] All fracture sites must be exposed widely to visualize and make the repairs adequately. All areas of critical defects receive primary bone grafts. Calvarial bone is preferred for most defects in the midface area. Larger defects associated with cranial vault injuries may require iliac crest, split rib, or split calvarial bone grafts. Dental impressions are taken for combined midface and mandibular fractures. The models are then cut, and bite wafers are prefabricated to ensure the proper occlusal relationships (Fig. 15–8). This aids in planning the steps needed to effect the repairs.

LeFort I Fracture

The LeFort I fracture is exposed widely, disimpacted, and placed in occlusion with the mandible acting as the principal guide in reestablishing the midfacial height. The mandible serves as the guide for establishing the correct height posteriorly, and the anterior buttresses establish the height anteriorly. The LeFort I pattern can usually be managed by open reduction, internal fixation, and mandibulomaxillary fixation (MMF). The timing of removal of the MMF is variable and must be determined on an individual basis.

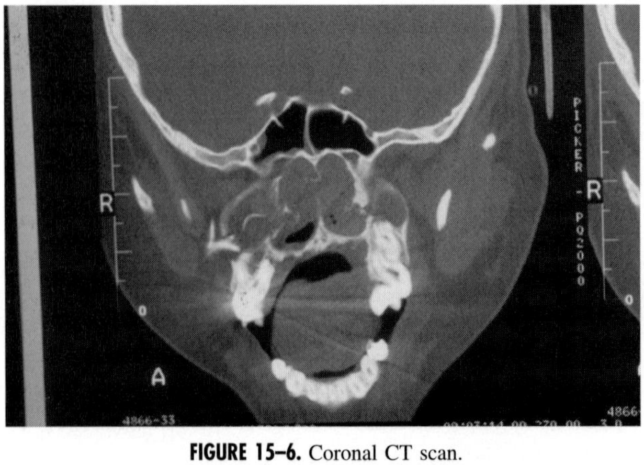

FIGURE 15–6. Coronal CT scan.

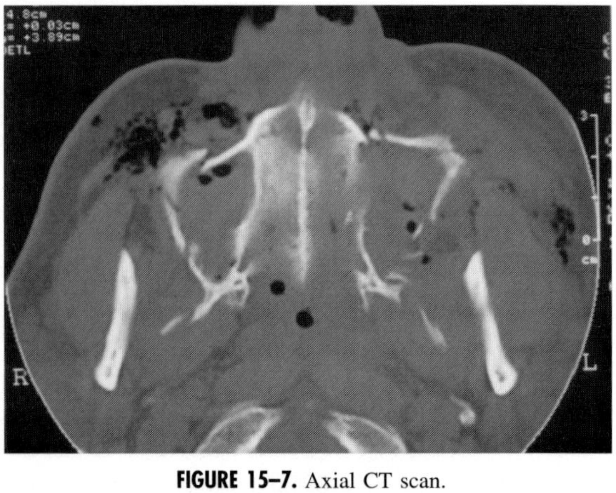

FIGURE 15–7. Axial CT scan.

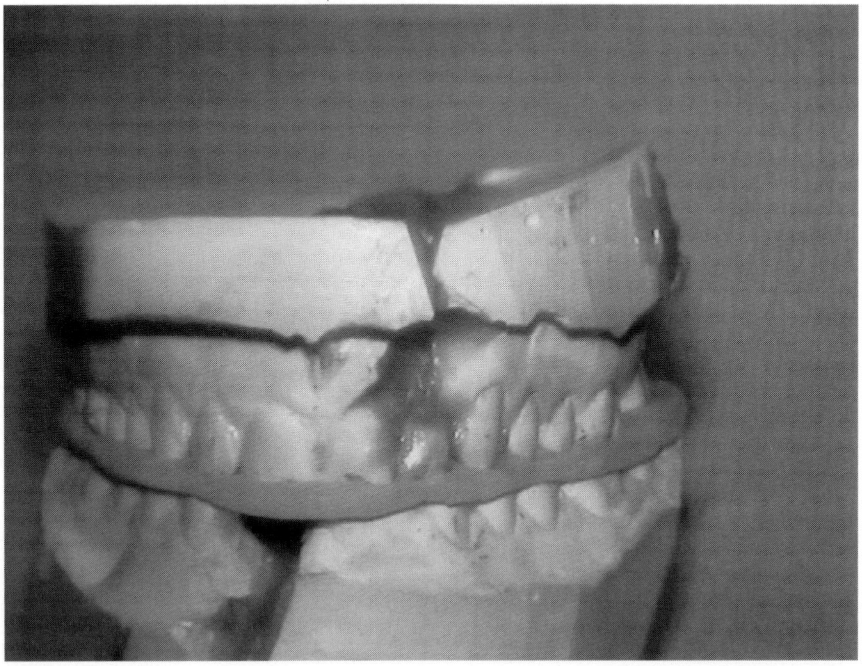

FIGURE 15–8. Dental model with prefabricated acrylic splint.

LeFort II Fracture

These injuries may involve considerable disruption of the orbit, of which both the floor and the medial wall may be severely damaged and require reconstruction. The fracture pattern is usually worse on one side than the other. These fractures can generally be exposed through a number of combined approaches. Subciliary or transconjunctival incisions can be used for exposure of the orbital floors and rims (Figs. 15–9 and 15–10). Midface exposure is achieved with a maxillary vestibular incision, which generally extends from first molar to first molar if both sides of the maxilla need exposure (Fig. 15–11). When both mandibular and maxillary fractures are present, the occlusal relationships are established first, and then the mandibular fractures are repaired, followed by the maxillary fractures. Patients with bilateral subcondylar fractures as well as midface fractures may require open reduction of those fractures first to reestablish the correct height of the posterior maxillary buttress. The various guidelines for absolute and relative indications for open reduction of subcondylar fractures should be applied as needed in the individual case. The side with the least amount of disruption of the pillar system can be used as a guide for correction of the anterior height discrepancy on the opposite side. Reestablishment of midfacial height sometimes requires immediate bone grafting of the fracture sites. I Prefer to use cranial bone grafts for areas of critical stability. These are held in place with rigid fixation where appropriate. Bone grafts are commonly used for reconstruction of the orbital floors and medial orbital walls. To effectively restore the proper amount of globe volume in severely comminuted orbital floor fractures, the bone grafts must be placed posterior to the axis of the globe. Exposure of the nasal fracture may be indicated to establish additional fixation.

LeFort III Fracture

This fracture is also referred to as craniofacial dysjunction due to the pattern of the fracture lines. It can occur unilaterally or bilaterally. The midface is disjoined from the skull base by a shearing force and remains attached by soft tissue only. This fracture requires multiple exposures to reduce and fix the fracture lines adequately. The fracture may be impacted and immobile; if so, it must be disimpacted first. The repair sequence is similar to that used with the LeFort II fracture with the addition of a bicoronal incision to expose the zygomatic arches as needed. The comminuted zygomatic arch must be fixed to ensure that malar flattening does not occur. This also allows forward support of the maxilla and ensures that the correct amount of anterior projection occurs. The nasal fracture may be severely comminuted and may require immediate bone grafting of the nasal dorsum. The medial canthal tendons may require realignment with fixation of the bony fragments.

Methods of Fixation

Rigid fixation is the standard employed by most specialists involved in the management of these fractures. This method of fixation withstands the deforming forces of contraction and muscle action. Miniplate and screw fixation provide rigid internal fixation and stability for the facial skeleton. Self-tapping screws can be used in areas of the midface where the bone is thin. Drill holes should be centrally placed to avoid compression. Primary bone grafting should be considered in defects measuring more than 5 mm. Rigid fixation of bone grafts inhibits resorption of the graft.

Malunited or Delayed Repair Fractures

Fractures in which there is a delay in repair for several weeks can be treated with the wide exposure and osteotomies

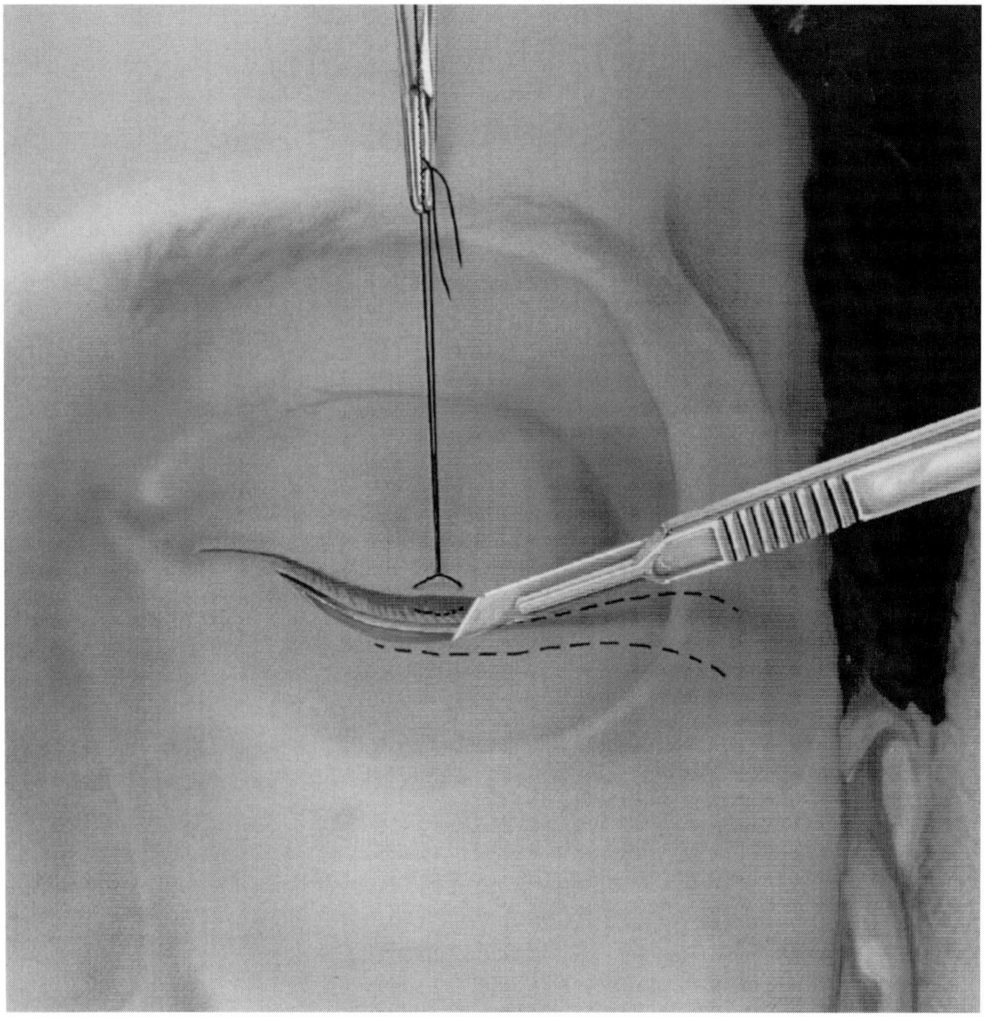

FIGURE 15–9. Transconjunctival approach (incision).

that are commonly used in today's craniofacial surgery for correction of congenital deformities. These techniques can be employed safely and effectively to correct the malunited and malpositioned fracture segments. Expectant soft tissue contraction mandates that wide exposure techniques be used to ensure adequate reduction.

The Edentulous Maxilla

In edentulous patients the patient's own denture or acrylic splints can be used to achieve the best relationship between the maxilla and the mandible. The mandibular denture is secured with a circumandibular wire, and the maxillary denture can be suspended from the zygoma or screwed into the palate. LeFort I fractures in edentulous patients may require no treatment if there is minimal evidence of displacement or disturbance of the mandibulomaxillary relationship. A soft diet is encouraged, and after the edema and hematoma have subsided a new denture can be made.

Sagittal Maxillary Fractures

Open reduction near or at the piriform aperture is necessary for sagittal maxillary fractures. Frequently the mucosa is torn, and the fracture site can be visualized. Exposure of the intraoral fracture line can be gained either through the torn mucosal edges or through direct incision and development of the mucosal edge flaps. An occlusal wafer aids in guiding the teeth into the proper relationship (Fig. 15–12). The palate can then be rigidly fixed. I typically place one or two small plates across the posterior extent of the fracture site. The posterior site can be reduced in a closed fashion, but this may prove difficult, and overtightening of the MMF wires to bring the teeth into occlusion may cause the maxillary teeth to become lingually tipped or may create a posterior crossbite.

POSTOPERATIVE MANAGEMENT

Vigorous oral hygiene is initiated in the early postoperative period. Mouth rinses and a pulsatile cleaning apparatus, when available, are the methods of choice. Adequate nutrition must be maintained; food can be supplied through a feeding or nasogastric tube placed at the time of surgery.

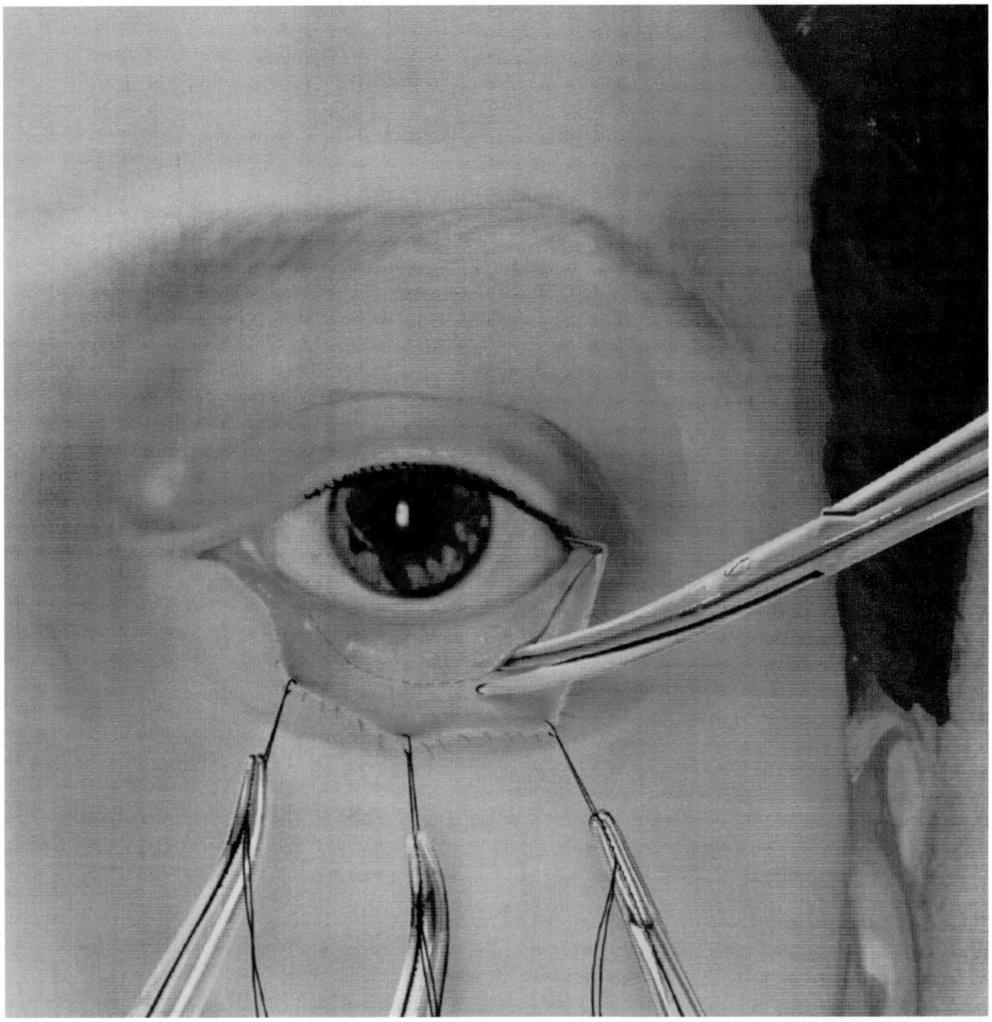

FIGURE 15–10. Subciliary approach (incision).

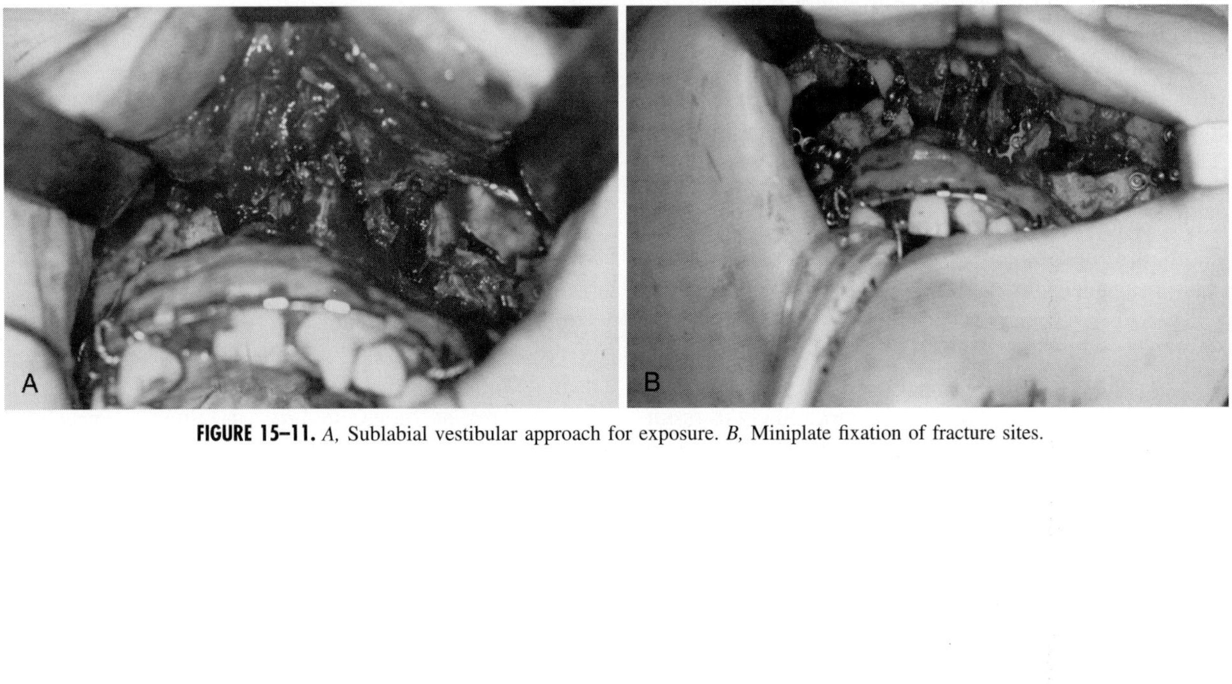

FIGURE 15–11. *A,* Sublabial vestibular approach for exposure. *B,* Miniplate fixation of fracture sites.

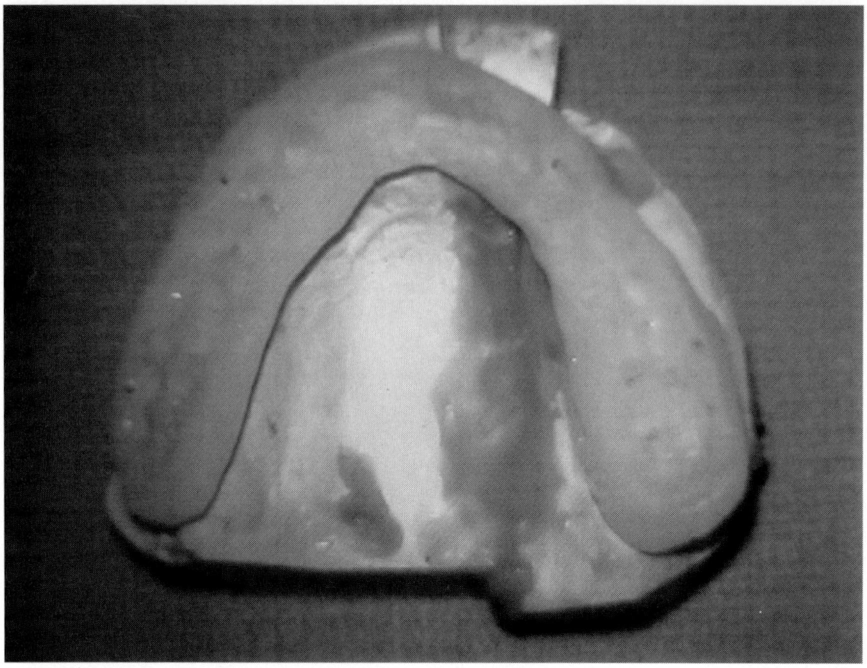

FIGURE 15–12. Occlusal view wafer helps to guide the teeth into the proper relationship with each other.

When the patient is alert and cooperative enough, oral feeding in the form of liquid foods can be introduced. The timing of release of the MMF is carried out on an individual basis. In a simple minimally displaced LeFort I fracture, the patient may be immediately released from MMF once the proper occlusion has been obtained. Wire cutters should be kept with the patient at all times for emergent release of the MMF in the event of potential emesis and aspiration.

COMPLICATIONS OF MIDFACE FRACTURES

Postoperative wound infections from midface injuries are less common than infections from mandibular fractures. Management of would infections is easily accomplished with local wound care. Complications associated with maxillary fractures are usually related to specific areas of the fracture sites. Orbital complications such as lacrimal apparatus injury, diplopia, enophthalmus, and blindness may occur. Facial height discrepancies may produce obvious facial asymmetries. Nasal obstruction, anosmia, and external deformities secondary to inadequate reduction or failure to use bone grafts may occur. Nonunion of the maxilla is extremely unusual. If any instability is noted at the time of removal of the MMF, usually an additional period of MMF will result in the occurrence of union. Nonunion is more likely to result from severe comminution and fragmentation in patients with extensive panfacial fractures or in those with bony discontinuity.[7] Bone grafting is encouraged in the initial repair of these injuries to avoid postoperative instability. The patient's occlusion may be slightly off, requiring some additional time in light elastic bands to help guide the teeth into the proper occlusal plane. Generally, when the patient is released from MMF the arch bars are left in place if additional fixation or the use of elastic traction is needed in the future.

Nasolacrimal duct injuries may occur with LeFort injuries. The duct may be transected or obstructed. If the canalicular system is intact and the patient has epiphora, a dacryocystorhinostomy should be performed. Injuries that cause comminution of the nasoethmoid region cause traumatic hypertelorism that should be corrected with direct repair at the initial operation. Injury of the extraocular muscle may result from either direct contusion of the muscle or the surgical repair. Blindness has been a reported complication of these fractures, mandating that the patient's vision and CT scan be reviewed carefully prior to repair attempts.[8]

SUMMARY

Midface fractures should be properly evaluated, studied with the aid of CT scans, and classified. Cervical spine injuries should be ruled out. Management of complex midface fractures requires a solid working knowledge of the anatomy of the facial skeleton. A multidisciplinary approach is required in a large percentage of cases. The surgical team's familiarity with midface injuries and other associated injuries can at times be life- and limb-saving. Titanium miniplating and intermaxillary fixation remain the gold standard for open reduction and internal fixation. A clear, concise approach to the individual patient is a must if these injuries are to be managed and reconstructed in the most anatomically beneficial manner. Such an approach helps to prevent or reduce the percentage of unfavorable results.

REFERENCES

1. LeFort R: Experimental study of fractures of the upper jaw, parts I and II. Rev Chir Paris 23:208, 1901. Translated by P Tessier. Reprinted Plast Reconstr Surg 50:497, 1972.
2. LeFort R: Experimental study of fractures of the upper jaw, part III. Rev Chir Paris 23:479, 1901. Translated by P Tessier. Reprinted Plast Reconstr Surg 50:600, 1972.
3. Manson PN, Hoopes JE, Su CT: Structural pillars of the facial skeleton: An approach to the management of LeFort fractures. Plast Reconstr Surg 66:54, 1980.
4. Sicher H: Oral Anatomy, 4th ed. St. Louis, CV Mosby, 1965, pp. 92–93.
5. Manson PN: Some thoughts on the classification and treatment of LeForte fractures. Ann Plast Surg 17:356–363, 1986.
6. Gruss JS, Mackinnon SE: Complex maxillary fractures: The role of buttress reconstruction and immediate bone grafting. Plast Reconstr Surg 78:9–16, 1986.
7. Thaller SR, Kawamoto HK: A histologic evaluation of fracture repair of the midface. Plast Reconstr Surg 85:196–201, 1990.
8. Manfredi SJ, Raji MR, Sprinkle PM, et al: Computerized tomographic scan findings in facial fractures associated with blindness. Plast Reconstr Surg. 68(4):479–490, 1981.

CHAPTER 16

Reconstructive Techniques of the Anterior Mandibular Arch

David W. Stepnick, M.D.
Alain Sabri, M.D.
Anthony J. Maniglia, M.D.

Anterior mandibular defects present a continuing challenge for the head and neck reconstructive surgeon despite the major advances that have been achieved in the field. Posttraumatic and postextirpative procedures for malignancies can leave patients with considerable cosmetic deformity and functional impairment including problems with speech, oral competence, mastication, deglutition, and the airway. In those with more extensive defects, soft tissue, muscular components, and motor and sensory nerves are lost as well as the architecture of the bony arch. Restoration of the lower facial contour and mandibular continuity alone does not automatically imply successful rehabilitation of the aforementioned functions.

Adding to the complexity of this surgical endeavor in many cases is the presence of an irradiated field, which predisposes the reconstruction to complications resulting from scarring, fibrosis, impairment of mucosal host-defense mechanisms, and poor vascularity of the recipient soft tissue bed. Additionally, the oral region is especially problematic and somewhat unique because of the risk of wound contamination by the normal oral flora. Potential complications include infection, tissue breakdown, fistula formation, and osteoradionecrosis. These problems can be devastating and can result in compromise of function, cosmesis, and loss of further reconstructive potential.

With the development of new reconstructive methods during the past two decades, ablative surgeons may be more willing to perform wider resections of the mandible and associated soft tissue. However, the prognosis of oromandibular carcinoma has not changed dramatically during the past few decades despite the possibility of more aggressive procedures, and the surgical focus has shifted to maintaining the quality of life. It is in this area that the major advances in treatment of this difficult problem have been achieved during the past few decades, and new techniques continue to evolve.

Defects of the anterior mandible present an especially difficult problem and are devastating to the patient. The nonreconstructed anterior mandibular arch results in the so-called Andy Gump deformity, which involves significant functional and cosmetic compromise (Fig. 16–1). The anterior arch is instrumental in maintaining the anatomic relationships of the tongue and suprahyoid muscles. These muscles insert on the lingual aspect of the anterior mandibular arch and play an important role in airway maintenance, articulation, and deglutition. Lateral mandibular defects are better tolerated and result in less morbidity than anterior ones, and many argue that these often do not need to be reconstructed.

Anterior mandibular defects can be generally divided into three major categories: (1) those limited to the anterior mandibular arch (the region between the mental foramina), (2) those that include one side (involving, in addition to the body, the angle or the ramus, or a combination of all three), and (3) total defects.

HISTORICAL NOTES

The obvious deformities and functional deficits posed by a missing jaw segment have prompted physicians to find innovative ways to replace what was lost by trauma, infection, or cancer. As one can imagine, mandibular defects were originally left unreconstructed. In some of the earliest documented cases in the literature, Dupuytren in 1833[1] and Heath in 1875[2] reported successful anterior mandibular re-

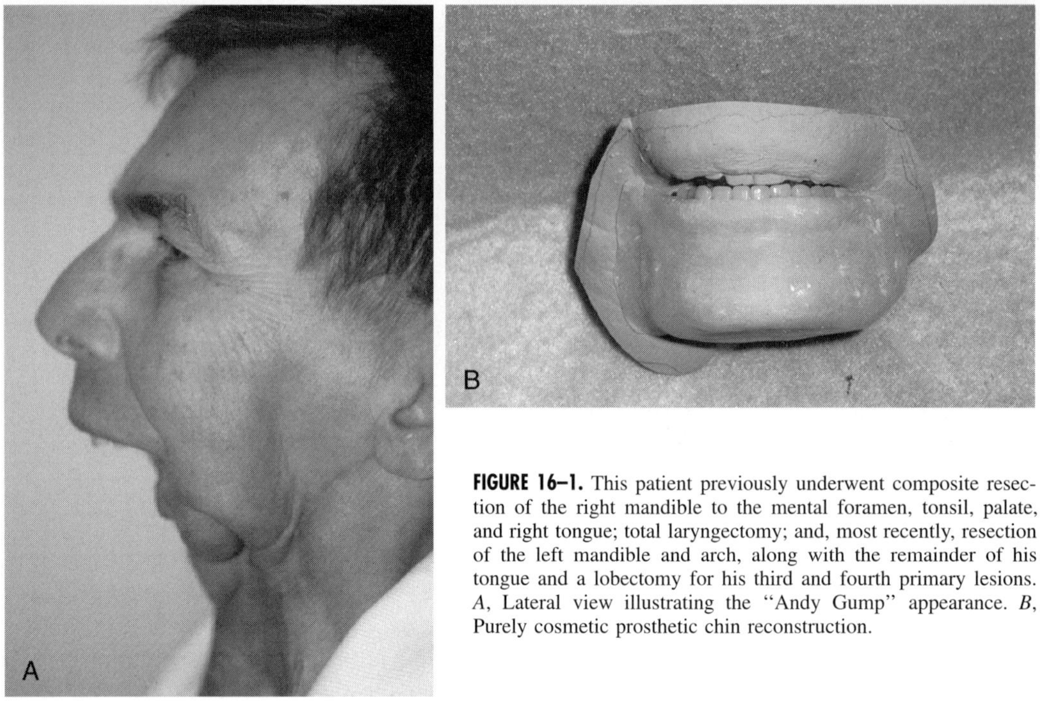

FIGURE 16–1. This patient previously underwent composite resection of the right mandible to the mental foramen, tonsil, palate, and right tongue; total laryngectomy; and, most recently, resection of the left mandible and arch, along with the remainder of his tongue and a lobectomy for his third and fourth primary lesions. *A*, Lateral view illustrating the "Andy Gump" appearance. *B*, Purely cosmetic prosthetic chin reconstruction.

sections, and these were left unreconstructed. Deadrick in 1910[3] also reported successful jaw resections that were left unreconstructed. Attempts to bridge these defects varied in technique, and a number of different materials were subsequently used. Partsch in 1897[4] used a metal band. Subsequently, different metals (steel, aluminum, brass, and magnesium) were used with little success.

Ollier, in 1816,[5] performed experimental work on bone physiology in animals and humans to investigate the potential for using bone grafts for osseous reconstruction. Bardenheuer, Sykoff, and others[6, 7] used bone grafts for mandibular reconstruction. Owing to a plethora of war-related mandibular injuries, World War I stimulated interest in this area, and bone grafting using segments of ribs and tibia became more popular. In 1918, Blair proposed use of the patient's own sterilized mandible to reconstruct missing mandibular segments.[8] Gillies (1920) reported on the British experience with iliac bone grafts.[9] A year later, Ivy reported a mandibular defect that was successfully grafted with iliac bone; he included details of long-term follow-up.[10, 11] Vitallium was used by Winter and colleagues in 1945.[12]

During World War II, another opportunity to develop new techniques resulted in the use of metal trays packed with cancellous bone (Fig. 16–2). Converse used such a tray packed with cancellous bone in 1945.[13] Subsequently, Dacron trays were used by Leake and Rappaport (1972),[14] and Boyne and Zarem (1976) used titanium trays.[15] Pike and Boyne, as well as others, used lyophilized mandibular allografts packed with cancellous bone.[16] For mandibles involved with tumor, Hamaker (1981)[17] used the patient's own mandible, first irradiating it with high-dose radiation to destroy viable tumor and then subsequently reimplanting it (Fig. 16–3). Others have used freezing to destroy tumor.[18] These methods, for the most part, were subsequently abandoned because better options became available. Indeed, high-dose radiation therapy destroyed not only viable cancer cells but osteocytes as well, essentially rendering the bone nonviable and making it no different than a cadaveric bone graft. Such grafts could not reliably support a denture and certainly would not support osseointegrated implants.

Another important landmark in the evolution of modern reconstructive techniques was the development earlier in this century of rigid internal fixation. Hansmann was the first to use and discuss the use of bone plates in 1886.[19] He applied a nickel-plated steel bar with holes to the bone and used screws to secure it in position. In 1949, Robert Danis published Theorie et Pratique de l'Ostéosynthèse,[20] which is the basis of modern understanding of the concepts of osteosynthesis as opposed to rigid internal fixation. In the 1950s, the

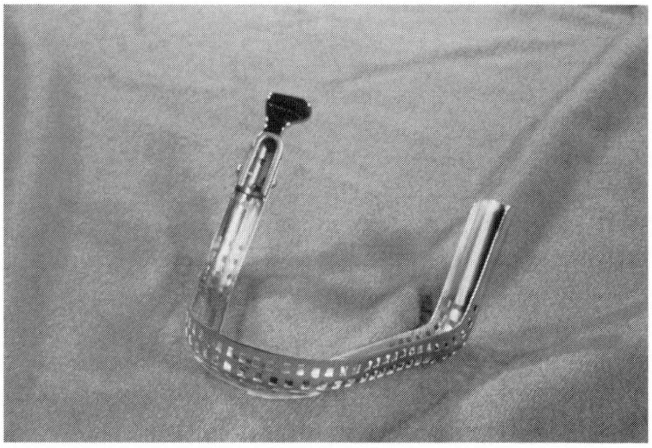

FIGURE 16–2. Stainless steel trays packed with cancellous bone were used by many for several years to replace mandibular segments.

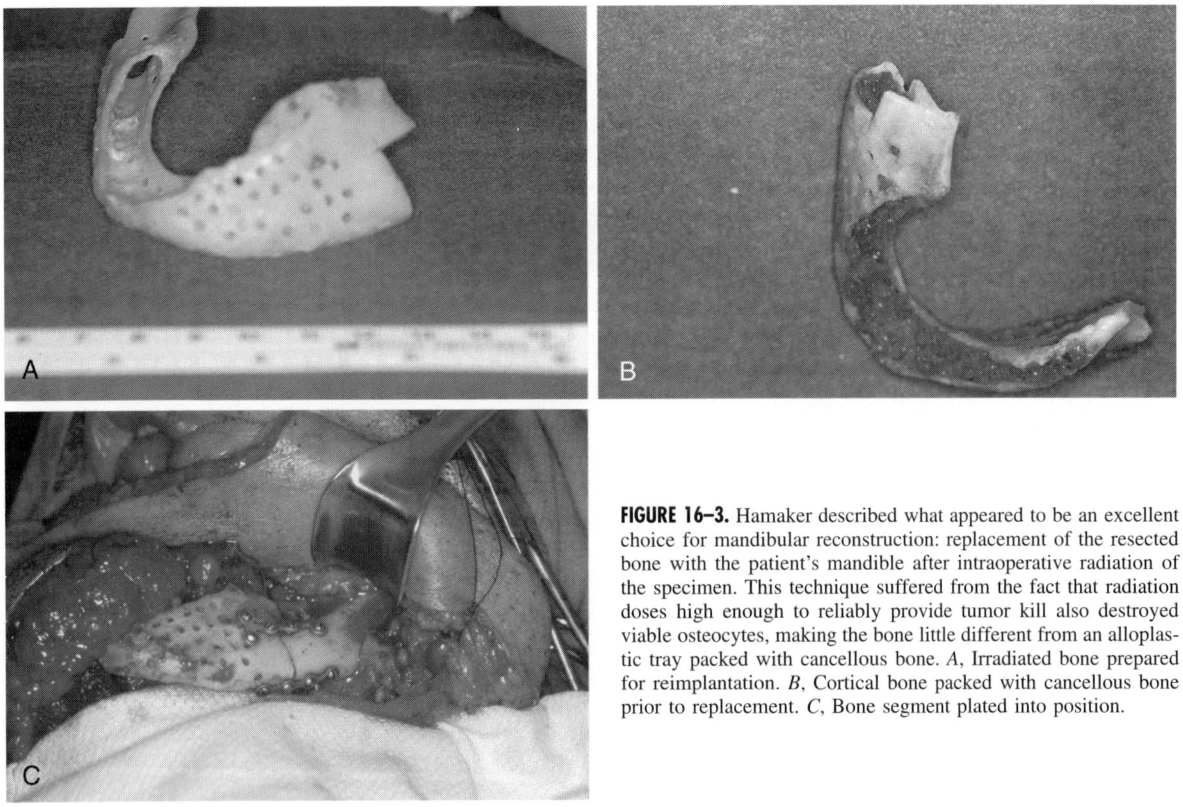

FIGURE 16–3. Hamaker described what appeared to be an excellent choice for mandibular reconstruction: replacement of the resected bone with the patient's mandible after intraoperative radiation of the specimen. This technique suffered from the fact that radiation doses high enough to reliably provide tumor kill also destroyed viable osteocytes, making the bone little different from an alloplastic tray packed with cancellous bone. *A*, Irradiated bone prepared for reimplantation. *B*, Cortical bone packed with cancellous bone prior to replacement. *C*, Bone segment plated into position.

Association for Osteosynthesis or Association for the Study of Internal Fixation (AO-ASIF) was founded by Morris Müller, who was greatly influenced by Danis's work. A great deal of information related to the physiology of bone healing and plating system design was generated by this group, who then practically applied it to the development of plating systems.[21]

Raveh and associates (1984) developed a plating system with several unique characteristics.[22] The THORP system (titanium-coated hollow screw and reconstruction plate system) utilized highly biocompatible titanium, hollow screws that allowed bone ingrowth, thereby maximizing screw integration, and, expandable screw heads that locked the screws to the plate through the pressure of the screw heads on the plate rather than compression on the underlying bone. This system was very thick and readily palpable when used for mandibular reconstruction, and a relatively high incidence of plate fractures occurred as a result of design. A second generation of locking screw plating systems has subsequently been developed that has a lower profile and is designed to eliminate such plate fractures. Although they are now used extensively to keep vascularized bone fragments that are part of free flaps in position during healing, the stronger (reconstruction) plates were used by many to bridge mandibular defects without replacing the bony component (Fig. 16–4). Still, some surgeons routinely use such plates to repair anterior defects despite better available options. The use of bridging plates, especially without adequate soft tissue coverage, more often than not eventually results in intraoral or external plate extrusion (Fig. 16–5). Early reports failed to recognize late failures and advocated bridging plates even for anterior defects. Now these authors add to the consensus that revascularized free tissue transfer is the treatment of choice for most of these patients.

All the methods mentioned previously were important stepping stones in the evolution of modern mandibular reconstruction, but they had an unacceptably high rate of complications and failures. The use of radiation therapy made reconstruction more difficult because of scarring, fibrosis, devascularization, and the absence of a healthy soft tissue bed, and complication rates were higher. It became apparent that transfer of vascularized tissue was needed for successful mandibular reconstruction, especially in patients in whom radiation therapy was part of the oncologic treatment. A variety of pedicled soft tissue flaps were used to solve oromandibular reconstructive dilemmas, improving the overall success rate of plate coverage. These flaps included the forehead and deltopectoral flaps as well as pectoralis major, trapezius, and latissimus dorsi myocutaneous flaps.

In 1972, Conley reported on the use of osteomyocutaneous flaps for mandibular reconstruction.[23] The flaps were intended to provide vascularized bone together with soft tissue, thereby eliminating the problems of bridging plates and ischemic radiation damage. The success rates were low, especially in irradiated fields (15%). Many flaps have been described in the literature since then, including the pectoralis major–fifth rib, the sternocleidomastoid with attached clavicle, the temporalis with outer calvarium, and the trapezius muscle with attached scapular spine.[24] These flaps achieved variable degrees of success, limited by the pedicle and the

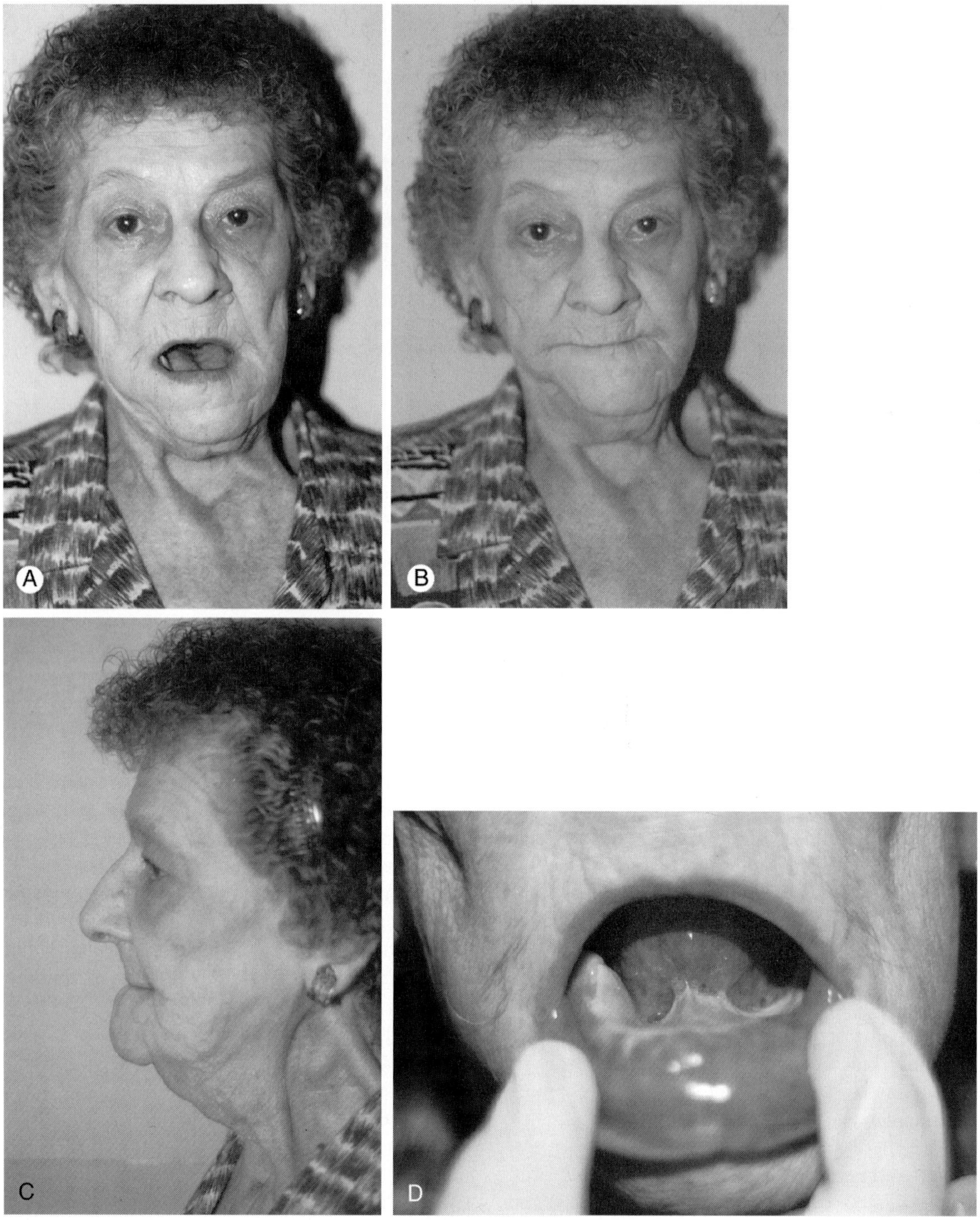

FIGURE 16–4. This patient, with severe emphysema, had a T_4 N_0 M_0 squamous cell carcinoma of the mandible. Preoperative assessment by a pulmonologist indicated that there was a significant risk that the patient would never come off a ventilator. Nonetheless, the patient and family, after careful thought and consideration, indicated that they would like to proceed with surgery. Mandible was excised from mental foramen to mental foramen, and a reconstruction plate was used to span the gap. A pectoralis major myocutaneous flap was used to cover the plate. Postoperatively, the patient eventually was weaned off the ventilator but remained in a nursing home for 6 months. Radiation therapy was not possible owing to logistic problems. At this time, the patient remains free of disease, is fully independent, and enjoys an excellent functional and cosmetic result. No plate extrusion has occurred to date. *A*, Frontal view 2 years postoperatively showing the patient's cosmetic appearance and ability to open and (*B*) close the mouth *C*, Profile showing excellent chin position. *D*, Intraoral view showing pectoralis major flap covering the plate in the floor of the mouth.

arc of rotation. In addition, the blood supply to the bony segment was variable. Anatomic studies by Reid and Taylor showed that the blood supply to the fifth to seventh ribs in the pectoralis "osteomyocutaneous flap" was tenuous and that the major supply was to the third and fourth ribs.[25] Only the trapezius-scapular osteomyocutaneous flap reliably provided vascularized bone, yet even it had limitations. Most notably, the configuration of the scapular spine was such that proper anatomic alignment was difficult after osteotomies had been performed to recreate a mandibular arch (Fig.

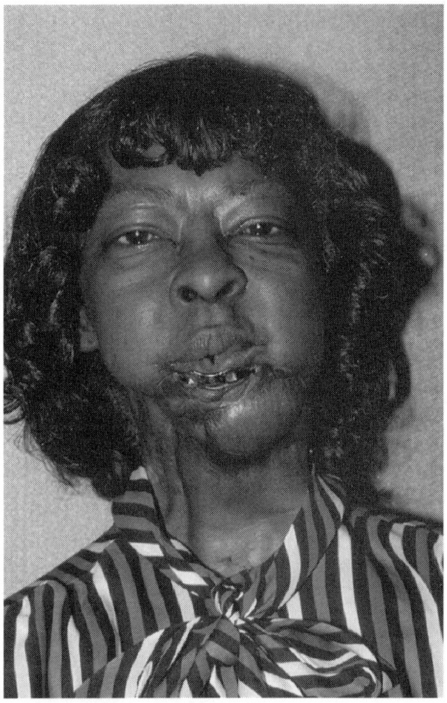

FIGURE 16–5. Alloplastic materials such as mandibular reconstruction plates almost invariably extrude, as shown in this woman who had a resection of the anterior mandible in the remote past.

16–6; see also Color plate). The bone thickness was marginal and allowed bony continuity but not a great deal of strength.

The advent of microvascular surgery has revolutionized mandibular reconstruction, especially in regard to the problem of the anterior arch. McKee in 1970 was the first to report on a free flap reconstruction of the mandible using a free rib graft.[26] Extensive work over the past two to three decades has led to the development of revascularized flaps with minimal donor morbidity and subsequent potential for good cosmetic results and oromandibular rehabilitation. Several of these flaps are discussed in more detail later in this chapter. Osseointegrated implants can reliably be incorporated into these richly vascularized neomandibles, providing excellent dental restoration. Sensate flaps allow reestablishment of sensation in this area, where such feedback plays an important role in oral competence. Together, these developments constitute today's state of the art in mandibular arch reconstruction.

GOALS OF RECONSTRUCTION

The ultimate goal of oromandibular reconstruction is to restore function and cosmesis to their premorbid status. This is rarely possible, however, and maintenance of a reasonable appearance and the ability to chew, swallow, and handle secretions properly are some of the basic results one should achieve.

The ideal oromandibular reconstruction should (1) maintain good mandibular contour with a good external skin color match, (2) maintain oral competence, (3) reconstruct the sulcus with adequate width and length, (4) provide a watertight closure between the oral cavity and the outside, (5) allow adequate tongue mobility for articulation and deglutition, (6) provide a strong bone stock to allow dental rehabilitation with dentures or with osseointegrated implants, (7) provide revascularized tissue to decrease the incidence of infections, wound breakdown, and fistulas, especially in irradiated patients, (8) provide a sensate flap both intraorally and externally, (9) create minimal donor site morbidity and deformity, (10) allow a simultaneous two-team approach to minimize operative time, (11) provide a soft tissue component that is pliable and maneuverable for the complex three-dimensional reconstruction often needed, and (12) restore proper occlusal relationships.

CLASSIFICATION OF DEFECTS

Generally, mandibular defects are classified into those involving lateral segments and those involving anterior segments; multiple classification schemes have been proposed. A classification system for oromandibular defects that accounts for bony, soft tissue, and neurologic defects was proposed by Urken and colleagues in 1991[27] and is used by many. Mandibular defects are categorized as involving the symphysis (S), hemisymphysis (SH) (central defects), body (B), ramus (R), or condyle (C) (lateral defects) (Fig. 16–7). Soft tissue defects are classified as mucosal, tongue, or cutaneous defects (Table 16–1). Neurologic deficits result from damage to the hypoglossal, lingual, facial, or inferior alveolar nerve (Table 16–2).

As with the TNM staging system for cancer, this classification scheme is helpful in accurately describing and categorizing the defects and deficits encountered thereby helping to standardize reporting among different surgeons. Additionally, this system ultimately should aid in the development of scientifically valid outcome measures for various defects. As mentioned earlier, anterior mandibular defects pose a far greater challenge in reconstruction and rehabilitation than lateral defects. The problem is compounded when there is, in addition to a bony defect, a soft tissue component. More extensive defects that include the anterior arch as well as the lateral segment pose an even greater challenge. As the size and complexity of the defect increases, the choice of a flap for reconstruction becomes more critical.

FREE FLAPS

The development of microvascular surgery and the subsequent use of free flaps has revolutionized mandibular recon-

TABLE 16–1. CLASSIFICATION OF SOFT TISSUE DEFECTS IN THE ORAL CAVITY

DEFECT	ABBREVIATION
Mucosa	
Labial	L
Buccal	B
Soft plate	SP
Hemi	SP^H
Total	SP^T
Floor of mouth	FOM
Anterior	FOM^A
Lateral	FOM^L
Pharynx	PH
Lateral	PH^L
Posterior	PH^P
Tongue	
Mobile	T^M
One quarter	$T^{M1/4}$
One half	$T^{M1/2}$
Three quarters	$T^{M3/4}$
Nonfunctional	T^M_{NF}
Tongue base	T^B
One quarter	$T^{B1/4}$
One half	$T^{B1/2}$
Three quarters	$T^{B3/4}$
Nonfunctional	T^B_{NF}
Total glossectomy	TG
Cutaneous defects	C
Cheek	C^{CH}
Neck	C^H
Mentum	C^M
Lips	C^L
Upper	C^{UL}; ¼, ½, ¾, and total
Lower	C^{UL}; ¼, ½, ¾, and total

struction. This technique allows surgeons bring composite flaps including flaps of bone, muscle and other soft tissue, and nerves from different sites of the body and incorporate them into a "hostile" field that in many instances has been (or will be) irradiated and contaminated, not only with normal microbial flora but also with deleterious organisms that thrive in the environment of the previously present necrotic tumor. The most commonly used free flaps used in mandibular reconstruction are discussed briefly below.

Radial Forearm Flap

Like its pedicled predecessor, the pectoralis major myocutaneous flap, the radial forearm flap probably deserves its designation as the soft tissue "workhorse" free flap for head and neck reconstruction. It may be harvested either as a fasciocutaneous flap, which is commonly done for oral cavity and oropharyngeal reconstruction, or as an osteocutaneous flap. This flap was first introduced in 1981 by Yang and colleagues in a military hospital in China and for many years was called the Chinese flap.[28] Its vascular supply is from the radial artery, and its venous return comes from either the venae comitantes or superficial veins of the forearm. The vascular pedicle is long (up to 20 cm), and most of the forearm skin may be harvested. It is supplied by 9 to 17 fasciocutaneous branches running in the lateral fasciocutaneous septum and separating the flexor carpi radialis from the brachioradialis (Fig. 16–8). The donor area is usually closed with a split-thickness skin graft; preservation of the paratenon during the dissection, meticulous attention to graft placement and fixation, and hand immobilization postoperatively are all important for successful skin take.

As noted previously, this flap may be used as a fasciocutaneous flap or an osteocutaneous flap with incorporation of the radius. As a fasciocutaneous flap, it is very popular for soft tissue restoration intraorally. It can also be used for lip reconstruction, skin replacement, and some times for circumferential pharyngeal defects. Some surgeons have used the flap as part of a "piggyback" flap. In this design, the distal radial artery (which normally is suture ligated) may be attached to another free flap so that blood flowing through the radial artery supplies both the radial forearm flap and whatever may be attached to it.

The flap is pliable and thin and offers a good color match with facial skin. Other modifications of the flap have included a bilobed design in patients who have undergone partial glossectomy. To maintain the mobility of the residual tongue, one lobe of the flap is used to line the floor of the mouth while the other replaces the remaining tongue. Another advantage of this flap is that it can be made sensate via the lateral antebrachial cutaneous nerve, which can be anastomosed to a recipient nerve. This characteristic offers an opportunity to reestablish intraoral or external sensation.

The radial forearm flap may also be harvested as an osteocutaneous flap and used for oromandibular reconstruction. A segment of radius 10 to 12 cm long harvested between the insertions of the pronator teres and the brachioradialis is used. However, no more than 40% of the circumference of the radius can be harvested to lessen the risk of pathologic fractures.

For anterior arch replacement, osteotomies must be performed to reconstitute the arch. As with other flaps, titanium plates are used to keep the segments together and to anchor the neomandible to the recipient mandible. Unfortunately, the osseous component of this flap has a smaller cross-sectional area than other flaps, resulting in a weaker reconstruction. This virtually precludes its use with osseointegrated implants for dental rehabilitation. Furthermore, pathologic fractures of the donor radius, which can result in significant morbidity, have been reported in up to 23% of cases.[29, 30] For these reasons, this reconstructive technique (for mandibular reconstruction) has, for the most part, been abandoned in North America.

TABLE 16–2. CLASSIFICATION OF NEUROLOGIC DEFECTS

DEFECT	ABBREVIATION
Neurologic	
Hypoglossal	N^H
Lingual	N^L
Facial	N^F
Inferior alveolar	N^{IA}
Bilateral defects	N_B

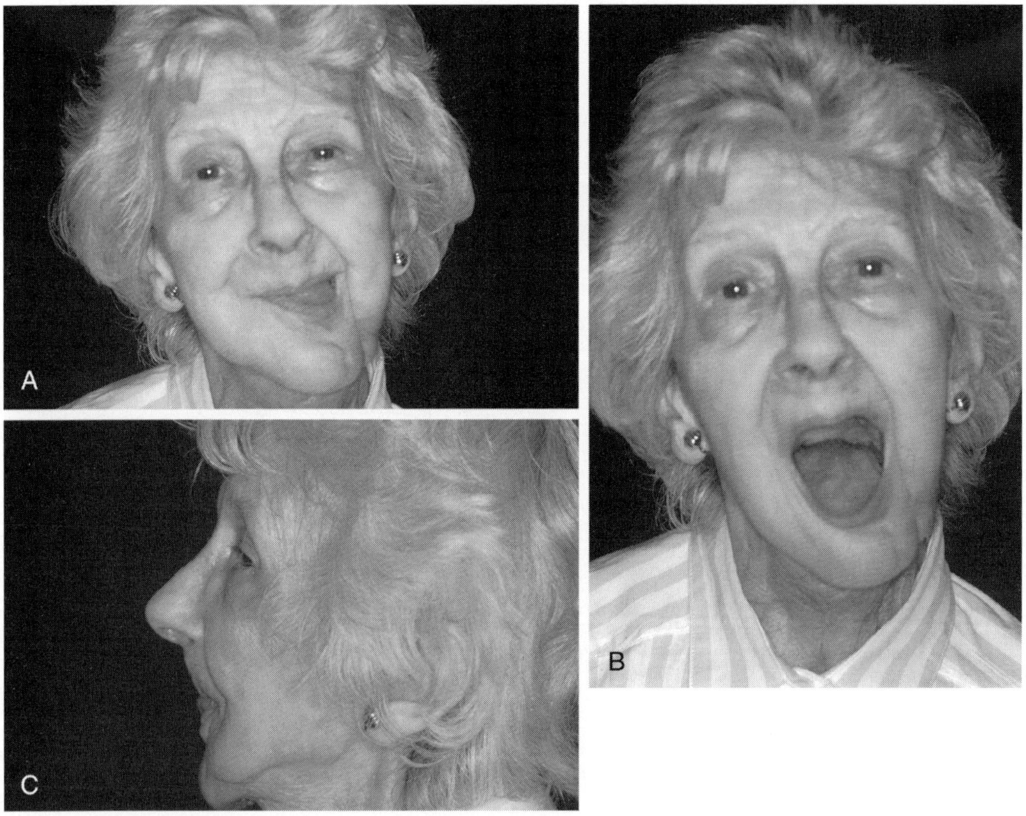

FIGURE 16–6. This patient underwent anterior mandibulectomy and trapezius-scapular spine mandibular reconstruction in 1987. Although she has a reasonable profile (*A*) and retains the ability to open her mouth and move her tongue (*B*), the frontal view (*C*) shows the typical appearance of such a patient in whom external fixation was used to secure relatively thin, oddly shaped bone fragments. This technique is primarily of historical interest because better techniques are available today. (See also Color plate.)

Dorsalis Pedis Flap

The dorsalis pedis flap was first described by McGraw and Furlow[31] and first used as an osteocutaneous flap by McLeod and Robinson.[32] This flap is based on the dorsalis pedis artery, and a 7- to 8-cm segment of bone may be taken from the second metatarsal. The skin component is harvested from the dorsum of the foot (Fig. 16–9). The flap is quite thin and pliable and is ideal for replacement of mucosal defects. Indeed, the main advantage of this flap is that it is not bulky and may readily be used for small defects. As

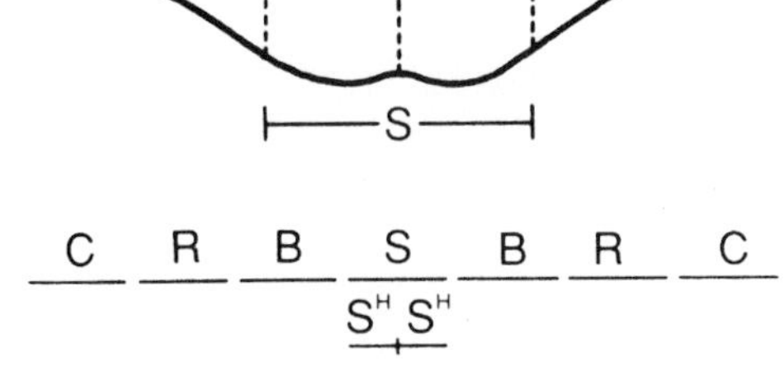

FIGURE 16–7. Classification of segmental bony defects. See text for explanation of symbols. (From Urken M, Weinberg H, Vickey C, et al: Oromandibular reconstruction using microvascular composite free flaps. Arch Otolaryngol Head Neck Surg 117: 733, 1991. Copyright 1991. American Medical Association.)

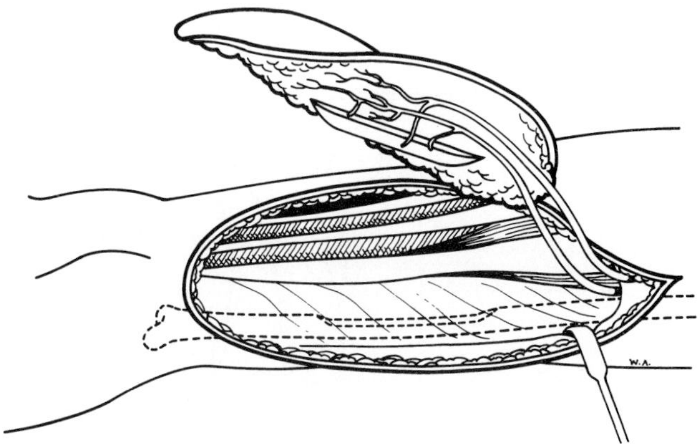

FIGURE 16–8. The radial forearm osteocutaneous flap. The vascular pedicle is taken from the lateral intermuscular septum. (From Paparella MM, et al: Otolaryngology Head and Neck. Philadelphia, W.B. Saunders Co., 1991.)

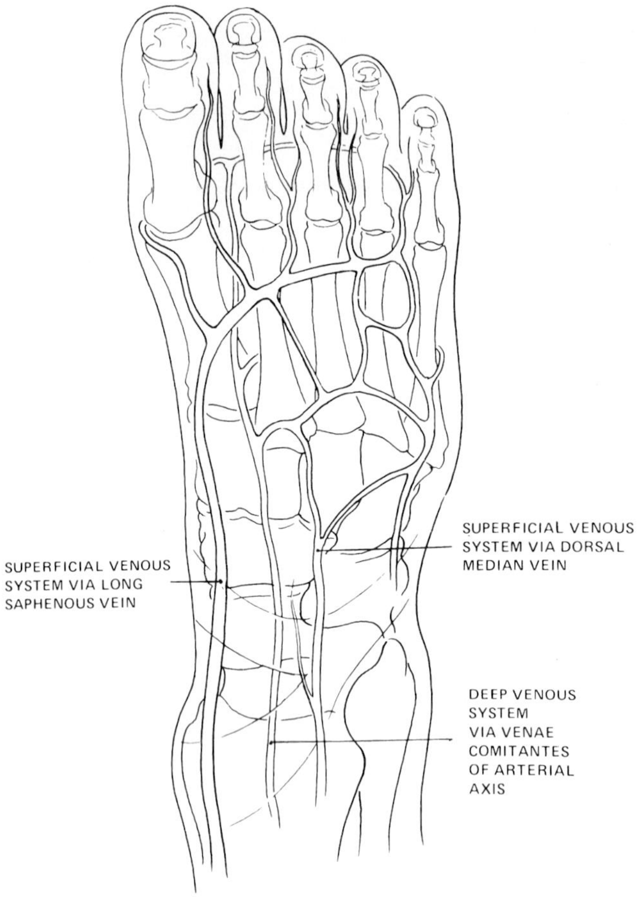

FIGURE 16–9. Vascular anatomy of the foot. The second metatarsal bone is used and is supplied by the first dorsal metatarsal artery. A skin paddle from the dorsum of the foot is part of this flap; it is supplied by branches from the dorsalis pedis and first dorsal metatarsal arteries. (From Baker S: Microsurgical Reconstruction of the Head and Neck. New York, Churchill Livingstone, 1989.)

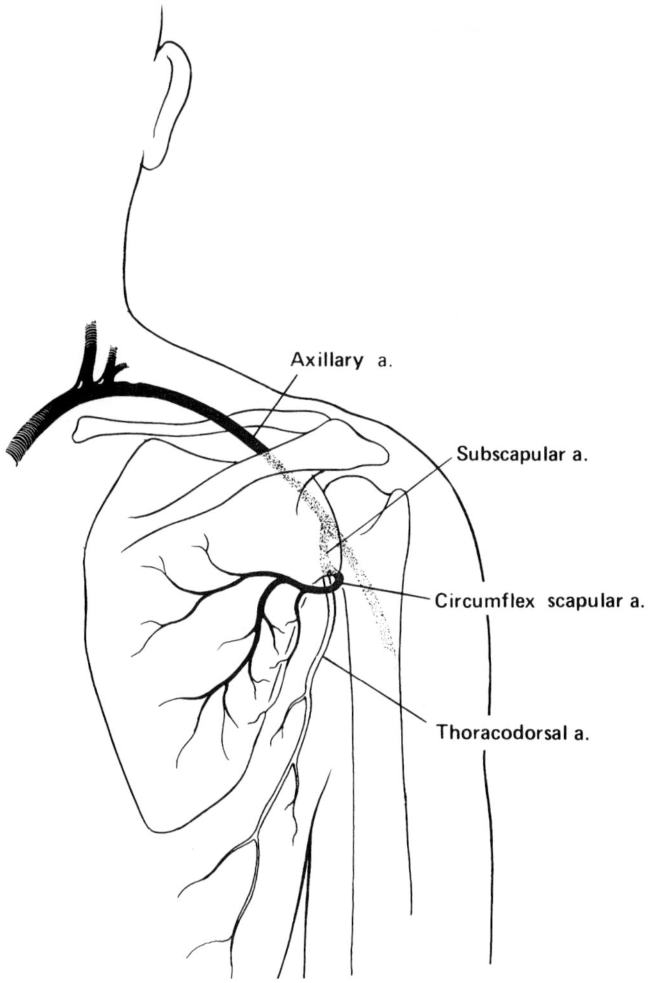

FIGURE 16–10. The vascular anatomy of the scapular flap. (From Baker S: Microsurgical Reconstruction of the Head and Neck. New York, Churchill Livingstone, 1989.)

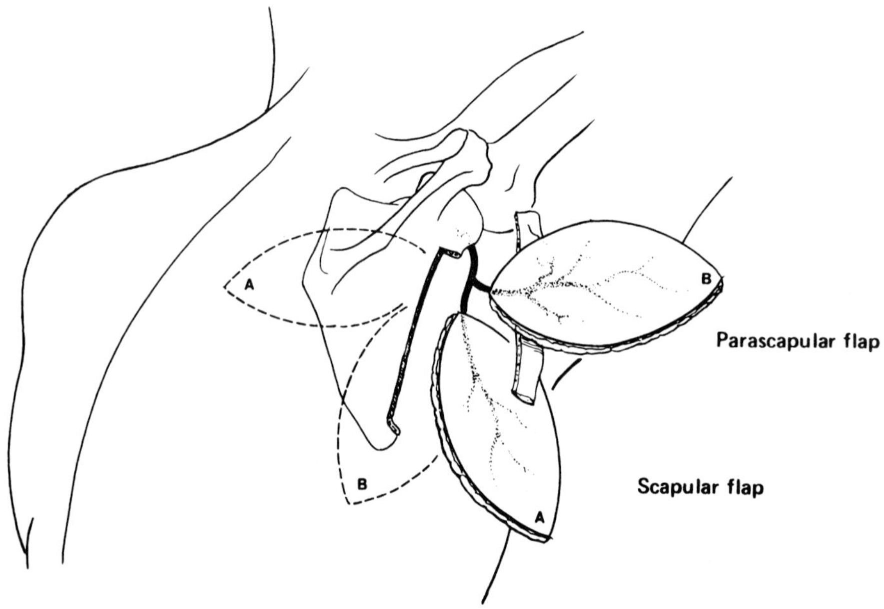

FIGURE 16–11. The skin paddles demonstrating the scapular and parascapular flaps with a portion of the scapular bone incorporated. (From Baker S: Microsurgical Reconstruction of the Head and Neck. New York, Churchill Livingstone, 1989.)

with other free flaps discussed in this chapter, osteotomies may be performed for contouring. The main disadvantages of this flap include its relative difficulty of harvesting, its short length, and its relatively weak bone when used for mandibular reconstruction. There are also frequent problems with the donor site, resulting in the additional morbidity of delay in ambulation and cosmetic deformity of the foot. Not only do the disadvantages outweigh the benefits, but other flaps that are clearly superior to this one for mandibular reconstruction are available as better alternatives.

Scapular Flaps

The subscapular artery, which arises from the third portion of the axillary artery, is the central vessel for several important flaps used in head and neck reconstruction (Fig. 16–10). "Subscapular system flaps" include the scapular and parascapular flaps (Fig. 16–11), the latissimus dorsi flap, the serratus anterior flap, and various combinations thereof. The scapular and parascapular flaps, which incorporate the lateral border of the scapula as their osseous component (as opposed to the scapular spine used in the trapezius osteomyocutaneous flap), together with the iliac crest flaps, were the most important free flaps for mandibular reconstruction from the late 1980s until the early to mid-1990s. These flaps, which differ only in horizontal versus vertical orientation of the skin paddle, were first developed in the 1980s by Saijo.[33] Swartz and associates[34] used and popularized this flap for mandibular reconstruction. It remained one of the most frequent flap choices until the fibular flap came into widespread use in the 1990s.

Both the scapular and parascapular flaps are based on the circumflex capillary artery, a branch of the subscapular artery, which has branches supplying the periosteum of the lateral border of the scapula. The vessel passes superficially through a muscular triangle bounded by the long head of the triceps and the teres major and minor muscles. It then bifurcates once in the subdermal plane, and one of the two branches courses horizontally, parallel to the scapular spine, while the other proceeds caudally, roughly parallel to the lateral border of the scapula.

The flap may be designed as a fasciocutaneous flap, an osseous flap, or a composite osteofasciocutaneous flap (Figs. 16–12 and 16–13). Twelve to fourteen centimeters of bone

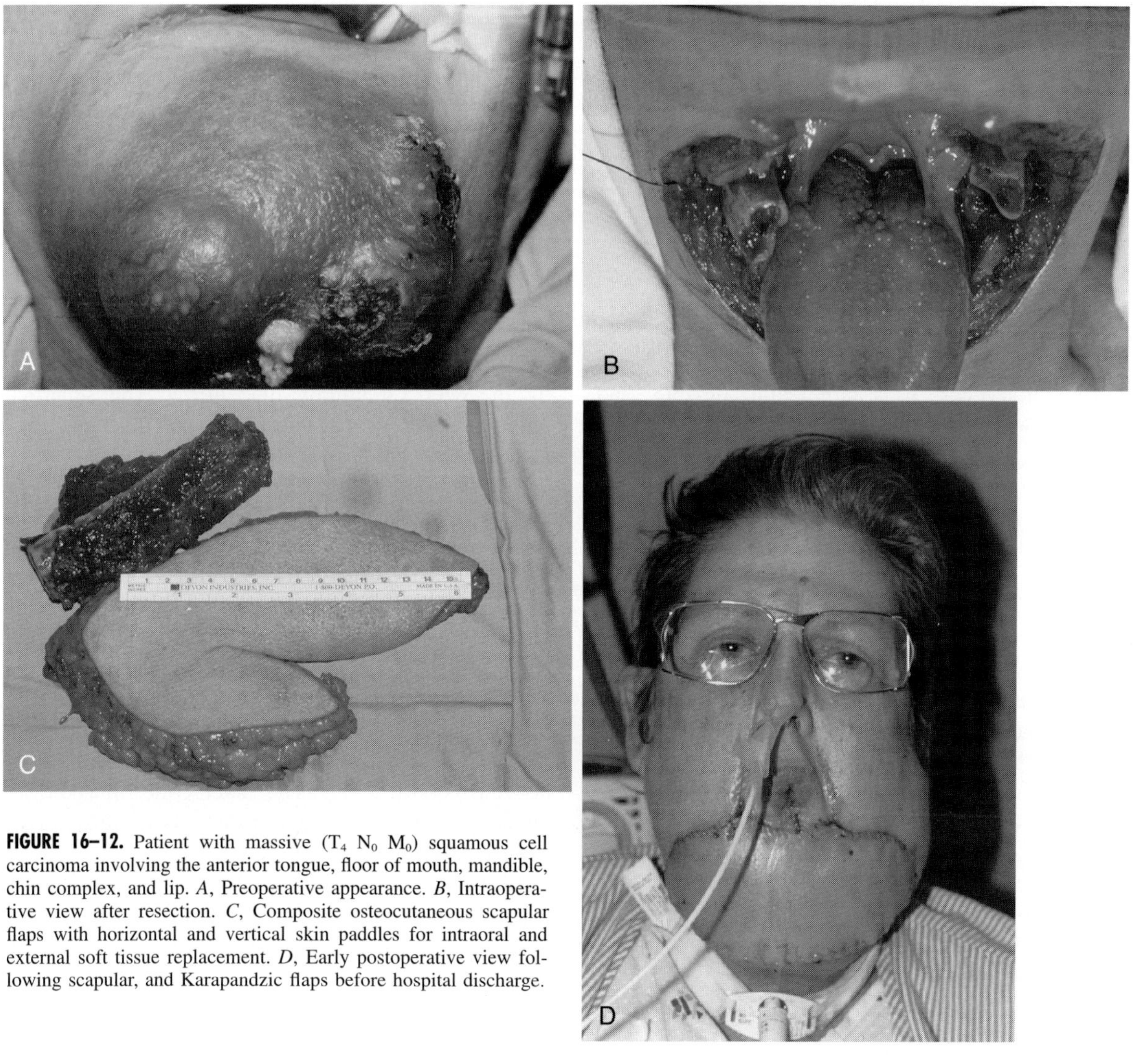

FIGURE 16–12. Patient with massive (T_4 N_0 M_0) squamous cell carcinoma involving the anterior tongue, floor of mouth, mandible, chin complex, and lip. *A*, Preoperative appearance. *B*, Intraoperative view after resection. *C*, Composite osteocutaneous scapular flaps with horizontal and vertical skin paddles for intraoral and external soft tissue replacement. *D*, Early postoperative view following scapular, and Karapandzic flaps before hospital discharge.

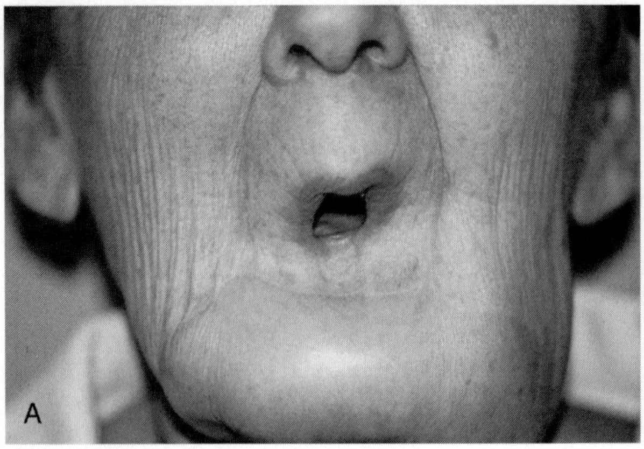

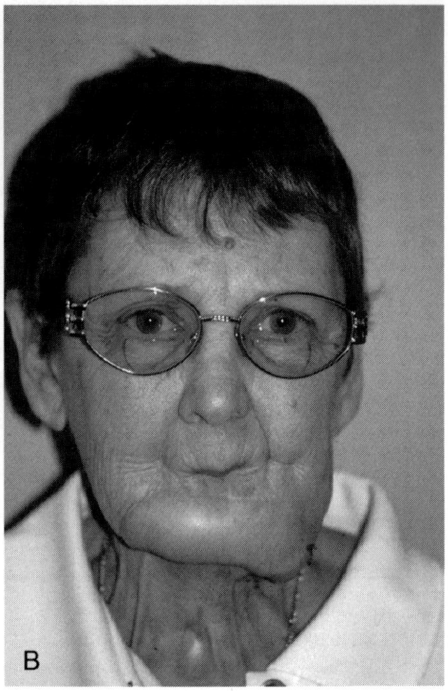

FIGURE 16–13. Same patient shown in Figure 16–12. *A*, Three-year follow-up view of competent but small mouth. *B*, Overall appearance following minor outpatient surgery flap debulking.

can usually be harvested. Almost always, the donor site can be closed primarily with minimal morbidity, leaving only a linear scar. Patients should undergo physical therapy to rehabilitate the shoulder and avoid potential postoperative morbidity.

The parascapular flap was described by Nassif and colleagues in 1982.[35] In this variation, the long axis of the skin paddle is oriented vertically and is perfused by the vertically oriented cutaneous branch. Thus, either a scapular or a parascapular skin flap may be utilized, or, as the defect requires, both may be harvested to provide separate internal and external skin paddles (Fig. 16–12*C*). Indeed, the size of the skin paddle is unique with respect to the currently used osteocutaneous free flaps. It is large, thin, flexible, and can be designed with two separate skin paddles. Moreover, because a single major vessel is between the bone and the skin (as opposed to a series of perforators, as with the iliac crest or fibular flap), the two components can be spatially oriented in virtually any direction and rotated in multiple dimensions.

In summary, the advantages of this flap include the following: (1) it provides a long vascular pedicle (up to 14 cm); (2) a large amount of skin can be harvested with separate skin paddles; (3) bone stock of sufficient thickness is available, allowing osteotomies to be made for contouring; and (4) the skin paddle and bony component can be separated by as much as 15 cm in certain cases, allowing for maneuverability of the soft tissue components with respect to the bone and modification of their orientation based on the reconstruction needed. Some of the disadvantages of this flap include: (1) the need to turn the patient to harvest the flap, which precludes a simultaneous two-team approach; (2) limited bone length for more extensive defects involving the anterior mandibular arch; (3) small size of the bone, which is too small to reliably support osseointegrated implants; and (4) absence of a cutaneous nerve for potential sensory rehabilitation.

Iliac Crest Osteocutaneous and Osteomyocutaneous Flap

Manchester in 1965[36] noted the resemblance of the anterior ilium to the mandible in shape and contour. Earlier, the iliac bone had been used as a free graft and as cortical or cancellous chips. It subsequently was used as a revascularized free flap (Fig. 16–14). Taylor and colleagues in 1979[37] reported on the reliability of blood supply to the bone by the deep circumflex iliac artery. The superficial iliac artery offered inconsistent supply to the bone but mainly supplied the skin paddle.

The flap can be used as revascularized bone alone or as an osteocutaneous flap. Its blood supply is the deep circumflex iliac artery, which is a branch of the external iliac artery. The deep circumflex iliac vein closely parallels the course of the artery, although there are some slight variations of vascular anatomy near the site where it empties into the iliac vein. Ten to sixteen centimeters of bone can be harvested, and the flap offers the strongest bone stock for mandibular reconstruction. It is bicortical with a thick cancellous component and can be harvested using different designs to fit the desired reconstruction. The inner cortex may be harvested alone, preserving the outer cortex. Osteotomies may be performed for contouring.

When harvested with its soft tissue component, the flap can be quite bulky and can be used for large defects. Urken has described a modification that increases its utility for combined internal and external soft tissue defects.[38] By incorporating the internal oblique muscle, which is supplied

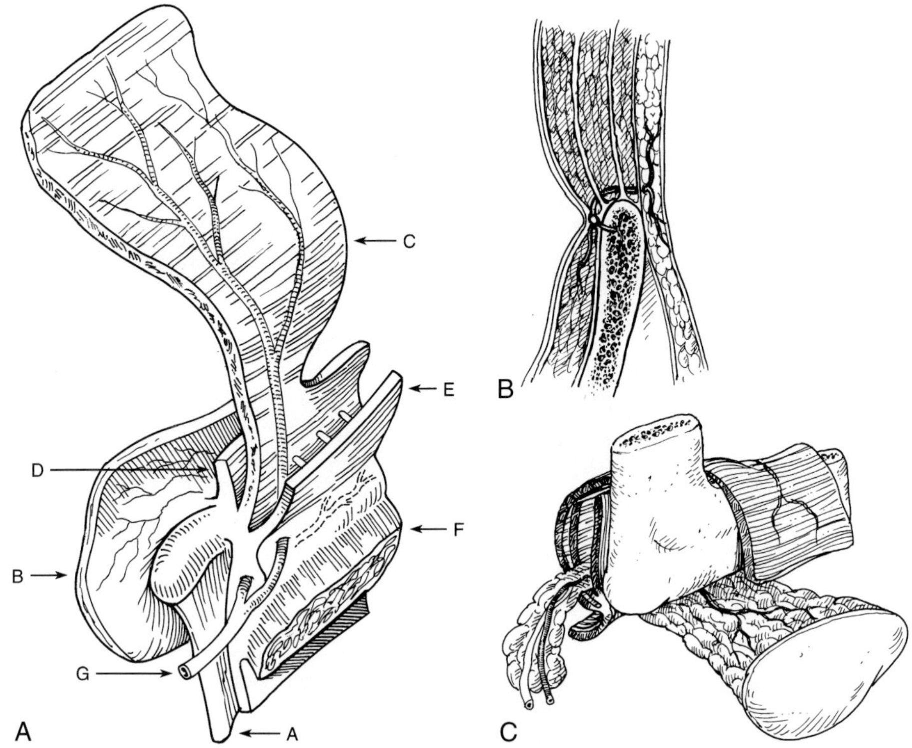

FIGURE 16–14. The iliac osteomyocutaneous flap. The iliac bone, pedicle, skin paddle, and cuffs of the iliacus, transversus abdominis, and internal oblique are shown. (*A* from Myers EN: Operative Otolaryngology Head and Neck Surgery. Philadelphia, W.B. Saunders Co, 1997. *B* and *C* from Myers EN, Suen JY: Cancer of the Head and Neck, 3rd ed. Philadelphia, W.B. Saunders Co., 1996.)

by the ascending branch of the deep circumflex iliac artery and remains attached to the medial aspect of the iliac bone, the flap can be used to line oral or pharyngeal defects and can be skin-grafted. The donor site is usually closed by approximation of the fascial layers. Possible complications of this flap include hernia formation, significant pain at the donor site, and delayed ambulation. Physical therapy is usually started a few days after surgery, and activity is gradually increased as tolerated. The primary limitations of the flap include the inability to use it in patients who have had hernia repair and its potential bulk when used with a soft tissue component.

Fibular Flap

The fibular osteocutaneous flap has increased in popularity and is now probably among the most commonly used free flaps in anterior mandibular reconstruction. The first successful fibular osteocutaneous flap was reported by Chen and Yan in 1983.[39] It was later used by Hidalgo for mandibular reconstruction in 1989 (Figs. 16–15 to 16–17).[40] (See also Color plate.) This flap includes the fibula, cuffs of muscle, and a skin paddle of the lateral leg (Fig. 16–18).

At the knee, the popliteal artery branches into the anterior and posterior tibial arteries, the latter of which gives rise to the peroneal artery, on which the vascular supply of this flap is based. The artery is accompanied by two venae comitantes, and the vascular pedicle courses between the tibialis posterior and the flexor hallucis longus muscles. A nutrient artery and musculoperiosteal vessels arise from the peroneal artery and supply the fibula. Because the blood supply is both periosteal and endosteal, osteotomies can be performed (thus disrupting the endosteal supply) to contour the bone to the shape of the resected mandible. The overlying skin paddle is supplied by musculocutaneous and septocutaneous perforators. As originally described, the osteocutaneous flap was harvested with bone and intermuscular septum. However, as reports of "skin flap unreliability" became more common, anatomic studies confirmed the presence not only of septocutaneous perforators but of musculocutaneous ones as well. For this reason, a cuff of soleus and flexor hallucis longus muscle should be incorporated into the flap. These muscles also provide additional bulk, which may be advantageous for the reconstruction.

The fibula is a long bone with a thick cortex. Up to 25 cm of it can be harvested. Care should be taken to leave 7 cm of bone proximally to avoid injury to the peroneal nerve, which is closely associated with the fibular neck, and to maintain knee joint stability. Similarly, 7 cm of bone are left in place distally to maintain ankle joint stability. Ambulation is usually resumed after a few days of immobility. Usually no problems are associated with harvesting this bone, since the fibula, unlike the tibia, is nonweight bearing. The donor site can occasionally be closed primarily or with a split-thickness skin graft.

The skin paddle is thin and pliable and is quite reliable when the flap is designed as described earlier. An elliptical skin paddle up to 20 × 10 cm can be harvested from the

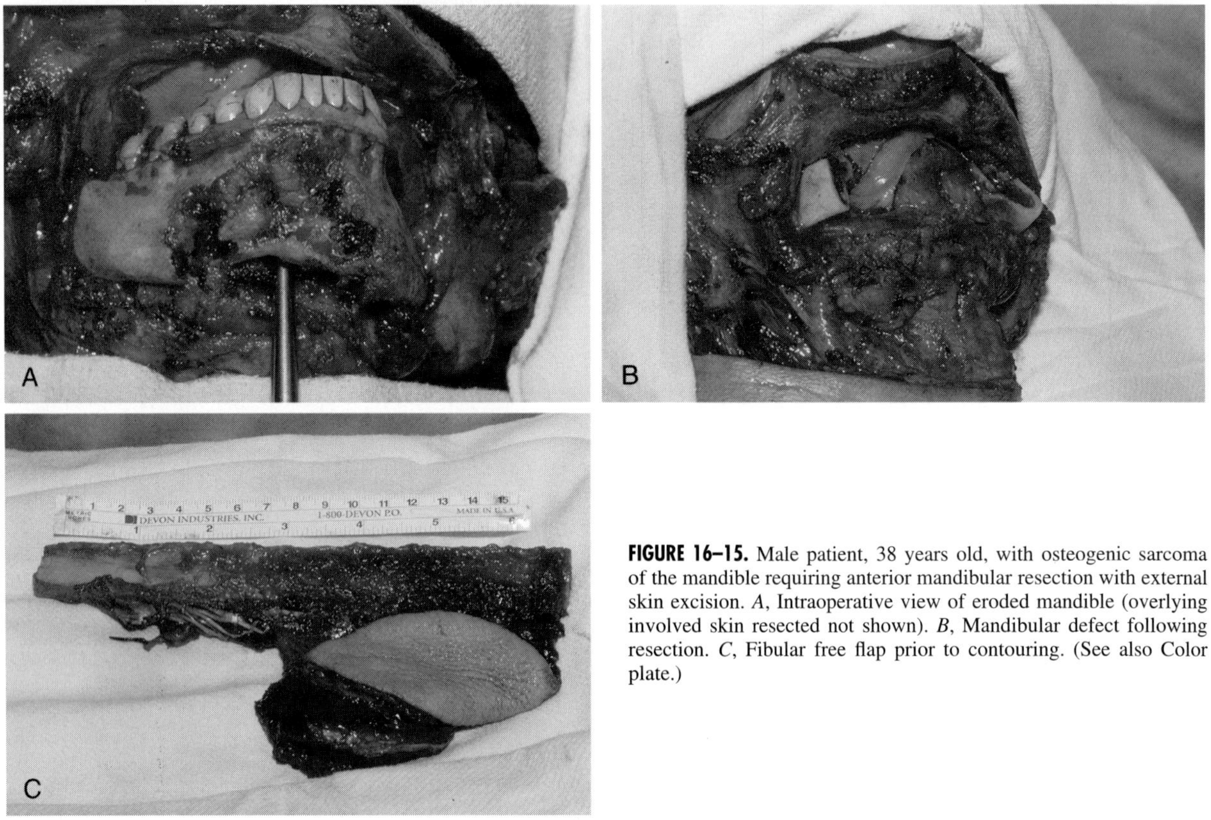

FIGURE 16–15. Male patient, 38 years old, with osteogenic sarcoma of the mandible requiring anterior mandibular resection with external skin excision. *A*, Intraoperative view of eroded mandible (overlying involved skin resected not shown). *B*, Mandibular defect following resection. *C*, Fibular free flap prior to contouring. (See also Color plate.)

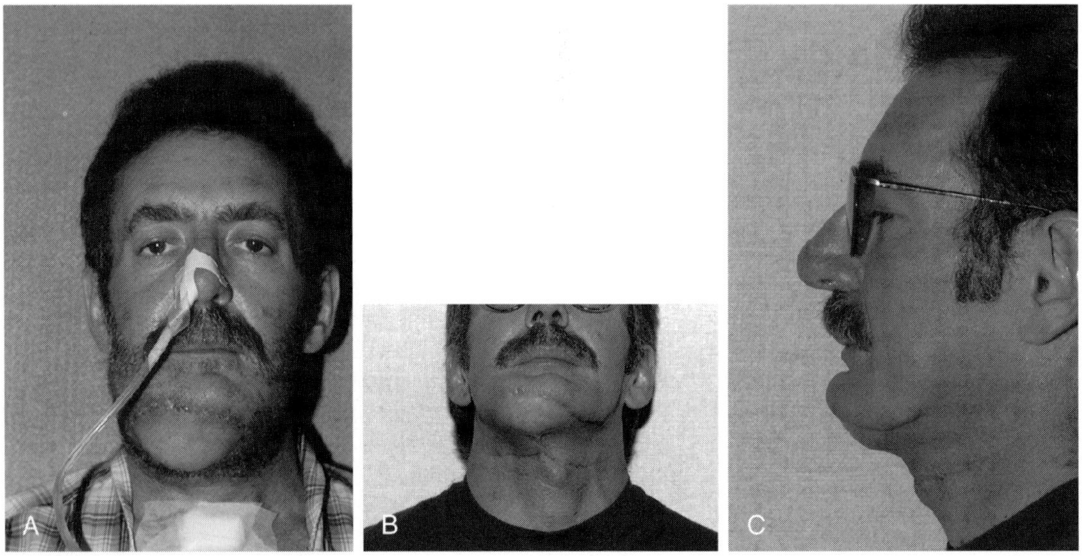

FIGURE 16–16. *A*, Early postoperative view. *B*, Frontal view. *C*, Lateral view showing excellent cosmetic results coinciding with similarly good functional results. (See also Color plate.)

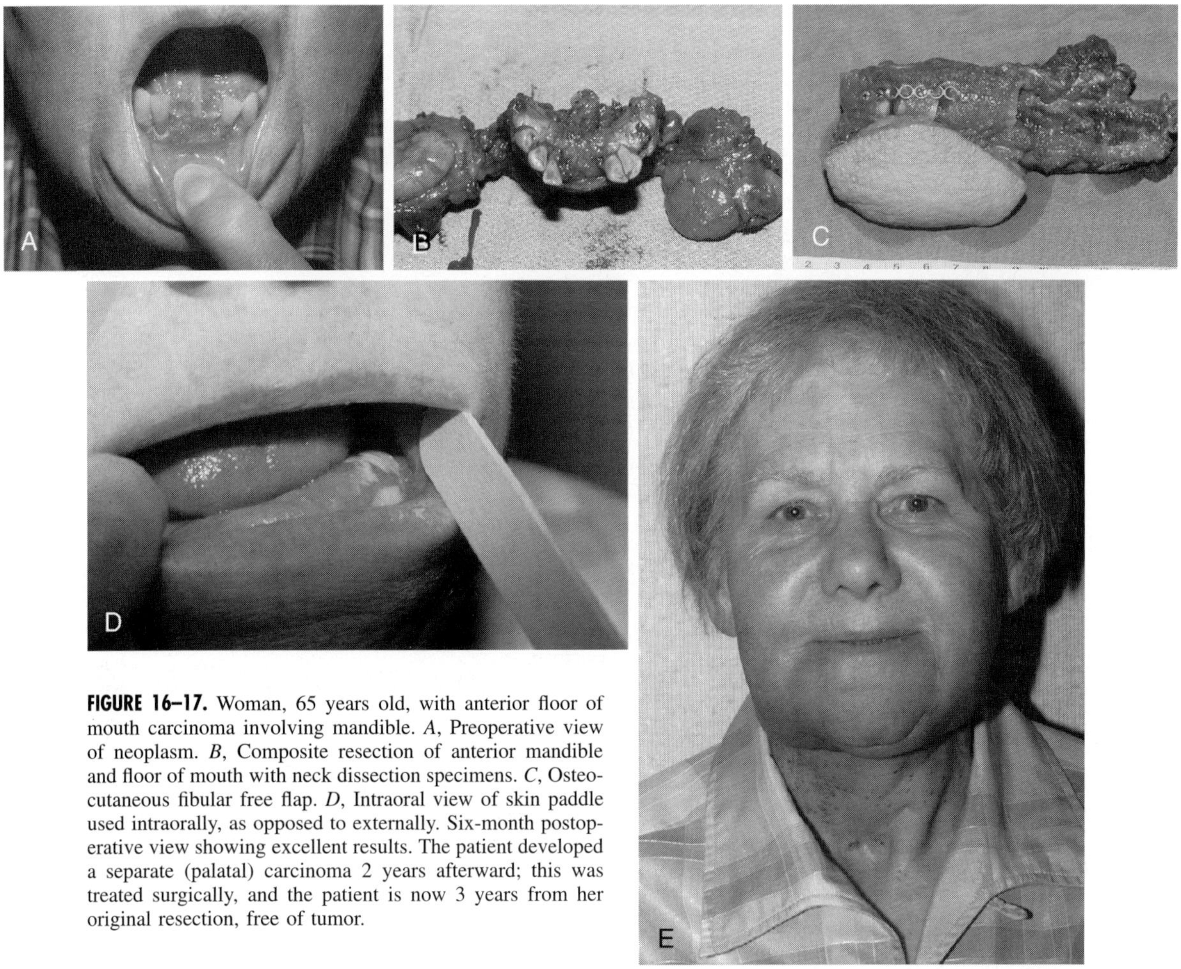

FIGURE 16–17. Woman, 65 years old, with anterior floor of mouth carcinoma involving mandible. *A*, Preoperative view of neoplasm. *B*, Composite resection of anterior mandible and floor of mouth with neck dissection specimens. *C*, Osteocutaneous fibular free flap. *D*, Intraoral view of skin paddle used intraorally, as opposed to externally. Six-month postoperative view showing excellent results. The patient developed a separate (palatal) carcinoma 2 years afterward; this was treated surgically, and the patient is now 3 years from her original resection, free of tumor.

lateral leg. It is centered over the intermuscular septum, which lies at the posterior aspect of the fibula, and is designed to encompass the region of the junction of the distal and middle thirds of the fibula because the number of perforators is highest in this region. Preoperative evaluation here should include lower extremity angiography to exclude the presence of significant compromise by atherosclerosis or vascular anomalies, which may lead to compromise of blood flow to the foot if the peroneal artery is harvested. Magnetic resonance angiography and duplex Doppler ultrasonography have been used by some.

This flap has been a significant addition to the armamentarium of flaps used in mandibular reconstruction. It is appealing mainly because it provides a long bone stock that has a strong cortex and allows reliable incorporation of osseointegrated implants. Multiple osteotomies can be performed close to each other, allow the surgeon to create a good mandibular contour. The flap is accessible by a two-team approach and results in minimal donor site morbidity. It also offers the potential for sensory rehabilitation with the use of the lateral sural cutaneous nerve. Potential complications of this flap include injury to the peroneal nerve, resulting in foot drop, ambulatory problems, neurovascular compromise to the lower extremity, cold intolerance, and pain. More recent reports have shown a failure rate of less than 5%, excellent dental rehabilitation with the use of osseointegrated implants, and good preservation of the fibular bone mass even in patients who received irradiation.[41, 42]

CASE REPORTS

Case 1

W. H. is an otherwise healthy 58-year-old white male who had a history of a squamous cell carcinoma of the oral cavity that was treated primarily with radiation therapy. Details of his past treatment, including specifics regarding the lesion and radiation dosimetry, were unavailable. He presented to our institution with osteoradionecrosis, osteomyelitis, and an orocutaneous fistula from the infected site. Despite perioperative antibiotics, he developed wound breakdown and purulent infection following debridement, mandibular resection, and an iliac crest free flap. A sizable fistula developed from the oral cavity in the mandibular arch to the neck (Fig. 16–19).

The patient was treated with saline wet-to-dry dressing changes, antibiotics, and hyperbaric oxygen. Granulation tissue from the revascularized iliac crest progressed, and the wound healed without further surgery. Ultimately, the patient underwent placement of osseointegrated implants and dental restoration, at which time good healing and rich vascularity of the reconstructed mandible were confirmed (Fig. 16–19*B–D*). This case illustrates the versatility and resistance to

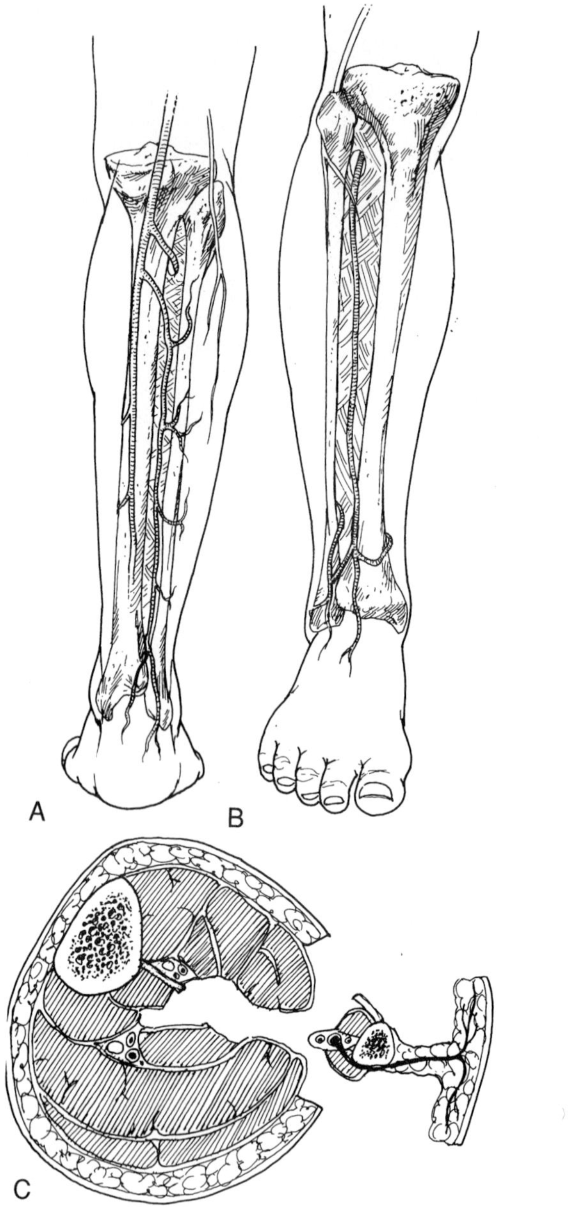

FIGURE 16–18. A cross-sectional view of the lower leg showing the neurovascular bundle, septocutaneous perforators, and related anatomic stuctures. As shown in these diagrams, cuffs of flexor hallucis longus and soleus muscles are harvested to preserve the musculocutaneous perforators. (From Myers EN, Suen JY: Cancer of the Head and Neck, 3rd ed. Philadelphia, W.B. Saunders Co., 1996.)

infection of revascularized free flaps. Not only did the flap in this case heal, it also provided the foundation for healing by secondary intention of a large infected fistula. Clearly, alloplastic devices such as a mandibular reconstruction plate or nonvascularized bone could not have provided such a result (Fig. 16–20).

Case 2

L. H. is a 65-year-old white female who presented with an extensive squamous cell carcinoma of the mandible, floor of mouth, and chin. No nodal disease was identified, nor was there evidence of distant metastases. Resection involved the anterior mandible, floor of mouth, anterior tongue, entire chin complex, lower lip, and about 10% of the upper lip. Clear margins were achieved, and reconstruction was performed with a bilobed composite osteocutaneous scapular flap and a Karapandzic flap (see Fig. 16–12). The patient was discharged on postoperative day 10 and healed uneventfully. She underwent full-course postoperative radiation therapy. She has survived more than 3 years free of disease and is happy with her appearance and function (see Fig. 16–13*A* and *B*). She has microstomia, but the oral sphincter is functional. A single revision of the bulky external scapular skin paddle was performed thus far to improve the cosmetic appearance and definition of the mandible.

This case illustrates the opportunity available to the reconstructive surgeon to replace dramatically different defects with the type and amount of tissue needed. There was no need to create two flaps, since the scapular flap provided the necessary amount of bone and soft tissue to repair this extensive defect. Furthermore, although the absence of nodal metastases is probably the single most important factor in the patient's cancer-free survival thus far, margins that are perhaps more liberal than would otherwise be possible can be used because of the availability of tissue for reconstruction. The illustrations of this case were discussed previously in the text to highlight the principles of this reconstructive technique.

Case 3

J. F. is a 38-year-old male who had a lesion in the anterior mandible. Originally the lesion was subjected to biopsy and thought to be a plasmacytoma. No other lesions were identified, and the patient was treated with radiation therapy for cure. Three years later the lesion recurred, and the patient presented to us. Metastatic work-up was negative, and the patient was taken to the operating room where he underwent an anterior segmental mandibulectomy with resection of the involved overlying skin. Reconstruction of the anterior arch defect with a fibular free flap was chosen to provide optimal bone stock with a thin skin paddle, which matched the resected skin in size, thickness, and overall consistency (see Fig. 16–15). The patient did well postoperatively and has had an excellent functional recovery. He resumed oral intake without difficulties such as loss of oral competence or drooling and ultimately chose to have a lower denture rather than undergo additional procedures for osseointegrated implants (see Fig. 16–16). The skin paddle was harvested from his densely hirsute leg and thus filled in the hair-bearing area of his chin very well.

DISCUSSION

During the past 10 years, free tissue transfer has become the option of choice for many reconstructive problems in the head and neck region instead of a novel alternative. Few defects in the head and neck region have so undeniably benefited from this technique as that of the anterior mandibular arch. Without question, a defect in this region causes tremendous functional and cosmetic impairment and leads to drastic changes in lifestyle. Also without question, the ability to reconstitute the bony mandibular arch with surrounding soft tissue using vascularized bone is current state-of-the-art allowing optimal functional and cosmetic rehabilitation. Nonetheless, it is important for the surgeon to have in his or her armamentarium a variety of techniques using composite materials from different anatomic sites so that he or she can use what is most suitable for each individual

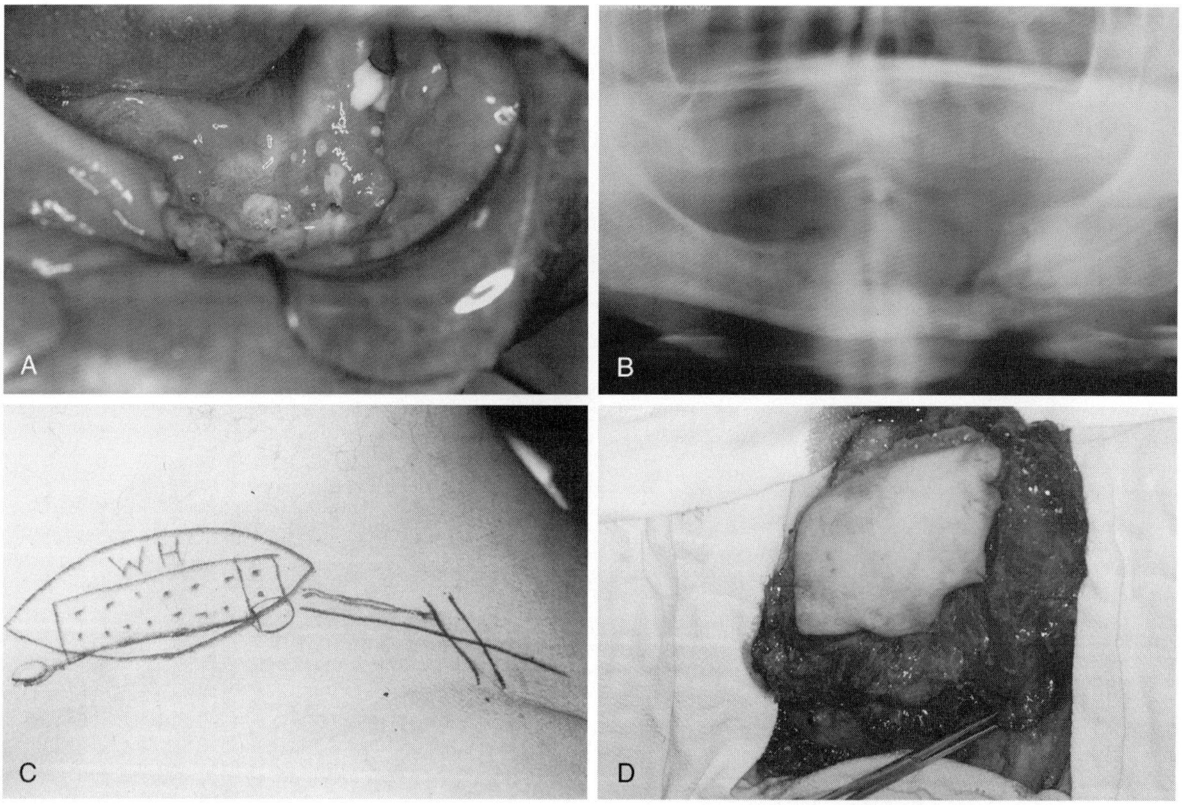

FIGURE 16–19. Patient with osteoradionecrosis of the mandible, osteomyelitis, and pathologic fracture resulting from radiation therapy for carcinoma of the oral cavity in the remote past. *A*, Preoperative view of chronic intraoral infection. *B*, Panorex view showing pathologic fracture and mandibular erosion. *C*, Outline of flap positioned over the iliac crest, showing perforators, intended ellipse of skin, and external iliac vessels. *D*, Bulky flap during harvest.

patient. Mandibular reconstruction using many of the techniques and materials discussed in the historical review was often plagued with failures and poor results. Free flap reconstruction constitutes the gold standard of reconstructive techniques today and has helped overcome many of the problems encountered with the earlier methods.

Occasionally, bony reconstruction of the mandible is not attempted following resection. These cases include those infrequent patients who refuse such treatment or other patients in whom the primary reason for the surgery is considered almost palliative. When the lateral mandibular segments are held in their native position for a period of time during the healing process (e.g., with arch bars or K-wires), a suboptimal but acceptable result can be achieved (Fig. 16–21).

In other cases, patients may not be good candidates for a free flap because of underlying medical problems or advanced vascular disease. Such operations can be quite lengthy and meticulous. In these cases, in which the surgery itself is considered to be a significant risk, better functional and cosmetic results can be achieved by utilizing a bridging reconstruction plate instead of leaving the mandibular segments free-floating. The patient shown in Figure 16–4 exemplifies the type of result that is possible. It is important to understand that despite coverage of such a plate with a myocutaneous flap, extrusion is likely to occur eventually. This type of reconstruction should *not* be advocated simply because the surgeon is not acquainted with or is unable to perform free flaps; in these cases, we believe that appropriate referral should be made to a center where revascularized tissue can be placed in the defect.

Osteomyocutaneous flaps offered surgeons the first real opportunity to place vascularized tissue in an anterior mandibular defect. However, most of the flaps described were either unreliable or did not truly incorporate vascularized bone. The only flap with consistent reliability in which the bone derived its blood supply from the accompanying muscle was the trapezius-scapular spine osteomyocutaneous flap. Unfortunately, the bone stock in this flap is relatively short, and the axis of greatest strength tends to "spiral" as one proceeds from medial to lateral. This resulted in difficult alignment of the segments and often led to a less than optimal cosmetic and functional outcome, especially in the era when external fixation devices were commonly used to keep the segments in position. These flap's are now of only historical interest because better options exist with free tissue transfer.

Free tissue transfer has dramatically changed the way anterior mandibular segment defects can be restored. The scapular flap and the iliac crest flap were the primary two flaps in widespread use from the mid-1980s until the early 1990s. As previously mentioned, the radial forearm and dorsalis pedis flaps were used by some but have largely been abandoned by most because of better options that now exist.

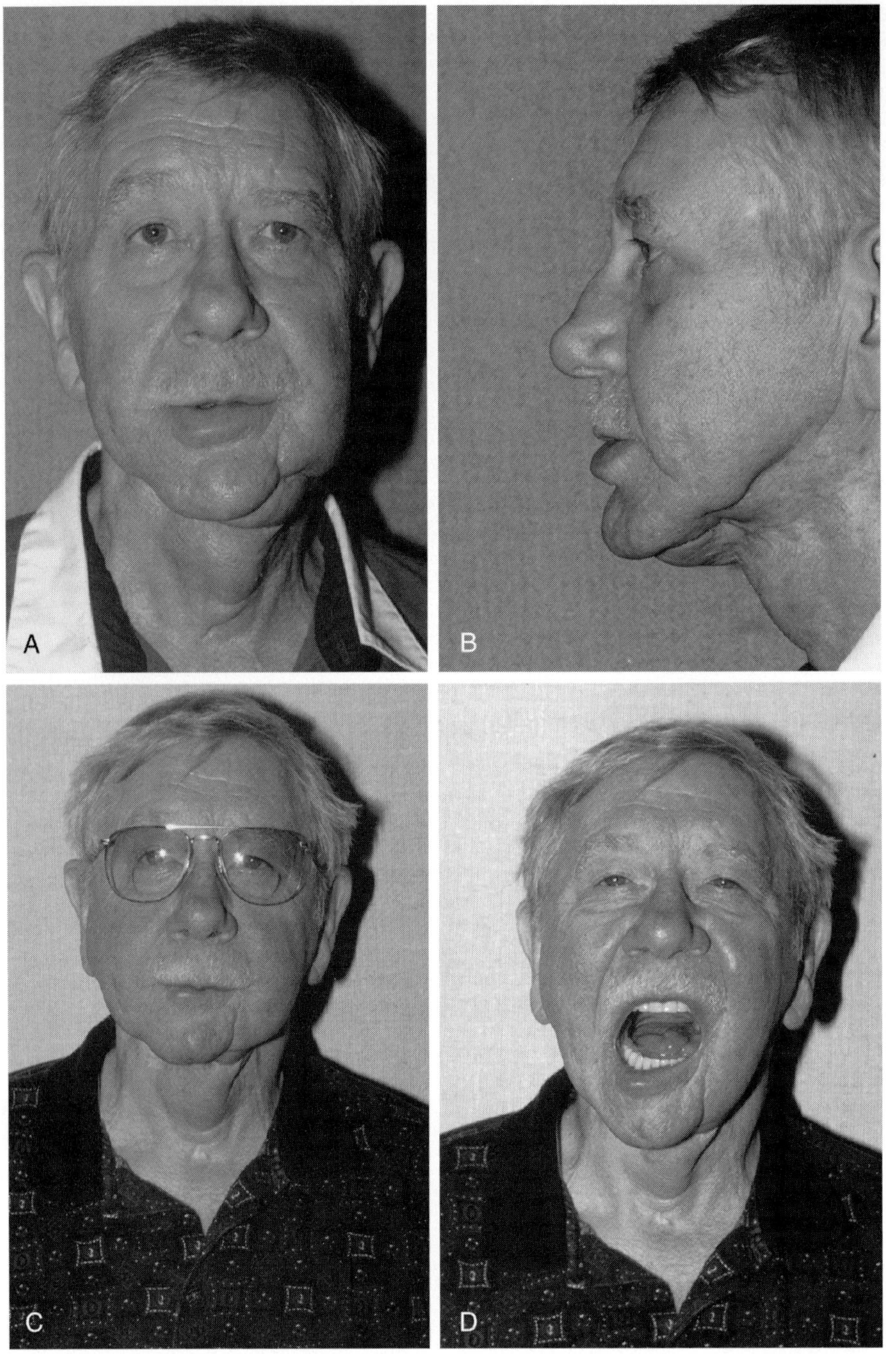

FIGURE 16–20. *A*, Frontal view at 5 month follow-up. *B*, Lateral view. *C*, Thirty-six months after free flap showing frontal appearance. *D*, Open-mouth view showing osseointegrated implants and implant-anchored denture.

For some surgeons, the choice between the scapular and the iliac crest flaps tended to be based on personal preference. However, these techniques offer distinctly different characteristics and for the most part are chosen based on defect requirements. The scapular flap has, as its primary advantage, a very large, thin skin paddle, which is especially useful for soft tissue defects with an extremely large surface area, especially those that are both intraoral and external. Although the iliac crest flap can be used in combination with a radial forearm flap or, incorporating Urken's internal oblique modification, for internal soft tissue coverage, it does not have the same flexibility for soft tissue replacement as the scapular flap. On the other hand, the iliac crest provides the best bone stock for osseointegration and thereby dental restoration and has been used extensively when dental restoration is important. Neither of these two flaps has sensate potential, and the scapula cannot be reliably osseointegrated. Furthermore, the scapula usually requires repositioning the patient for harvesting and eventual insetting and revascularization. The iliac crest flap, on the other hand, often is quite painful, and delayed ambulation is possible. Its skin component often is very thick because of the obligatory

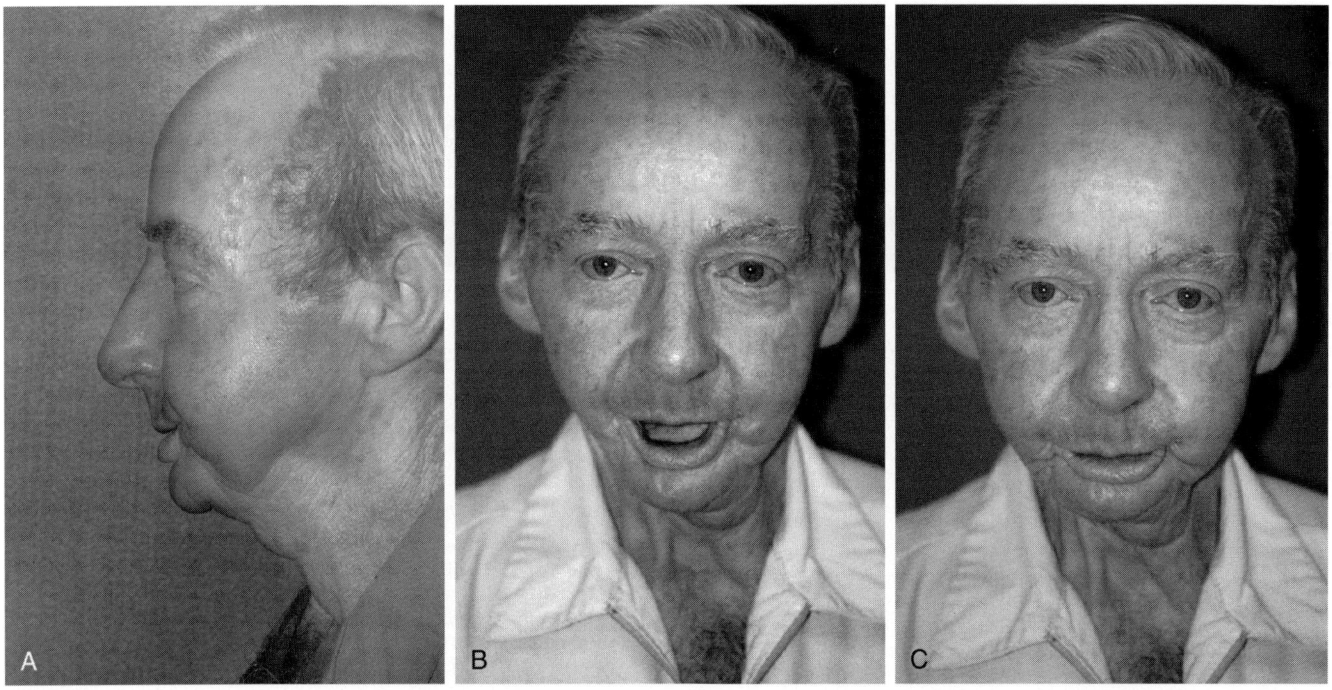

FIGURE 16–21. This patient had had anterior mandibular resection with excision of the anterior third of the tongue. A pectoralis major flap was used to fill in the tongue and floor of mouth defect, and the mandibular segments were held in normal position by K-wires. The wires required removal because of pain and extrusion. *A*, Lateral view of patient missing anterior mandible from mid-body to mid-body. *B*, Mouth open. *C*, Mouth closed.

muscle cuff and the typically generous amount of subcutaneous fat.

The fibular free flap has become the most popular flap for mandibular reconstruction during the past several years because it offers several distinct advantages. It provides excellent bone stock that can be reliably osseointegrated. This allows the patient to chew foods sometimes even better than when the native mandible was in place, because many tumors of the mandible loosen the teeth or occur in patients with significant dental disease. The flap can be harvested with a skin component that is thin and pliable. The initial problems encountered with skin paddle reliability have been for the most part overcome by incorporating a cuff of soleus muscle with the bone. A very long piece of bone can be used with minimal or no morbidity; patients do not seem to have a great deal of pain and walk early. Because of its location, the flap can be easily harvested using a two-team approach, thereby minimizing operating room time.

Hayden and associates recognized the sensate potential of the skin paddle and demonstrated that not only could the bone of the mandible be replaced and osseointegrated but also sensation of the skin paddle could be achieved, thereby providing additional sensory input to an area normally devoid of such sensation following cancer resection.[43] To date, this flap allows the surgeon to most closely achieve the goals mentioned earlier in this chapter for oromandibular reconstruction. Indeed, as long as the treatment of cancer involves as one of its primary options ablative surgery that destroys cosmesis and function, every attempt should be made to restore the patient to his or her premorbid condition.

OUTCOME STUDIES AND QUALITY OF LIFE

It is only recently that attention has shifted to the quality of life after mandibular reconstruction. There have been scattered reports on this issue, and, as one may imagine, it is quite difficult to standardize outcomes with the often complex and variable resection and reconstructive surgeries. In a recent analysis of 50 fibular free flap reconstructions, swallowing was normal in 64% of patients, oral continence was normal in 67%, speech was normal or easily intelligible in 90%, and aesthetic results were excellent or acceptable in 95%.[44] As more focus is directed toward quality of life, a standardized way of assessing these patients is helpful in comparing the different reconstructive techniques. This is made easier with a standardized classification system such as the one described earlier in this chapter.

SUMMARY

Some of the major milestones in the development of mandibular reconstruction have been reviewed. Such reconstruction is obviously a formidable task, and significant advances have been made that allow surgeons to restore the patient's appearance and function close to their premorbid status. A wide range of reconstructive techniques is available to us today. The most recent ones include microvascular free tissue transfer. This, we believe, constitutes the state of the art in oromandibular reconstruction, especially when defects involve the anterior arch. Free osteocutaneous flaps offer vascularized bone and soft tissue that are very useful in reconstructing composite complex defects and are quite reliable in hostile environments such as the irradiated fields often encountered in these patients. Great progress has been made as well in dental rehabilitation in the form of osseointegrated implants that allow patients to chew their food.

It is important to keep in mind, however, that not all patients are good candidates for free flaps because of poor general health, advanced disease, or poor tissue conditions. These patients may be reconstructed with plates and soft tissue flaps, bone grafts, or pedicled osteomyocutaneous flaps.

References

1. Dupuytren G: On amputation and resection of the lower jaw. Lancet 1: 56, 1833.
2. Heath C: A case of epithelioma of the tongue: Survival for over 23 years after removal of the growth. Lancet 1: 1354, 1899.
3. Deadrick WH: A case of removal of the lower maxillary bone. Am Med Recorder 6: 516, 1823.
4. Partsch H: Prosthesis of lower jaw after resection. Arch Klin Chir 55: 746, 1897.
5. Ollier L: Recherches éxperimentales sur les greffes osseuses. J Physiol 3: 88, 1860.
6. Bardenheuer P: Veber Unterkiefer-und Oberkiefer-Resection. Arch Klin Chir 44: 604, 1892.
7. Sykoff V: Zur Frage der Knocken-plastic am. Unterkiefer Zbl Chir 27: 881, 1900.
8. Blair VP: Surgery and Diseases of the Mouth and Jaws. St. Louis, CV Mosby, 1918.
9. Gillies HD: Plastic Surgery of the Face. London, Oxford University Press, 1920.
10. Ivy RH: Extensive loss of substance of mandible due to removal of sarcoma, replaced by bone graft from crest of ilium. Int J Orthodont 7: 483, 1921.
11. Ivy RH: Iliac bone graft to bridge a mandibular defect: 49 year clinical and radiologic follow up. Plast Reconstr Surg 50: 483, 1972.
12. Winter L, Lifton JC, McQuilan AS: Embedment of a vitallium mandibular prosthesis as an integral part of the operation for removal of an adamantinoma. Am J Surg 69: 318, 1945.
13. Converse JM, Campbell RM: Bone grafting in surgery of the face. Surg Clin North Am 34: 375, 1954.
14. Leake DL, Rappaport M: Mandibular reconstruction: Bone induction in an alloplastic tray. Surgery 72: 332, 1972.
15. Boyne PJ, Zarem H: Osseous reconstruction of the resected mandible. Am J Surg 132: 49, 1976.
16. Pike RL, Boyne PJ: Composite autogenous marrow and surface decalcified implants in mandibular defects. J Oral Surg 31: 905, 1973.
17. Hamaker RC: Irradiated autogenous mandibular grafts in primary reconstructions. Laryngoscope 91: 1031, 1981.
18. Cummings CW, Leipzig B: Replacement of tumor-involved mandible by cryosurgically devitalized autograft. Human experience. Arch Otolaryngol 106: 252, 1980.
19. Hansmann A: A new method of fixation of fragments in complicated fractures. Ver Deutsch Aes Chir 15: 134, 1886.
20. Danis R: Theorie et Pratique de l'Ostéosynthèse. Paris, Librairies de l'Academie de Medecine, 1949.
21. Müller ME, Allgöer M, Willenegger H: Manual of Internal Fixation. New York, Springer-Verlag, 1970.
22. Raveh Y, Stitch H, Sutter F: The use of titanium-coated hollow screw and reconstruction plate system in bridging of lower jaw defects. J Oral Maxillofac Surg 42: 281, 1984.
23. Conley J: Use of composite flaps containing bone for major repairs in the head and neck. Plast Reconstr Surg 49: 522, 1972.
24. Panje W, Cutting C: Trapezius osteomyocutaneous island flap for reconstruction of the anterior floor of the mouth and the mandible. Head Neck Surg 3: 66, 1980.
25. Reid C, Taylor GI: The vascular territory of the acromiothoracic axis. Br J Plast Surg 37: 194, 1984.
26. McKee D: Microvascular rib transposition of the mandible. Presented at the annual meeting of the American Society of Plastic and Reconstructive Surgeons, Toronto, Ontario, 1971.
27. Urken M, Weinberg H, Vickery C, et al: Oromandibular reconstruction using microvascular composite free flaps. Arch Otolaryngol Head Neck Surg 117: 733, 1991.
28. Yang G, Chen B, Gao Y, et al: Forearm free skin flap transplantation. Nat Med J China 61: 139, 1981.
29. Urken M: Composite free flaps in oromandibular reconstruction: Review of the literature. Arch Otolaryngol Head Neck Surg 117: 724, 1991.
30. Boorman J, Brown J, Sykes P: Morbidity in the forearm donor arm. Br J Plast Surg 40: 207, 1982.
31. McGraw G, Furlow L: The dorsalis pedis arterialized flap. Plast Reconstr Surg 55: 177, 1975.
32. McLeod A, Robinson D: Reconstruction of defects involving the mandible and floor of mouth by free osteocutaneous flaps derived from the foot. Br J Plast Surg 35: 239, 1982.
33. Saijo M: The vascular territories of the dorsal trunk: A reappraisal for potential flap donor sites. Br J Plast Surg 31: 200, 1978.
34. Swartz W, Barris J, Newton D, et al: The osteocutaneous scapular flap for mandibular and maxillary reconstruction. Plast Reconstr Surg 77: 530, 1986.
35. Nassif T, Vidal L, Boset J, et al: The parascapular flap: A new cutaneous microsurgical free flap. Plast Reconstr Surg 69: 591, 1982.
36. Manchester W: Immediate reconstruction of the mandible and temporomandibular joint. Br J Plast Surg 18: 291, 1965.
37. Taylor G, Townsend P, Corlett R: Superiority of the deep circumflex iliac vessels as the supply for free groin flaps: Experimental work. Plast Reconstr Surg 64: 595, 1979.
38. Urken M, Weinberg H, Vickery C, et al: The internal oblique-iliac crest free flap in composite defects of the oral cavity involving bone, skin, and mucosa. Laryngoscope 101: 257, 1991.
39. Chen Z, Yan W: The study and clinical application of the osteocutaneous flap of fibula. Microsurgery 4: 11, 1983.
40. Hidalgo D: Fibular free flap: A new method of mandible reconstruction. Plast Reconstr Surg 86: 71, 1989.
41. Urken M, Buchbinder D, Costantino P, et al: Oromandibular reconstruction using microvascular free flaps. Report of 210 cases. Arch Otolaryngol Head Neck Surg 124: 46, 1998.
42. Disa JJ, Winters RM, Hidalgo DA: Long term evaluation of bone mass in free fibula mandible reconstruction. Am J Surg 174(5): 503, 1997.
43. Hayden R, O'Leary M: A neurosensory fibula flap: Anatomical description and clinical applications. Presented at the 94th Annual Meeting of the Americal Laryngological, Rhinological, and Otological Society Meeting, Hawaii, May 1991.
44. Shpitzer T, Nelligan P, Gullane P, et al: Oromandibular reconstruction with the fibular free flap: An analysis of 50 consecutive flaps. Arch Otolaryngol Head Neck Surg; 123: 939, 1997.

Bibliography

Baker S: Microsurgical Reconstruction of the Head and Neck. New York, Churchill Livingstone, 1989.

Boyd JB, Morris S, Rosen I, et al: The through-and-through oromandibular defect rationale for aggressive reconstruction. Plast Reconstr Surg 93: 44, 1994.

Boyd JB, Rosen I, Rotstein L, et al: The iliac crest and the radial forearm flap in vascularized oromandibular reconstruction. Am J Surg 159: 301, 1990.

Cheung S, Anthony J, Singer M: Restoration of anterior mandible with the free fibula osseocutaneous flap. Laryngoscope 104: 105, 1994.

Cuono C, Ariyam S: Immediate reconstruction of a composite mandibular defect with a regional osteomyocutaneous flap. Plast Reconstr Surg 65: 477, 1980.

Garrison F: History of Medicine, 4th ed. Philadelphia, W. B. Saunders, 1928.

Gullane P: Primary mandibular reconstruction: Analysis of 64 cases and evaluation of interface radiation dosimetry on bridging plates. Laryngoscope 101: 1, 1991.

Hidalgo D: Aesthetic improvements in free-flap mandible reconstruction. Plast Reconstr Surg 84: 71, 1989.

Lawson W, Baek SM, Loscalzo L, et al: Experience with immediate and delayed mandibular reconstruction. Laryngoscope 92: 5, 1982.

McCarthy J (ed): Plastic Surgery, Vol 2. The Face, part 1. Philadelphia, W. B. Saunders, 1990.

Papel I, Price J, Kashima H, et al: Compression plates in the treatment of advanced anterior floor of mouth carcinoma. Laryngoscope 96: 722, 1986.

Shockley W, Weissler M, Pillsbury H: Immediate mandibular replacement using reconstruction plates. Arch Otolaryngol Head Neck Surg 117: 745, 1991.

Tucker M, Terry B, White R, et al: Rigid Fixation for Maxillofacial Surgery. Philadelphia, J.B. Lippincott, 1991.

Urken M, Cheney N, Sullivan M, et al: Atlas of Regional and Free Flaps for Head and Neck Reconstruction. New York, Raven Press, 1995.

CHAPTER 17

Reconstructive Techniques for Defects After Resection of Carcinoma of the Lip

David W. Stepnick, M.D.

Carcinoma of the lip is the most common malignancy of the oral cavity, accounting for approximately 30% of malignant tumors of this region. Actinic radiation is believed to be the most important etiologic factor in the development of lip cancers, although other causes such as pipe smoking, periodontitis, poor oral hygiene, and even ill-fitting dentures have been implicated by association. Lip cancers tend to be well differentiated and slow growing. Squamous cell carcinomas are the most common malignancy; basal cell carcinomas are the next in frequency. The latter is sometimes locally aggressive but is less likely to metastasize. Most lip cancers arise at the vermilion border of the lower lip and are often painless or are preceded by visible premalignant lesions. Five percent arise from the upper lip. Only 1% arise primarily from the commissure regions, although another 2% extend to involve this area. The incidence of lip cancer peaks in midlife. These cancers are more commonly seen in men and those with fair skin.

Tumors involving the commissure regions are more likely to produce regional metastases owing to the richer lymphatic supply in this area. They behave more aggressively than carcinomas arising from either the upper or lower lip. Overall survival of patients with carcinoma of the lip is 90%, but the chances for cure are much decreased when regional nodes are affected.

Although much less common than either squamous cell or basal cell carcinoma of the lip, melanomas may also occur in this region. Aggressive treatment including primary excision and lymph node dissection is sometimes combined with other modalities of therapy such as chemotherapy, immunotherapy, or biologic response modifiers. Other unusual histopathologic types include malignant fibrous xanthoma, mucoepidermoid carcinoma, adenocarcinoma, and adenoid cystic carcinomas.

EXTIRPATION OF THE TUMOR

Cautery, astringents, phenol or acid application, radiation therapy, and surgical excision have all been used to treat malignant neoplasms of the lip. Leukoplakia and actinic cheilitis are clinical findings that are seen in association with carcinoma of the lip in nearly 50% of cases. Lip shave, designed to remove all of the damaged mucosa, is the treatment of choice for lips with these clinical findings, which are histologically determined to be severe dysplasia, atypia, or carcinoma in situ. Because carcinomas evolve histologically from dysplasia to frank malignancy, vermilionectomy can succeed in removing areas of premalignancy that may eventually evolve into invasive carcinoma. If invasive cancer is confirmed histopathologically, treatment by surgical excision (in most cases) or radiation therapy must be considered. If the former is chosen, reconstruction of the resultant defect is needed to restore the form and function of the lip.

Although reconstructive options must be considered prior to resection of the primary tumor, ablation should be guided by sound oncologic principles rather than by a desire to aid an easier and less complicated reconstruction by compromising margins and preserving tissue. Depending on the histopathology of the tumor and the technique of margin assessment used (standard pathologic sampling versus total margin control), adequate margins must be taken including what appears to be clinically uninvolved tissue. For squamous cell carcinoma, many cite 5 mm as an ideal clinical margin. Palpation can often reveal induration indicative of tumor involvement in tissue that otherwise appears to be normal, and this should be used in combination with inspection to assess the true limit of tumor extension. Because frozen section often reveals tumor that has extended beyond that which is clinically apparent, additional tissue may have to be taken to achieve clear margins. In some cases, an entirely different technique of reconstruction than that originally planned must be chosen if additional tissue is resected as a result of positive results on frozen section. This demands flexibility on the part of the reconstructive surgeon, who must necessarily consider the potential size of the defect and have several reconstructive options in mind prior to initiating the excision. Immediate reconstruction is almost always performed once clear margins have been obtained.

For T_1 and T_2 lesions, elective neck dissection or therapeutic neck irradiation is generally not considered necessary, especially if close follow-up of the patient is possible. If these patients with N_0 necks ultimately develop neck disease, appropriate surgical therapy, generally neck dissection of some sort, can achieve survival rates that are statistically similar to those of patients who may have had elective neck dissection at the time of primary tumor resection. T_3 N_0 and T_4 N_0 patients generally receive a suprahyoid or, in some cases, a supraomohyoid neck dissection with formal modified neck dissection if positive nodes are encountered in the course of the dissection. Patients with poorly differentiated carcinomas and those with commissure involvement generally receive elective neck dissection or radiation because of the higher propensity for occult metastases from these tumors.

Needless to say, patients with clinically apparent nodal disease are appropriately treated with either surgical neck dissection or radiation therapy. Generally, if surgical excision of the primary tumor is chosen, the neck should be addressed through neck dissection unless the node or nodes are fixed. Radiation offers another treatment modality in selected patients.

GOALS OF RECONSTRUCTION

The ideal reconstructive procedure accomplishes a variety of goals. These should be considered when choosing a technique to repair any particular defect. Goals include:

- Reestablishment of oral competence
- Creation of an adequate lip sulcus
- Restoration of contour
- Adequate oral aperture
- Good sensation
- Adequate support for the lower lip
- A normal-looking lip—not "too tight"
- One-stage reconstruction
- Ability to perform reconstruction at the time of primary tumor excision

ANATOMY OF THE LIPS

The muscle primarily responsible for a competent oral sphincter is the orbicularis oris muscle with minor functional contributions from the extended fibers of the buccinator muscle. The muscles surrounding the orbicularis, such as the quadratus labii do not play a role in this sphincteric action. These muscles primarily have a positional role and are responsible for the essentially infinite variety of facial expressions. The muscles of facial expression, as positional muscles, can be detached from the orbicularis oris without jeopardizing its sphincteric action. Both the orbicularis oris and the surrounding muscles of facial expression derive their motor supply from branches of the facial nerve. The infraorbital and mental nerves provide sensation to the upper and lower lips, respectively.

Other than these critical muscles, the remainder of the anatomic unit comprising the lips consists of skin, mucosa, submucosal glands, and fat. Blood supply to the area is derived primarily from the facial artery, which approaches the lips from an inferolateral position and continues on toward the lips as the superior and inferior labial arteries. Mobilization of a myocutaneous flap (i.e., the Karapandzic flap, discussed below) by dissection of these vessels from the surrounding tissue is facilitated by the tangential approach of these vessels to the lips.

HISTORY OF LIP RECONSTRUCTION

Amid continuing refinements in functional and cosmetic reconstruction of the lip and ongoing reports of these advances in the contemporary literature, it is useful to recognize that reconstruction of this anatomic region has a rich history, with principles developed as early as 1000 BC guiding our surgical approaches even today. The first published report of these techniques is credited to Celsus in 60 AD. In the sixteenth century, Gaspare Tagliacozzi brought many principles from the secret and hidden atmosphere of the barber-surgeon workshops of the Middle Ages to early "modern" medicine and deserves great credit for applying these principles to reconstructive surgery. Tagliacozzi used local sliding flaps and tissue from the forearm for reconstruction of the lip.

Transfer of tissue from the lower to the upper lip was described by Sabattini (1838) and Abbé (1898); Stein (1848) transferred tissue from the upper to the lower lip. Estlander (1872) is credited for his description of reconstruction of the commissure using a rotation flap. Dieffenbach was among the first to recognize regional flaps as a viable source of tissue for lip reconstruction. He described a lower lip repair using two inferiorly based cheek flaps lined with mucosa (1834) and upper lip reconstruction using the nasolabial flap (1845).

SURGICAL TECHNIQUES

Numerous surgeons, many of whom earned fame for various contributions to medical science, played significant roles in the development of techniques for lip reconstruction and have developed a multitude of procedures that provide solutions for the problems encountered. Indeed, the neophyte trying to decide upon a technique of reconstruction can easily become confused by the myriad of surgical options available. The remainder of this chapter focuses on what are in my view the most important and practical of these procedures.

As with any surgical reconstruction, the location and size of a lip defect dictate the available options for surgery. Oncologic principles must not be violated to allow a less complicated reconstruction. Compromise of these principles results in an increased chance of recurrence of the tumor, thereby (possibly) eventually requiring an even larger resection. "Bridges may be burned" in that certain repairs may not be feasible in the face of previous surgical intervention due to disruption of the vascular supply. A thorough understanding of the expected defect, including the limits of excision with adequate margins, is essential during preoperative planning of the surgical reconstruction. However, flexibility and an armamentarium of various techniques must be available when unexpected positive margins are found intraoperatively, requiring additional excision and resulting in a larger defect than anticipated.

Fortunately, due to the elasticity of the lips, primary closure of fairly large defects is possible. The elasticity of the lip, combined with the patient's dentition, helps to determine the final aesthetic result. The cupid's bow of the upper lip is anatomically more complex than the corresponding area of the lower lip and is difficult if not impossible to recreate. More so than in the lower lip, the anatomy of the upper lip limits the ability of the surgeon to close it primarily without distortion. In any case, defects of up to 33% of the upper lip and 50% of the lower lip length may be closed primarily. Localized defects of the vermilion may be closed with a mucomuscular advancement flap (Fig. 17–1). Another option

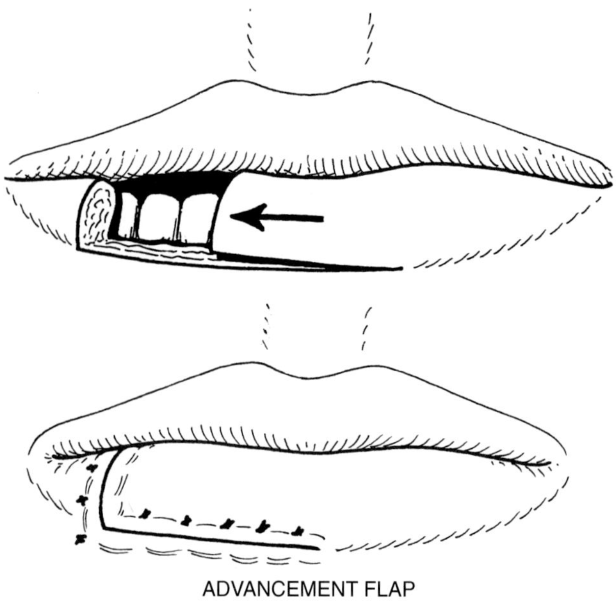

FIGURE 17–1. Relatively small defects of the vermilion can be closed by developing and advancing a mucomuscular flap based on the labial artery.

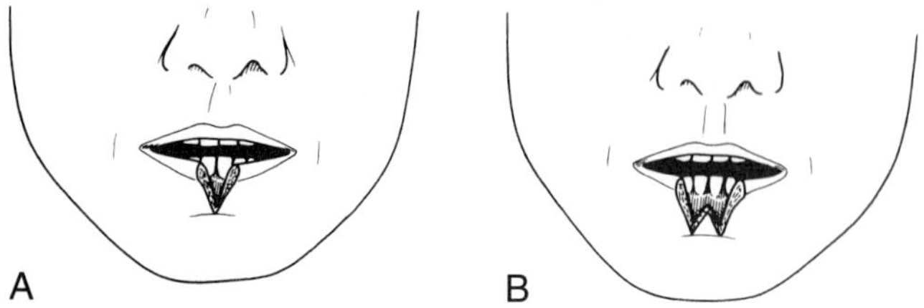

FIGURE 17–2. The V excision (*A*) is the treatment of choice for defects not extending beyond the labiomental sulcus. The W excision (*B*) is used to excise larger lesions without having the incisions cross the anatomic boundary. (From Stepnick D: Cancer of the lip. *In* Gates G (ed): Current Therapies in Otolaryngology, 5th ed. St Louis, CV Mosby, 1993.)

is a V lip excision (Fig. 17–2), which is often the reconstructive technique of choice. A number of modifications such as W-plasty, M-plasty, or shield designs allow primary closure without crossing into another anatomic subunit by limiting the length of the required excision with minimal distortion. These techniques should be considered when the planned excision extends (as a result of the planned reconstruction) inferiorly beyond the labial-mental crease. When the planned W-plasty itself crosses this anatomic boundary, modifications such as the flared W-plasty or single- or double-barreled excisions should be considered (Fig. 17–3).

Schuchardt Flaps

For defects involving one third to three quarters of the lower lip, a variety of options are available. An extension of the double-barreled excision, the Schuchardt flap (1954), allows further mobilization of the lower lip to close these larger defects (Fig. 17–4). This procedure is actually a rotation advancement flap that preserves neuromuscular and neurosensory function at the expense of creating relative microstomia. Patients with dentures may be unable to insert them when this reconstruction is used for defects greater than 50% of the lip. In addition, a "tight-appearing" lip results as increasingly large segments of it are removed.

Johansen Technique

Johansen (1974) described another modification that employs a staircase or stepladder incision to advance tissue from the chin upward to allow closure of defects of up to two thirds of the lower lip (Fig. 17–5). Its disadvantages are the same as those of the Schuchardt flaps, but like it, neuromuscular and neurosensory innervation is preserved. Its biggest drawback is that the resultant scar on the chin is quite apparent and is difficult to camouflage.

Abbé Flaps

An entirely different surgical principle is the basis for the Abbé flaps, described in 1898. Instead of advancing tissue to close extirpative defects, a small vascularized island flap is developed from the unaffected lip and transferred, with its pedicle attached, to the defect. Complete transection of

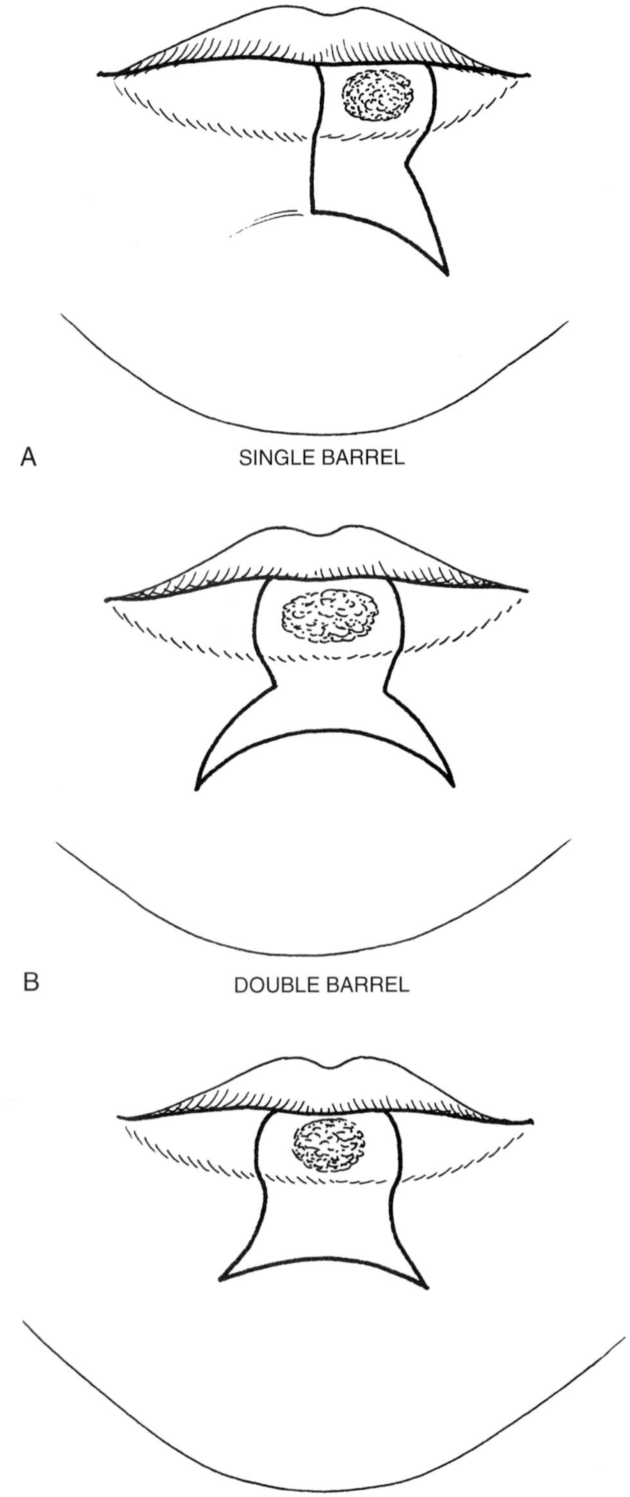

FIGURE 17–3. When a W-plasty design crosses the labiomental fold, a conspicuous scar can be avoided by modifications such as (*A*) the single-barreled excision, (*B*) the double-barreled excision, and (*C*) the flared W.

the lip occurs on one side of the flap; the other side is incised only to within 6 mm of the vermilion (Fig. 17–6) to preserve the vascular pedicle (labial artery). The flap can be based either medially or laterally. The length of the borrowed lip is equal to approximately half the length of the defect and the vertical heights of the two flaps are the same. This procedure allows lip to be replaced with lip; hence, the tissue match is excellent. Microstomia occurs to a lesser degree than with many of the other techniques presented herein. The donor site heals well, and the scar is inconspicuous. The Abbé flap may be used singly or in combination with a contralateral flap to repair larger defects. It can be developed to reconstruct either the upper or the lower lip.

The Abbé flap, a lip-switch operation, is necessarily a two-stage procedure, and for 2 or more weeks, the upper and lower lips are physically connected. A liquid diet is necessary during this period, and wound care can be difficult. Revision is usually unnecessary for the donor site but is often required for the recipient site. The lip-switch procedure

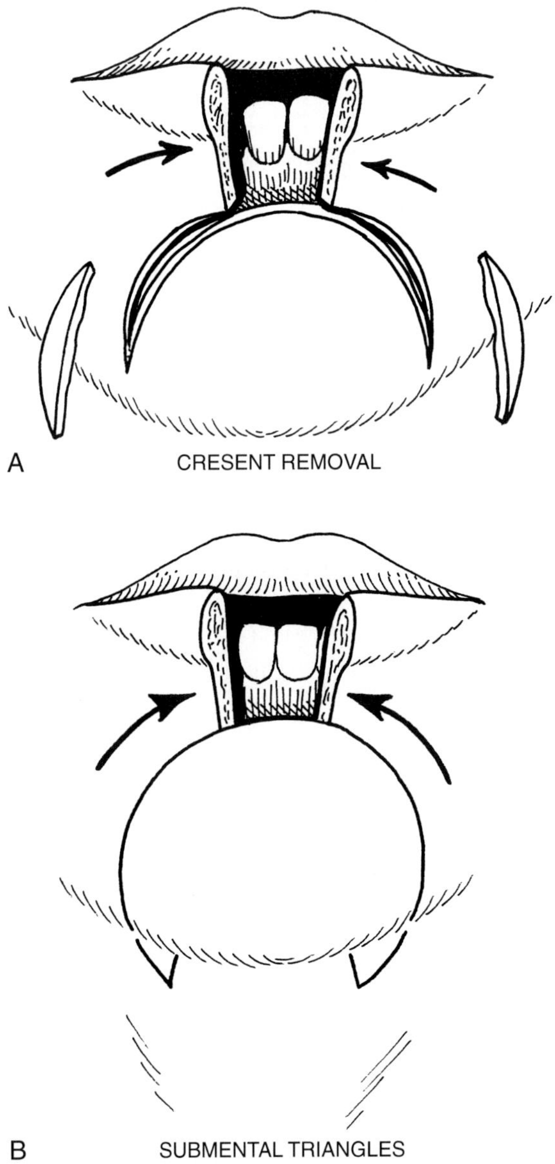

FIGURE 17–4. Moderate-sized defects of the lower lip can be reconstructed by a cheek/lip rotation-advancement flap. This procedure, developed by Schuchardt, removes (*A*) crescents or (*B*) submental triangles and uses the cheek/lip complex for closure.

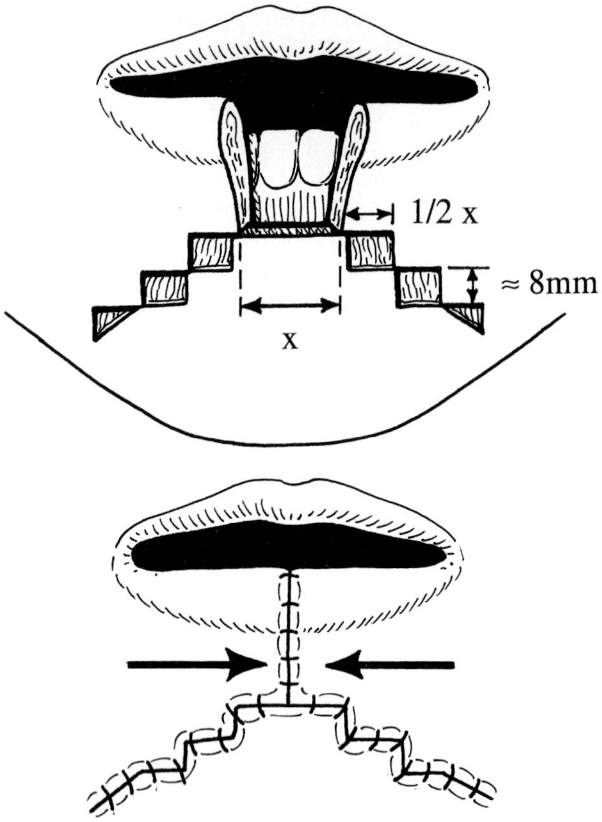

FIGURE 17–5. Johansen's staircase technique preserves oral function and sensation. It allows reconstruction of central or lateral defects at the expense of cosmetically undesirable incisors.

is an important and useful technique for reconstructing defects that are too large to be closed primarily when microstomia must be avoided. By virtue of the technique used to create the flap, total denervation occurs at the time of transfer. Electrosystagmography (ENG) studies demonstrate that at least partial motor function returns in most patients. Partial return of sensation typically occurs as well, probably due to the relatively small piece of tissue typically transferred.

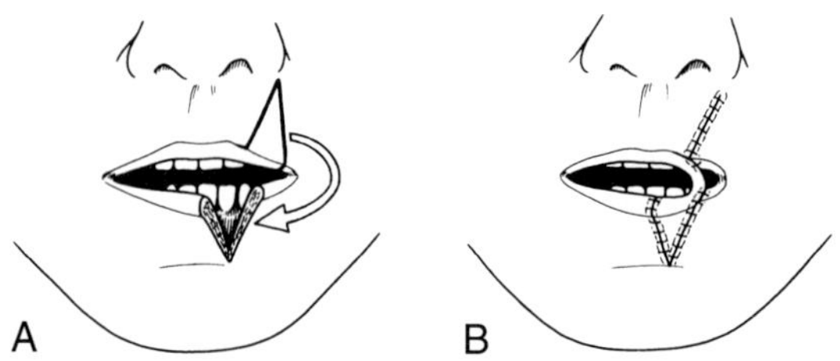

FIGURE 17–6. The Abbé flap, also known as the lip-switch procedure, utilizes a vascularized wedge of upper lip tissue to reconstruct the lower lip, or vice versa. It can be medially or laterally based and can be used in tandem with a second flap (when laterally based) to reconstruct larger defects. It is particularly useful for reconstruction of the region of the philtrum of the upper lip. The donor site generally heals with excellent cosmetic results. (From Stepnick D: Cancer of the lip. *In* Gates G (ed): Current Therapies in Otolaryngology, 5th ed. St Louis, CV Mosby, 1993.)

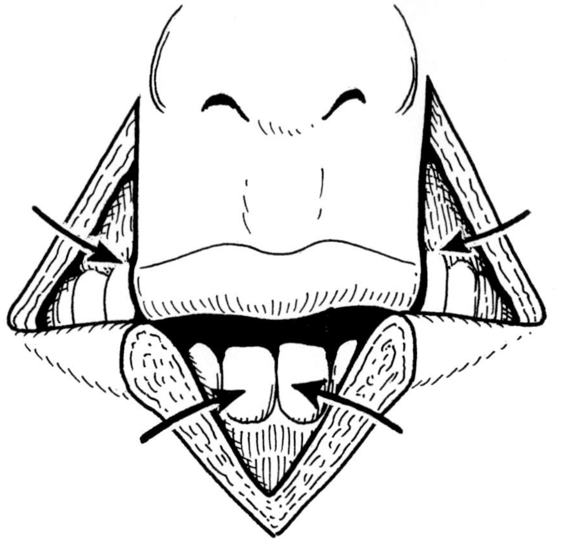

FIGURE 17–7. A through-and-through full-thickness triangular excision with a wedge-shaped lower lip excision was the hallmark of Bernard's original lower lip repair.

Bernard Technique

As the defect size approaches the length of the entire lower lip, other techniques must be applied. Bernard (1853) removed the tumor as a wedge from the central lower lip and then recruited remaining lip together with cheek tissue to recreate the lip.[1] Incisions extending outward from the commissure (Fig. 17–7) were combined with through-and-through full-thickness triangles excised lateral to the upper lip to advance bilateral cheek flaps inward. Although it was an important development in the history of lip reconstruction, the Bernard procedure had a number of drawbacks including denervation (motor and sensory) of the upper lip, distortion of the commissure, and absence of the vermilion when the excision involved the entire lower lip.

A variety of modifications have been proposed over the years that enhanced the acceptability and utility of this procedure, one of which was proposed by Webster in 1960 (Fig. 17–8). Webster excised the tumor as a quadrilateral segment rather than as a wedge. Skin and subcutaneous tissue rather than full-thickness tissue is excised, thus preserving the neurovascular supply to the upper lip. The natural crease of the nasolabial fold is used to hide the triangular excisions by placing them more laterally than originally described by Bernard. A new vermilion is recreated from bilateral buccal mucosal advancement flaps, which are preserved for this purpose. The lower lip cheek flap incisions are extended inferiorly using the Schuchardt principle. The lower lip, thus reconstructed, is watertight, sensate, functional, and cosmetically superior to that in the originally described reconstruction.

Estlander Flap and Fan Flap

Lateral defects near to or involving the commissure may be repaired by the Estlander flap (1872) (Fig. 17–9). This

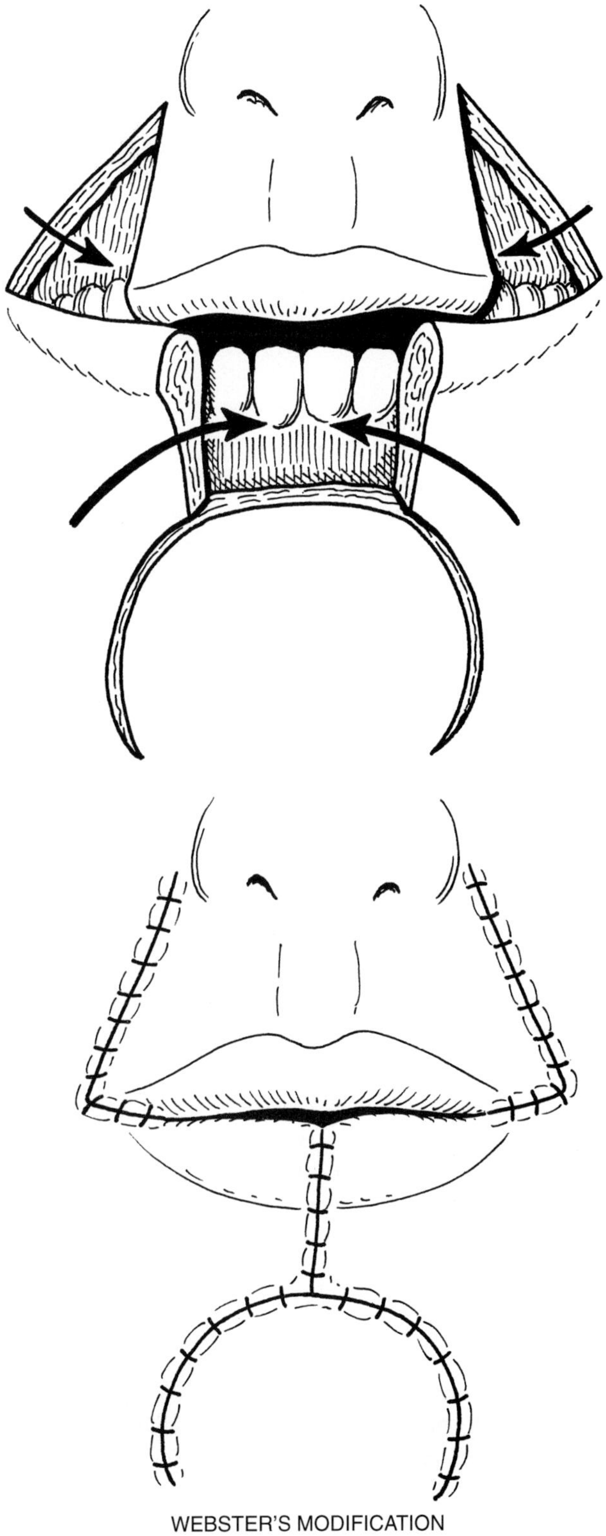

FIGURE 17–8. Improvements in Bernard's technique allowed preservation of upper lip sensory and motor function and reconstruction of the vermilion; these were accomplished with Webster's modification (1960) of Bernard's original procedure. Closure was facilitated by Schuchardt flaps.

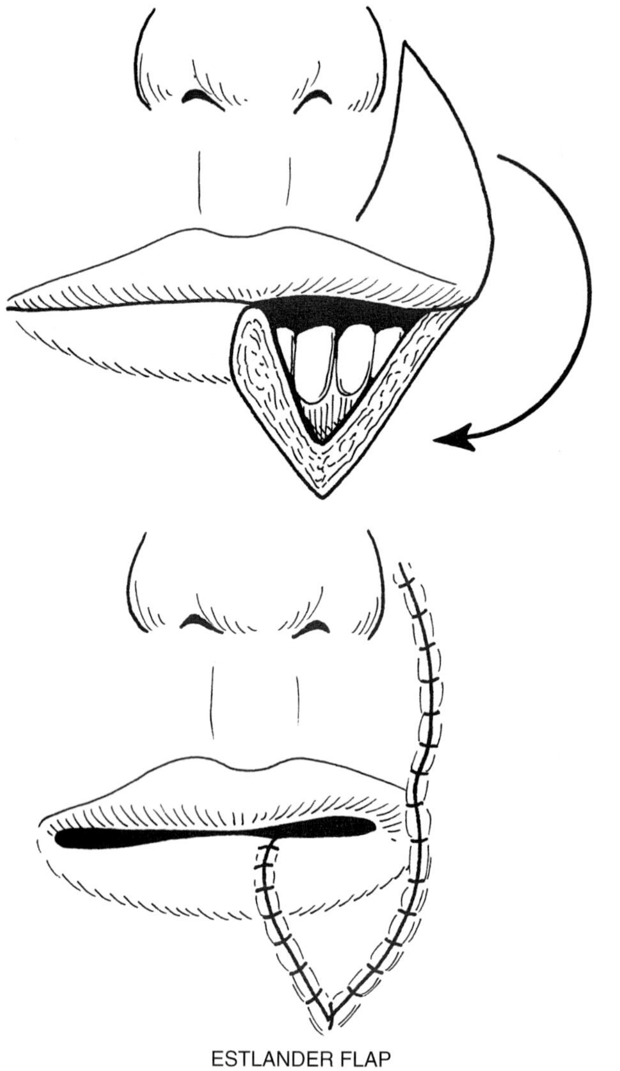

FIGURE 17–9. Like the Abbé flap, the Estlander flap is a lip-switch procedure designed to repair lateral or commissure defects. It produces a rounded commissure that may require secondary revision.

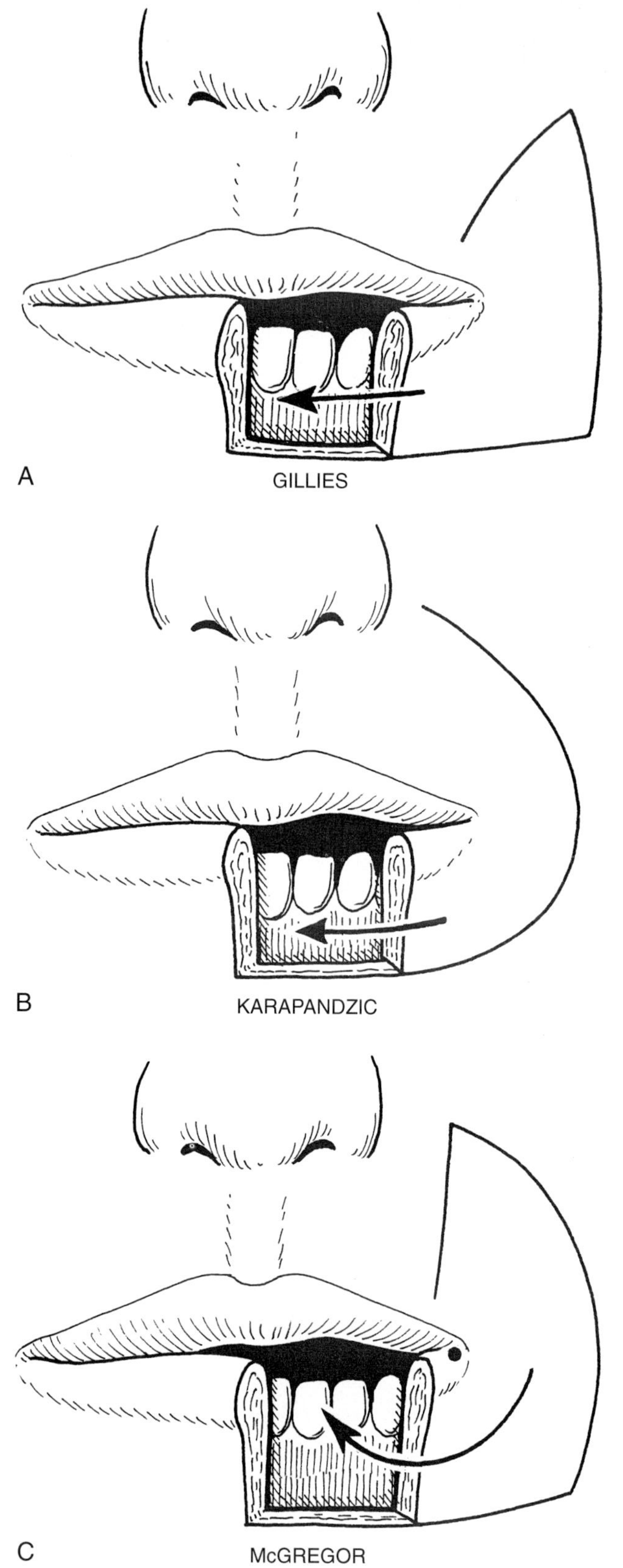

FIGURE 17–10. *A*, The Gillies advancement flap is useful for large lip defects but tends to distort the commissure. *B*, The Karapandzic myocutaneous flap is advanced with an intact neurovascular pedicle, thereby preserving sensation and oral competence. The oral aperture is narrowed. *C*, The McGregor and Nakajima procedures pivot tissue around the commissure, thereby producing less distortion than other methods. These techniques maintain the intercommissure distance; however, new vermilion is required and muscle fiber direction is changed. The difference between these two techniques is that the Nakajima method maintains the facial vessels supplying the flap.

lip-switch technique employs a medially based full-thickness triangular upper lip flap to reconstruct the lower lateral lip and commissure. Although the sphincter is maintained, rounding of the commissure is common and usually requires secondary revision. The fan flap of Gillies and Millard[2] (1957) (Fig. 17–10*A*) is an extension of the Estlander flap that is designed to repair larger defects; when used bilaterally, this procedure can be used to repair defects that involve the majority of the lower lip. The commissure and lower lateral lip are carried inward to reconstruct the more medially located lower lip defect.[3] The procedure is designed to reconstruct a rectangular defect on one side of which a flap is created in the outline of a fan that encircles and is centered on the angle of the mouth.[4] It is designed with a final backcut toward the vermilion but spares the narrow pedicle in which is contained the superior labial vessels.[5] According to McGregor, the fan flap, together with the Bernard procedure and its modifications, is probably the flap most commonly used for reconstruction of large defects of the lips.[5] Transection of the motor and sensory nerves, however, leaves the lip devoid of sensation and sphincteric control, potentially resulting in troublesome drooling and oral incompetence.

McGregor criticized this flap, however, as well as the subsequent modifications that preserved the neurovascular pedicle because it did not include resection of the remaining vermilion that had malignant potential. His modification (Fig. 17–10*C*) pivots around the commissure and allows removal of the vermilion. The cut edge is transposed upward and sewn to the remaining "normal" lip; thus, the medial margin of the flap becomes the superior margin of the lip, obviously devoid of vermilion. The vermilion is separately reconstructed with a tongue flap. This technique causes less distortion of the commissure but results in redirection of the muscle fibers (hence a less competent sphincter), an asensate lip (potentially causing drooling), and the need for vermilion reconstruction. Although there is less microstomia with this technique than with the Karapandzic flap, it changes the direction of the muscle fibers and thus creates a weaker sphincter. McGregor has reported spontaneous return of (primarily) sensory but also motor function and claims that drooling has not been a common problem in patients undergoing this reconstruction.

Other modifications of the fan flaps include the Karapandzic procedure, discussed in detail below, and the Nakajima procedure.[6] The latter is similar to the McGregor procedure except that the facial vessels supplying the flap are dissected and carefully preserved (see Fig. 17–10*C*).

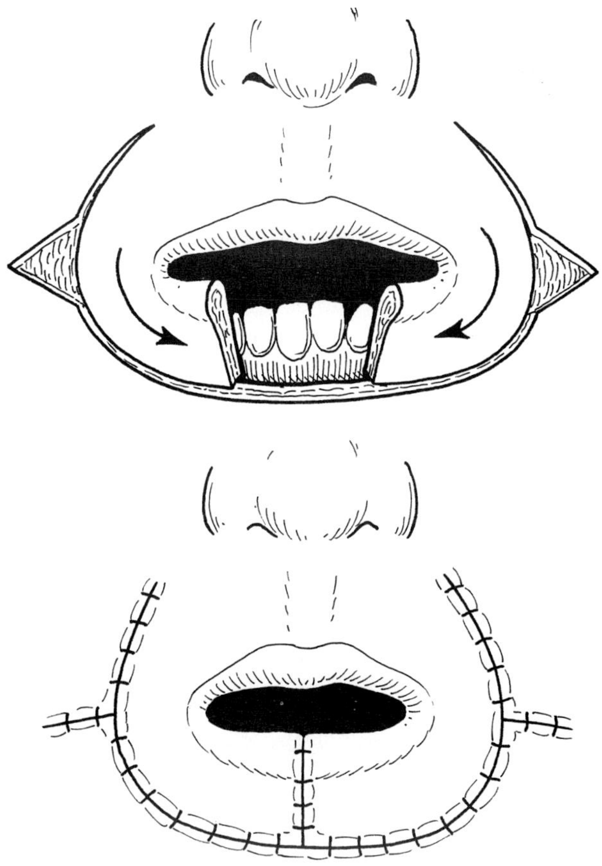

KARAPANDZIC TECHNIQUE

FIGURE 17–11. The Karapandzic technique (1974), essentially an orbicularis oris myocutaneous flap, provides a strong, sensate sphincter that preserves optimal oral competence. The literature supports use of this technique for up to 80% of the lip; I have used it successfully to reconstruct as much as the entire lower lip together with 5% to 10% of the upper lip.

Karapandzic Flap (Orbicularis Oris Myocutaneous Flap)

Unlike other popular myocutaneous flaps (e.g., the pectoralis major flap) that have multiple potential reconstructive applications, the Karapandzic flap has one specific application: it is used to reconstruct large defects of the lips with specific emphasis on functional restoration of the oral sphincter. Because the Karapandzic flap is a myocutaneous flap designed to preserve the neurovascular structures, sensation in the resultant reconstructed lip is maintained as is sphincteric competence, preventing drooling (Fig. 17–11).

The flap was first described in 1974 by Miodrag Karapandzic from the University of Belgrade, Yugoslavia.[7] Karapandzic used this technique in 58 patients from 1967 to 1972 to reconstruct defects ranging from 3.5 to 7 cm in size. Occasionally the entire lower lip was involved. Because the technique necessarily created a smaller oral commissure, one might think that secondary correction of microstomia would be a frequent occurrence. However, only 13 of Karapandzic's original patients required such correction.

Karapandzic, and subsequently Jabaley,[8] by developing a true myocutaneous flap that preserves both the vascular and neural connections to the orbicularis oris muscle and lips, created a technique that allows functional recreation of the oral sphincter. Not only is muscle function is preserved, but also a deep, untethered sulcus is retained. A lip is constructed that has normal height and does not have a tendency to sag.

Radial Forearm Flap

Early attempts to reconstruct the total lower lip defect utilized regional tissues that closed the defect but did not reestablish a sensate, dynamic, competent stoma. Oral competence can be maintained or achieved when the reconstruction allows interdigitation of the muscle fibers around the oral commissure. Examples of such flaps include the Webster-Bernard, Van Bruns, and Karapandzic procedures. Unfortunately, although these procedures reestablish oral competence, they require rearrangement of much of the lower half of the face. Although it produces an innervated lip with strong sphincteric action, the Karapandzic procedure used for near-total lower lip reconstruction has the considerable disadvantage of also producing significant microstomia. Chest flaps such as the deltopectoral and pectoralis major flaps have been used for this repair as well, but these are less ideally suited than the distant flaps that are now available with revascularized free tissue transfer techniques.

The radial forearm free flap has become increasingly popular in head and neck reconstruction, especially for defects of the oral cavity. It is useful for reconstruction of large defects involving the lower lip and chin as well. The flap is reliable, quickly and easily harvested, and results in minimal donor site morbidity. It allow a one-stage operation that appears to be functionally superior to the aforementioned chest flaps and reduces further scarring by sparing the remaining tissues of the face. The flap is extremely thin and pliable. As such, it can reestablish complex contours and readily be folded on itself to reestablish both external and internal epithelial surfaces. A major disadvantage of using this thin fasciocutaneous portion alone is the lack of support it provides across the lip, which potentially limits competence of the neosphincter.

Sakai and colleagues[9] first described the successful use of this flap combined with the palmaris longus tendon to reconstruct the entire lower lip and chin. The fasciocutaneous portion of the flap was used to provide both internal and external coverage, while the vascularized palmaris longus tendon was used to provide the necessary lower lip suspension. Sadove and colleagues[10] reported the first series of four patients in whom this technique was used. Despite an absence of muscle in the flap, their patients apparently did not suffer from drooling. Animation of the tissue appeared to be transferred passively owing to continuity with the remaining facial muscles, although fine motor function could not be restored (Fig. 17–12). The authors reported a high degree of patient satisfaction with this technique.

Because the upper border of this flap is devoid of a vermilion, immediate or subsequent procedures are needed to create a more normal appearance of this aesthetic unit. A tongue flap, as reported by McGregor,[4] is useful for this purpose. Patients who refuse subsequent procedures may benefit from medical tattooing of the vermilion. Minor revisions to improve the labiobuccal sulcus were necessary in 50% of Sadove's cases.[10] Combining a radial forearm flap with a ventral tongue flap and then reinnervating the tissue by performing a lateral antebrachial cutaneous nerve to men-

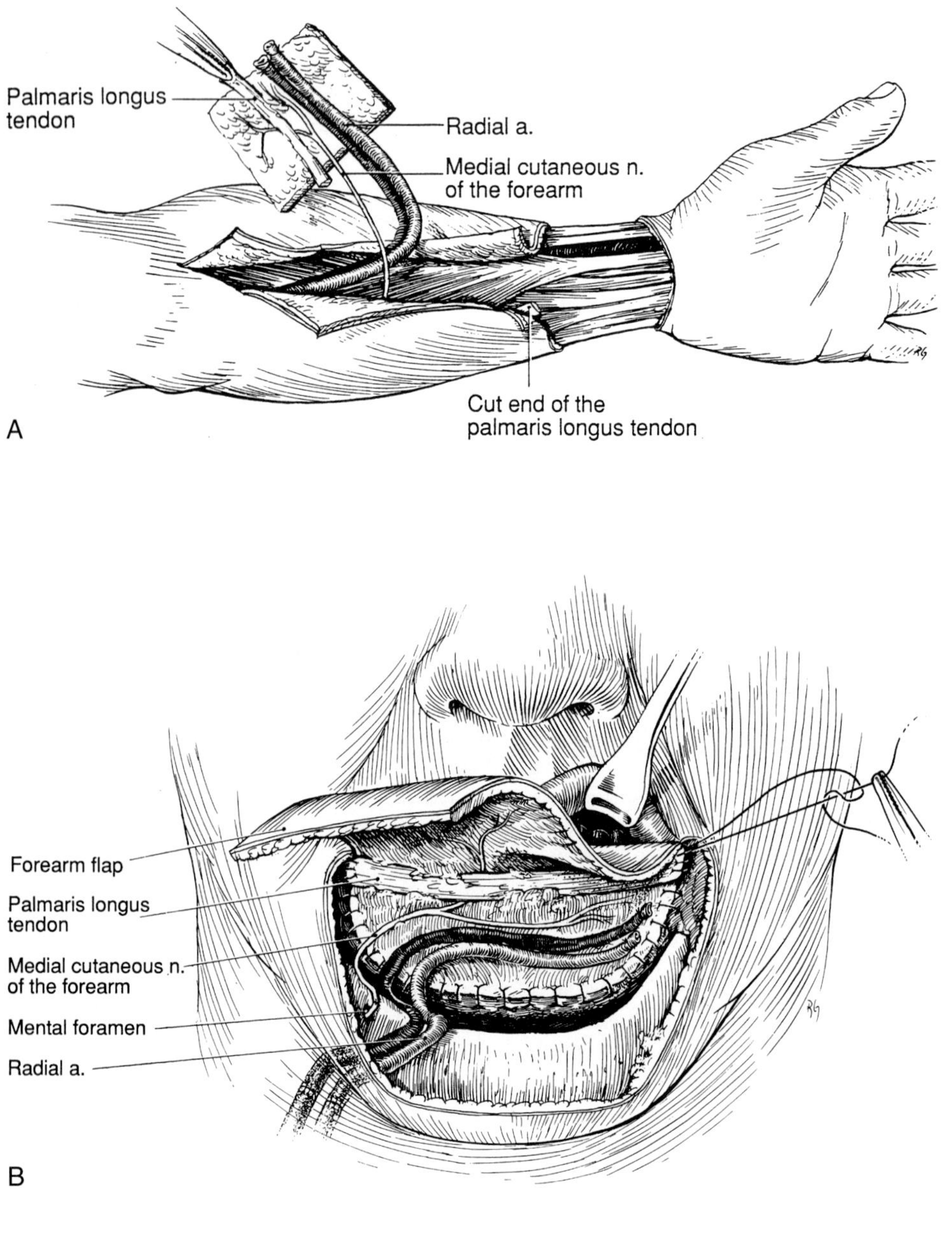

FIGURE 17–12. *A*, Schematic illustration demonstrating dissection of the radial forearm–palmaris longus flap prior to transfer. *B*, Schematic illustration demonstrating total lower lip and chin reconstruction. The intraoral closure, revascularization, nerve repair, and suture of the palmaris longus tendon to the modiolus have been completed. (From Sadove RC, Luce EA, McGrath PC: Reconstruction of the lower lip and chin with the composite radial forearm–palmaris longus free flap. Plast Reconstr Surg 88: 209–214, 1991.)

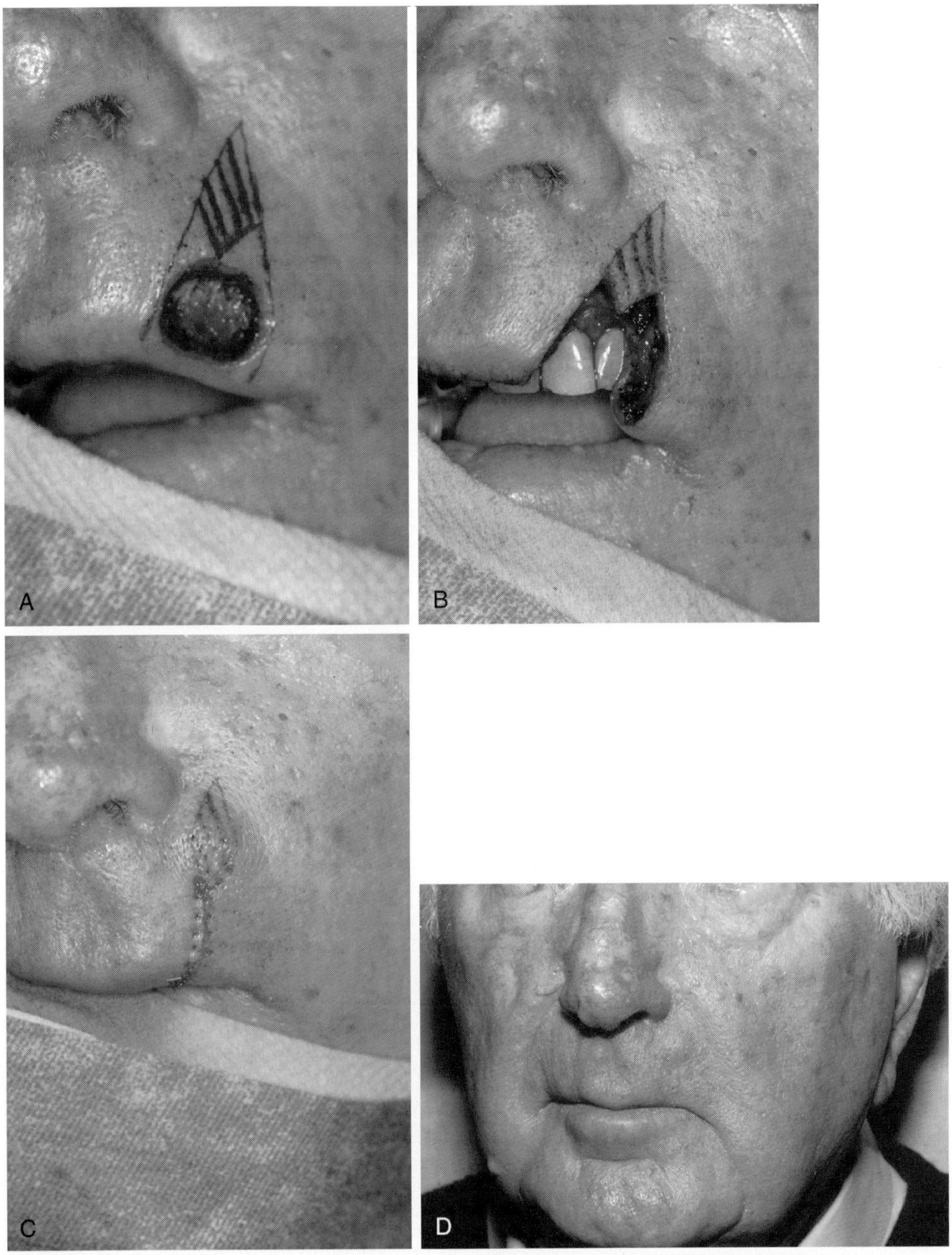

FIGURE 17–13. Many of the same techniques applicable to lower lip reconstruction can be used in the upper lip. *A*, Patient whose carcinoma was excised using total margin control; clear margins are present prior to reconstruction. *B*, W excision is used to facilitate closure and is designed to prevent the scar from crossing the nasolabial crease. *C*, Intraoperative view of the closed incision. *D*, Postoperative appearance several months later.

tal nerve neurorrhaphy currently appears to be the most advanced technique of restoring appearance and function to the maximum degree in patients with total lower lip defects.[11]

Upper Lip Defects

As previously noted, the great majority of cancers occur on the lower lip, and reconstruction of upper lip defects is consequently required less frequently. Many of the procedures described for lower lip reconstruction are applicable to the upper lip as well and will not be discussed again herein. As with the lower lip, among the most useful techniques for the upper lip are primary closure, V and W closures (Fig. 17–13), the Karapandzic procedure, and the Abbé flaps. The use of advancement flaps combined with perialar crescentic excisions is noteworthy in that this procedure is specifically designed for the upper lip. The technique is useful for small to moderate sized upper lip defects, especially defects in the central lip where the mobility of the lip is limited due to the structural support provided by attachments to the nasal base. For mobilization of this area, it is necessary to detach the lip from the nose and mobilize the lip using bilateral perialar crescentic excisions to facilitate tension-free closure. Distortion of the cupid's bow must be anticipated, but results are usually quite acceptable (Fig. 17–14). When cosmesis is of utmost importance, advancement flaps using perialar crescentic excisions may be

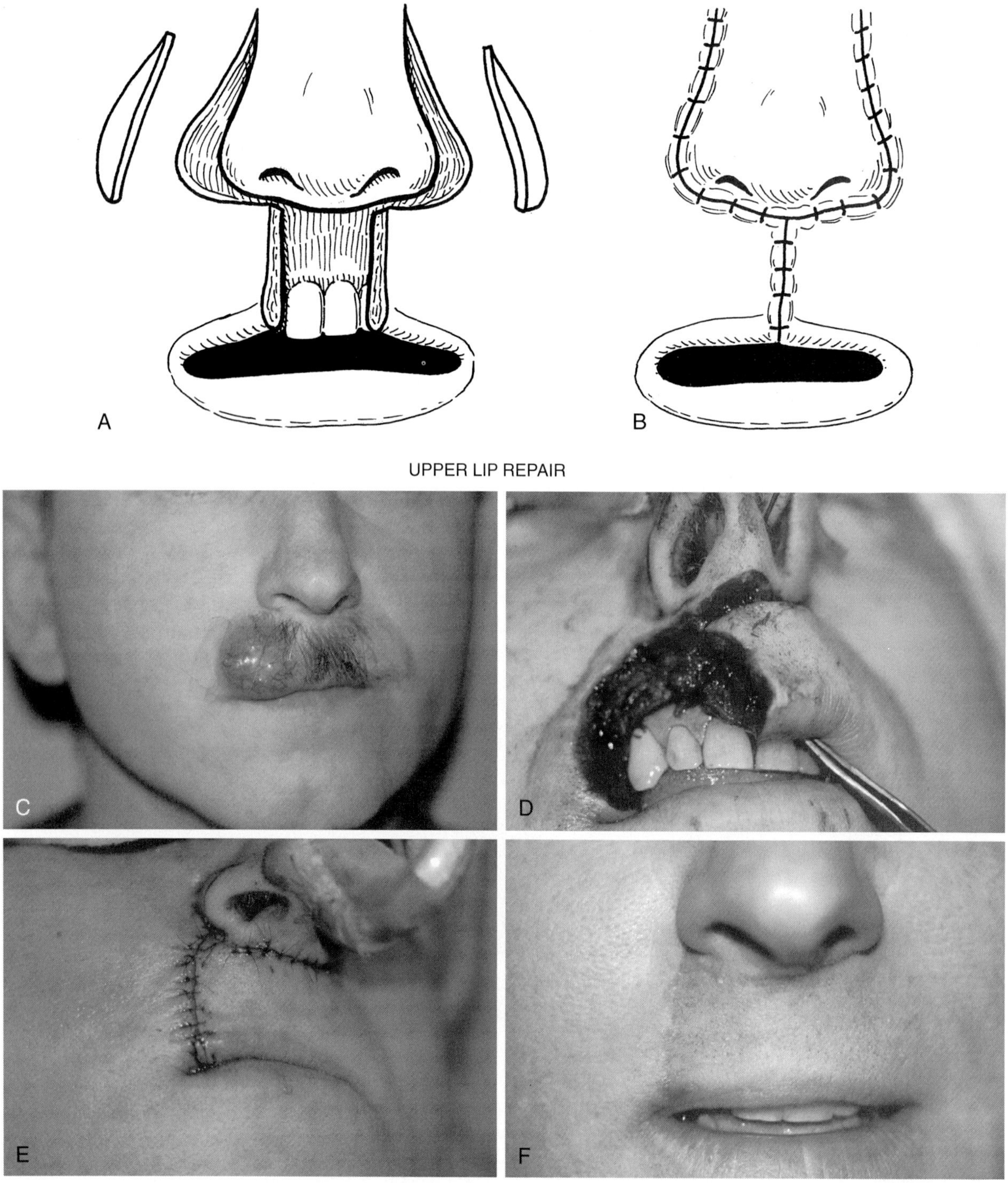

FIGURE 17–14. Central defects of the upper lip may not be appropriate for V or W excisions and closure. In this area, perialar crescentic excisions (*A*) may facilitate closure of such defects. *B*, Cupid's bow is lost, but the results are cosmetically acceptable. *C*, This patient with limited metastatic sarcoma presented with a lip metastasis that was both a functional and cosmetic problem. A rapid, low-morbidity treatment was desired. *D*, Intraoperative view showing defect and incision beneath columella. *E*, Closure of defect with minimal tension, using a contralateral perialar excision. Note absence of cupid's bow. *F*, Early postoperative result (see text).

combined with lower lip-switch flaps to create a philtral dimple.

Large Through-and-Through Cheek Defects Involving the Commissure

An especially difficult area for lip reconstruction is the area of the oral commissure. Much has been written about techniques to recreate this region. There are a number of options for requiring small defects of the commissure, but choices are limited in patients with large defects involving significant portions of the upper and lower lips, especially when these are combined with through-and-through tissue loss through the cheek and buccal mucosa. In the past, pedicled myocutaneous flaps have been used to reconstruct this area with reasonable results. However, revascularized tissue probably provides a better repair. The radial forearm flap is too thin to be used for reconstruction of full-thickness cheek defects and can result in concavity or tightening and loss of all pliability over a period of months. Thicker flaps must be chosen to provide a better match for the excised tissue and to minimize the chances of such complications. The scapular fasciocutaneous flap is useful for this reconstructive challenge (Fig. 17–15). More commonly used as an osteocutaneous flap incorporating the lateral border of the scapula, this flap, based on the circumflex scapular artery, may be harvested without the bony component. The moderately thin, fasciocutaneous portion can either be skin grafted on the inner surface or folded and turned in on itself. Secondary revisions may help to achieve the precise shape and thickness desired (see Fig. 17–16*D* and *E*). Oral mucosal grafting or tattooing can help improve its final appearance.

Other free tissue transfer options exist, including the lateral thigh flap and the upper arm flap. As with any reconstructive problem, flap choice must be based on the anatomy, size, and function of the resected structures. Larger defects involving the lips generally require more ingenuity on the part of the reconstructive surgeon to ensure optimum restoration of form and function.

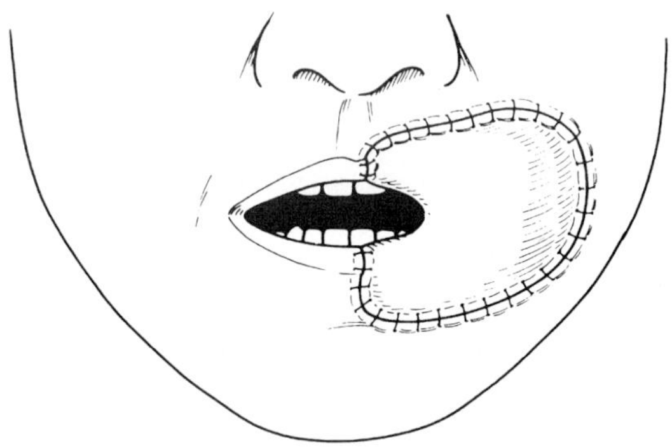

FIGURE 17–15. Relatively thin fasciocutaneous flaps can be useful for reconstruction of the commissure when the remaining lip will not provide suitable tissue for reconstruction and a major rearrangement of the lower face is not desired. The scapular flap, upper arm flap, or lateral thigh flap may be considered for this purpose. The surgeon should anticipate changes that will occur as the flap matures and not be hasty when planning subsequent procedures to improve the commissure. (From Stepnick D: Cancer of the lip. *In* Gates G (ed): Current Therapies in Otolaryngology, 5th ed. St. Louis, CV Mosby, 1993.)

CASE REPORTS

Case 1

A. R., a 35-year-old white male, had undergone treatment previously with chemotherapy and radiation for a poorly differentiated soft tissue sarcoma in the inguinal region. The treatment had been effective in limiting disease progression. The patient then developed a mass lesion of the right upper lip that was initially treated at another institution by incising the overlying mucosa on the inside of the dental aspect of the lesion and essentially "coring it out." Not surprisingly, the lesion recurred. No evidence of other metastases could be identified.

Because the lesion was cosmetically unappealing and caused some minor difficulty with eating, the patient sought advice about treatment options. Consultation with a radiation oncologist elicited the opinion that surgical excision would, in all likelihood, provide better palliation ("quicker" treatment with less long-term morbidity) than radiation therapy. After a thorough discussion of the treatment options available, the patient requested surgery. His goals, though, were to have the lesion excised with minimal morbidity and without the need for subsequent revision procedures. The lesion was excised, free margins were obtained, and the defect was closed with an advancement flap consisting of the remainder of the upper lip.

An incision was carried along the base of the columella and into the contralateral perialar region, where a small crescent was removed to facilitate closure (Fig. 17–14). The wound healed without difficulty, and the patient returned to normal oral function within days. One year later, despite continued problems with sarcoma outside of the head and neck region, there has been no evidence of local recurrence.

Case 2

D. P is a 54-year-old white male who has had significant (and ongoing) exposure to the sun as a result of outdoor activity, especially golfing. He was diagnosed with a basal cell carcinoma of the oral commissure region a number of years prior to referral to us. Initially, small local excisions were performed, and the disease was thought to be under control. However, because the patient had irregular follow-up owing to poor compliance with recommendations by his physicians, tumor progression occurred.

Eventually, he again sought care, but by this time the tumor extensively infiltrated the tissues of the commissure and cheek, causing dimpling and external deformity (Fig. 17–16*A*) (see also Color Plate). It became apparent that resection would be extensive and would involve soft tissue from the mouth, chin, cheek, and buccal mucosa. A large defect resulted from the through-and-through excision (Fig. 17–16*B*). A fasciocutaneous scapular flap was designed to repair the defect. The distal portion of the ellipse was folded intraorally and used to replace the buccal mucosa. An intervening segment of epithelium "at the fold" was removed, effectively deepithelializing a linear band of dermis, which was buried alongside the remaining lip and orbicularis. Edges were reapproximated, and the tissue was revascularized.

Postoperatively, the patient underwent radiation therapy and now has no evidence of disease, 4 years after surgery (Fig. 17–16*D* and *E*). Two minor revisions were performed in an ambulatory setting, one of which was designed to improve the "valley" between the scapular flap and the chin, and the other to defat that portion of the flap inferior to the mandible to improve mandibular

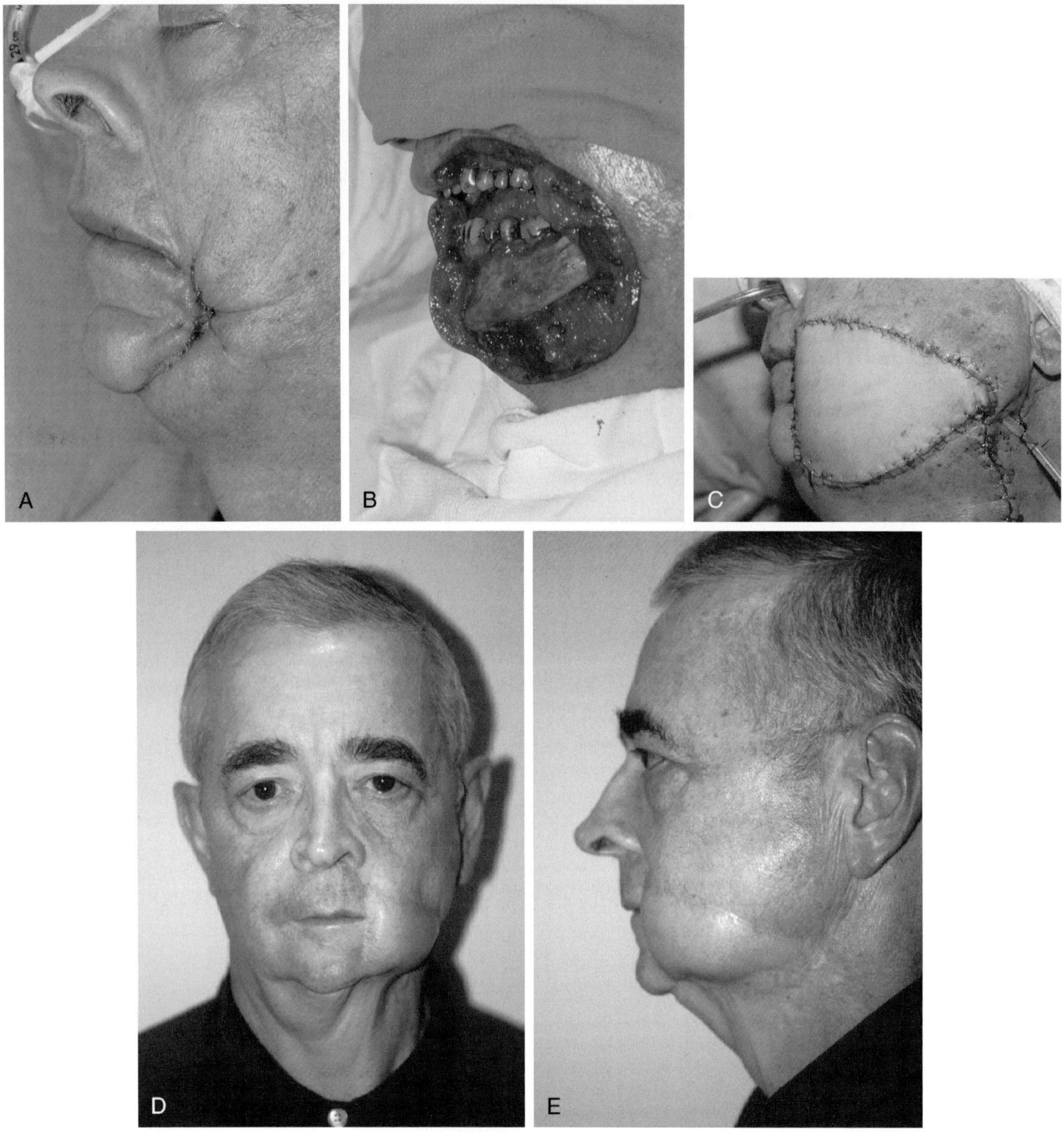

FIGURE 17–16. *A*, Preoperative view of patient showing retraction and skin changes as a result of carcinoma in the commissure region. *B*, Intraoperative view, following excision after clear margins were obtained. *C*, Intraoperative view of scapular free flap in position. Note that the flap has been turned in on itself to create an epithelial lining inside the mouth as well. The intervening segment, now attached to the remaining lip, has been deepithelialized. *D* and *E*, Postoperative views, following radiation and eventual secondary revision, 36 months later. The patient is now free of disease at 4 years. (See also Color Plate)

contour. The patient eats a normal diet, has no speech problems, and is delighted with his appearance.

SUMMARY

As the worldwide incidence of skin cancer continues to rise, one can expect the number of cancers of the lip to do the same. Since surgery is generally the treatment of choice for such lesions, the need for reconstruction of these defects will become increasingly important. Perhaps no other area of the body has had as many techniques described for its reconstruction as the lip. Every plastic surgery textbook is replete with a sometimes bafflingly large number of options, and the novice surgeon can easily become confused about which might the best choice.

As with any surgical procedure, whenever there are many ways to perform an operation, no one technique is always best for achieving one's goals. Indeed, for reconstruction of the lip, the wide variety of described techniques provides the surgeon with a powerful armamentarium for dealing with this problem. However, it is my opinion that one need not be confused by the myriad of procedures available; developing skill and expertise in only a few will allow successful reconstruction of almost any defect.

Small defects of the lips can be closed primarily, and V or W excisions can be used in the lower lip and lateral upper lip for small to moderately large lesions. Advancement flaps can also be useful for these small to moderate sized lesions, using the technique of perialar crescentic excisions when upper lip defects are encountered.

Moderate sized defects can be closed effectively with the Karapandzic flap, which effectively maintains oral sensory and motor function. The resultant microstomia is rarely a problem, and most patients are delighted to have oral competence returned following removal of such a large section of the mouth. The lip-switch operations can also be effective in repairing these moderate sized defects, although these can be time-consuming, difficult to care for, may require a secondary procedure, and rely on nerve regrowth for any sensory or motor function that may recover.

Large defects are effectively treated with Karapandzic flaps as well and can provide a functioning oral sphincter to patients who otherwise would be severely handicapped. The reinnervated radial forearm–palmaris longus flap is another option for these huge defects involving the entire lower lip and chin and probably represent the state of the art as it exists at the time of writing. Other free flap options should be considered for complex defects that include significant portions of the lip, cheek, buccal mucosa, and even the mandible. Indeed, flexibility and choice are powerful allies of the reconstructive surgeon in dealing with defects of the lip.

References

1. Bernard C: Cancer de la levre inferieure opere par un procede nouveau. Gazette Hopitaux 44, 1853.
2. Gillies HD, Millard DR: The Principles and Art of Plastic Surgery. London, Butterworth, 1957.
3. Zide B: Deformities of the lips and cheeks. *In* McCarthy JG (ed): Plastic Surgery, Vol 3, The Face, Part 2. Philadelphia, WB Saunders, 1990.
4. McGregor IA: Reconstruction of the lower lip. Br J Plast Surg 36: 40–47, 1983.
5. McGregor IA: Fundamental Techniques of Plastic Surgery and Their Surgical Applications. New York, Churchill Livingstone, 1989, pp. 138–142.
6. Nakajima T, Yoshimura Y, Kami T: Reconstruction of the lower lip with a fan-shaped flap based on the facial artery. Br J Plast Surg 37: 52–54, 1984.
7. Karapandzic M.: Reconstruction of lip defects by local arterial flaps. Br J Plast Surg 27: 93–97, 1974.
8. Jabaley ME, Clement RL, Orcutt TW: Myocutaneous flaps in lip reconstruction: Applications of the Karapandzic principle. Plast Reconstr Surg 59: 680–688, 1977.
9. Sakai S, Soeda S, Endo T, Ishii M, Uchiumi E: A compound radial artery forearm flap for the reconstruction of lip and chin defect. Br J Plast Surg 42: 337, 1989.
10. Sadove RC, Luce EA, McGrath PC: Reconstruction of the lower lip and chin with the composite radial forearm–palmaris longus free flap. Plast Reconstr Surg 88: 209–214, 1991.
11. Serletti JM, Tavin E, Moran SL, Coniglio JU: Total lower lip reconstruction with a sensate composite radial forearm–palmaris longus free flap and a tongue flap. Plast Reconstr Surg 99: 559–561, 1997.

CHAPTER 18

Osseointegrated Percutaneous Titanium Implants

Anders Tjellström, M.D., Ph.D.
David Proops, M.D., B.D.S.
Gösta Granström, M.D., D.D.S., Ph.D.

Defects in the craniofacial region have an enormous impact on the quality of life for the patient and his or her family as well as the general public. Many of these patients withdraw from society, and it is not uncommon for patients to leave their homes only after dark. Plastic surgery may be successful in many cases, but in some conditions such procedures do not give a good result or cannot be carried out at all. In this chapter we will discuss how to establish a lasting anchorage of components in the facial skeleton to be used for the retention of prosthetic devices.

HISTORICAL BACKGROUND

The use of prostheses to cover facial defects has a long tradition. In an interesting review, Conroy[1] found that as early as 2000 BC facial prostheses were used in China. Silver, gold, and copper prostheses dating from this time have been found. It is not known whether other materials were used, but it does not seem unlikely that if these were used they have degraded over time, and only those made of precious metals have remained. Enamel and ceramics came into use in the nineteenth century, and some made of leather have been preserved from the latter part of that period.

In those days the defects covered with prostheses were often due to trauma and infectious diseases such as leprosy. Tumors of the face were probably only covered with bandages because surgery was performed rarely and was seldom curative. During World War I the handling of battle casualties reached a level at which many of the soldiers survived despite major injuries, including facial defects. This situation became the starting point of a new era in craniofacial rehabilitation using prosthetic devices.

The first modern textbook on facial prostheses was published in 1945 by Bubulian, a dentist working at the Mayo Clinic in Rochester, Minnesota.[2] During the first part of the twentieth century gutta percha and papier mâché had been used, but Bubulian introduced the new compound latex for facial prostheses. Development of various prostheses since then has been very rapid, and soon acrylic resin became widely used. Acrylic is still used and has the advantage of being stable and keeping its shape. The color of an acrylic prosthesis is also fairly stable, but the appearance is "hard," and the normal complexion is difficult to imitate in acrylic. Another disadvantage is that the prosthesis is very hard and its edges cannot be made thin, so that it will not follow any movement of the surrounding tissue. In 1978 Jani and Schaaf reported their experiences with acrylic facial prostheses at the well-established and renowned Rosswell Park Clinic in Buffalo, New York.[3] In their survey of patients' opinions of their prostheses, only 50% of the mailed surveys were answered, and of those who did respond, only every second patient used his or her prosthesis every day. One common complaint was skin irritation due to the adhesive used and the lack of comfort caused by the hard acrylic material. The poor appearance was, however, the main reason for dissatisfaction, even among those who used their prostheses.

The introduction of permanent skin-penetrating, bone-anchored implants in 1977 opened new possibilities in the rehabilitation of patients with facial defects. The technique of retaining facial prostheses with implants made it possible to use softer materials, and the need to make the edges thin became the next important step in development.

OSSEOINTEGRATION

The new treatment modality of osseointegration was made possible by the creation of a stable and lasting fixation for implants in bone tissue. This concept was introduced by Professor Per-Ingvar Brånemark in 1977 and was termed osseointegration.[4] The original definition of osseointegration by Brånemark was "a direct contact between living bone tissue and a loaded implant surface." This definition has been questioned. On what level is this "direct" contact? Do all implants need this direct contact to be called osseointegrated? Some have claimed that the term is too vague and have abandoned it. However, we believe that it is a well-established term, and from the clinical point of view it expresses a lasting anchorage in bone tissue of an implant that can bear a load.

Albrektsson and co-workers have identified six important factors in the establishment of osseointegration.[5] These will be briefly discussed here, but for an understanding in depth, the textbook on this topic edited by Worthington and Brånemark[6] is recommended.

Implant Material. The implant material used by the authors is commercially pure titanium (cpTi), manufactured by Nobel Biocare AB, Sweden. Titanium is a common and very light metal with an atomic number of 48. In its refined form it is soft, which is of clinical importance when handling implants. When cpTi is machined in a normal atmospheric environment the surface within milliseconds becomes covered with an oxide layer. This oxide layer is very corrosion resistant and has physical properties that are important in its contact with bone and soft tissues. One of the most common titanium alloys in the medical field is Ti6Al4V, composed of 90% titanium, 6% aluminum, and 4% vanadium. It is possible to achieve osseointegration with this alloy, but the quality of the contact is not as good as that with cpTi.[7] In the short run this may not be of clinical significance, but the long-term effects are not known.

Macro Structure. The implant is screw-shaped and has a flange. The design has not been changed since clinical usage began in 1977. The reason for the screw shape is the importance of achieving initial stability during the healing phase. It has been shown that even minor movements during the healing phase can cause fibrous encapsulation instead of osseointegration.[8] The flange contributes further to this stability. The diameter of the implant is 3.75 mm, and the flange is 5.5 mm. It comes in three lengths—3, 4, and 5.5 mm. About 90% of the implants used by the authors are 4 mm long.

Micro Structure. The surface of the implant has a high di-electrical constant, which is one reason for its good biologic properties. The surface also has a great affinity for other material, and this is why the implant is never touched by anything except titanium-clad instruments and never by the gloved hand directly. Minor contamination even of sterile particles may jeopardize osseointegration. It has been shown that if the implant has a polished surface osseointegration is not as good as if the surface were slightly rough.[9] On the other hand, a surface that is too rough could release fragments into the tissue and even cause ionic leakage. Not only will osseointegration be less than optimal but also the long-term effect is not known. This is of special importance for implants placed in children and for implants containing toxic components such as aluminum.

Surgical Technique. The surgical technique is described in some detail below. One of the most important details is to reduce the inevitable tissue trauma caused by any surgical procedure. If the bony tissue is damaged too much, there is a risk that healing will result in fibrous tissue encapsulation instead of bony contact. Best results are achieved by strictly following the surgical protocol. Sharp drills, controlled drilling speeds, adequate cooling during drilling, and proper handling of the components to avoid contaminating their active surfaces are some of the important points.

Quality and Quantity of Tissue at Implant Site. Irradiation interferes with soft as well as with calcified tissues. The skin reaction after irradiation is often settled after some months. In bone the opposite situation applies. The quality of bone deteriorates as time goes on owing to several factors. The result is a gradual decrease in oxygen tension in the tissue. This process will continue unless the patient is treated with hyperbaric oxygen as described later. Sometimes the amount of bone remaining is not enough to accommodate an implant. This occurs frequently in young children but occasionally also in adults. This situation can be solved by using free bone grafts from the iliac crest[6] or by using membrane techniques.[10]

Loading Conditions. Implants for the retention of dentures in the edentulous jaw have been used by oral surgeons for many years. However, not until Brånemark introduced the two-stage procedure was the failure rate brought down to an acceptable level. It has been shown that even small movements of an implant during the initial healing phase can result in fibrous encapsulation.[8] Such implants were thus left unloaded for 3 to 4 months before they were loaded, and the success rate with this technique was very high and is well documented.[11] The forces to which implants are exposed in mastication are, however, of a much higher magnitude than those encountered in craniofacial prosthetics, and based on a study that began in 1989 a modified one-stage procedure is used today in the nonirradiated adult mastoid process.[12] In the orbit and midface as well as in the irradiated mastoid process a two-stage procedure is still recommended.

SURGERY

Preoperative Evaluation

Before describing the details of the different steps of this procedure it is important to be aware that placing the implant is only one, and not seldom the easiest, part of the total rehabilitation program. A well-integrated implant with a prosthesis of poor quality is not a good treatment. As discussed in more detail in Chapter 20. The team approach to this treatment modality is more important than it is in many other treatments. This team approach should be in place and functioning when the patient comes in for the first consultation. Are there other treatment possibilities? What will the plastic surgeon be able to do? If a good result can be achieved with autogenous material, this is of course preferable. How many procedures will that take? Are the results predictable? What are the needs of the patient? The next person on the team to have input in the planning is the prosthodontist or anaplastologist or technician who is responsible for making the prosthesis. What are the optimum positions of the implants? How many will be needed? What is the direction of the implants? The surgeon must evaluate the bone available at the site of the defect. Is a bone transplant necessary? Will bone regeneration using a membrane technique be needed?

Most important is the information given to the patient that this is a prosthetic procedure and that he or she has must return for regular check-ups. The importance of good hygiene is stressed. During presurgical planning the team must determine whether the patient has realistic expectations for the treatment. Is he or she well motivated? One of the few contraindications to this treatment is psychiatric disease or drug abuse, and these should also be evaluated before surgery.

Surgical Technique

The technique described in some detail here is implant surgery for an auricular prosthesis, but the process is very much the same for other prosthetic appliances. In the nonirradiated mastoid it is often possible to perform the surgery in one stage. In irradiated tissue and in the orbit and midface, irradiated or not, a two-stage procedure is recommended with an interval of 3 to 6 months between operations. This important issue is discussed in more detail under the heading Implants in Irradiated Tissue.

The artist's view of this procedure is presented in Figures 18–1 to 18–19, and these figures can be followed in this step-by-step presentation. The optimum position and direction of the implants should be marked before the patient is taken to the operating theater (Fig. 18–1). This is especially important in patients with congenital defects in whom landmarks may be difficult to identify when the patient is draped. For an auricular prosthesis, the implant should be placed 20 to 22 mm from the center of the external ear canal opening or, if this is absent, from its anticipated position. The reason for this position is that the bar construction should be under the anthelix ridge to enable the anaplastologist to make a prosthesis that is deep enough to produce a good cosmetic result. In our experience this positioning is one of the main difficulties in plastic surgical reconstruction. As shown in Figure 18–1, not only is the distance from the meatus indicated but also the relative position. For the caudal implant on the right side this corresponds to 1 to 2 o'clock and to about 3:30 to 4:30 o'clock for the most cranial implant.

The surgical area is covered with plastic draping because even sterile foreign material present at the implant site may jeopardize osseointegration. Ten mL of 2% Xylocaine with 12.5 μg/mL adrenaline is injected into the surgical field. The incision is made 7 to 10 mm behind the intended implant site down to but not through the periosteum. A hole about 6 mm in diameter is made in the periosteum at the intended site of the implant closest to the mastoid tip (Fig. 18–2). The reason for this is that sometimes the large air cell in the tip area may force the surgeon to choose another site more cranially located. If the cranial implant has already been placed, the distance between the implants could then be too short. It is suggested that there should be at least 15 mm between the two implants. In placing the cranial implant there is often a greater degree of freedom because the bone in the linea temporalis area is generally fairly thick. How-

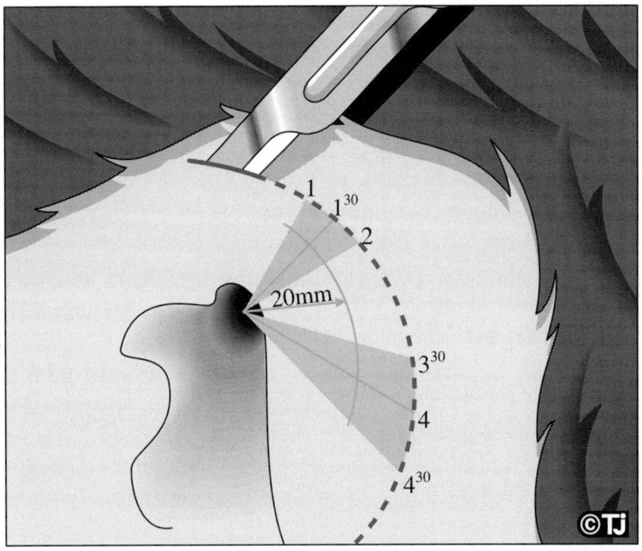

FIGURE 18–1. The position of the ideal implant sites is marked in relation to the external ear canal opening on this left side defect.

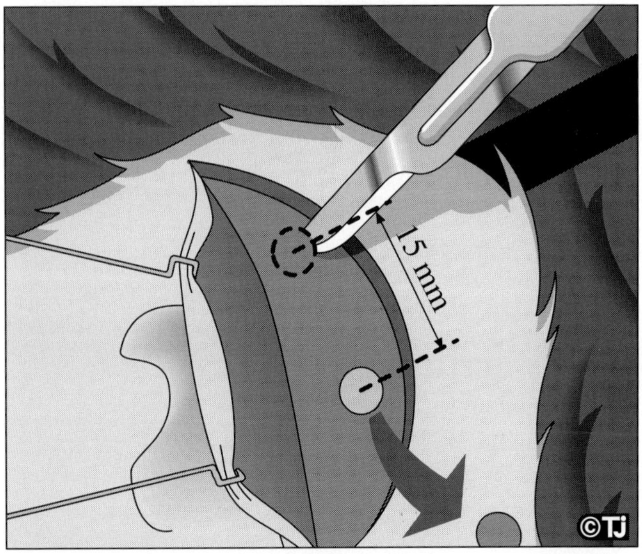

FIGURE 18–2. The skin flap has been elevated, and 6-mm wide holes in the periosteum are made.

ever, above the linea temporalis the bone can be very thin, especially in patients with defects due to congenital malformations.

The drilling starts with a cutting-guide drill made of steel, which is 2 mm in diameter (Fig. 18–3). These drills have shields that allow the drill to penetrate 3 or 4 mm. During all drilling adequate cooling is essential to reduce tissue trauma. An osteocyte can stand a temperature of 44° to 47°C for only 1 minute, and if the inevitable trauma to the bone tissue is too extensive, there is a risk that healing will result in fibrous tissue encapsulation instead of bony contact. During this drilling the hole is widened slightly to gain a good view of the bottom of the implant site. This is important to avoid damaging the wall of the sigmoid sinus or the dura of the middle cranial fossa. Widening the hole also allows the cooling fluid to reach the place where the cutting really takes place.

The next step is also performed with a stainless steel drill. A spiral drill with a countersink will give the implant site its final and exact diameter and direction before tapping takes place (Fig. 18–4). The drill speed during these first two steps is 2000 to 3000 revolutions per minute (rpm).

At this time the surgeon changes to titanium components and to low speed (15 to 20 rpm). The tap comes sterile-packed in a glass cylinder. The cylinder is broken, and the tap is placed in the titanium organizer. It is important not to touch the tap with the gloved hand or anything else except titanium-clad instruments. A stainless steel adapter is placed in the low-speed hand-piece, and the tap is picked up from the organizer. The tapping procedure starts by locating the tap immediately over the prepared hole in the bone (Fig. 18–5). It is important to achieve the correct angle when starting the tapping; if not, the tap could get stuck, and tissue trauma will increase. This may not be as important in the

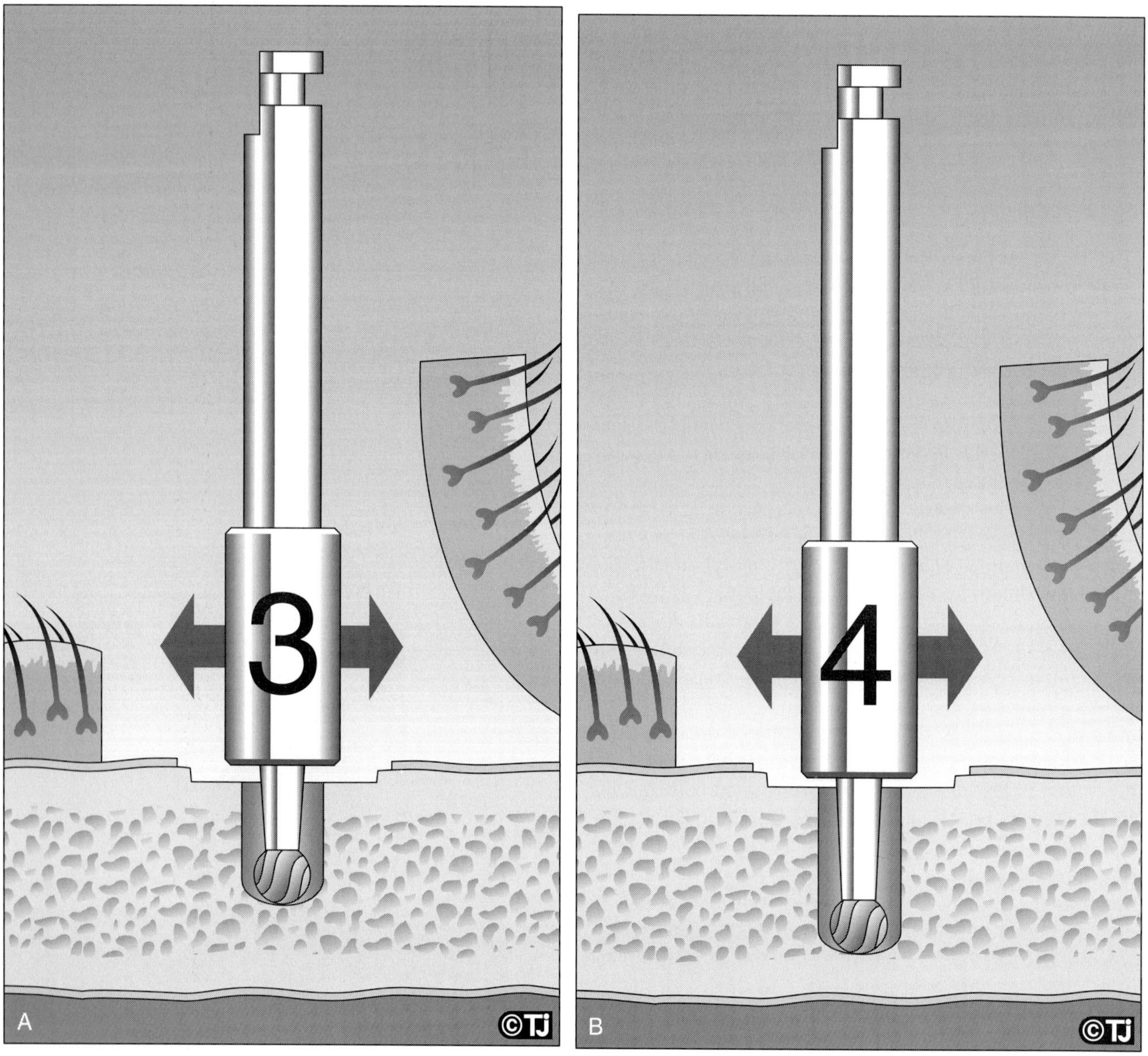

FIGURE 18–3. *A* and *B*, The drilling is started with a guide drill with a protecting shield, which allows only 3 or 4 mm of penetration.

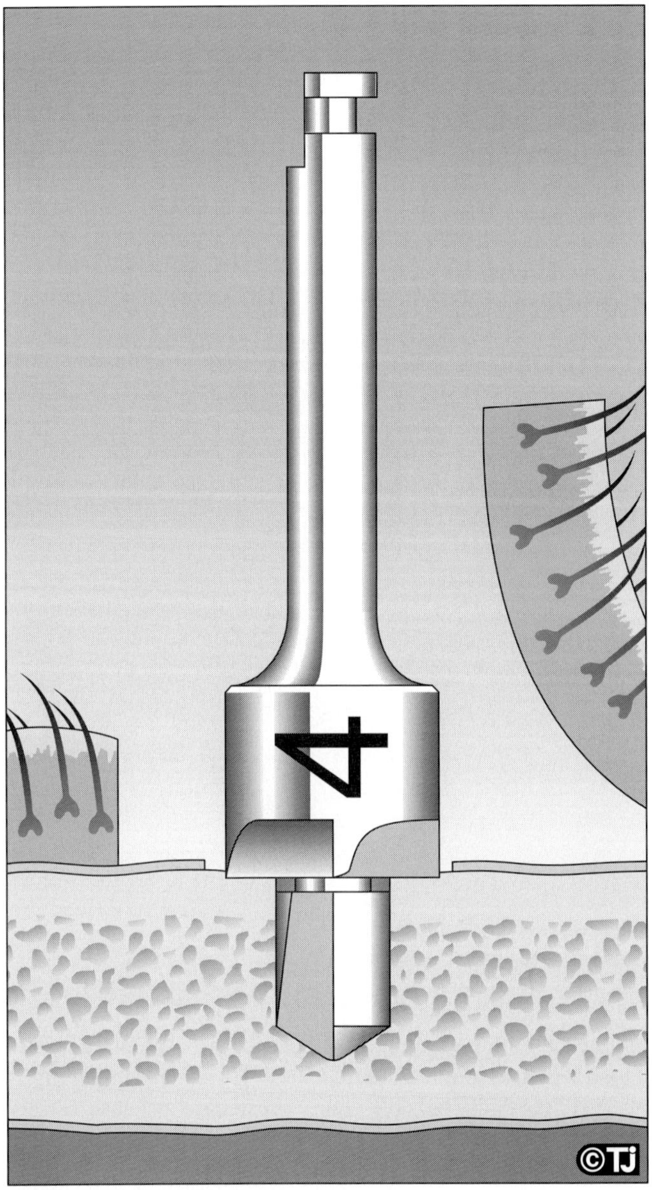

FIGURE 18–4. A spiral drill with countersink will give the final diameter and direction of the implant site.

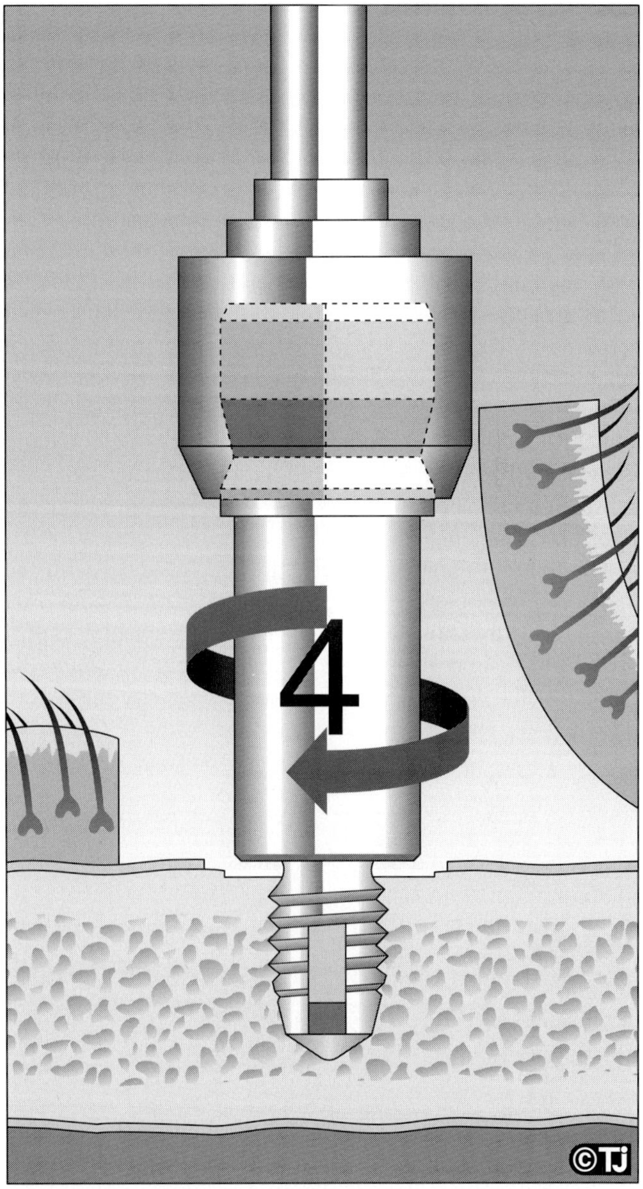

FIGURE 18–5. The titanium tap is picked up with a connector fitted on the low speed hand-piece. Tapping is made with 8 to 15 rpm.

good-quality cortical bone of the mastoid as in irradiated orbital bone. When the tapping is done the grooves on the side of the tap are cleaned of bone fragments with a titanium needle, and the tap is replaced in the organizer ready for the second hole.

The implant, the fixture, also comes sterile-packed in a glass cylinder. When the cylinder is broken it should be kept vertical and over the titanium organizer. If this is not done, the short fixture could easily be dislodged and dropped on the cloth, in which case it could not be used before being properly cleaned according to a fairly complicated procedure, including the use of strong chemical baths and ultrasonic vibrations. The titanium fixture is placed in the titanium organizer with titanium-clad tweezers. A titanium fixture mount is picked up with a fork-shaped instrument (Fig. 18–6). The internal screw of the fixture mount is then secured to the fixture, thus avoiding contact of the fixture with anything but titanium instruments. When the fixture is secured to the mount it is important to tighten the internal screw according to the quality of the bone. In the normal adult mastoid bone this tightening may be fairly hard; if it is not, the hexagon on the top of the fixture could be damaged because the cpTi is soft. In the soft bone of a child tightening should be less firm to avoid damaging the bone at the implant site when removing the mount from the implant.

The fixture mount with the fixture is picked up with the low-speed hand-piece and kept above the prepared hole (Fig. 18–7). The direction is checked, and the implant is introduced with a light pressure. When the implant has found the threads of the hole no pressure is needed because the fixture will find its way by itself. When the fixture is down the engine will stop automatically because it is torque-adjusted. The adapter is removed (Fig. 18–8). If manual tightening is needed it should be done with great care because a very high torque can be reached with the ratchet wrench (Fig. 18–9). A high torque on insertion will result in tension on the bone tissue, which could interfere with the microcirculation at the interface. In soft bone it is important to maintain a low torque because otherwise the threads in the bone could be damaged. When the implant is down the screw of the fixture mount is loosened, and the fixture mount is removed.

If a two-stage procedure is scheduled, the internal threaded hole of the fixture is protected with a cover screw (Fig. 18–10). The skin flap is sutured in place, and a normal mastoid dressing is applied for one day (Fig. 18–11). The second stage is then delayed for 3 to 6 months. However, in most cases it is possible to continue directly to make the

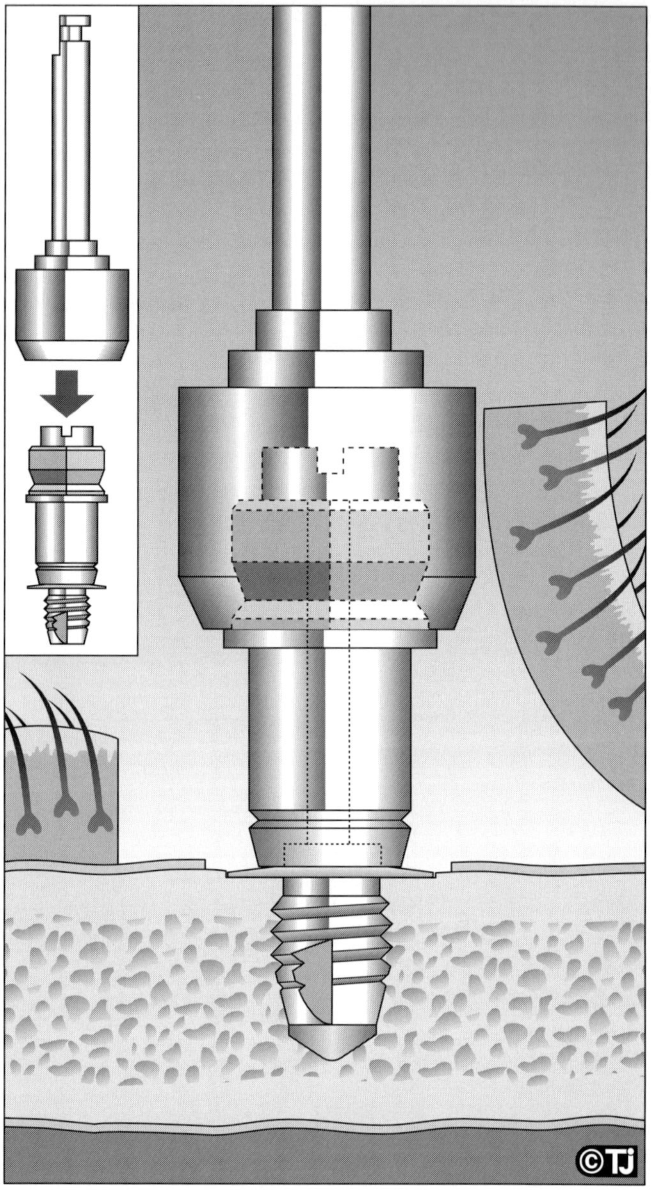

FIGURE 18–7. The mount with fixture is picked up with the adapter of the hand-piece. The fixture is thus never touched by the surgeon.

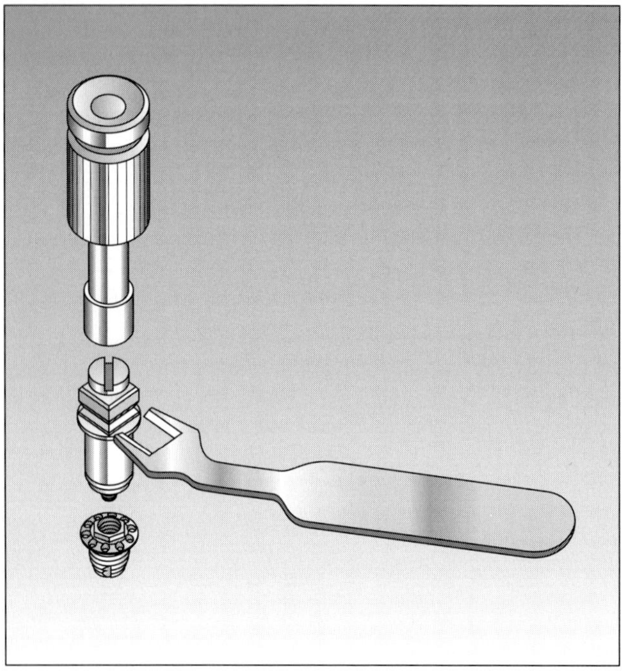

FIGURE 18–6. The implant, the fixture, is secured to the mount with an internal screw.

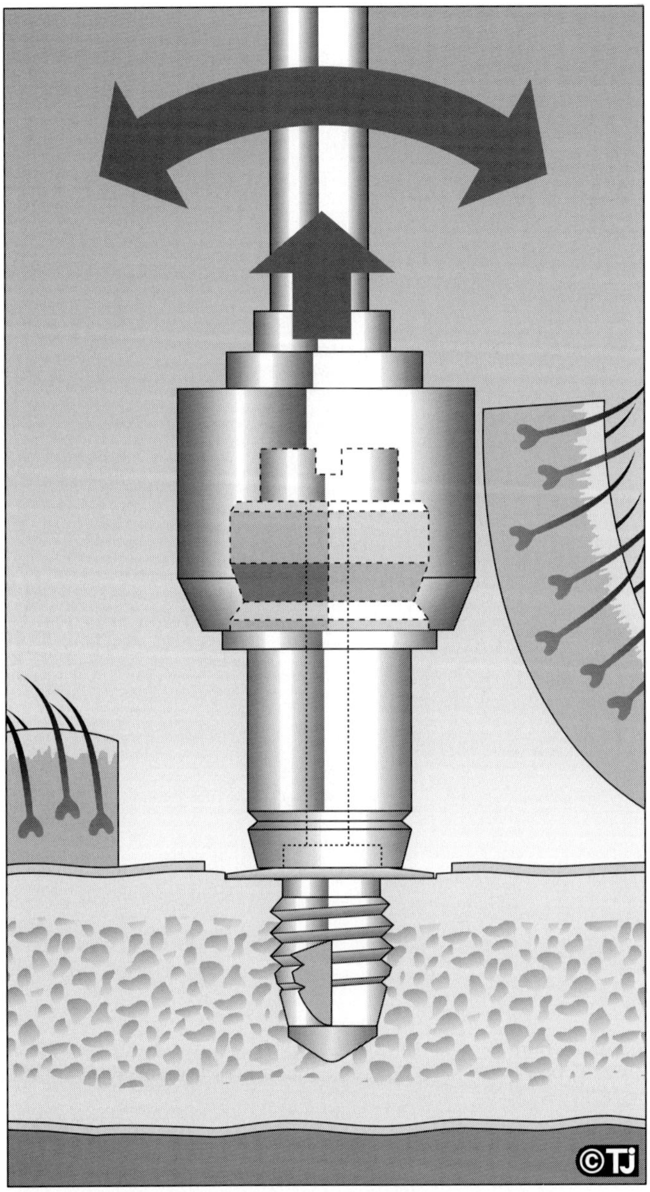

FIGURE 18–8. When the fixture is seated the adapter is released from the mount by turning the hand-piece slightly counterclockwise.

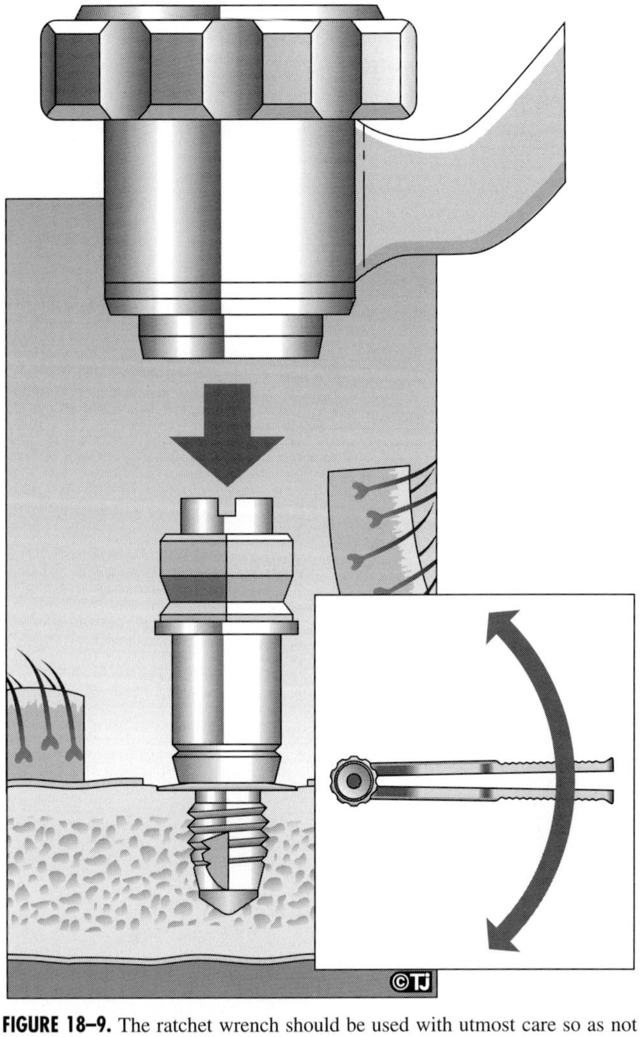

FIGURE 18–9. The ratchet wrench should be used with utmost care so as not to induce excessive trauma to the bone tissue.

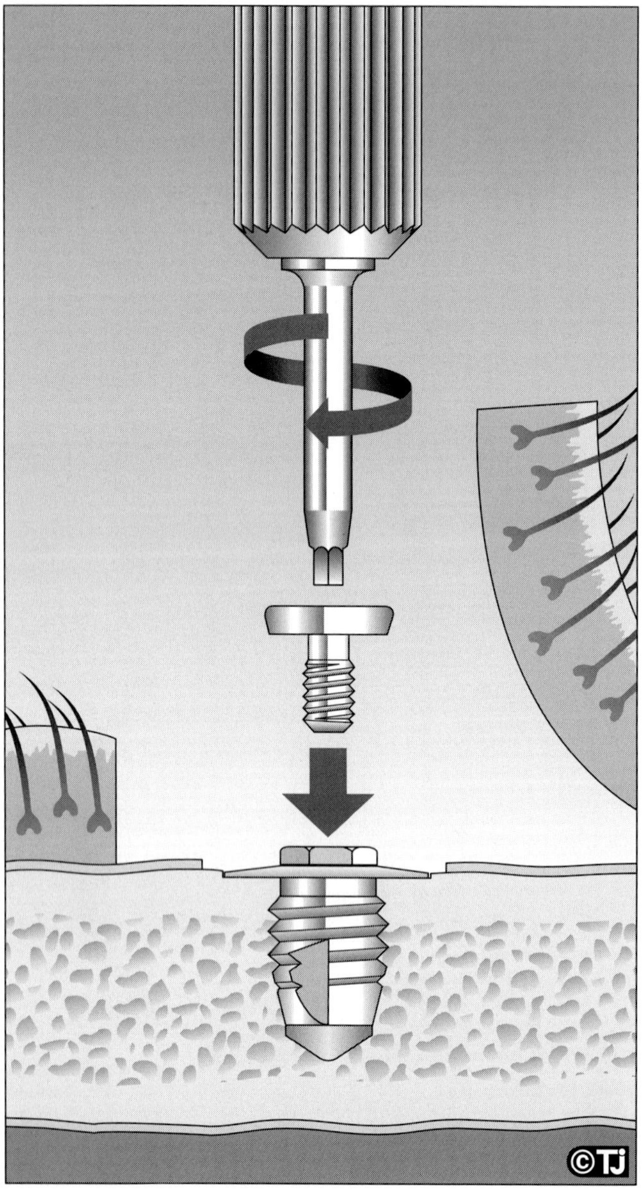

FIGURE 18–10. On a two-stage procedure a cover screw is placed to protect the internal threading and the hexagon of the fixture.

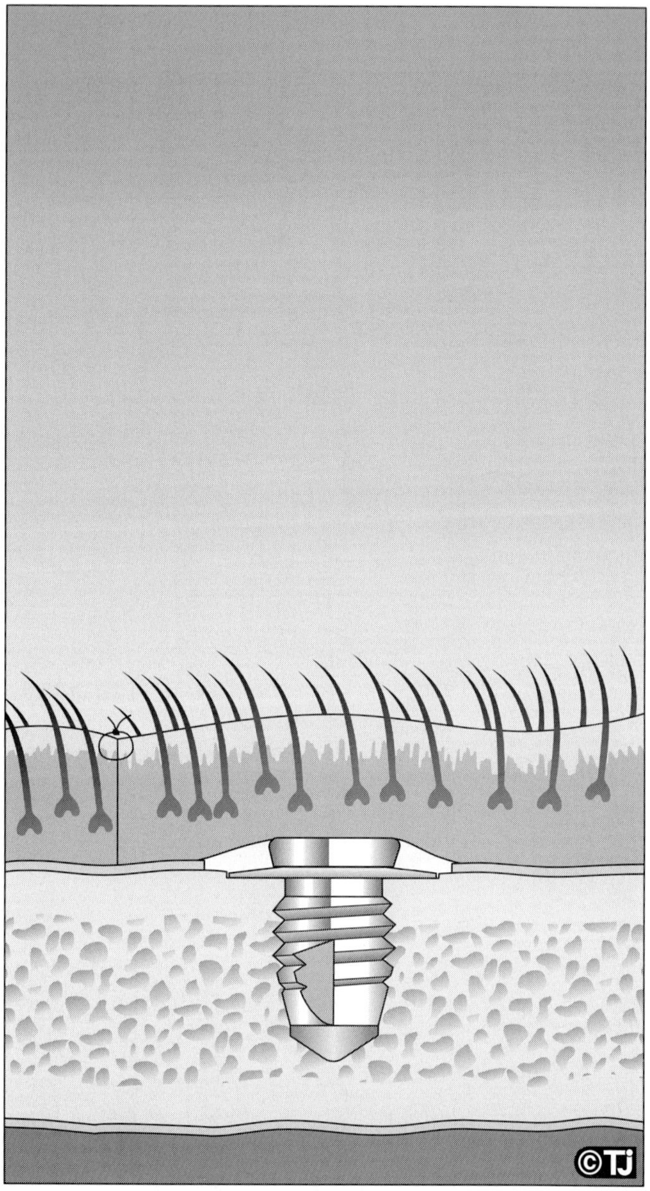

FIGURE 18–11. The skin flap is put in place.

skin penetration. To minimize the risk of later skin irritation there are two prerequisites. Movement at the interface between the skin and the implant should be minimized as much as possible. This is achieved by performing a subcutaneous tissue reduction (Fig. 18–12). Either the flap can be thinned out extremely or a split-thickness skin graft can be placed over the implants. The size of this thinned area should be at least 10 mm from the implants, and the edges of the surrounding tissue should slope gently down toward this area. The second prerequisite to avoid hair follicles at the implant site. In thinning the flap or harvesting a thin graft with a dermatome this goal can often be achieved at the same time (Fig. 18–13). This hairless situation will facilitate the most important daily cleaning routines.

When the flap or graft has been sutured in place, holes are made over the fixtures with a dermatologist's disposable punch 4 mm in diameter (Fig. 18–14). Two 4-mm-long skin-penetrating abutments are secured to the fixtures (Fig. 18–15). Two plastic healing caps are screwed onto the abutments. These caps serve to keep an ointment-soaked gauze patch down, protecting the site from postoperative hematoma and swelling (Fig. 18–16). Finally an ordinary mastoid dressing is applied until the next day, when it is removed; only a light patch is needed after this. The patient very seldom has any postoperative pain. Some experience numbness in and around the surgical area depending on how wide an area was subjected to subcutaneous tissue reduction.

Five to seven days later the healing caps are temporarily removed, and the gauze is taken off. The area is cleaned, and every second stitch can often be removed. The healing caps are put back, and a new gauze patch is placed for another 5 to 7 days, after which the gauze and the caps are permanently removed, and the remaining stitches are removed. The patient is asked to clean the area gently with soap and water every day. A mild antibiotic ointment is prescribed to be used should there be any minor irritation. Some patients do not need to use any ointment at all, whereas some use it more routinely. Patients find their own everyday treatment protocol that best suits their individual needs.

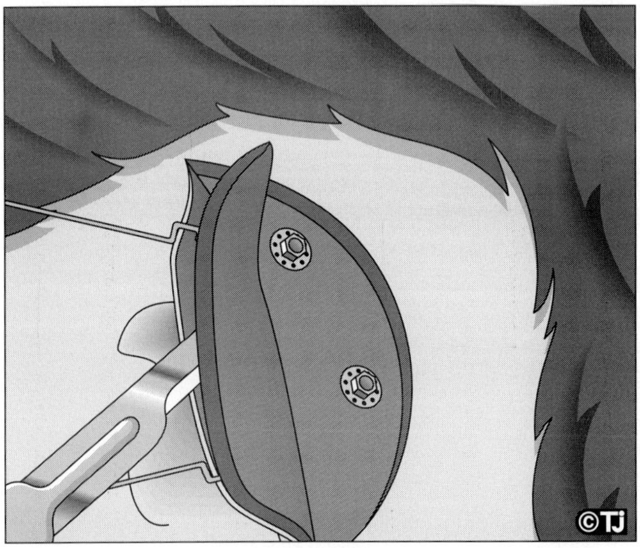

FIGURE 18–12. If a one-stage procedure is performed, or at the second stage, the flap is thinned out.

Three to four months after surgery the implants often have been integrated so well that it is possible to load them without losing them. At this time the swelling of the soft tissues has often disappeared, and the prosthodontist or anaplastologist can start to make the prosthesis by taking an impression of the defect area with the implants (Figs. 18–17, 18–18, and 18–19). This procedure and the steps following it are described in Chapter 20.

IMPLANTS IN IRRADIATED TISSUE

Implants in irradiated tissue present a special problem.[13] Soft tissue and calcified tissue react differently on irradiation. In soft tissue the reaction is often apparent early as a dermatitis or mucositis due to the sensitivity of tissue with a high cellular turnover. This reaction often becomes less pronounced after some months. The reaction of hard tissue is completely different and has a much longer time perspective. In hard tissue vasculitis is often seen with fibrosis, demineralization, and an increased risk of bone infection and ultimate necrosis. Due to the poor blood supply in bone, infections are often of long-standing and are hard to treat. This deterioration of bone quality continues as time goes on, and there seems to be no time at which this deterioration levels off. Time is thus a most important factor in the patient who receive radiotherapy. The dosage also influences the reaction in bone tissue toward an implant and consequently the survival of that implant. Osteoradionecroses is not as common with doses of less than 49 Gy compared with those of more than 65 Gy. Superfractionation causes more damage to bone tissue than normal fractionation. Low-energy irradiation is likewise more deleterious than high-energy irradiation such as that delivered with cobalt devices.

To overcome these problems hyperbaric oxygen (HBO) therapy has been introduced in the treatment protocol. The rationale for this is the knowledge that irradiated bone is hypoxic.[14] By placing the patient in an HBO chamber the oxygen tension in the bone tissue can be increased to about 80% of the value of nonirradiated bone. The following protocol has been used. The patient is placed in the HBO chamber, and the pressure is increased to 2.5 atmospheres. Once a day for 20 days pure oxygen is presented through a face mask for 90 minutes. Implant surgery is performed on day 21. The day after surgery the patient continues with another ten treatments according to the same protocol

The issue of how to handle patients who already have implants and must be iradiated is of special concern. The tissue in front of the implant will receive an increased dosage due to the backscatter effect, whereas the tissue behind will

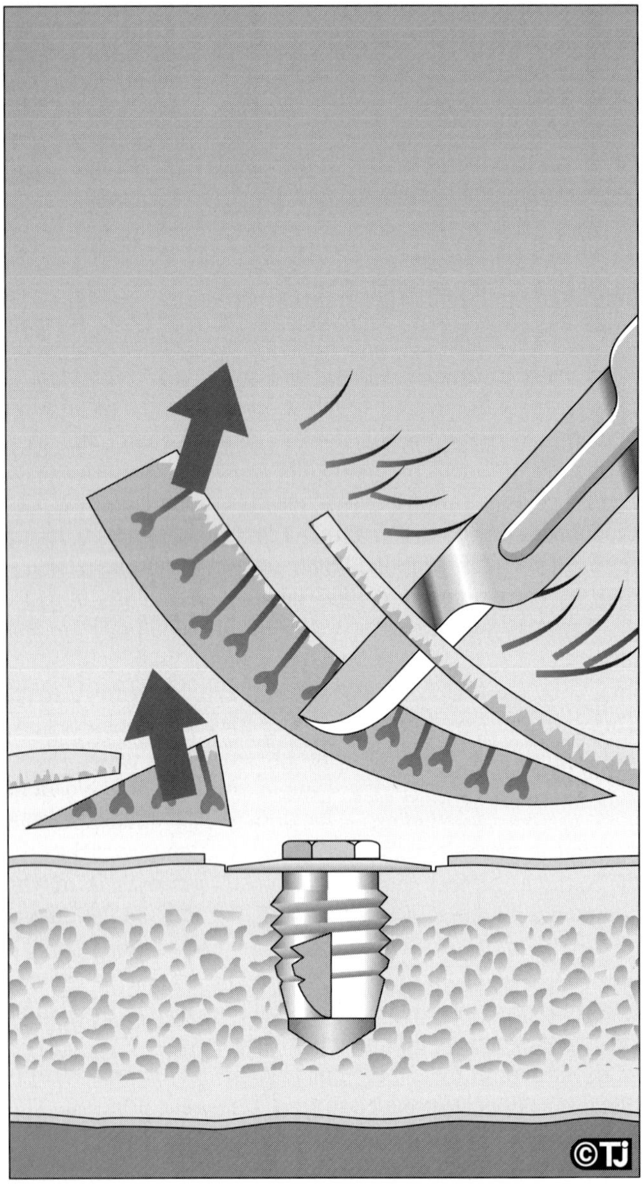

FIGURE 18–13. All hair follicles at the implant site should be removed.

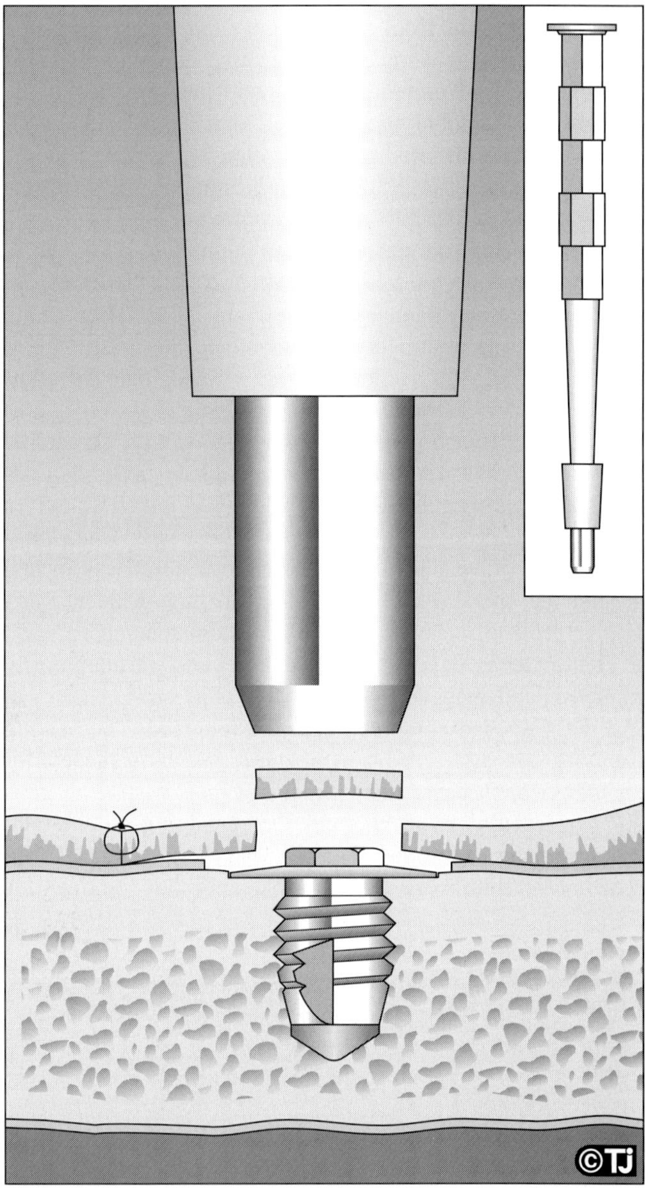

FIGURE 18–14. A hole is made with a punch in the hairless thin skin flap.

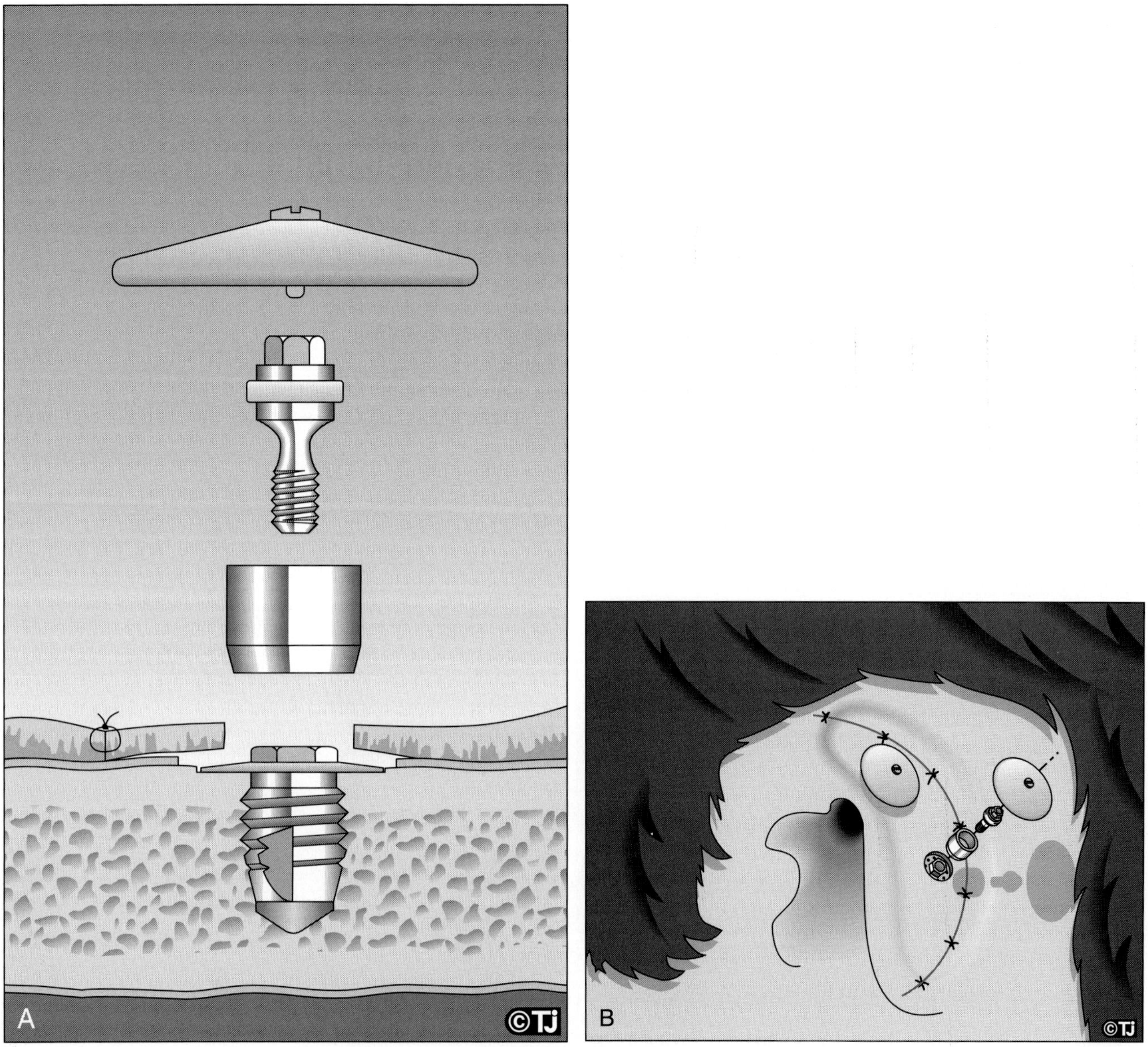

FIGURE 18–15. *A* and *B,* Plastic healing caps are put in place.

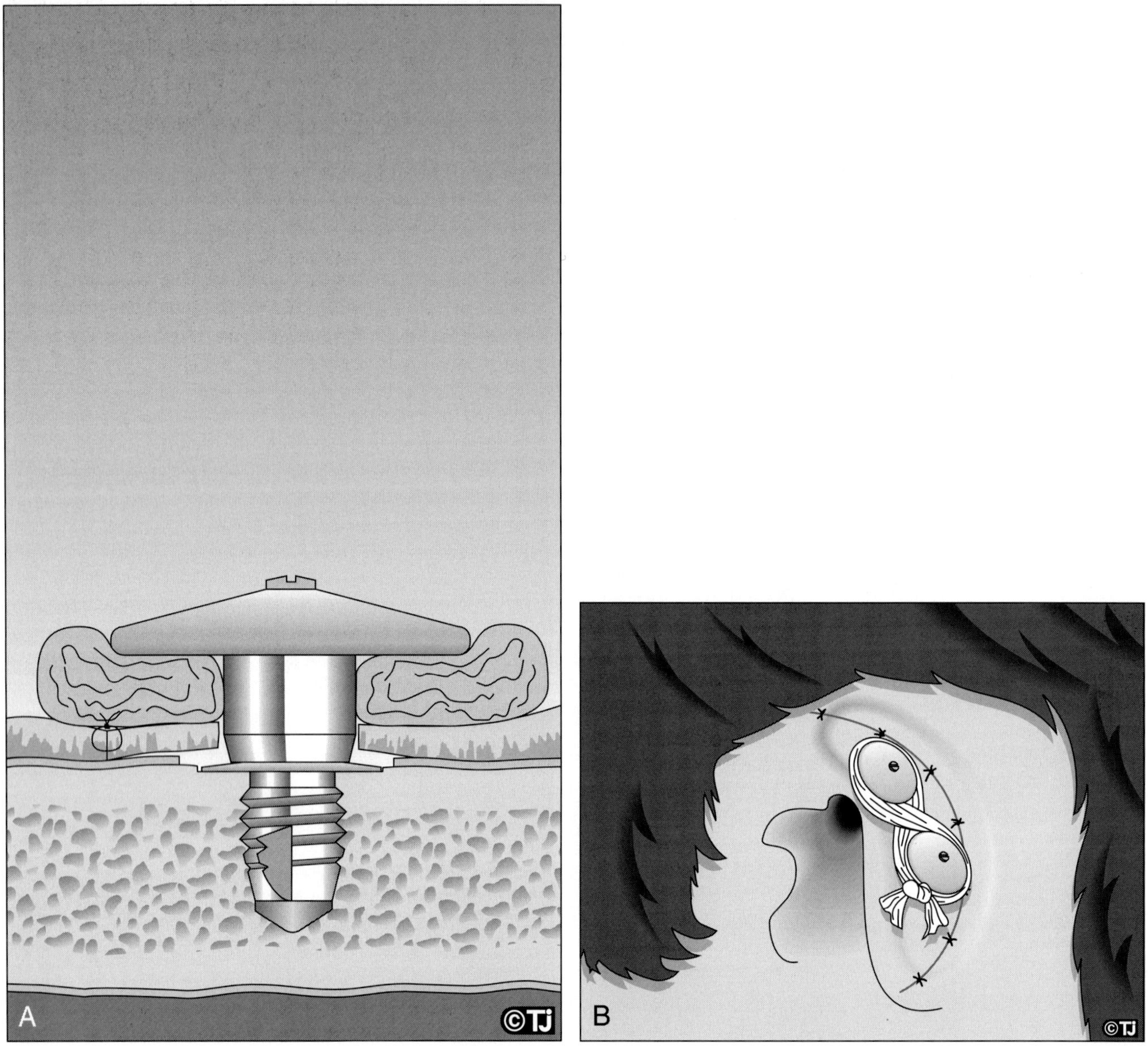

FIGURE 18–16. *A* and *B,* An ointment-soaked gauze protects from postoperative hematoma and swelling.

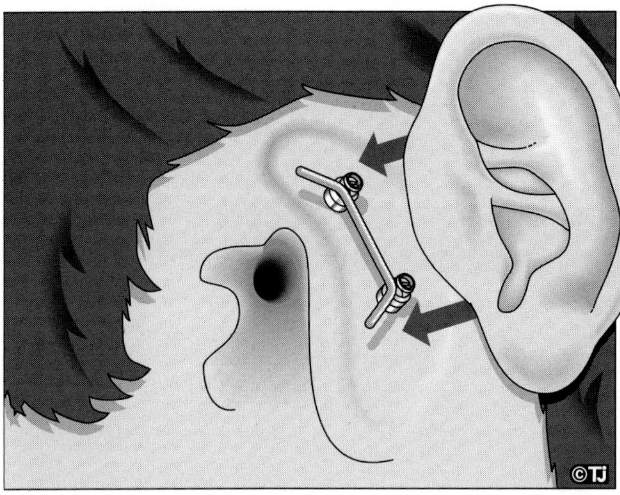

FIGURE 18–17. Three to four months after implant surgery, a bar construction is made and attached to the percutaneous implants. The external ear is sculptured.

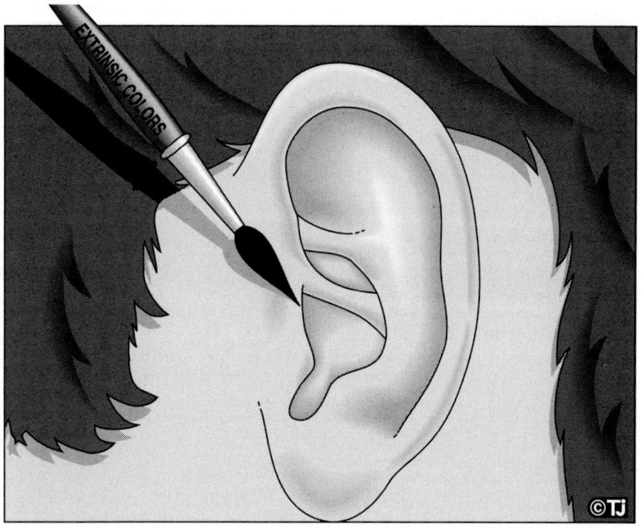

FIGURE 18–19. Most of the coloration is intrinsic, but a final touch with extrinsic coloration could be made to perfect the appearance.

receive a lower dose due to the shadow effect of the implants. The degree of these effects depends on the size of the implant and the atomic number of the implant material. Because titanium is a light metal the effect will, however, be relatively small, and it has been estimated that the backscatter effect of an implant made of cpTi will increase the dosage by 10% 0 to 3 mm from the implant. The shadow effect will be of the same magnitude.[14]

In this group of patients the authors have noted an increased frequency of adverse skin reactions. The clinical routine is thus to remove the superstructures and cover the bony implants with a not too thin flap or graft. Healing is allowed to take place for 2 to 3 weeks before irradiation therapy is started. The new abutments can generally be fitted 6 months after termination of irradiation.[14]

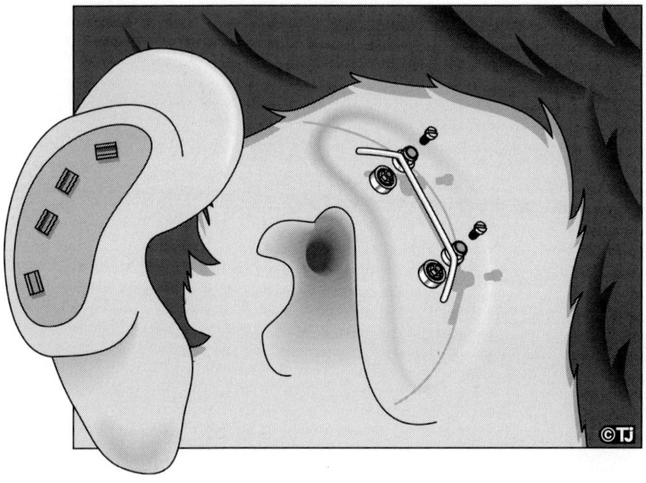

FIGURE 18–18. The fitting side of the prosthesis is shown with the retention clips in the acrylic base plate.

REFERENCES

1. Conroy B: The history of facial prostheses. Clin Plast Surg 10:701, 1983.
2. Bubulian AH: Facial Prostheses. Philadelphia, WB Saunders, 1945.
3. Jani RM, Schaaf NG: An evaluation of facial prostheses. J Prosthet Dent 39:546, 1945.
4. Brånemark PI, Hansson BO, Adell R, et al: Osseointegrated implants in the treatment of the edentulous jaw. Experience from a 10-year period. Sand J Plast Reconstr Surg 16 (Suppl):1–132, 1977.
5. Albrektsson T, Brånemark PI, Hansson BO: Osseointegrated titanium implants: Requirements for a long-lasting, direct bone-to-implant anchorage in man. Acta Orthop Scand 52:155, 1981.
6. Worthington P, Brånemark PI (eds): Advanced Osseointegration Surgery: Applications in the Maxillofacial Region. Chicago, Quintessence Publishing, 1992.
7. Johansson C, Albrektsson T: Integration of screw implants in the rabbit. A 1-year follow up of removal torque of titanium implants. Int J Oral Maxillofac Implants 2:69, 1987.
8. Aspenberg P, Goodman S, Toksvig-Larsen S, et al: Intermittent micro motion inhibits bone in growth. Acta Othop Scand 63:141, 1992.
9. Wennerberg A: On surface roughness and implant incorporation. Thesis, Göteborg University, Göteborg, Sweden, 1996.
10. Granström GPB, Tjellström A: Guided tissue generation in the temporal bone. Ann Otol Rhinol Laryngol 1996.
11. Adell R, Lekholm U, Rockler B, Brånemark PI: A 15-year study of osseointegrated implants in the treatment of the edentulous jaw. Int Oral Surg 10:387, 1981.
12. Tjellström A, Granström G: One-stage procedure to establish osseointegration. A zero to five years follow-up report. J Laryngol Otol 109:593, 1995.
13. Granström G: The use of hyperbaric oxygen to prevent implant fixture loss in the irradiated patient. *In* Worthington P, Brånemark PI. (eds): Advanced Osseointegration Surgery. Chicago, Quintessence Publishing, 1992.
14. Granström G, Tjellström A, Brånemark PI, et al: Bone-anchored reconstruction of the irradiated head and neck cancer patient. Otolaryngol Head Neck Surg 108(4):334, 1993.

CHAPTER 19

Maxillofacial Prosthetics

Glenn E. Turner, D.M.D., M.S.D.
Nicholas J. Cassisi, D.D.S., M.D.

The treatment of cancer can no longer be undertaken unilaterally but must be multidisciplinary in nature. This "team" concept includes surgeons, radiation oncologists, medical oncologists, pathologists, imagers, general dentists, and maxillofacial prosthodontists. To "cure" a patient of head and neck cancer is no longer enough because function, cosmetics, and quality of life are equally important.

In general, surgical reconstruction is preferred by both the patient and the surgeon. Often, however, as in the case of patients undergoing maxillectomy with or without orbital exenteration or total rhinectomy, this is not possible or even desired. In these cases the maxillofacial prosthodontist is an invaluable member of the team. As a general rule, dentists who have not had specialized training in maxillofacial prosthetics do not have the expertise to help these patients, and such patients require a tremendous amount of postoperative follow-up.

PREOPERATIVE PLANNING AND PREPARATION

After a work-up has been completed and a treatment plan formulated that includes a need for a maxillofacial prosthesis, the patient should be seen by the prosthodontist so that he or she can identify the extent of the lesion, make some impressions, and offer some preoperative counseling. Prior to surgery a planning conference that includes the surgeon and the maxillofacial prosthodontist is held to determine the extent of resection, the teeth that are to be saved, if any, and the best method of securing the temporary prosthesis at the time of surgery. The prosthetic device is then constructed and is placed by the maxillofacial prosthodontist at the time of surgery. Any corrections that may be necessary are made at the operating table.

MAXILLOFACIAL PROSTHESES

Most patients generally prefer surgical reconstruction with autogenous grafts to a prosthesis. A prosthesis will not function as well as the patient's own tissue. However, in some situations a prosthetic device is the treatment of choice. The most common benefits of a prosthesis are: (1) It allows early detection of recurrences because the prosthesis can be removed to examine the defect; (2) elderly patients who are medically compromised may not be able to endure the increased operating time or the multiple surgical procedures that may be required to reconstruct the defect with tissue; and (3) radiation therapy, when used, increases the risk of complications associated with reconstruction and may preclude successful surgical reconstruction. Today, many patients require postoperative radiation therapy following cancer surgery. These are a few of the conditions in which a prosthesis is the treatment of choice.

The key to successful prosthetic reconstruction is coordinated planning between the surgeon and the prosthodontist. This planning should begin before surgery and continue during the surgical procedure.[1] Which trained professional is best qualified to work with the surgeon in planning surgical resection before and during the surgical procedure and then reconstruct the defect with artificial materials? This professional naturally comes from the discipline of dentistry. Dentists have the basic medical-dental science background to understand the pathology and the resultant disabilities that occur following ablative surgery. With the widespread use of implants to stabilize and support intraoral and extraoral prostheses, dental specialists are required to monitor these implants on a regular basis and maintain the health of the tissue surrounding the implants. Dental specialists are also able to detect any recurrence of tumor in the defect as

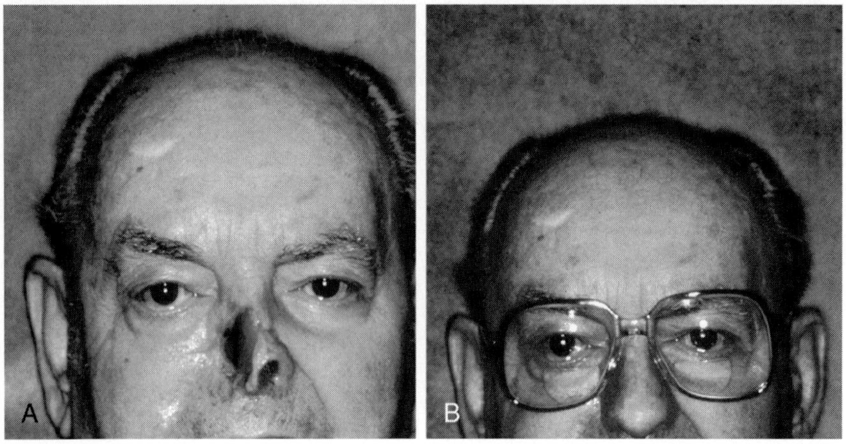

FIGURE 19–1. Partial rhinectomy. *A*, Nasal defect (see Color plate). *B*, Full face with prosthesis and eyeglasses in place (see Color plate).

well as early changes associated with osteoradionecrosis. Construction of a functional and cosmetic prosthesis requires making an accurate impression and sculpting and coloring the prosthesis in a life-like manner to match the surrounding tissue. The maxillofacial prosthodontist is the best qualified individual to provide these services. He is a dental specialist with a certificate or masters degree in prosthodontics and an additional 1-year certificate in treating patients with maxillofacial defects.

NASAL DEFECTS

Tissue left at the surgical site after subtotal and total rhinectomy procedures may be used in surgical reconstructions performed at a later date. However, these tissues frequently present problems in prosthetic reconstruction. They do not form a stable base and frequently force the prosthodontist to construct the prosthesis larger than the original anatomic structure (Figs. 19–1 and 19–2) (see Color plate). When the team, including the surgeon, prosthodontist, and patient, have decided prior to surgery that prosthetic reconstruction is the preferred method, surgical guidelines should be applied at the time of the primary surgery. Use of this team approach reduces the number of operations needed for reconstruction. The patient is always reluctant to undergo secondary procedures for prosthetic reconstruction. With the increasing use of radiation therapy there is not time for secondary procedures before such radiation therapy begins, and they are frequently contraindicated after radiation therapy.

Once the nasal lesion has been surgically excised, the alae, columella, anterior portion of the nasal septum, and the nasal bones should be removed even if the tumor does not extend into these structures. Care should be taken to avoid distortion of the adjacent facial contours.[2] Figure 19–2*A* shows an 80-year-old patient who was treated with high-dose radiation therapy. The nasal bones, alae, and nasal septum are still present. Although a prosthesis was constructed (Fig. 19–2*B*), it was too large and thin in the area of the nasal bones, too thin over the nasal septum, and too wide at the inferior border, since it must cover the alae. The nasolabial fold area has healed quite well. The following steps will improve the prosthetic results for patients with nasal defects:[2–4]

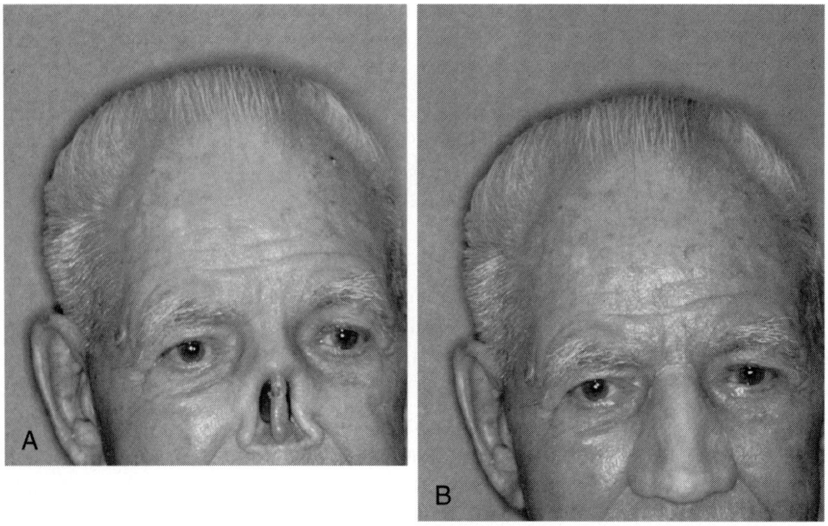

FIGURE 19–2. Rhinectomy with alae and nasal septum remaining. *A*, Full face showing defect (see Color plate). *B*, Prosthesis is too wide (see Color plate).

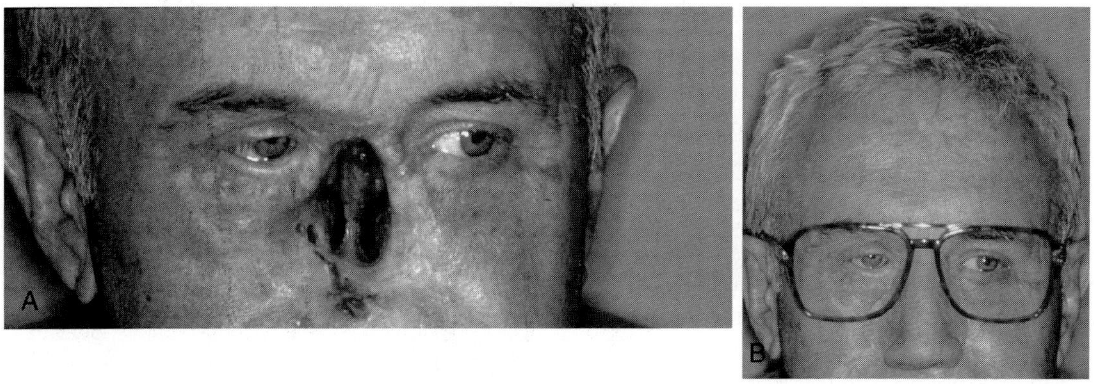

FIGURE 19–3. Good tissue base. *A*, Full face showing the defect (see Color plate). *B*, Prosthesis in place with eyeglasses (see Color plate).

1. The nasal bones should be removed.
2. Split-thickness skin grafts prevent displacement or distortion of the upper lip.
3. Primary closure of margins should be avoided because of the possibility of distorting the midfacial contours.
4. Distortion of the nasolabial folds should be avoided when these are uninvolved by tumor.
5. The nasal septum is trimmed back when a total rhinectomy is performed.
6. The anterior nasal spine is preserved when it is not involved with tumor.

In Figure 19–3 (see Color plate) the defect is well designed, and the prosthesis is proportional to the patient's face. The bridge of the nose is of normal size, and the eyeglasses fit well. The eyeglasses also cover the superior half of the nasolabial folds. The upper lip has a split-thickness skin graft that prevents its distortion (Fig. 19–3*A*). The anterior nasal spine was preserved and the nasal septum was resected; therefore, the inferior portion of the prosthesis has adequate support. Since the alae were removed, the tip of the prosthesis has normal width (Fig. 19–3*B*).

ORBITAL DEFECTS

Restoration of an orbital defect presents a special problem. The normal eye moves constantly, whereas the artificial eye is fixed; the eyelids do not move, and the gaze does not change direction. The orbital prosthesis can be camouflaged by means of eyeglass frames. The cosmetic success of an orbital prosthesis differs, however, from that of a nasal or auricular prosthesis. All three prostheses appear natural in a photograph; in real life, however, ear and nasal prostheses appear life-like, but orbital prostheses may not.

The orbital prosthesis is the most difficult to construct and may be poorly accepted by the patient if the artificial eye, or ocular, does not line up accurately with the normal eye when the patient gazes straight ahead. Lack of alignment calls attention to the side with the defect because during conversation it is normal to glance at the speaker's eyes. Proper placement must be verified at the second sculpting appointment. At this appointment, placement of the ocular is again verified, and the patient is instructed to turn the head to the side when looking at an object so that the ocular tracks with the normal eye.

Before construction of the prosthesis, the patient should understand its cosmetic advantages and disadvantages. It is helpful if patients can talk with other patients who have had similar treatment. Demonstrations and audiovisual aids also are valuable.

The surgeon can greatly enhance the prosthetic result by preparing the surgical defect during the primary surgery. After consulting with the prosthodontist, the surgeon should plan to:

1. Remove the eyelids[2-4] when the orbital contents are resected (Fig. 19–4).
2. Line the orbital defect with split-thickness skin grafts.[2-4]
3. Leave the eyebrow undisturbed when possible (Fig. 19–4). Skin grafting or use of the upper lid to cover the superior bony wall should be done carefully so that scar contraction does not pull the eyebrow into the defect. This greatly alters the appearance of the defect, and the skin adhesive used to attach the prosthesis will not adhere very

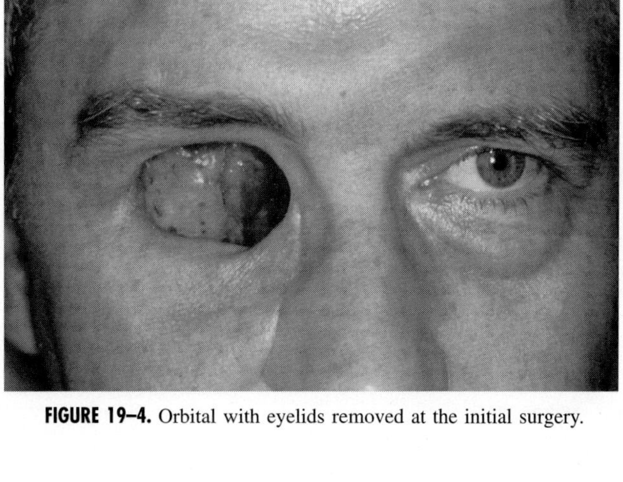

FIGURE 19–4. Orbital with eyelids removed at the initial surgery.

well to the hair follicles of the eyebrow. Surgical defects that extend into the skull base make it very difficult to hide the margins of the prosthesis (Fig. 19–5). It is understood that the surgical team may not be able to limit extension of the defect into the anterior skull base when they are establishing appropriate tumor margins.

4. Discourage pedicle grafts. The most important drawback of pedicle grafts is that they limit the ability of the surgical team to adequately visualize recurrent disease at the primary site. The prosthesis is frequently compromised owing to the reduced depth of the defect, which limits placement of the ocular prosthesis within the orbital prosthesis (Fig. 19–6).

Extraoral implants can provide support and retention for prostheses that are far superior to those achieved with skin adhesives. However, radiation therapy compromises the healing of bone around the implants. Extraoral implants placed in irradiated tissue have a much lower success rate than implants placed in nonirradiated tissue. The patient in Figure 19–6 received 5000 rads to the right orbit, and two Brånemark extraoral implants were placed 15 months after radiation therapy was completed. The supraorbital and infraorbital rims are the usual sites considered for implant placement. When a maxillectomy is performed along with orbital exenteration, the infraorbital rim is also sacrificed. In the supraorbital rim there are air cells that should be avoided when placing implants. In the patient shown in Figure 19–6, the lateral implant began to show tissue irritation after 1 year. The patient was meticulous with her implant hygiene, but 2 years after placement of the implant the tissue had broken down around the lateral implant, exposing the metal flange. This implant was rejected 3 years after placement. The tissue healed normally, and there was no evidence of osteoradionecrosis. The other implant has remained healthy and functional for more than 5 years. The patient still uses the original prosthesis, but now she places a small amount of skin adhesive on its medial aspect.

We have discussed the benefits of a team approach to surgical and prosthetic management of facial defects. The complexities of craniofacial implants used in intraoral and extraoral sites require even more coordination than before.

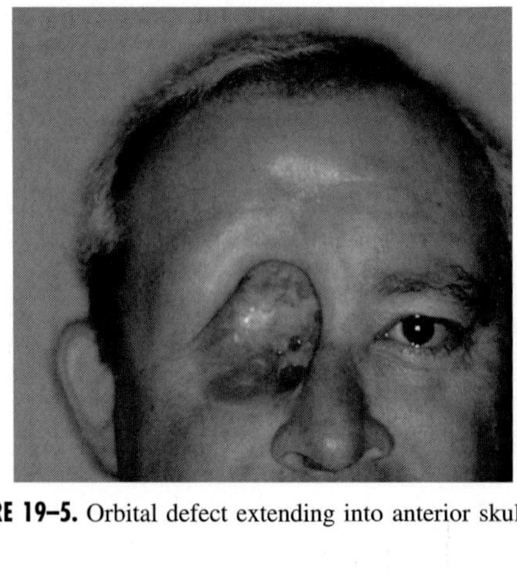

FIGURE 19–5. Orbital defect extending into anterior skull base.

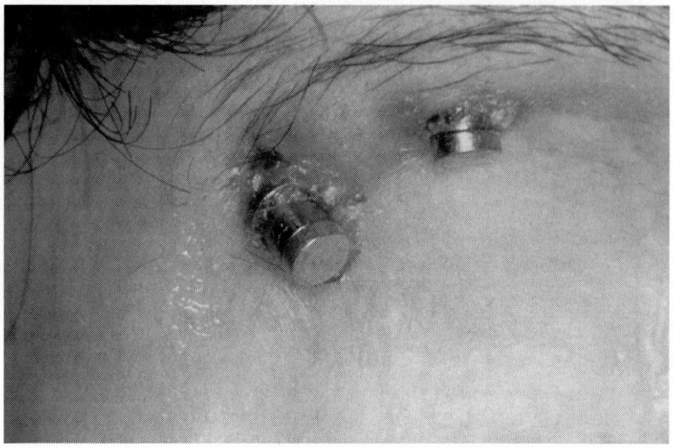

FIGURE 19–6. Orbital with implants. *A*, Defect reconstructed with a pedicle graft and tissue breakdown in radiation port.

Only multidisciplinary teams who have the clinical, scientific, and academic background to deal with this type of surgery should follow these patients over the long term to report and document the outcomes.[7]

AURICULAR DEFECTS

When the helix of the ear must be surgically excised to remove a carcinoma and a prosthesis is planned, a preoperative consultation is arranged by the surgeon with a prosthodontist. The following procedures are discussed:

1. Residual tissue tags should be removed except the tragus, which hides the anterior margin of the prosthesis.[2] Since tissue tags, including the ear lobe, provide no support or retention, it is important that the remaining tags be removed to give the auricular prosthesis a stable base. Figure 19–7*A* shows a healed surgical site in which the middle third of the auricle was removed. The superior cartilage does serve a purpose in supporting eyeglasses. However, it can be seen in Figure 19–7*B* that the superior tip is pulled away from the head owing to scar contraction. The inferior portion of the remaining cartilage is moveable and provides no support. The margins of the finished auricular prosthesis are visible at both top and bottom. Because the remaining cartilage of the ear moves slightly, the margins of the prosthesis can separate from the underlying tissue.

2. Split-thickness skin grafts without hair should be used to cover the surgical defect (Fig. 19–8*A* and *B*).

3. Scalp flaps containing hair follicles should be avoided. Skin adhesive does not stick well to hair.[4] Also, proper hygiene is difficult to maintain around such a prosthetic area because hair holds grease and bacteria in the area.

Surgical reconstruction of auricular defects with autologous tissue is usually preferred by patients because a prosthesis cannot compete with the patient's own skin for function. Surgical reconstruction of an ear is a very difficult

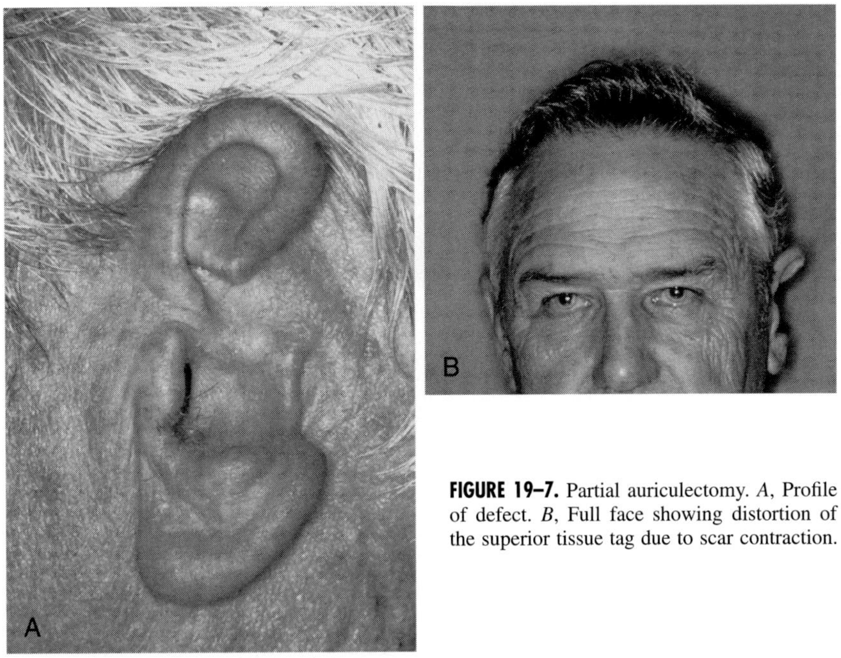

FIGURE 19–7. Partial auriculectomy. *A*, Profile of defect. *B*, Full face showing distortion of the superior tissue tag due to scar contraction.

process that requires many surgical procedures. In some situations the grafts do not retain their contour owing to a reduced blood supply from a restricted base. The patient shown in Figure 19–9 lost her ear in an auto accident. She had undergone several attempts at placing cartilage in the area, including cartilage from a rib (Fig. 19–9*A*). To place extraoral implants in this area all the residual cartilage must be removed down to the periosteum, and a very thin skin graft must be placed (Fig. 19–9*B*). The patient must be handled carefully at the evaluation appointment because both the patient and the family have invested a great deal of time and effort in the previous surgeries.

The right ear of the patient in Figure 19–10 (see Color plate) was surgically excised to remove a carcinoma. The surgeon, after consultation with the prosthodontist, created an ideal defect. In radiation therapy following surgery the superior margin of the port was placed at the level of the external auditory meatus. Implants were placed 4 months after radiation therapy. Six months after placement, the implants were uncovered, and an implant-supported prosthesis was placed (Fig. 19–10*B* and *C*).

Fourteen months after placement of the implant the patient returned for a routine follow-up visit. It was noted that the inferior implant had bloody exudate around it. The connect-

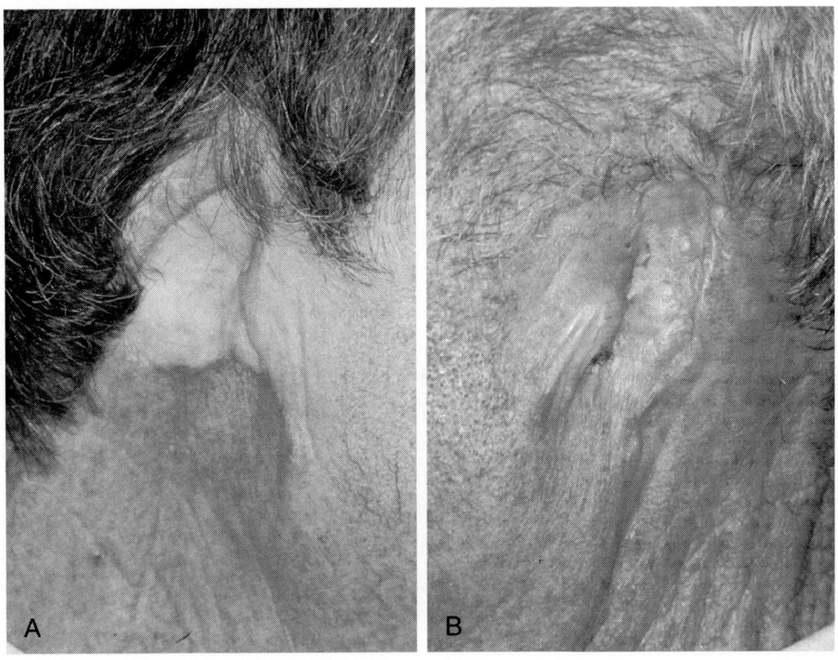

FIGURE 19–8. Split-thickness skin graft in retaining the tragus. *A*, Skin graft without hair to provide a stable base for a prosthesis. *B*, Skin graft for implants must be thin.

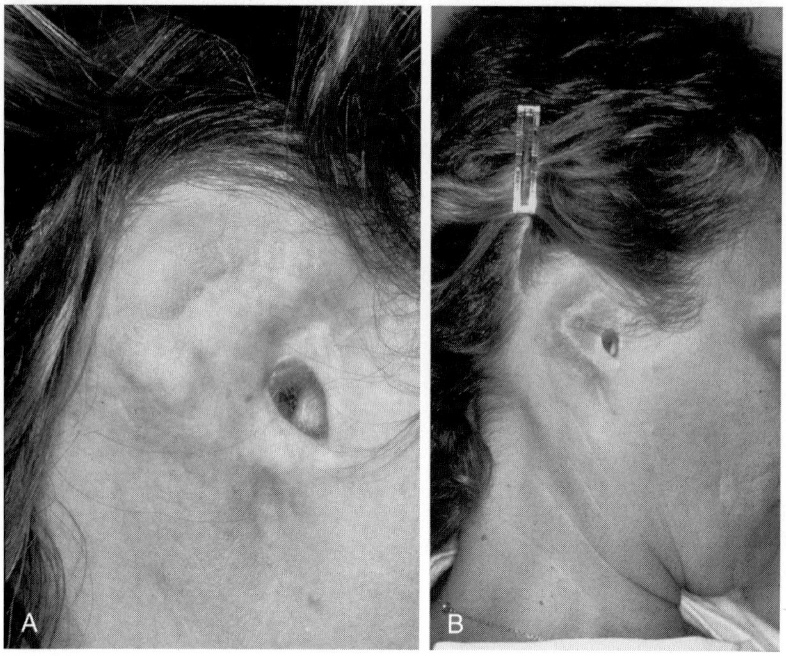

FIGURE 19–9. Attempt at surgical reconstruction following trauma. *A*, Defect with cartilage from previous surgeries *B*, Cartilage removed.

ing bar was removed, and the inferior implant easily separated from the skin. Note the granulation tissue covering the defect (Fig. 19–10*D*). There has been no evidence of osteoradionecrosis. The bar was replaced on the two implants, and the prosthesis continues to function. The plan is to redesign the bar for two implants and reconstruct the prosthesis. It has been suggested that patients who receive postoperative radiation therapy should be treated with hyperbaric oxygen prior to receiving an implant. There have been no large series showing that patients treated in this way have a lower incidence of extrusion. In general, hyperbaric oxygen should be reserved for treatment of osteoradionecrosis should it occur.

MIDFACE DEFECTS OR COMBINED INTRAORAL-EXTRAORAL DEFECTS

The high risk of tumor recurrence and a poor long-term survival rate have been the primary reasons why many head and neck surgeons prefer a prosthesis to autologous reconstruction for these patients. A prosthesis can be constructed relatively quickly. The surgical interventions needed to facilitate the use of a prosthesis can be done at the same time as the primary surgical resection. The prosthesis can be removed to inspect the cranial base for recurrent disease without the need for computed tomography or magnetic resonance imaging.[8]

Prior to primary tumor resection the surgical and prosthodontic team should consider the following:

1. All teeth should be retained provided they are not involved with surgical margins. These teeth can be used to support the combined facial and intraoral prostheses.
2. A soft tissue bed should be prepared to create undercut areas to facilitate retention.
3. Split-thickness skin grafts must be placed on the tissue bed and especially on the undercut areas in the tissue bed created for retention. The grafts prevent excessive scar contraction and possible loss of the undercut areas. Without grafts, much of the denuded tissue will become epithelialized with nonkeratinized squamous or respiratory epithelium. Nonkeratinized epithelium will not bear the pressure of a prosthesis.
4. Skin grafting of the nasal floor allows this area to be used to retain a midfacial prosthesis.
5. Osseointegrated implants are used to supply needed support for prostheses that replace a large volume of resected tissue. Implants should be placed at the time of the primary tumor resection, thereby reducing the number of surgical procedures needed for patients who are frequently medically compromised.[4]

Some sources state that small amounts of remaining upper lip are of little value. For most defects, surgical reconstruction of the upper lip is contraindicated. The reconstructed lip is frequently improperly placed posteriorly, is immobile, and restricts access to the oral cavity because of a greatly decreased circumference of the oral stoma. The decreased size of the oral stoma may prevent fabrication of an oral prosthesis. The reconstructed lip, if it contracts posteriorly, may prevent lip valving during speech and is frequently aesthetically displeasing and draws attention to the defect and the midfacial prosthesis.[2, 4]

Although reconstructing a totally resected upper lip has many problems, a small rim of the patient's lip when a surgical obturator is placed during surgery[4] supports the obturator and maintains the length of the lip. The surgical obturator retains the facial contours so that an intraoral

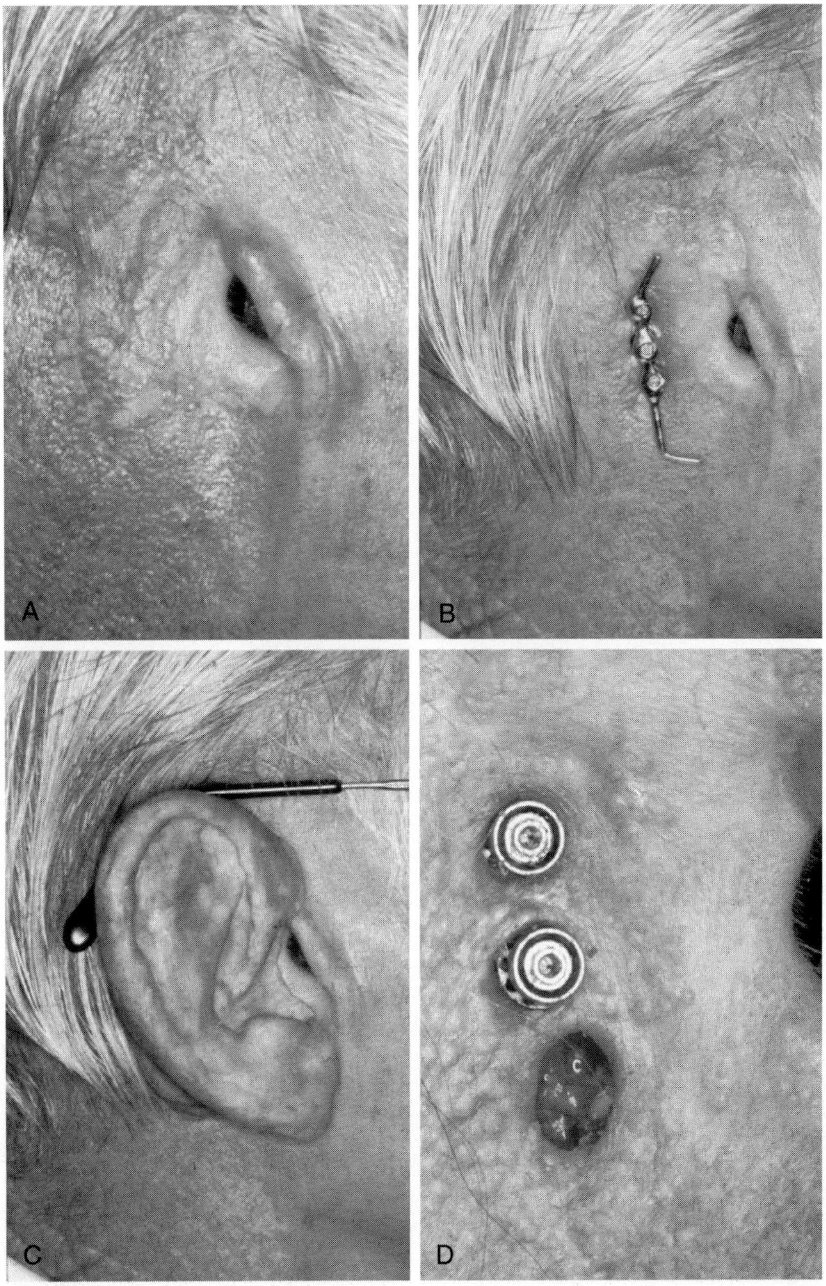

FIGURE 19–10. Excellent result following auriculectomy with a skin graft. *A*, Skin graft and tragus; radiation therapy port stopped at the level of the external auditory meatus (see Color plate). *B*, Implants and gold bar (see Color plate). *C*, Prosthesis clipped in place (see Color plate). *D*, Bar removed; inferior implant was very mobile and separated easily from the granulation tissues.

prosthesis can be fabricated later (Fig. 19–11). This remaining portion of lip is as important for support and anterior retention of an oral prosthesis as the retained teeth. A better situation would be to retain both lip and teeth, but, as in this case, that is not always possible.

The patient shown in Figure 19–12 (see Color plate) was 80 years old when she underwent bilateral maxillectomy and total rhinectomy. Figure 19–12*B* shows the two-piece prosthesis constructed for the obturator and maxillary prosthesis. Since a skin graft had not been placed on the floor of the remaining nasal cavity, the tissue on the floor of the nose would not bear the pressure of an acrylic prosthesis. Therefore, a silicone plug for the nasal cavity was constructed. The silicone plug snaps onto acrylic studs on the maxillary obturator, as shown in Figure 19–12*B*. Note that the vermilion border of the upper lip is rigidly attached to the obturator and acts like a shelf to support the facial prosthesis. All three intraoral segments are shown in place in Figure 19–12*C*. Note the positive tissue stop in the glabella area and two small horizontal studs onto which the facial prosthesis snaps. After using the prosthesis for some time the patient's speech became understandable, but eating was still difficult; however, her grandchildren would sit in her lap, whereas before they were frightened (Fig. 19–12*D*).

As stated previously, reconstruction of the upper lip with autologous tissue has many potential problems for the pros-

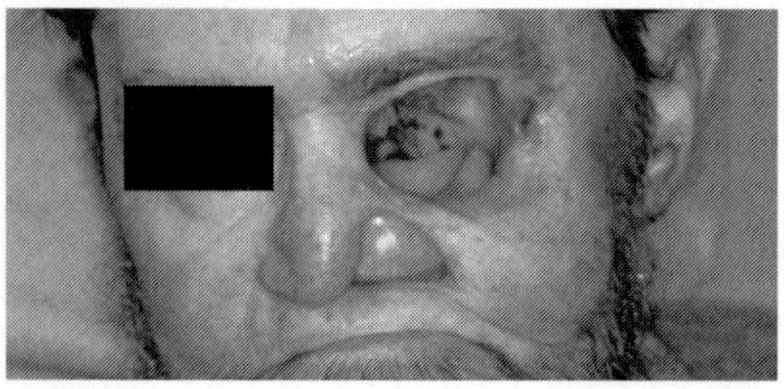

FIGURE 19–11. Rim of the lip supports the obturator.

thodontist.[2] However, prosthetic reconstruction of midface defects is very difficult when there is no lip tissue remaining to retain and support the prosthesis. As prosthodontists and surgeons plan reconstructions, they have begun to explore the use of autologous flaps and grafts, either free grafts or microvascular flaps, in conjunction with the placement of osseointegrated implants.[8, 9]

MAXILLECTOMY DEFECTS

Treatment planning includes a thorough preoperative dental evaluation and the obtainment of maxillary and mandibular impressions to determine which teeth and structures will be retained after surgery.[10] The surgeon outlines the surgical

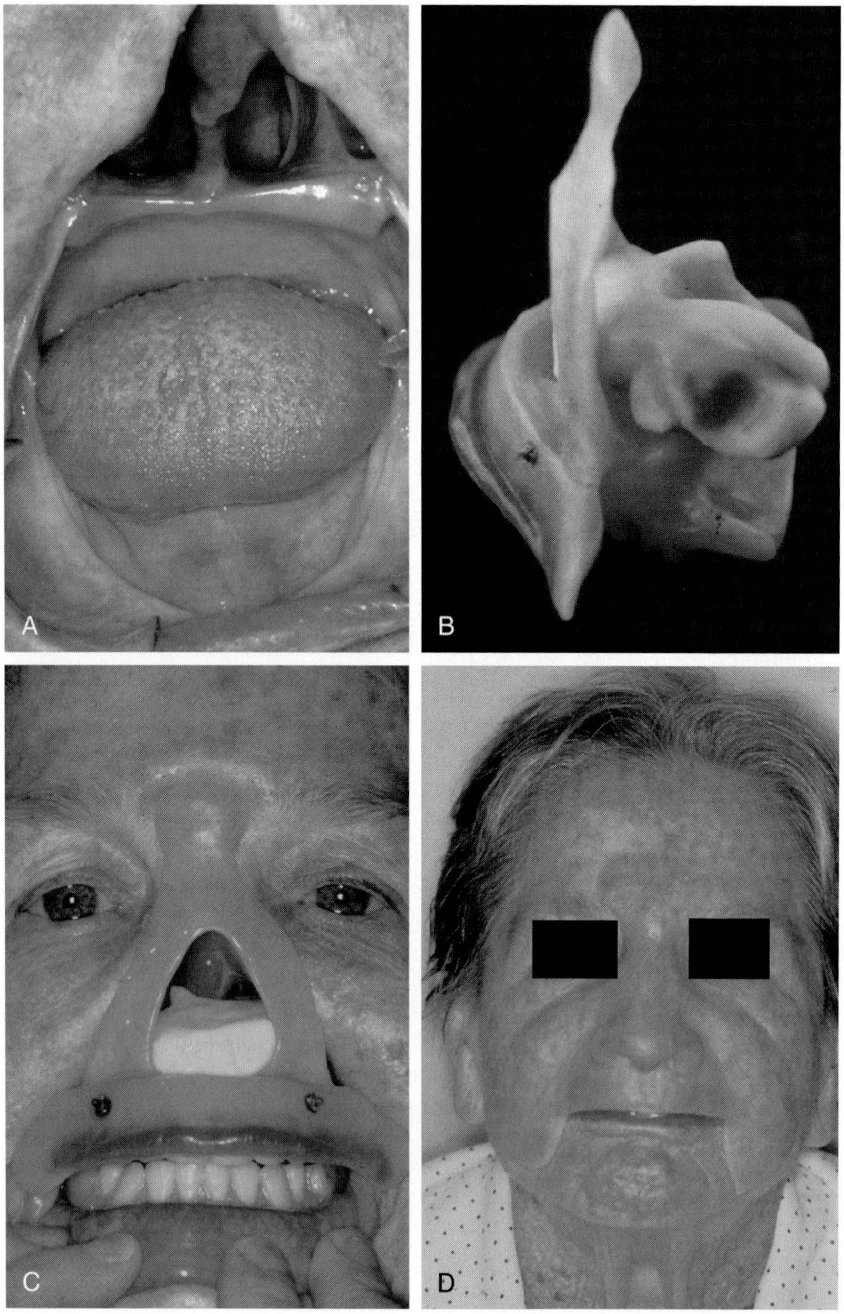

FIGURE 19–12. Bilateral maxillectomy, rhinectomy, and removal of the upper lip. *A*, Close-up of the defect. *B*, Silicone sinus bulb snapped onto obturator. *C*, Obturator in the patient's mouth; note the two horizontal projections and upper lip in acrylic to support the silicone facial prothesis (see Color plate). *D*, All prostheses in place (see Color plate).

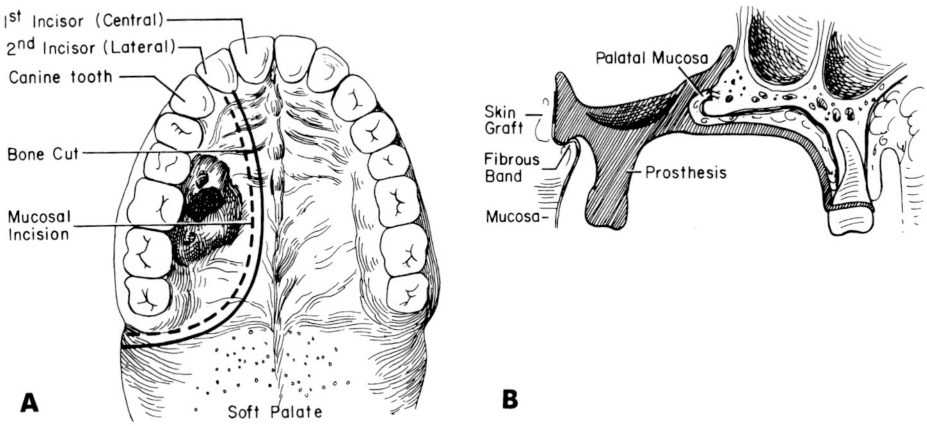

FIGURE 19–13. Diagram of surgical procedures that support the construction of a prosthesis. *A*, The mucosal incision is 4 to 5 mm lateral to the bony incision. The bone incision is placed through the socket of the extracted tooth and as far away from the retained tooth as possible. *B*, The prosthesis should be made to engage the undercut on the palatal shelf and the soft tissue of the buccal mucosa above the fibrous scar band. (From Turner G: Maxillofacial Prosthetics. Management of Head and Neck Cancer, 2nd ed. J.B. Lippincott, Co.: Philadelphia, p. 172, 1994.)

margin on a diagnostic cast of the maxilla, from which the extent of the surgical obturator is determined.

The following surgical guidelines will facilitate the use of an obturator prosthesis:

1. As much maxilla as possible should be saved within the realm of adequate margins.
2. Retention of the premaxilla improves function in both dentulous and edentulous patients. The premaxilla is the most effective site for implant placement.
3. Key teeth should be retained with the maximum amount of bone on the defect side of the tooth adjacent to the defect. That is, the tooth adjacent to the retained tooth should be extracted, and the bone cuts are made as far away from the retained tooth as possible (Fig. 19–13*A*). The strongest teeth are the canines and then the molars, and these should be retained if possible.
4. Four to five mm of palatal mucosa should be saved to cover the medial bony margin. This can be achieved by making the mucosal incision 5 mm toward the defect from which the bone cut will be made and then wrapping the mucosa around the bone margin (Fig. 19–13*B*). The bone margin must be rounded using a bur and drill. If there is insufficient palatal mucosa, a skin graft should be used.
5. Cheek flaps should be lined with split-thickness skin grafts. These limit scar contraction, increase flexibility of the cheek, and create a sizable lateral undercut superior to the scar band formed by the junction of the skin graft and oral mucosal junction. This result allows the prosthodontist to develop stability, support, and retention intraorally and to achieve relatively normal midfacial symmetry extraorally.
6. If a total maxillectomy is planned, the surgeon should consider stripping the mucosa from the sinus side of the floor of the orbit and placing a skin graft.[11]
7. The distal third of the soft palate remaining after tumor removal should be retained. This rim of soft palate (Fig. 19–14) is used to support the obturator. Contact with the lateral and inferior bones of the floor of the orbit provides support for the obturator. However, structures such as the turbinates may block access to this area, compromising the function of the prosthesis (Fig. 19–14). In patients with large maxillectomies the turbinates should be removed and a skin graft placed.[12]
8. Large maxillectomy defects should not be closed using flaps if a prosthesis is planned. Although flaps will close or partially close the surgical defect, the available space for a prosthesis is severely compromised, and midface contours, speech articulation, and swallowing are greatly diminished. In addition, the ability to recognize recurrent disease is diminished when flaps are used.
9. Flaps designed to restore significant amounts of cheek tissue, however, are very effective. Whenever a maxillectomy with orbital exenteration and resection of the skin of the cheek has been performed, flaps should be used to restore the cheek. The radial forearm flap has been very useful in restoring the cheek.[11] A flap in this area does not interfere with the fitting of a palatal prosthesis, especially if a surgical obturator is used to support the flap at the time of surgery.

Most of the surgical procedures that have been discussed under maxillectomy procedures will cause trismus. Severe trismus can prevent the use of an intraoral prosthesis. Trismus is worst in patients who do not perform any jaw-stretching exercises postoperatively for fear that they will

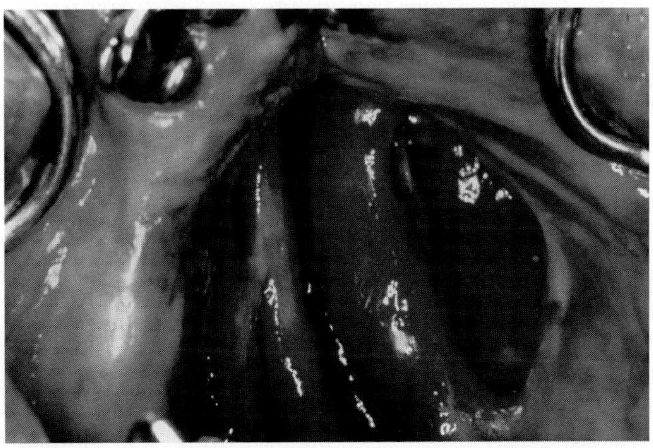

FIGURE 19–14. Large maxillectomy defect in an edentulous patient. A large defect created by maxillectomy with the retention of a small band of soft palate can greatly enhance the posterior retention of the prosthesis and the nasal bones that block access to the floor of the orbit.

interfere with healing by doing exercises to open the jaw. But it is this lack of movement that contributes most to trismus. The surgeon, prosthodontist, and other members of the surgical team must explain to the patient that the earlier stretching begins, the greater the recovery. Patients must begin stretching exercises at 2 weeks postoperatively. They must begin to *open* the mouth to stretch the scar bands, and this should be done four or more times daily. The patient can use tongue blades or other devices to measure the degree of success and to assist in the stretching. These stretching exercises are performed every day throughout the healing period. Since radiation therapy can increase trismus, stretching should be continued through radiation therapy until the last 2 to 3 weeks of therapy. Then it must be resumed 2 to 3 weeks following the completion of radiation therapy and continued for a few months.

Prosthetic Reconstruction of Maxillectomy Defects

Maxillectomy, including removal of the hard palate, partial removal of the soft palate, and/or orbital exenteration, is the most common operation for cancer that creates an intraoral defect. Patients with this defect have an excellent prognosis for rehabilitation. The materials and technique used result in a durable, functionally satisfying, and aesthetically pleasing prosthesis that camouflages the presence of the surgical defect.

The initial prosthesis should be placed at the time of the operation. Patients need an intraoral prosthesis to continue swallowing and speaking. The prosthesis used in this situation is termed the *surgical obturator* (Fig. 19–15*A*). The surgical obturator is replaced by the *interim obturator* (see Fig. 19–15*B*), and when healing is complete (see Fig. 19–15*C*), the *definitive obturator* is constructed (see Fig. 19–15*D*).

The main objectives of the surgical prosthesis are to seal off the maxillary defect created between the oral and nasal cavities and to hold the packing close to the split-thickness skin graft that lines the inner aspect of the cheek. Patients are able to speak and swallow immediately after surgery, and the nasogastric tube can be removed 1 to 2 days postoperatively and often is not necessary at all. The prosthesis also has a psychological effect that makes the postoperative course easier: Patients are aware that their rehabilitation has begun. The quality of the result depends on the location and size of the defect, the presence of prior radiation therapy, the quality of the remaining tissue, surgical complications, and whether any teeth remain.

The definitive prosthesis is made after healing is complete and remodeling of the defect has stabilized, usually 4 to 6 months after surgery, radiation therapy, or both. Dental preparation of the mouth and teeth should be completed or be planned as an integral part of the fitting of the definitive prosthesis (see Fig. 19–15*C*). Figure 19–15*C* also shows the healed skin graft located on the medial bone margin and across the superior bone cuts. This squamous epithelium provides support and a positive stop vertically for the obturator. The skin graft was placed during the initial surgery and was stented with gauze packing supported by a surgical obturator wired to the remaining teeth. This definitive obturator restores mastication, speech, and swallowing intraorally and restores the symmetry of the midface extraorally. Figure 19–15*E*, showing the prosthesis in place, demonstrates the return of midface symmetry.

MANDIBULAR DEFECTS

A rim resection of the mandible used in place of a segmental mandibulectomy greatly reduces the patient's morbidity. However, if the rim resection is done without consulting a prosthodontist unnecessary postoperative complications can result. In Figure 19–16 a mandibular rim resection was done to remove an anterior floor-of-mouth lesion. The lesion was totally removed, and the surgical site was closed primarily. That is, the buccal vestibule was sutured to the lingual vestibule, which covered the exposed bone, and excellent healing of the surgical defect occurred. The patient was referred for evaluation for a mandibular prosthesis after intraoral healing had occurred. Intraoral examination revealed that the tongue and floor of the mouth were continuous with the cheek. This tissue was very mobile and would not tolerate long-term contact with a prosthesis. There was more than enough height of mandible left to perform a vestibuloplasty using a skin graft and a mandibular surgical stent.

Both the cancer surgery and the restorative surgery can and should be performed at the same time. This reduces the total number of operations, and patients rarely accept a second surgery for restorative reasons alone; also, with the use of radiation therapy, there is rarely enough time for healing to occur before radiation therapy is begun. Figure 19–17*A* shows a patient with a diagnosis of squamous cell carcinoma of the mandibular right alveolar ridge who was referred preoperatively to the maxillofacial prosthetic service for construction of a surgical stent. The proposed surgery was a right mandibular rim resection and extraction of the remaining teeth followed by postoperative radiation therapy. The surgical stent was fabricated before surgery. In the operating room, after the tumor was removed and the skin graft had been sutured in place, the fit of the surgical stent was corrected by using a modeling-plastic impression compound. This impression was relined with a soft lining material and ligated in place with circummandibular wires. When the stent was removed (10 to 21 days after surgery), the healed surgical site had attached mucosa on the superior portion of the mandible (Fig. 19–17*B*). This provided a stable base for a prosthesis without the need for a second procedure.

The philosophy of treating patients who have had segmental mandibulectomy must be based on the priorities of function and appearance. Even if only a few of the priorities can

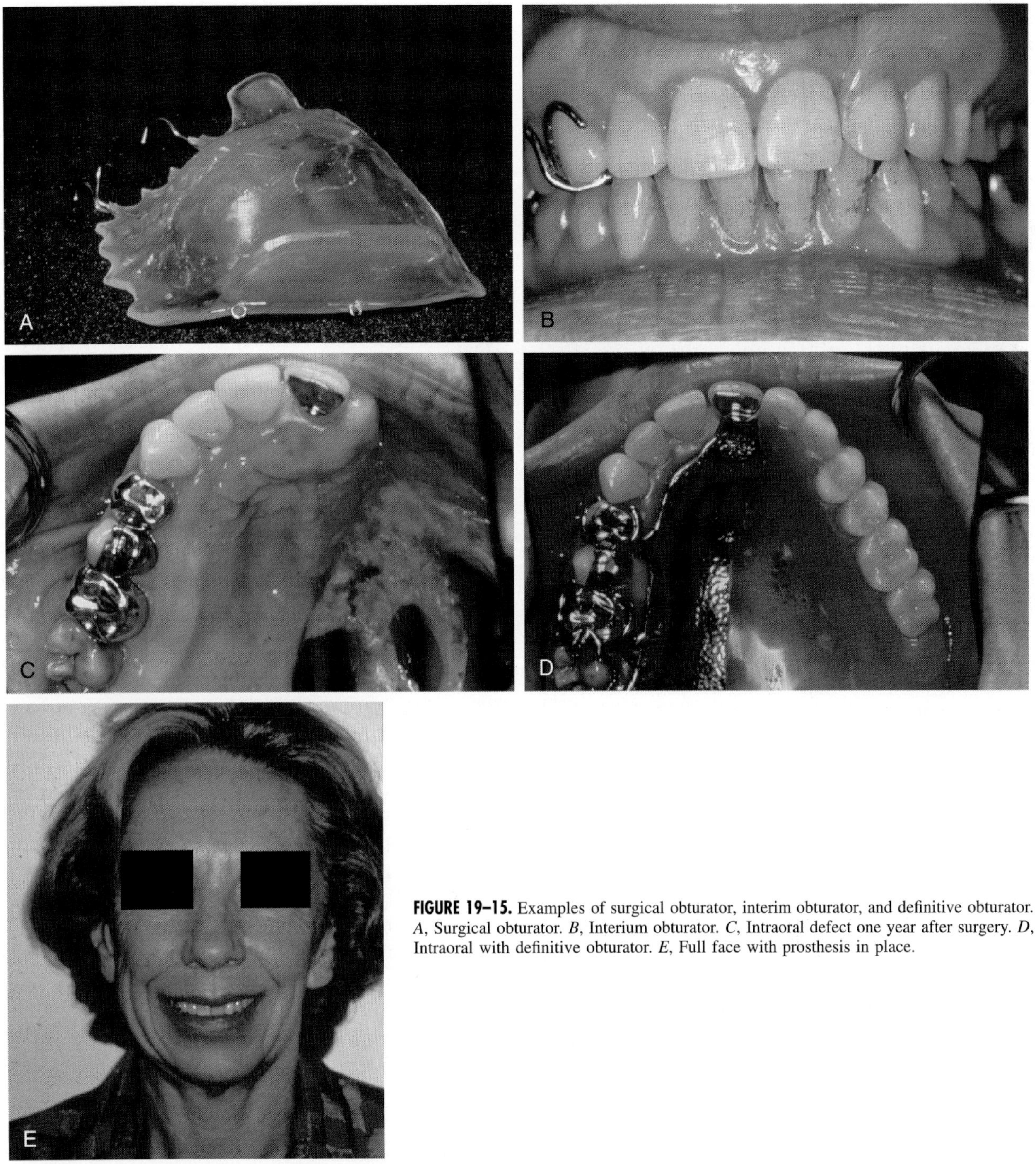

FIGURE 19–15. Examples of surgical obturator, interim obturator, and definitive obturator. *A*, Surgical obturator. *B*, Interium obturator. *C*, Intraoral defect one year after surgery. *D*, Intraoral with definitive obturator. *E*, Full face with prosthesis in place.

be satisfied by using a prosthesis, patients benefit significantly. These priorities, in order of importance, are swallowing and control of saliva, speech, cosmetic appearance, and masticatory efficiency.

Resection of a portion of the mandible is usually associated with soft tissue defects of the floor of the mouth and tongue. The prognosis for prosthetic reconstruction deteriorates rapidly as the amount of tissue removed increases. Problems that result after mandibulectomy without surgical reconstruction include an unaesthetic defect, deviation of the mandible to the side of the defect, and functional loss proportional to the amount of tongue and soft tissue removed. Surgical reconstruction of the bony mandible is preferable to prosthetic management alone. Surgical management restores the continuity of the mandible and greatly reduces distortion of the face. Removal of a large amount of tongue tissue may not allow restoration of normal speech by either surgical or prosthetic means. However, even with greatly reduced tongue volume, patients can learn to swallow.

Trismus was discussed in the earlier section on maxillectomy defects. It was stressed that patients must be told to

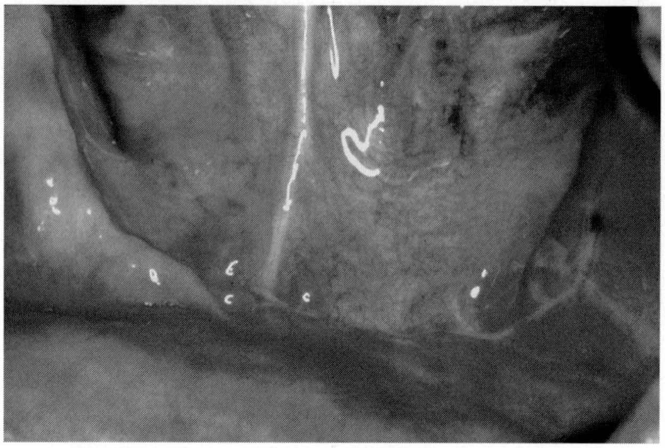

FIGURE 19–16. Rim mandibulectomy with primary closure.

begin stretching exercises 2 weeks after surgery if they are to regain some of their previous ability to open the jaw. For patients who have had a segmental mandibulectomy there is an additional consideration besides vertical opening—these patients must also be instructed to move the remaining mandible laterally. If the surgically removed segment was on the right side, the patient is instructed to push toward the left with the palm of the right hand against the remaining mandible until the teeth or alveolar ridge lines up horizontally with the maxillary ridge. Thus the mandibulectomy patient must stretch the jaw both vertically and horizontally.

When surgical restoration is not planned, prosthetic management must be instituted immediately. Placement of an inclined plane or guide flange prosthesis trains the patient to center the mandible, which minimizes facial distortion. The initial inclined plane prosthesis is modified during the healing phase, and after healing a definitive guide prosthesis is fabricated.

Speech and swallowing problems occur after major tongue resection. A partially successful method of improving tongue function in both speech and swallowing is a palatal augmentation prosthesis. This involves lowering the palate by means of a thickened prosthesis to enable the remaining portions of the tongue to touch the palate and aid in swallowing. Speech articulation involving the tongue and palate can also be improved in this manner.

In edentulous patients, the situation must be viewed in perspective: Wearing a full lower denture is difficult even for edentulous patients who have an intact mandible. In patients who have had a mandibulectomy, there is a greater potential for difficulties. Prosthetic restoration after segmental mandibulectomy requires the construction of a complete denture on the reduced basal seat provided by the residual mandibular alveolus. The denture should not extend into the defect area where no bony support is available.

Edentulous patients have little chance of regaining their preoperative level of function after a mandibulectomy without surgical reconstruction. The reasons for this bleak prospect include decreased neuromuscular control resulting from denervation of the tissues surrounding the denture, decreased basal seat for support of the denture, altered mucosal surface resulting from radiation therapy, altered saliva output due to radiation with its higher mucin content, and altered pathway of mandibular closure after a partial mandibulectomy.

Surgical reconstruction after a hemimandibulectomy and radiation therapy is very challenging and requires several surgical procedures. Before surgery the patient shown in Figure 19–18 was treated with hyperbaric oxygen. The body and ramus of the mandible were reconstructed using freeze-dried bone and autogenous corticocancellous bone. Vestibuloplasty was done as a separate procedure to avoid compromising the blood supply to the bone graft. After the skin graft had healed, a prosthesis was constructed, and the patient returned to his full-time job.

The patient in Figure 19–18 has been carefully followed by the maxillofacial prosthetic service and otolaryngology department. During this time the patient has had root canal therapy and the placement of crowns and an anterior bar bridge, and many decayed teeth have been restored. He is not compliant with the use of fluoride carriers and a toothbrush, but we have been able to maintain most of his teeth during an 11-year period (Fig. 19–18*D*).

The patient shown in Figure 19–19 underwent a segmental hemimandibulectomy and radiation therapy. Because the ra-

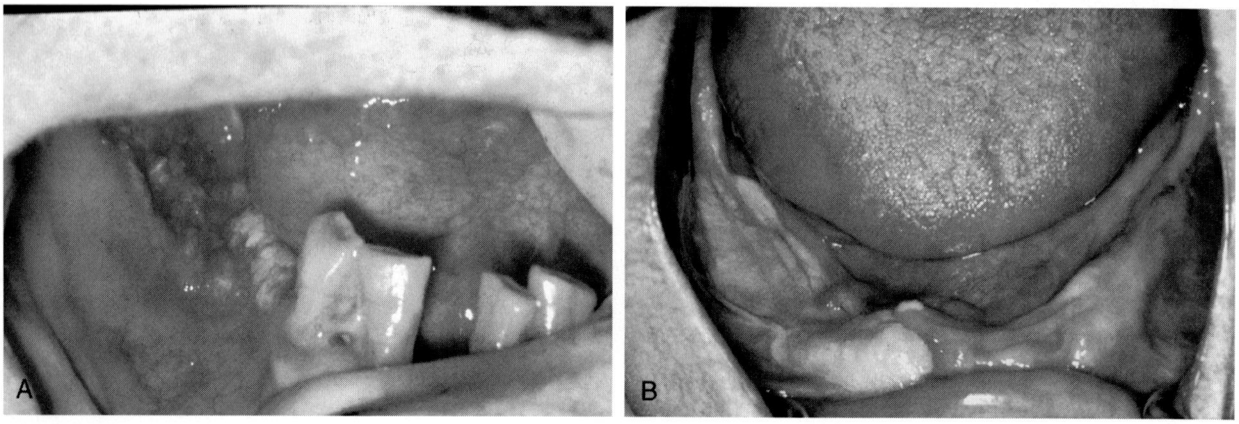

FIGURE 19–17. Multidisciplinary plan. *A*, Patient referred for maxillofacial prosthetics and a multdisciplinary plan prior to cancer surgery. *B*, Intraoral view of healed skin graft.

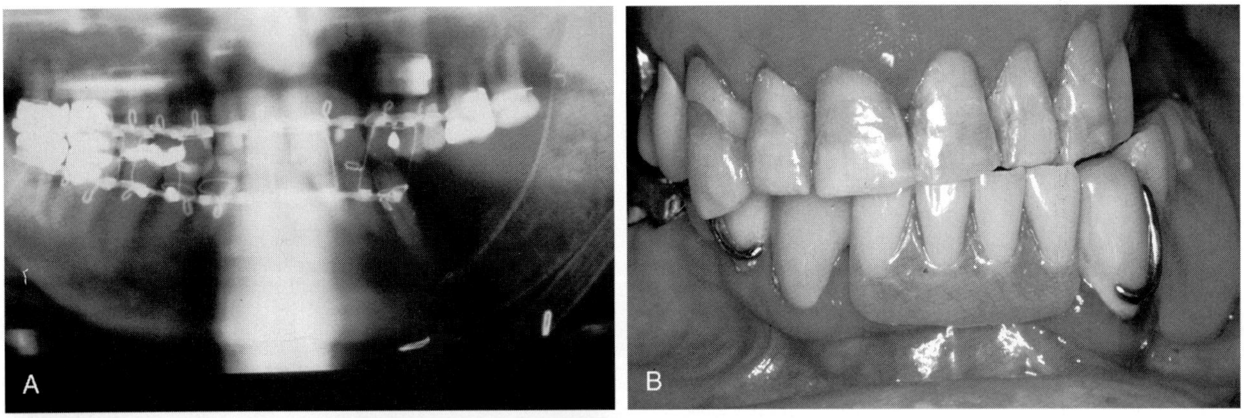

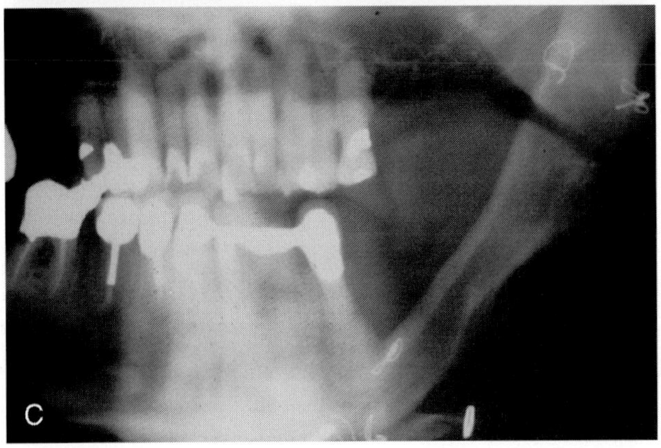

FIGURE 19–18. Mandibular reconstruction. *A*, Radiograph following surgical reconstruction with freeze-dried rib after hyperbaric oxygen. *B*, Intraoral view with resection prosthesis in occlusion. *C*, Radiograph taken 11 years postoperatively.

diation dose was less than 5000 rads, hyperbaric oxygen was not required. Mandibular reconstruction was performed with freeze-dried bone and marrow from the iliac crest. At a subsequent surgery a left mandibular vestibuloplasty was done with dissection of scar bands from the tongue and placement of a skin graft. A mandibular surgical stent was modified with modeling plastic and a soft liner. This surgical stent was ligated with circummandibular wires to prevent a blood clot forming under the skin graft. A few months later three Brånemark implants were placed; after being covered with tissue for 6 months, they were then uncovered. A four-unit fixed bridge made from precious alloy and porcelain was then fabricated (Fig. 18–19*A* and *B*). This bridge has remained functional for over 6 years.

SUMMARY

It takes a team approach to coordinate and provide comprehensive treatment for the patients' needing reconstructive surgery, radiation therapy, and prosthodontic rehabilitation. The team of trained specialists from each discipline must

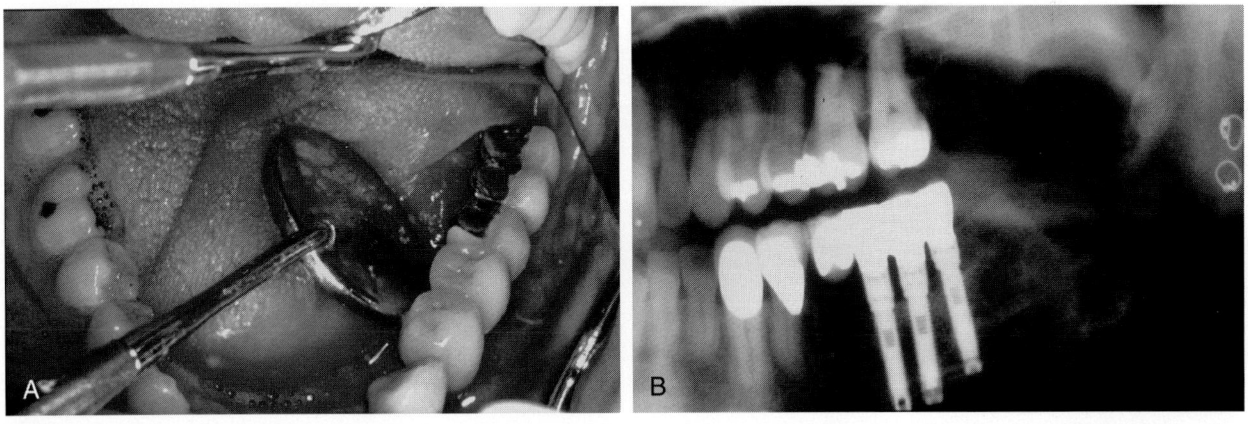

FIGURE 19–19. Mandibular reconstruction and dental implants. *A*, Mirror view of implant-supported fixed bridge. *B*, Radiograph taken 6½ years postoperatively.

participate in the planning phase so that the most effective treatment can be provided. The importance of maxillofacial prosthetics in the treatment of head and neck defects is intimately related to the patient's quality of life following surgery and/or radiation therapy. Quality of life is affected by the functional effect of an illness and its therapy upon a patient. Surgeons and radiation oncologists provide primary treatment and follow-up management for detection of recurrent cancer. The patient's self-esteem and socialization continue to be affected by problems related to speech, deglutition, and facial deformity. Prosthodontic rehabilitation restores many of the lost functions and allows the patient to return to a more normal life style. Since continued maintenance of a prosthesis is required, the prosthodontist has a continuing influence on the patient's quality of life.

REFERENCES

1. Turner G: Maxillofacial prosthetics. *In* Management of Head and Neck Cancer, 2nd ed. Philadelphia, J.B. Lippincott, 1994, pp. 169–183.
2. Buemer J, et al: Facial defects, alterations at surgery to enhance the prosthetic prognosis. *In* Zlotolow I, Esposito S, Beumer J (eds). Proceedings of the First International Congress on Maxillofacial Prosthetics, April 27–30, 1994, pp. 105–107.
3. Vergo T: Nasal Prosthesis. Fundamentals of Facial Prosthetics. ABI Professional Publications, Arlington, VA, 1995, pp. 137–138.
4. Beumer J, Ma T, Marenick M, et al: Restoration of facial defects: Maxillofacial Rehabilitation. Tokyo, Ishaiyaku EuroAmerica, Inc., 1996, pp. 385–453.
5. Thomas K: Compromise in prosthetic treatment of orofacial defects. J Prosthet Dent 76(2):115–118, 1996.
6. Van-Doorne J: Extra-oral prosthetics: Past and present. J Invest Surg 7(4):267–274, 1994.
7. Wolfaardt J, Wilkes G: Craniofacial osseointegration. J Can Dent Assoc 60(9):805–809, 1994.
8. Reece G, Lemon J, Jacob R, et al: Total midface reconstruction after radical tumor resection: A case report and overview of the problem. Ann Plast Surg 36(5):551–557, 1996.
9. LaVelle W. Arcuri M, Panje W, et al: Transmolar pin and magnetic carrier for midfacial reconstruction: A clinical report. J Prosthet Dent 70(3):204–206, 1993.
10. Rahn A, Goldman B, Parr G: Prosthetic principles in surgical planning for maxillary and mandibular resection patients. J Prosthet Dent 42:429, 1979.
11. Curtis T, Beumer J: Restoration of acquired hard palate defects. Maxillofacial Rehabilitation. Tokyo, Ishiyaku EuroAmerica, Inc., 1996, pp. 225–284.
12. Beumer J, Nishimura R, Roumanas E: Maxillary defects: Alterations at surgery to enhance the prosthetic prognosis. *In* Zlotolow I, Esposito S, Beumer J (eds). Proceedings of the First International Congress on Maxillofacial Prosthetics, April 27–30, 1994, pp. 22–26.

CHAPTER 20

Anaplastology and Its Application to Facial Rehabilitation

David W. Proops, M.B., B.D.S., F.R.C.S.
Michael J. Wake, M.B., B.D.S., F.D.S.
Steven Worrollo, M.I.M.T.
Lindsey Morgan-Lundie, M.I.M.T.

Facial disfigurement devastates lives. It may be either congenital—that is, the individual is born with the condition—or acquired as the result of trauma or surgical intervention, usually for malignant disease. The effect on observers is curiosity manifest either as fascination or revulsion. The immediate effect on the afflicted individual depends on the personality, but almost always it results in a negative self-image. The severity of this reaction depends on both the personality and the person's coping mechanisms.

The whole beauty industry is based on enhancing or disguising facial characteristics. Conventional and plastic surgical techniques have been employed for centuries. These well-tried techniques remain unchallenged in certain situations such as cleft palate. However, the results of plastic surgery in other situations do not fulfill the patient's requirements or should not be undertaken until the patient is free from disease, and in these cases anaplastology can offer alternatives. Anaplastology has been defined by the American Anaplastology Association as "the art and science of restoring a malformed or absent part of the human body through artificial means." Facial replacements have traditionally been retained by attaching them to spectacles or by using medical adhesives.[1, 2]

The development of extraoral osseointegration has revolutionized prosthetic facial rehabilitation. The primary aim of extraoral prostheses is cosmetic, but functional aspects are developing such as hearing aids built into ear prostheses. However, at the moment functional prostheses such as bone-anchored hearing aids are offered separately even though they may be an integral part of the rehabilitative package for that patient. Osseointegration was discovered and the name coined by Brånemark.[3] The details of the science and the surgical methods are outside the scope of this chapter but are well covered in Chapter 18. The complications associated with osseointegration are very much the concern of this chapter because they affect the planning and long-term life of the prostheses, and they will be discussed later.

METHOD

Those undertaking this work should aim to practice with a well-based team that should be composed of anaplastologists, otolaryngologists, plastic surgeons, and maxillofacial surgeons with support from other disciplines such as audiology, speech pathology, psychology, and clinical genetics.[4, 5]

Patients are divided roughly into a younger group who have congenital abnormalities and an older group who have acquired facial losses mainly as a result of surgical ablation of cancer or trauma. The needs of these two groups are very different, and their only common feature is their facial disfigurement. Needless to say, they should be handled sensitively and if possible discreetly. Special clinics in which all team members can be present to meet and assess the patients are ideal. An examination and treatment area designed to respect these patients' anxieties about privacy should also be available. It is helpful if new patients can meet and discuss their problems with already treated patients because this enhances the confidence of those seeking the advice and care of the team.

At the end of the assessment, which will also include information gathering about previous treatments and other new investigations such as radiology, a treatment plan is formulated. This should be agreed on by all team members, of course including the patient. If a patient is due to have or has already undergone radiotherapy and/or adjuvant chemotherapy as part of the management of the primary disease process, this should be considered in formulating the treatment plan. Implants can be placed at the time of ablative surgery if it is undertaken before radiotherapy. When the patient has received radiotherapy and is later referred for prosthetic rehabilitation, pre- and postimplantation hyperbaric oxygen therapy is mandatory.[6, 7] The extra effort, time, and expense needed for this treatment may dissuade some potential patients, illustrating the need for multidisciplinary team decision making.

The surgery itself requires two stages—first, to place the titanium fixtures, and second, after several months, to allow osseointegration to take place, at which time the skin-penetrating abutment is secured to the fixture, and the overlying soft tissues are thinned. When the soft tissues have healed the prosthetic aspect of surgery can commence, and indeed this may already have started if interim adhesive-retained prostheses are employed while the surgical component is completed.

In patients undergoing ablative surgery, it may be possible to place the fixtures at the time of surgery if this does not prejudice complementary treatment such as radiotherapy. The classic example of this is pinnectomy in an elderly patient with a small lesion and no sign of metastatic disease. Uncomplicated prothetic rehabilitation for pinnectomy in older patients may safely be undertaken as a single-stage procedure.[8]

The construction and method of fitting the prosthesis to the abutments are completed with the anaplastologist in full-time attendance. This is valuable time spent with the patient because the patient and family often reveal many of the worries, psychological scars, and guilty feelings that almost always beset them.

Good pre- and post-treatment clinical photographs are essential not only as good practice but as a reminder to the team and the patient of the starting point of treatment, the goals of reconstruction, and whether these goals were achieved.

Long-term maintenance must be a concern. One of the problems of the prosthetic method is that patients require lifelong maintenance, which involves periodic remaking of the prosthesis, and the patient and family need to participate in maintaining the cleanliness and health of the skin and soft tissues around the skin-penetrating abutments. Plastic surgical reconstruction does not carry this burden. Funds and time must be identified for this long-term commitment, and every team will become bigger and busier as their ongoing patient load increases.

The method therefore can be summarized as follows:

1. Patient referral
2. Team assessment
3. Formulation of treatment plan
4. Staged surgery
5. Construction and fitting of prosthesis
6. Other support as required
7. Long-term maintenance and support

THE FABRICATION OF FACIAL PROSTHESES AND MEANS OF RETENTION

Facial prostheses have been documented as far back as Egyptian times. These early prostheses were fashioned out of various materials including metal and wood. Through the ages different materials and methods have been used to construct such prostheses, eventually leading to today's most commonly used material, silicone elastomer. This material is favored because of its elastic properties, which make the prosthesis feel more lifelike. Today anaplastologists or maxillofacial prosthetists custom-make facial prostheses for each individual.

Construction

Various construction processes are involved in the fabrication of a silicone elastomer facial prosthesis. These include taking an impression of the area of the defect and then sculpting the prosthesis directly onto the patient. This is followed by the use of the lost wax technique to create a two- or three-part mold. Layers of silicone that have been individually color-matched to the person's skin tone can then be placed on the mold.

Retention

Methods of retaining facial prostheses have also developed over the ages, and now there are three main types. These are spectacle retention, adhesive retention, and the best method, osseointegrated implant retention.

Spectacle Retention

There are two main disadvantages of spectacle retention. The first is that whenever the spectacles are taken off the prosthesis is also removed. Second, it is difficult for the anaplastologist to achieve an inconspicuous thin edge on the prosthesis because of the slight movement of the spectacle frame. This form of retention is still useful for patients with poor manual dexterity or as a temporary measure until osseointegration can be achieved.

Adhesive Retention

Adhesive retention works well for highly motivated patients with good manual dexterity. Its disadvantages include the time needed to apply and remove the adhesive, the allergic reaction of some patients to medical adhesives, problems with positioning the prostheses, and concerns about day-long stability. The adhesive can also tear the thin edge of the prosthesis. The main advantage of this system is that it does not require surgery, and the patient can begin to wear a prosthesis almost immediately following surgery.

Both spectacle and adhesive retention still have indications and should always be considered. The most important aspect of retention of facial prostheses is making the correct choice by means of multidisciplinary consultation.

Osseointegrated Implant Retention

This form of retention has revolutionized the treatment of many patients with a facial disfigurement who require a facial prosthesis. The prosthesis is extremely secure and can be fabricated with a very thin and inconspicuous edge, which blends into the face.

Once healing has taken place after the second stage of surgery, the patient is seen again by the prosthetist. An impression is taken of the area of the defect to reflect the implant position. Impression copings are used for this process. When a working model of the implant site has been made, the type of retention method to be linked into the implant can be chosen. There are two main forms of retention: bar-clip retention and magnet retention.

Bar-Clip Retention. The bar-clip is the most common form of retention for auricular prostheses. Gold collars of either 3 or 4 mm in height are placed on the abutments. The length is chosen by the prosthetist and depends on the space available. A gold bar is then soldered to the collars in a position that will not interfere with the aesthetic appearance of the prosthesis. It is important to construct the bar so that it will prevent rotation of the prosthesis (see Fig. 20–4*A*). Clips can then be applied to the bar construction; these are incorporated within an acrylic base plate onto which the silicone elastomer is bonded.

This form of retention can also be used in other defect areas, but skin irritation can occur if there is not sufficient room for the patient to clean behind the bar. This can be a particular problem in orbital defects because access is poor and the patient's visibility is already reduced. The bar retention method can also hinder placement of the eye unit, which will compromise the final aesthetic result.

Magnet Retention. Magnet retention is mainly used with orbital prostheses because it provides a secure prosthesis that can offer flexibility when positioning the eye unit. The magnets also allow access to the implant area so that the patient can clean it easily and effectively. Magnet caps are screwed directly into the abutment, and the opposing magnet is then incorporated into an acrylic base plate onto which the prosthesis is eventually bonded.

Other abutments and attachments such as console abutments and ball and socket attachments can be used in particular cases if other more routine components are insufficient.

COMPLICATIONS AND HOW TO AVOID THEM

Surgical Complications

The first requirement is correct placement of the fixtures for the best cosmetic result. This can only be achieved by careful preplanning by both the surgeon and the anaplastologist with the patient present. Ideally, templates are constructed by the anaplastologist for use by the surgeon during surgery with the ideal position for the fixtures marked.[9] The presence of the anaplastologist in the operating room is very helpful because the ideal placement may not be possible owing to insufficient bone or underlying structures. In this situation the anaplastologist can advise an alternative site, and the surgeon can then attempt to find adequate bone to ensure secure placement of the fixtures.

The second problem is that of inadequate bone. Ideally, the longer 4-mm extraoral titanium fixture should be used, but occasionally, especially in children, only 3 mm or less of bone may be available. When inadequate bone is encountered, there are several options. First, the fixture may be left proud, and in this situation it is best covered with Gore-Tex membrane, which facilitates osteoneogenesis. Second, if dura is encountered it may be gently pushed away, allowing full seating of the fixture.

Some important underlying structures may be encountered. Usually, in this situation one places further guide holes in adjacent areas until a noncomplicated site is discovered. The exception to this is the lateral venous sinus, where placement of the fixture will obviously stop the bleeding from this low-pressure system.

In all other sites except the unaerated adult temporal bone it is helpful to place more fixtures than are needed for planned requirements. The reason for this is the expected fixture failure rate. There may be either early failures owing to nonosseointegration or unexplained late failures. The presence of these extra "sleeping" fixtures permits prompt return of full function of the prosthesis despite the failure of one of the retainers. Late failures are more common in some sites. The best results are achieved in the temporal bone followed by the orbit; prostheses in the nasal area have the poorest results. The reasons are multifactorial: the quality of the bone is one, and the load that each fixture carries subsequently is another.

Nonsurgical Complications

Radiation therapy decreases the survival of the fixtures dramatically and always necessitates hyperbaric oxygen therapy.[6, 7] *Local hygiene* is important, and this is facilitated by gross soft tissue reduction, rendering the skin surrounding the fixture and abutment relatively immobile. Chronic sepsis undoubtedly reduces the life of the fixtures, and if the patient is unable to maintain meticulous hygiene, a family member must undertake it for them. If the patient's personal hygiene is very poor, it is probably better not to use this method of rehabilitation. Elderly men who live alone must be particularly carefully evaluated in regard to their motivation and hygiene.

In children *trauma* is surprisingly common. This is probably just a reflection of the constant traumas of childhood but is another good reason for providing the prosthesis as late in childhood as possible. Trauma may result simply in damage to the prosthesis, but it may also damage the superstructure and even the screws holding the abutment to the fixture. Rarely, the fixture may be removed from the bone, in which case the only recourse is to replace it. Spare prostheses are often provided in case of loss or damage, and summer and winter prostheses may be necessary for individuals who have marked skin color changes with the seasons.

Coping with Failures

It is demoralizing for the patient to experience problems with the prosthesis. The team should obviously maintain a positive and hopeful approach and should have prearranged protocols available to handle each type of difficulty.

The most common problem is soft tissue reaction around the abutment. This is best dealt with by regular cleaning and the application of an antibiotic or steroid cream. If this is unsuccessful, the abutment may not be correctly seated on the fixture, producing a dead space that can become contaminated and can form a nidus for an inflammatory reaction. Alternatively, if the skin is too thick or too mobile around the abutment problems will result. In the latter case, a revision is required. The skin is surgically reduced so that thick skin and periosteum are all that remain, producing an immobile skin area around the abutment. When pediatric patients enter their teenage years extra skin growth can be a particular problem that may necessitate a reduction.

Loss of a Fixture

Loss of a fixture may be primary if the failure occurs soon after loading, which implies that inadequate osseointegration has taken place. Secondary failures occur later, often much later, and are usually preceded by pain when the fixture is loaded. This type of failure is more difficult to explain. Previous radiotherapy results in loss of fixtures, but in nonirradiated cases there appears to be a steady loss of bone from the flange of the fixture downward accompanied by granulation tissue. This type of failure most closely resembles periodontal disease of the dentition. If the parallel is maintained for prevention, then the answer similarly lies in maintaining meticulous hygiene.

If a fixture fails and there are parked "sleeping" implants, they can be brought through and the original prosthesis adapted as a temporary measure. If there are no parked implants, medical adhesive can be used as an extra form of retention on a temporary basis.

Prostheses deteriorate with age, partly from the wear and tear of everyday usage and partly from the lack of stability of the materials. Children and those working in dirty environments accelerate this process and require replacement prostheses more regularly. Those who smoke or live with a smoker experience less color stability and early yellowing of the prosthesis.

Growth

Growth is a key consideration, particularly in patients with unilateral aural atresia. The child continually grows and changes shape, and therefore the prosthesis has to be resculpted every 2 to 3 years in children up to 16 years of age, after that it should be remade every 4 years up to the age of 30 and then approximately every 6 years thereafter. Patients should be made aware of these issues. In those with bilateral aural atresia the prostheses have to be resculpted to keep up with facial growth but do not pose such an obvious problem.[10]

Children who have undergone orbital exenteration followed by extensive radiotherapy also present problems to the prosthetist because the defect on the treated side does not develop and grow at the same rate as the normal side. Compromise has to be accepted.

Implant technology has revolutionized the treatment that can be offered to people with facial disfigurements. With close liaison between multidisciplinary team members a high-quality, aesthetically pleasing, and efficient service can be delivered. The importance of this liaison cannot be stressed enough, and it must always be remembered that rehabilitating such patients in a holistic manner is the key to true rehabilitation.

CASE STUDIES

The best illustration of this method of overall management is provided by discussion of specific cases. These are divided into the four major types of cases that are amenable to this method and are regularly treated by the team approach to anaplastology. In order of frequency of occurrence and in reverse order of difficulty, these categories are the ear, the orbit, the nose, and combined complex cases. When appropriate, cases of congenital and acquired problems and young and old patients are discussed to highlight the different priorities in management.

CASE 1: CONGENITAL EAR DISORDER AFTER PLASTIC SURGERY

R. J. S., aged 16, was born with a congenitally atreatic right ear. He had undergone 16 operations, one to create a meatus and 15 to fashion a pinna. Both he and his parents were very unhappy with the result. Preoperatively, infected Silastic was found to be extruding from the ear (Fig. 20–1*A*).

The approach was as follows:

Operation 1: Silastic removed; 3 months recovery.
Operation 2: Three fixtures placed; 3 months recovery.
Operation 3: Fixtures uncovered, soft tissues thinned, ear remnants removed.
Stage 4: Fabrication of prosthesis (Fig. 20–1*B*).

One year later further soft tissue reduction was performed. The patient has had five prostheses over a 10-year period and is very happy and well adjusted.

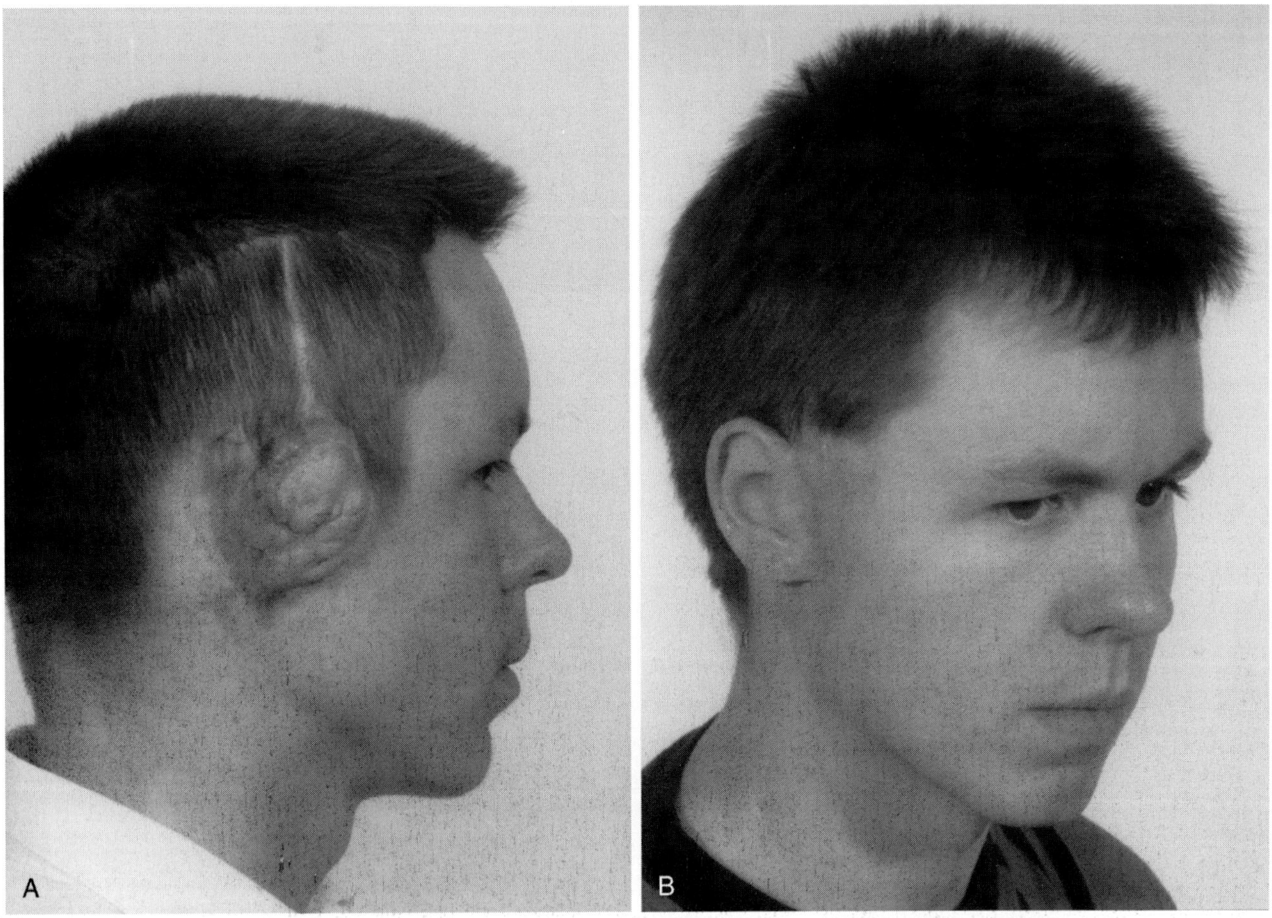

FIGURE 20–1. Case 1: Congenital atreatic right ear. *A,* Preoperative view. Note extruding Silastic. *B,* After placement of osseointegrated retained auricular prosthesis.

CASE 2: BILATERAL CONGENITAL EAR DISORDER (SYNDROMAL CHILD)

K. W., aged 4, was born with severe Treacher Collins syndrome. She needed a tracheostomy in the first few months of life for airway problems, and later pharyngoplasty was performed to allow gross nasal escape. Severe conductive hearing loss was managed initially with a conventional headband bone-conduction hearing aid. She was seen at 4 years of age, and a treatment plan was formulated.

A bone-anchored hearing aid on the right side was placed at 4 years of age in a staged procedure (Fig. 20–2*A* and *B*). This was very successful, but complications occurred 1 year later when the hearing aid was loosened by trauma and had to be replaced.

At 9 years of age an auricular prosthesis was fitted in a staged procedure (Fig. 20–2*C* and *D;* see also Color plate). Because her speech was still markedly hypernasal, speech therapy was given throughout the treatment time.

CASE 3: BILATERAL CONGENITAL EAR DISORDER (SYNDROMAL ADULT)

D. G., aged 27, had severe Treacher Collins syndrome (Fig. 20–3*A*). She had been fitted with a conventional bone-conduction hearing aid at an early age and had attended a school for the physically handicapped. Her speech was very poor, and at 17 years she was very depressed because of her appearance.

At 20 years she underwent a maxillary osteotomy and then genioplasty with good effect. At 27 years of age bilateral osseointegrated retained prostheses and a bone-anchored hearing aid were placed in a staged procedure (Fig. 20–3*B*). A large input of specialized speech and language therapy resulted in a marked improvement in the clarity of the patient's speech. Following treatment the patient's confidence improved dramatically, and a naturally outgoing personality emerged. The patient married, received genetic counseling, and has mothered a nonaffected son.

CASE 4: SINGLE-STAGE AURICULAR REPLACEMENT FOLLOWING NONIRRADIATED PINNECTOMY

C. O., aged 68, had undergone a total pinnectomy for carcinoma and was initially provided with a spectacle-attached prosthesis. Two years following pinnectomy a single-stage procedure was performed for placement of two 4-mm fixtures (Fig. 20–4*A–C;* see also Color plate). Four months later the abutments were loaded and the prosthesis was fitted; it provided 2 years of trouble-free usage. This case demonstrates that single-stage surgery in the nonirradiated patient can be successful and speeds rehabilitation.

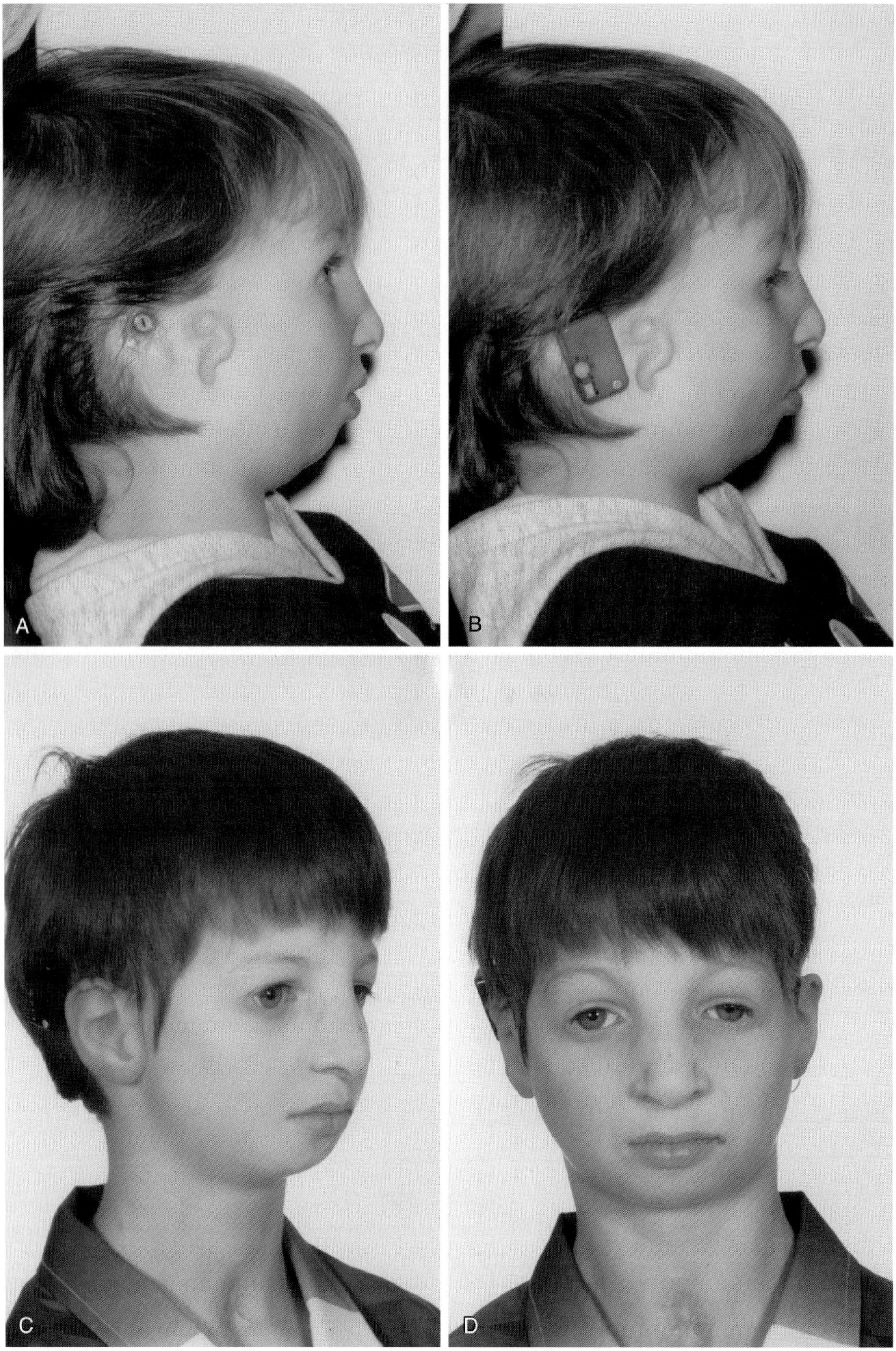

FIGURE 20–2. Case 2: Treacher Collins syndrome. *A,* Bone-anchored abutment. *B,* Bone-anchored hearing aid. *C,* Auricular prosthesis and bone-anchored hearing aid. *D,* Full-face view of bilateral auricular prostheses (see also Color plate).

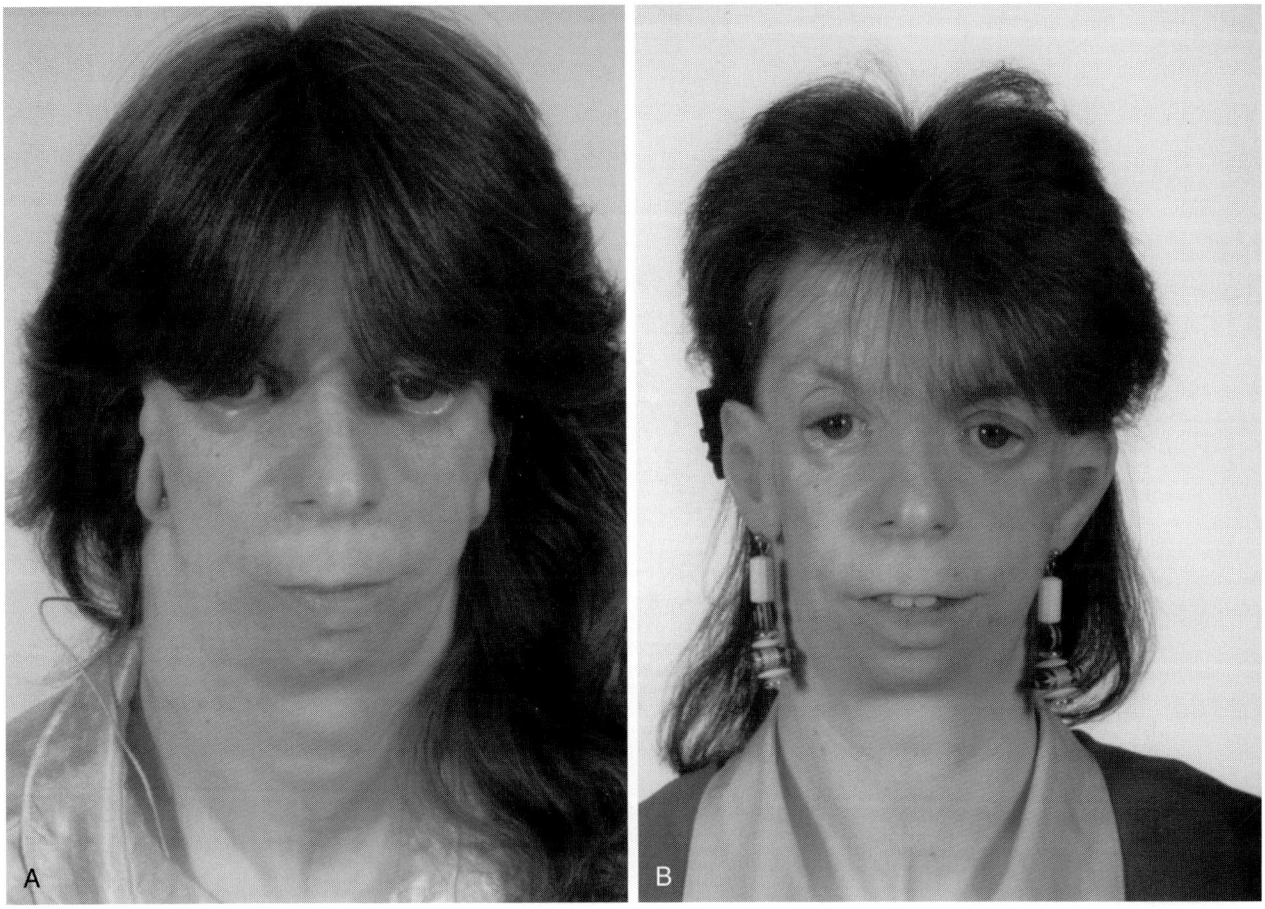

FIGURE 20–3. Case 3: Treacher Collins syndrome in an adult. *A,* Presentation at age 27. *B,* Appearance following provision of osseointegrated auricular prostheses and bone-anchored hearing aid; note the outrageous earrings.

CASE 5: TRAUMATIC ORBITAL DEFECT

M. D., aged 58, had lost her right eye in a traffic accident 20 years previously. Her spectacle prosthesis was found to be unsatisfactory when she became a grandmother and her young grandchildren attempted to remove it. An osseointegrated-retained prosthesis was provided after five fixtures were placed; three were used with magnet retention (Fig. 20–5*A–C*).

Ten years after the implantation two fixtures were lost to unknown causes. The sleeping fixtures were then exposed and loaded successfully.

CASE 6: BILATERAL ORBITAL AND NASAL LOSS AS A RESULT OF GUNSHOT WOUND

O. B., aged 41. An accidental gunshot wound at age 16 had led to loss of the eyes, orbits, and bridge of the nose (Fig. 20–6*A* and *B;* see also Color plate). The patient developed a frontal sinus mucocele. Via a bicoronal flap the mucocele was excised, and fixtures were placed in both supraorbital rims. Eight months later the fixtures were exposed and found to be well integrated. A midface prosthesis was constructed as a single unit and is retained with magnets (Fig. 20–6*C–F;* see also Color plate).

CASE 7: COMPLEX CRANIOFACIAL RESECTION FOR ANTRAL CARCINOMA INCLUDING LEFT ORBIT

D. M., aged 69, had carcinoma of the left antrum. In 1989 he underwent maxillectomy followed by radical radiation therapy at a dose of 62 cGy in 31 fractions. In 1990 a recurrent squamous cell carcinoma was treated with a local implant. Further recurrence in 1991 required orbital exenteration. The treatment plan was for an orbital prosthesis secured by osseointegration with pre- and postimplant hyperbaric oxygen therapy. A course of 25 hyperbaric dives was followed by the insertion of five titanium fixtures to the orbital rim, which was followed by 15 further hyperbaric dives. After a 6-month delay the fixtures were uncovered. Three of them were used for the orbital prosthesis, which is secured by magnet adhesion (Fig. 20–7*A–D*). A separate conventional maxillary obturator was also constructed. No complications have occurred after 3 years of follow-up.

CASE 8: RHINECTOMY FOR AGGRESSIVE POSTRADIOTHERAPY RECURRENCE OF BASAL CELL CARCINOMA

P. C., aged 64, had recurrent basal cell carcinoma of the nasal tip. A partial rhinectomy was followed by placement of a nasal prosthesis using spectacle

Text continued on page 273

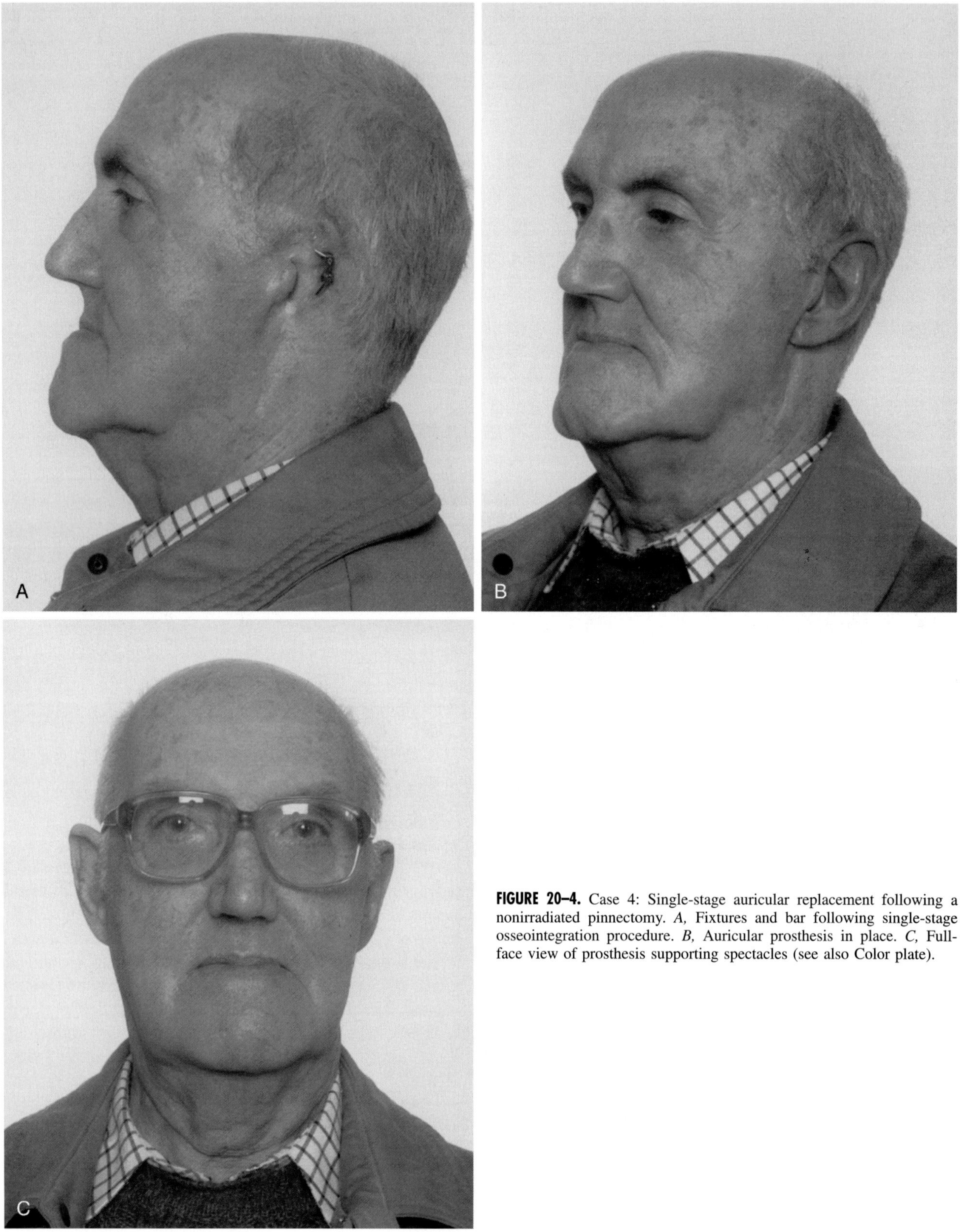

FIGURE 20–4. Case 4: Single-stage auricular replacement following a nonirradiated pinnectomy. *A,* Fixtures and bar following single-stage osseointegration procedure. *B,* Auricular prosthesis in place. *C,* Full-face view of prosthesis supporting spectacles (see also Color plate).

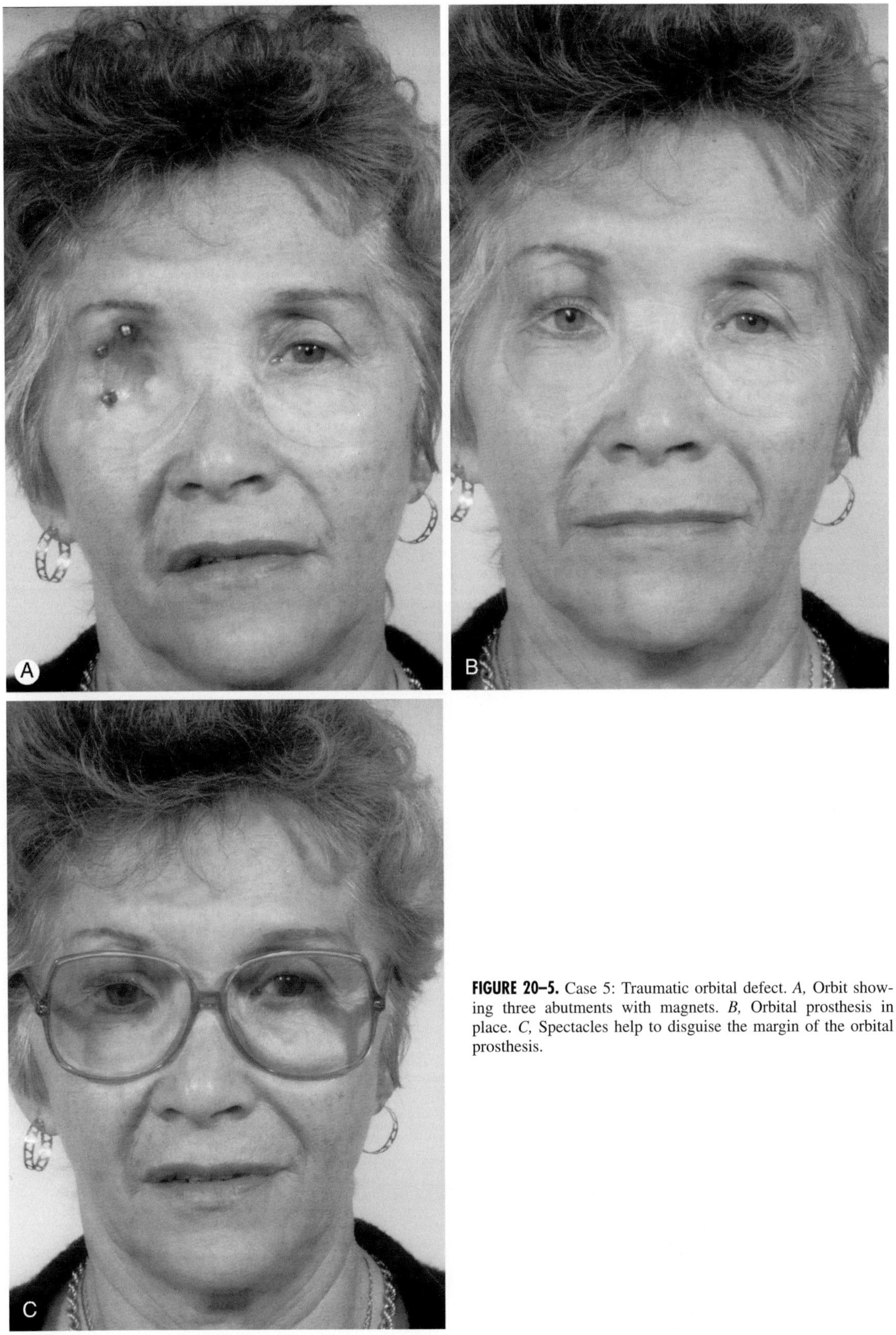

FIGURE 20–5. Case 5: Traumatic orbital defect. *A,* Orbit showing three abutments with magnets. *B,* Orbital prosthesis in place. *C,* Spectacles help to disguise the margin of the orbital prosthesis.

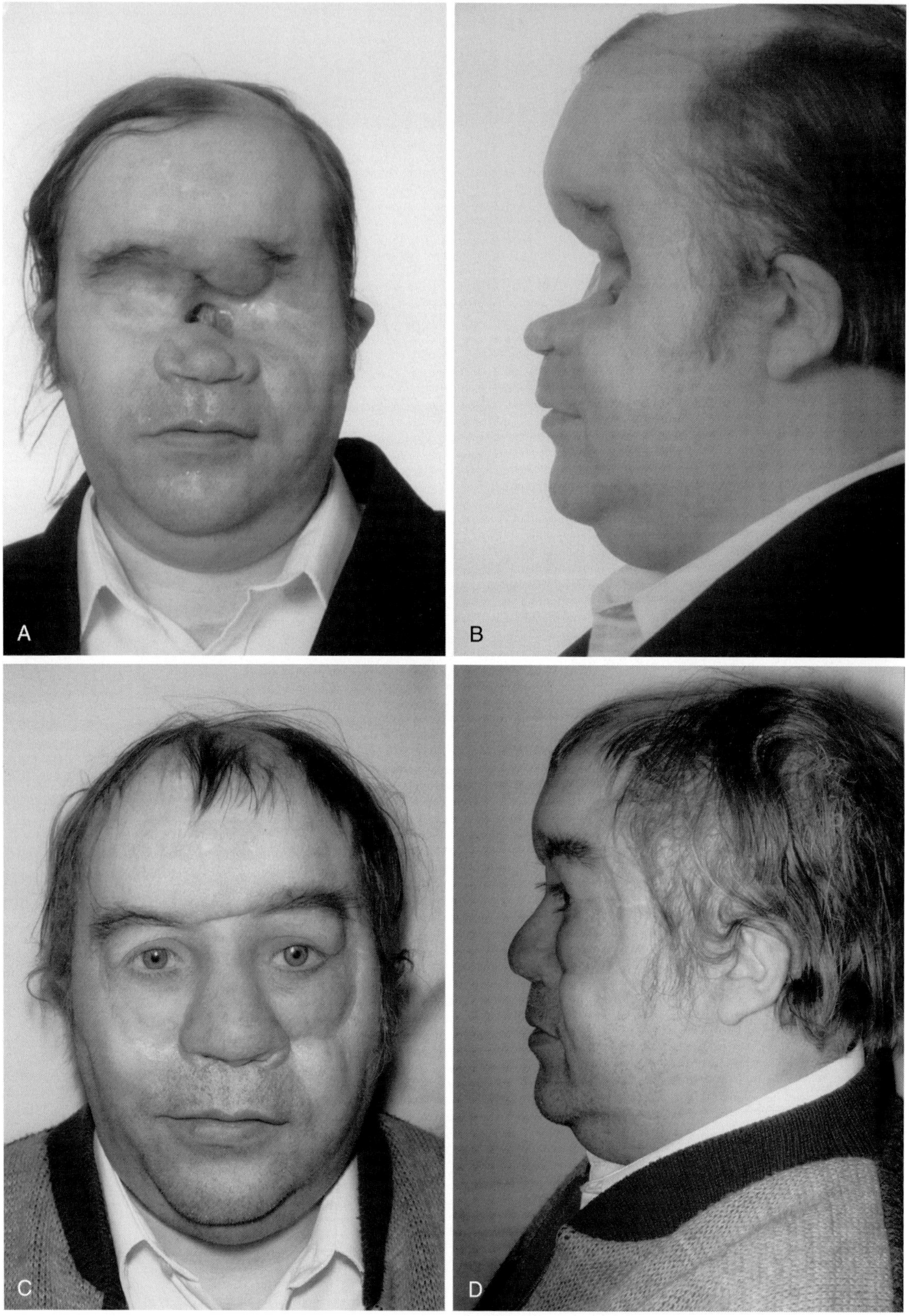

FIGURE 20–6. Case 6: Bilateral orbital and nasal loss due to gunshot wound. *A,* Preoperative frontal view. *B,* Preoperative lateral view. *C,* Postoperative frontal view. *D,* Postoperative lateral view.

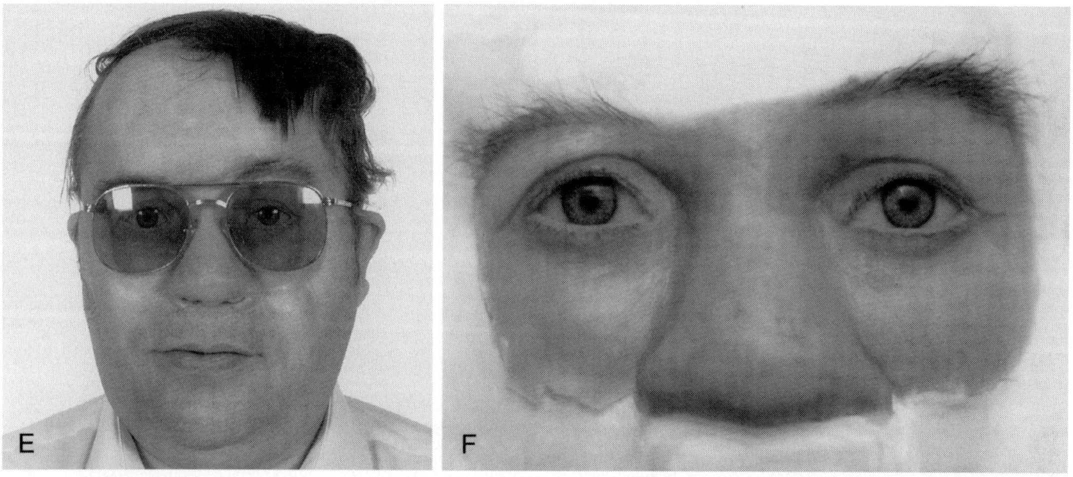

FIGURE 20–6 *Continued. E,* Postoperative view with spectacles. *F,* Midface prosthesis (see also Color plate).

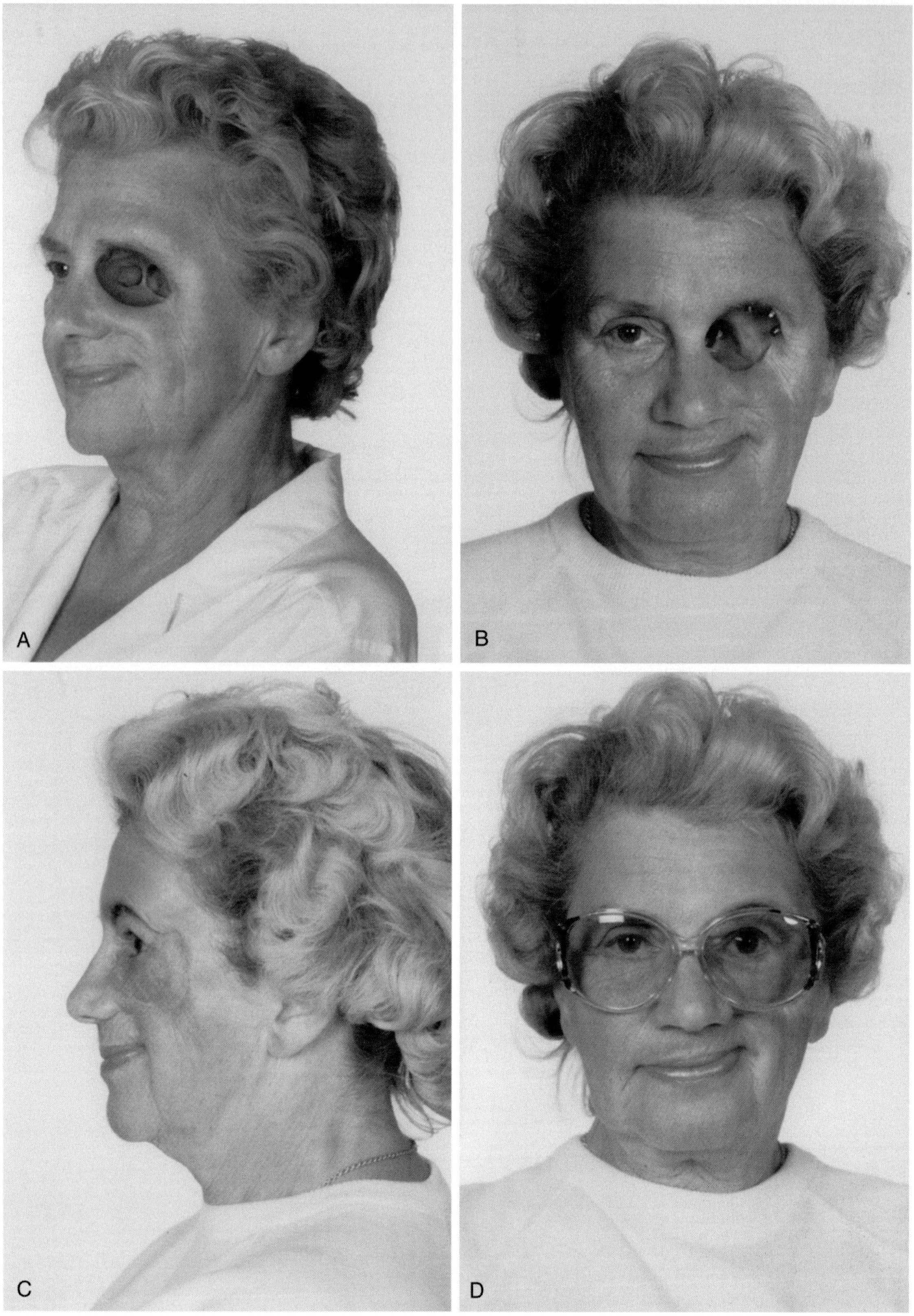

FIGURE 20–7. Case 7: Craniofacial resection for antral carcinoma. *A,* Preoperative view of defect. *B,* Postoperative view of magnetic abutments on the loaded orbital fixtures; note maxillary obturation. *C,* Lateral view without spectacles. *D,* Frontal view with spectacles, which help to disguise the margin of the prosthesis.

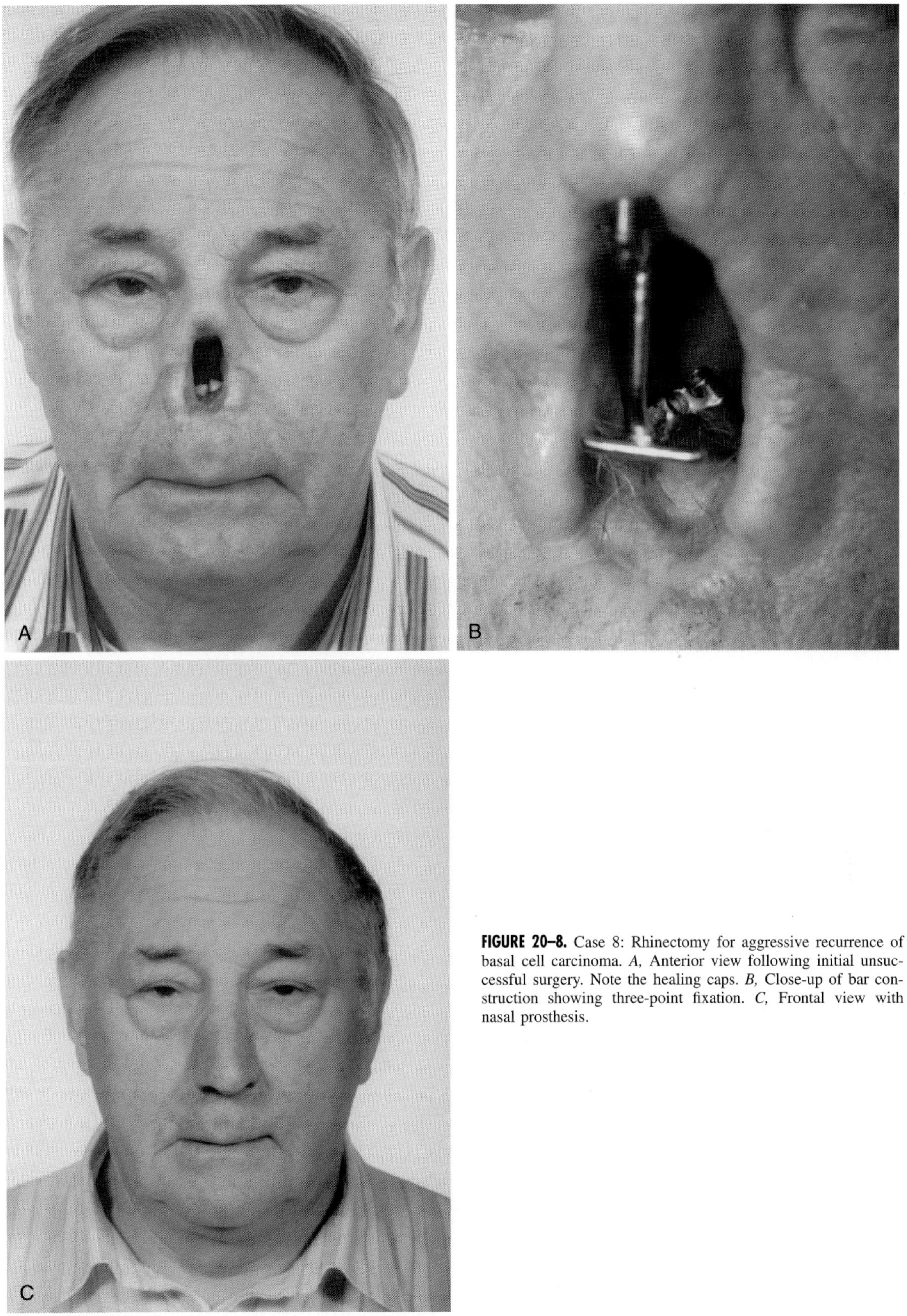

FIGURE 20–8. Case 8: Rhinectomy for aggressive recurrence of basal cell carcinoma. *A,* Anterior view following initial unsuccessful surgery. Note the healing caps. *B,* Close-up of bar construction showing three-point fixation. *C,* Frontal view with nasal prosthesis.

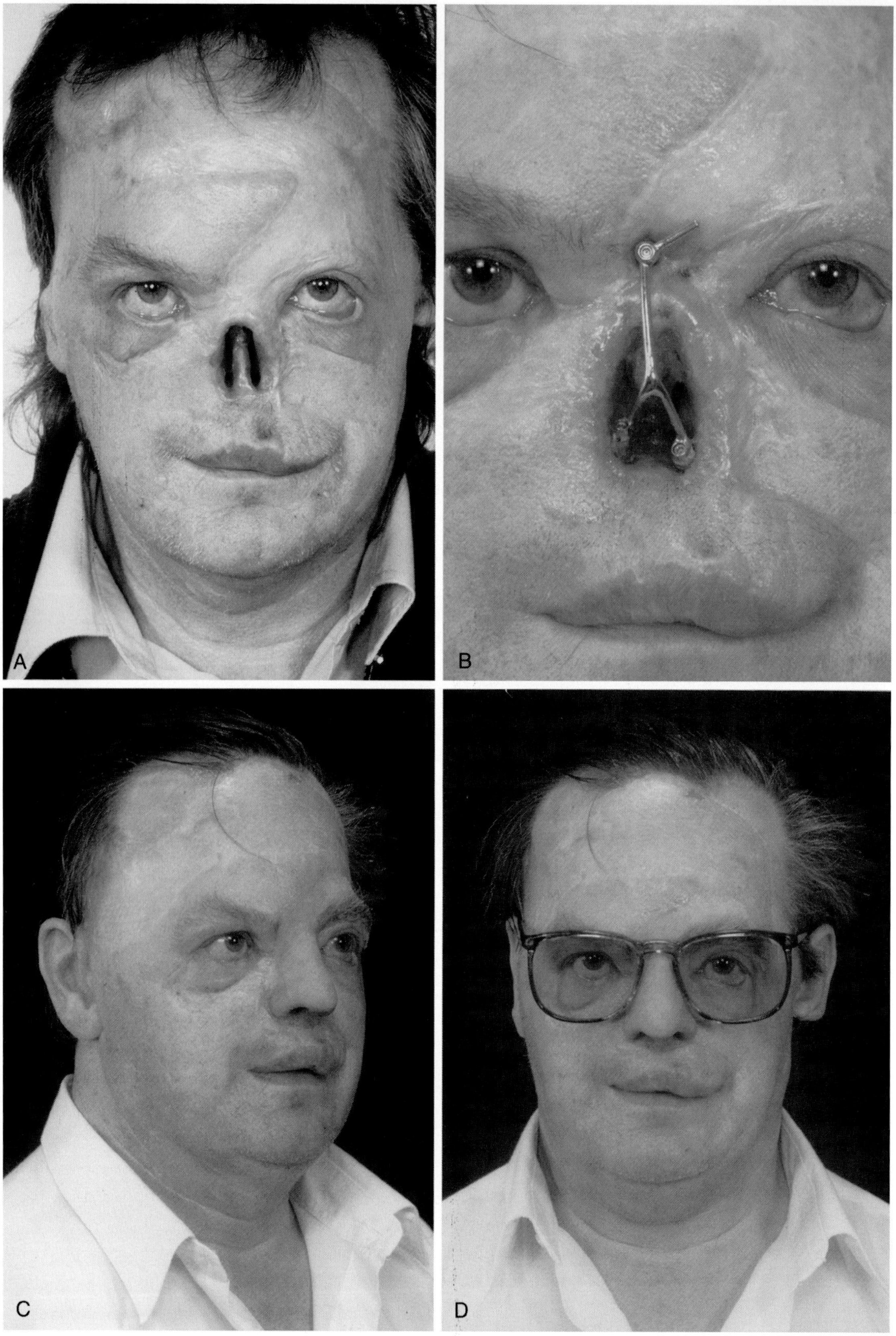

FIGURE 20–9. Case 9: Facial injuries due to dog attack. *A,* View of patient several weeks following injury and completion of plastic surgery procedures. *B,* Three-point fixation and bar for nasal prosthesis. *C,* Patient fitted with right auricular and nasal left brow prosthesis. *D,* Full-face view. Spectacles disguise the scars and margins of the nasal prosthesis (see also Color plate).

retention. Three 4-mm extraoral fixtures were placed, all of which failed to integrate (Fig. 20–8*A*). Subsequently, bone grafts with two intraoral fixtures were placed into the maxilla from the nose, and one extraoral fixture was placed in the nasium. Bar construction was used for the nasal prosthesis (Fig. 20–8*B* and *C*). The nasium fixture failed after 3 years. P. C. enjoyed good rehabilitation for 5 years until he died from an unrelated carcinoma.

CASE 9: SEVERE FACIAL INJURIES CAUSED BY DOG ATTACK

F. T., aged 54, was attacked by two pit bull terriers who inflicted terrible facial injuries. Extensive plastic surgery was performed, but the nose and right ear were avulsed (Fig. 20–9*A*; see also Color plate.) A treatment plan was devised that included rehabilitation with an osseointegrated retained nasal prosthesis that also carried a right eyebrow and right ear prosthesis.

Two intraoral and three extraoral fixtures for the nose, only three of which were loaded, and two fixtures for the ear prosthesis were placed in a two-stage procedure (Fig. 20–9*B–D*; see also Color plate). The results have been excellent, and the patient has requested further surgery for ectropion. As a result of this case the law in the United Kingdom was amended to prohibit the keeping of pit bull terriers.

REFERENCES

1. Conroy B: The history of facial prostheses. Clin Plast Surg 10: 701, 1983.
2. Bubulian AH: Facial Prostheses. Philadelphia, WB Saunders, 1995.
3. Albrektsson T, Brånemark PI, Hanson BO: Osseointegrated titanium implants: Requirements for long-lasting, direct bone implant anchorage in man. Acta Orthop Scand 52: 155, 1981.
4. Jani RM, Schaaf NG: An evaluation of facial prostheses. J Prosth Dent 39: 546, 1945.
5. Worthington P, Brånemark PI (eds): Advanced Osseointegration Surgery: Applications in the Maxillofacial Region. Chicago, Quintessence Publishing, 1992.
6. Ganstrom GI: The use of hyperbaric oxygen to prevent implant fixture loss in the irradiated patient. *In* Worthington P, Brånemark PI (eds): Advanced Osseointegration Surgery. Chicago, Quintessence Publishing 1992.
7. Ganstrom G, Tjellstrom A, Brånemark PI, et al: Bone-anchored reconstruction of the irradiated head and neck cancer patient. Otolaryngol Head Neck Surg 108 (4): 334, 1993.
8. Tjellstrom A, Ganstrom G: One-stage procedure to establish osseointegration. A zero to five year follow up report. J Laryngol Otolaryngol 109: 593, 1995.
9. Waterfield LJ, Worrollo SJ, Wake MJC, Proops DW: The position of the bone-anchored hearing aid in relation to the bone-anchored auricular prosthesis. J Maxillofac Prosthet Technol 1: 9–12, 1997.
10. Watson VJ, Waterfield LJ: The growth of the pinna in unilateral aural atresia patients. J Maxillofac Prosthet Technol 2(1):17–19, in print.

CHAPTER 21

Evolution of the Management of Rhinophyma and Related Diseases

Fred J. Stucker, M.D.
Denis Hoasjoe, M.D.
Paul E. Goco, M.D.

Rhinophyma was first described in the Greek literature as early as 2000 BC[1–3] Modern descriptions of the condition have been credited to Hebra in the first part of the nineteenth century.[3] Falsely, the disease has been considered a stigma of uninhibited alcoholic consumption, but there is no proof of any relationship between rhinophyma and alcohol use. This facial deformity has been the trademark of more than a few famous men in history, including W.C. Fields and J.P. Morgan. The disfiguring aspect of rhinophyma was depicted in art as early as the fifteenth century in Domenico (Bigordi) Ghirlandajo's painting, "Old Man with a Child." Popular names for this condition have included references to the plant and animal kingdom such as potato nose and elephantiasis.

Rhinophyma is a condition that affects the nasal skin. It is a localized form of rosacea that causes hyperplasia of the overlying nasal soft tissue components. Nasal airway obstruction and an irregular erythematous deformity of the nose gradually ensue. The resulting deformity affects an individual both cosmetically and functionally. Because of the gradual onset of this condition, most patients seek help because of the cosmetic deformity rather than the nasal obstructive symptoms.

Medical therapy has had limited success, and surgery is the accepted treatment modality. Numerous surgical techniques have been developed with varying success. The senior author (FJS) has had experience in performing multiple surgical resection techniques and is familiar with their various inherent deficiencies. In managing more than 150 cases he has developed a surgical technique over the years that is quick, simple, and has minimum morbidity.

EPIDEMIOLOGY

The etiology of this condition is unknown. Rhinophyma is a form of rosacea. With progressive hyperplasia of the overlying nasal soft tissue,[4] the acne rosacea progresses to rhinophyma. The thinner skin area of the upper nasal dorsum is rarely involved by rhinophyma. Acne rosacea has a strong genetic predisposition and is seen primarily in people of English and Irish descendants; it is less commonly seen in blacks.[5] It usually occurs between the ages of 30 and 50.[4]

Unlike acne rosacea, rhinophyma is more common in males than females; the reported ratio ranges from 5:1 to as high as 30:1.[2,6] The reason for the male preponderance can be explained by two factors: (1) females lack the overlying thick nasal skin that progresses to rhinophyma; (2) females also lack the long-term stimulation of androgenic hormones, which may cause irreversible hypertrophy of the nasal sebaceous glands.

Various other etiologic factors have been proposed. Rhinophyma has been linked to the presence of the mite, *Demodex folliculorum.* However, this parasite is also found in normal follicles, and therefore this etiologic correlation is doubtful. Other associated factors such as facial infection, vitamin deficiencies, stress, and endocrine abnormalities have been proposed, but there is no conclusive evidence to support any specific etiologic cause.[4]

PATHOLOGY

Rhinophyma affects primarily the nasal tip area and spreads gradually to other areas of the nose. Two different types of progression are noted: (1) Proliferative growth of sebaceous glands with development of comedones and inspissated sebum that is frequently infected and foul smelling, and (2) scarring and fibrosis that has a solid character and feel.[6] The progression of the disease is clinically and pathologically indistinguishable from acne rosacea and includes involvement of other facial regions such as the cheeks, glabella, and chin (Fig. 21–1).

Histologically, vascular dilatation and nonspecific dermal lymphatic infiltrates are seen in erythematous areas. There is hyperplasia of the sebaceous glands, connective tissue, and vascular structures.[4] Distributed throughout the rhinophymatous lesions are foci of epithelioid and giant cells. The giant cells are a result of an inflammatory reaction to the excess keratin produced by the sebaceous follicles. This inflammatory reaction leads to vascular dilatation and nonspecific dermal lymphatic infiltrates. The clinical presentation of erythema and tissue hypertrophy is secondary to the hyperplasia of sebaceous glands, connective tissue, and the vascular bed.

A clinical classification of rhinophyma was proposed by Clark and Hanke.[10] However, this classification does not correlate well with the treatment options. The site of the rhinophyma (the nose) is of more importance than its size. A lesion around the nasal alae must be managed more carefully than one at the nasal tip. The potential for scarring is much greater in the alar region because of the shallow basal appendage. Alar retraction often occurs in the alar region from underlying scarring prior to any treatment.

In the older dermatologic literature, rhinophyma was noted to have a higher association with basal cell carcinoma.[11–13] These reports were based on small patient series with poor statistical correlation. It is important to point out that the incidence of basal cell carcinoma has been reported to be as high as 27.6% in normal nasal skin. The concept of basal cell carcinoma arising from rhinophyma is questionable.[14] The presumed etiologic factors of rosacea can be treated; these include poor local hygiene, stress, and infections. Similarly, the aggravating factors for the condition can be treated. Steroids to prevent scarring, and/or antibiotics to prevent infection can be tried. In the older dermatologic literature isotretinoin oil (13-*cis*-retinoic acid [Accutane]) was reported to reduce the volume of the sebaceous glands,[8, 15] but the use of this medication has not been shown to reduce the size of the rhinophymatous nasal tumor. In the first half of this century, radiotherapy was employed for many benign lesions, and its use in rhinophyma was successful; however, the potential carcinogenic effect on the surrounding tissue later precluded use for treatment of most nonmalignant lesions.

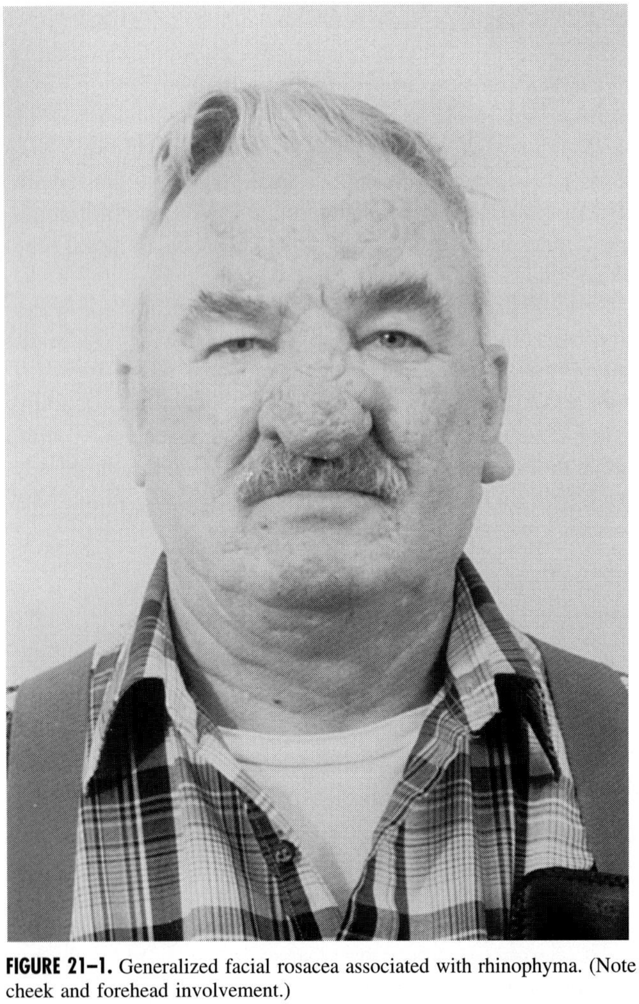

FIGURE 21–1. Generalized facial rosacea associated with rhinophyma. (Note cheek and forehead involvement.)

SURGICAL THERAPIES

Surgical excision is the primary modality used for the treatment of rhinophyma. Different excisional techniques have been proposed, and as new technology develops, new surgical tools are added to the armamentarium. The basic principles of the excision have not changed. The surgical techniques can be classified as (1) total removal of the rhinophymatous tissue with repair of the tissue defect, usually with grafting or flaps (total excision of the tumor with skin grafting or local flap closure is only applicable for small lesions) and (2) partial excision of the tumor, leaving the basal appendages in place for eventual re-epithelialization.

Rhinophyma usually involves multiple nasal subunits. The reconstructive aspects of total excision are not very satisfactory. For disease that involves only one aesthetic subunit, excision without grafting gives very satisfactory results. For most rhinophymatous lesions, partial excision and re-epithelialization provides the best result. Many different decortication techniques have been described. All, if properly carried out, provide an acceptable outcome. The different techniques include: scalpel excision,[11] cryosurgery,[16] electrocautery,[10, 17] dermabrasion,[6, 11] and laser therapy; both carbon dioxide[17, 18] and argon laser therapy[19] have been proposed. Various combinations of these treatments have also been reported.[20–23] A brief outline of the techniques along with their potential for complications will be presented. The senior author's 30 years of experience with all these techniques has led to the development of a surgical treatment that yields good cosmetic and functional results. This technique consists of the use of a Weck blade for the excision and sculpting and the argon laser beam coagulator for hemostasis.

Cryosurgery

Cryosurgery is a popular technique with older dermatologists. Sebaceous tissue is easily destroyed by low temperatures. Liquid nitrogen, supplied in a spray gun, is the most common cryogen used. The rhinophyma is treated with a freeze–thaw cycle. Two cycles are generally used; the freeze time of 30 seconds is followed by a 4-minute thaw time. Bulk reduction of the tumor can be achieved with this technique. This method is easy to use and produces good hemostasis. Nasal cartilage has been reported to be more resistant to freeze injury than the rhinophymatous tissue; therefore, there is a lower incidence of scarring and other structural damage with this technique. Even though cryosurgery is relatively inexpensive, the lack of proper control in regard to the depth of injury has precluded its wide acceptance. There is no ability to contour the nose. The associated hypopigmentary changes that occur with cryotherapy are also a concern in a region as cosmetically prominent as the nose.

Dermabrasion

Dermabrasion has been used extensively in the treatment of rhinophyma but primarily as an adjuvant to other surgical modalities. This method is a good tool for contouring the nose. The technical problem associated with this surgical method is the difficulty of obtaining hemostasis, both intraoperatively and postoperatively. Vascular dilatation is a common pathologic feature of rhinophyma. Bleeding from the hypervascular tissue during the surgery makes it very difficult to determine the depth of penetration of the dermabrasion. Postexcision bleeding is also a problem. After dermabrasion, the thinned tissue does not lend itself to hemostasis, and further tissue destruction is likely to occur with electrocautery.

Electrocautery

Electrocautery has been in use sine the 1950s.[26] This technique has been reported to work best with lesions isolated to the nasal tip. The electrocautery hand-piece utilizes a bipolar loop attachment in the cutting mode with maximum power. The tissue is removed in thin layers. Because of the potential for heat transmission, tissue damage can be quite extensive. Intraoperative bleeding impairs visualization, and the thermal damage inhibits postoperative re-epithelialization. The underlying structural cartilage can be thermally damaged, resulting in significant scarring of the nasal soft tissues. In the literature, more than half of patients treated solely with this technique had scarring,[7] most commonly around the alar rims. The process of achieving hemostasis with cauterization results in deeper and significant damage to the underlying tissue. The length of the contact time between the cautery and the tissue bed is also a factor; a prolonged period of cautery-tissue contact can increase the depth of the damage. Owing to these characteristics and the advances in surgical technology, electrocautery is a relatively unappealing alternative for rhinophyma excision.

Scalpel Excision

Scalpel excision was the first and for many years the primary surgical technique used to treat rhinophyma. The difficulty of achieving hemostasis is the main drawback to this method. An instrument that combines the scalpel with cautery such as the Shaw blade has been used with reasonable success. This scalpel is heated to a temperature of 130° to 180°C by an electric current. It is able to control small and medium-sized vessels.[9] The heated blade produces a narrower area of tissue destruction compared to other cauterization-cutting instruments, but the extent of tissue destruction is still not controllable.[27] Full-thickness injury is possible. Some authors have recommended the use of ice application to the area of excision to achieve hemostasis, but this has not been particularly effective when used on such vascular areas as the nasal tip.

Laser Therapy

Different types of lasers have been used for the excision of rhinophymatous lesions. Proponents of each can provide good arguments for their choice of laser. Argon laser has been used because (1) it selectively coagulates the blood capillaries because of oxyhemoglobin absorption in the blue-green wavelength spectrum (488 to 514.5 nm) and (2) it diverts coagulation shrinkage of the hypertrophic connective tissue. Dermal necrosis of up to 0.5 mm has been reported with the argon laser.[10] This laser has been used without any local anesthesia.[10] The bulk of the tumor is removed with the laser after a trial of medical therapy with tetracycline and resorcinol. The effectiveness of the argon laser as a cutting and debulking tool is questionable, and this laser has few proponents for its use in rhinophyma patients.

The carbon dioxide laser has been the most popular surgical tool for the treatment of rhinophyma for the past decade (Fig. 21–2). When using this laser most surgeons use a cutting spot size of 0.2 mm for the resection of exuberant tissue. The spot size is increased or the beam is defocused for hemostasis. There is less chance of permanent scarring, compared with cautery because of the limited depth of thermal damage. The carbon dioxide laser can seal off blood vessels as small as 0.3 mm in diameter.[11] In the rhinophymatous nose, the vascular dilatation associated with the disease process far exceeds this size and makes hemostasis difficult. This is the major disadvantage of the carbon dioxide laser in treating this condition. The operating time usually averages 50 minutes or more with this method—another distinct disadvantage. The special safety precautions and expenses for the equipment are also inhibiting factors.

TWA Technique

Different combinations of the above techniques have been proposed, such as scalpel excision and cautery, and scalpel

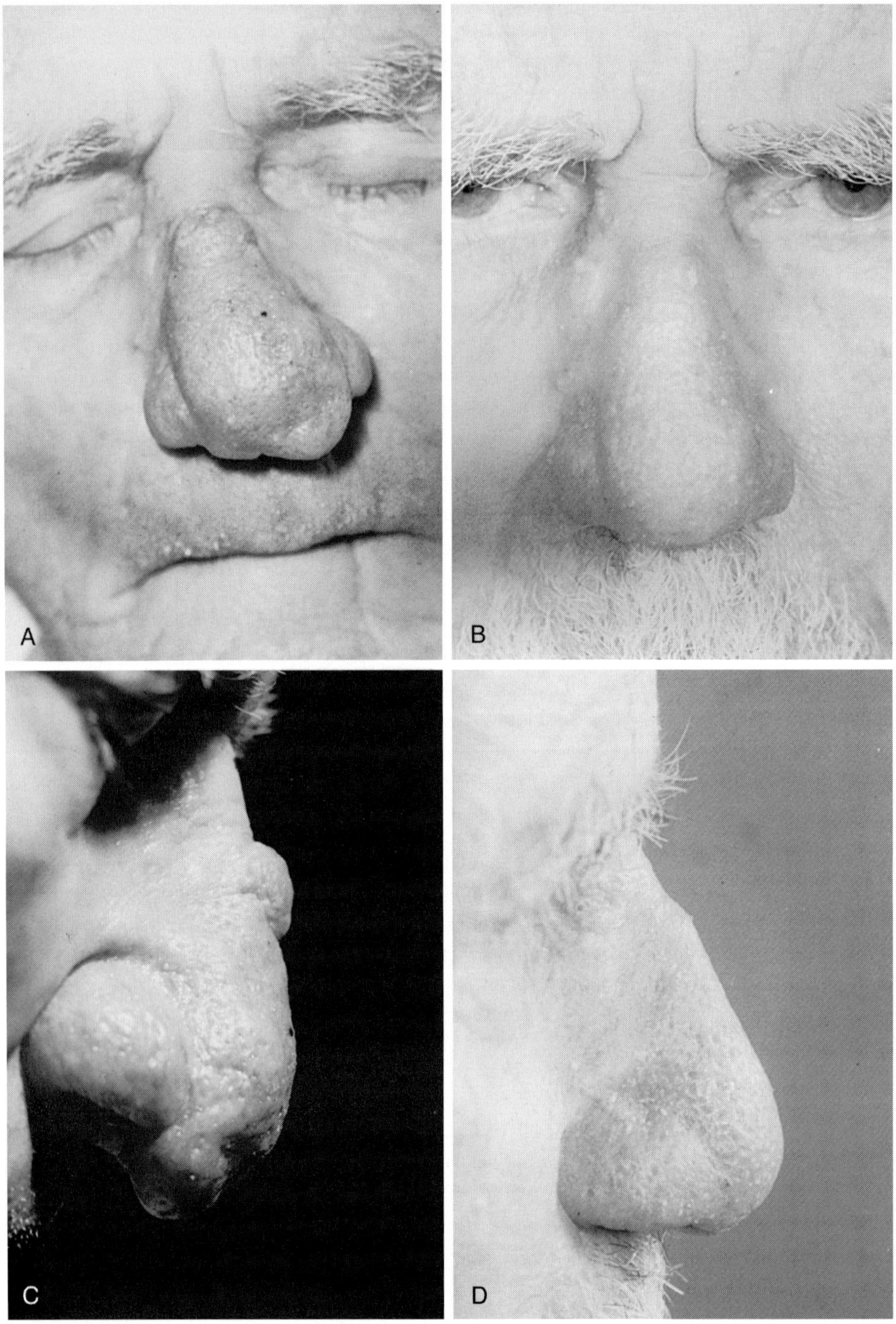

FIGURE 21–2. *A,* Preoperative full face view of patient with rhinophyma. *B,* One-year postoperative view after treatment with the CO_2 laser (operating time 57 minutes). *C,* Preoperative lateral view of patient with rhinophyma. *D,* One-year postoperative view after management with CO_2 laser.

excision and carbon dioxide laser vaporization. One of the techniques that has been shown to be beneficial during the past few years is the TWA technique (tumescent anesthesia, Weck blade, with argon beam coagulation). This method involves: (1) large amounts of local anesthetic agent injected into the nasal soft tissue to provide vessel tamponade (tumescent anesthesia); (2) scalpel contouring of the rhinphymatous lesion with the Weck blade to a desirable depth; and (3) use of the argon beam coagulator (ABC) for hemostasis.[12] The ABC uses a beam of argon gas as a medium to transmit radiofrequency energy of between 40 W and 150 W. The ABC can coagulate vessels up to 2 to 3 mm in diameter,[13] allowing control of vessels up to 10 times the size of those that can be controlled by the carbon dioxide laser. The depth of tissue destruction has been shown to be less than 10.5 μm.[14] The simplicity of this method has reduced the operating time for the rhinophyma excision to less than 10 minutes in all 57 cases handled to date. The cosmetic results are good to excellent, although not superior to those achieved with other techniques (Fig. 21–3).

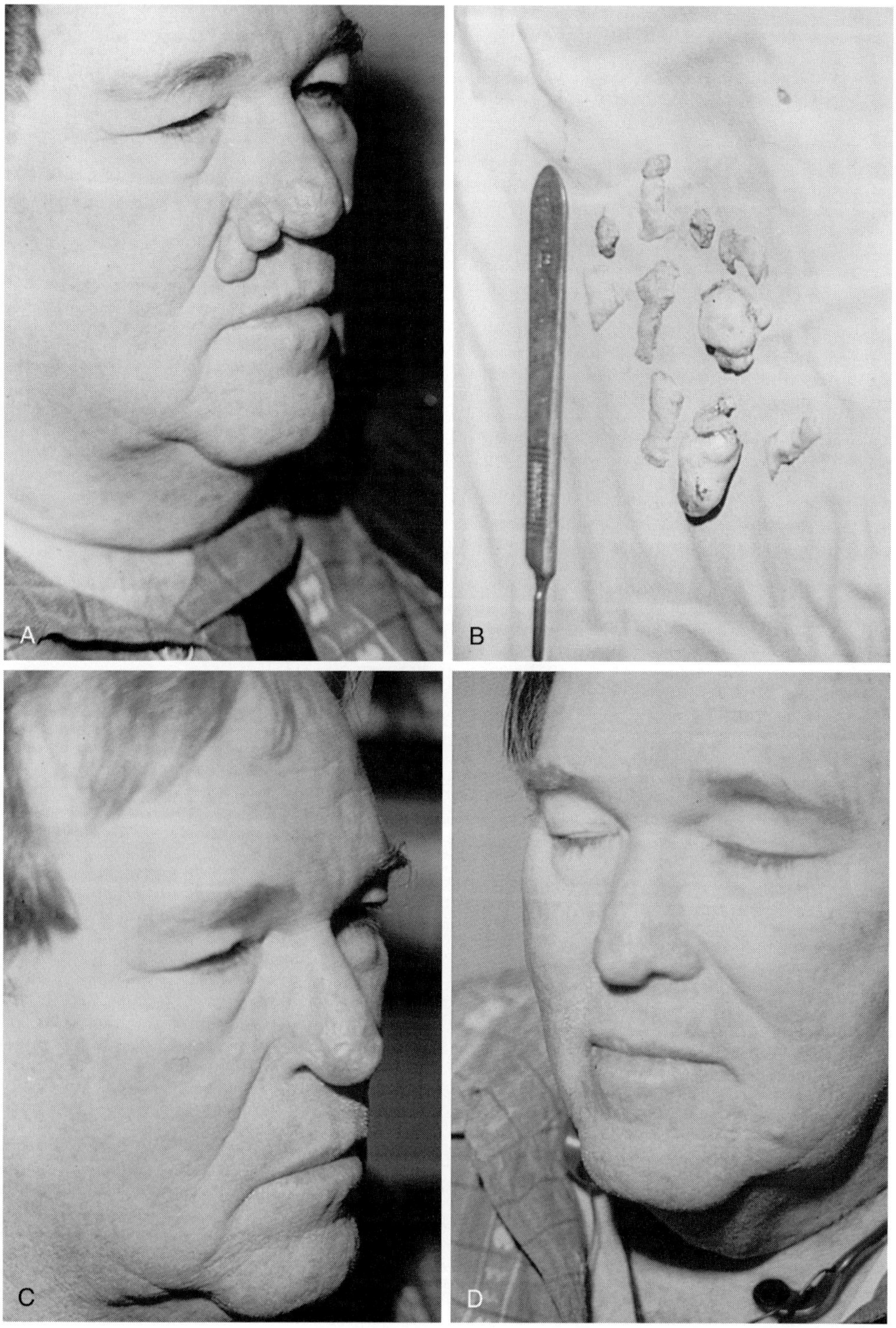

FIGURE 21–3. *A,* Preoperative right oblique view of patient with right-sided only rhinophmya. *B,* Diseased tissue removed with Weck blade. *C,* Postoperative right oblique view at 1 year (operating time 5 minutes). *D,* Postoperative left oblique view; disease was essentially confined to right side.

The value of the TWA technique is that it combines the advantages of surgical resection with elimination of the problem inherent in this vascular lesion, which is primarily bleeding. The chronic inflammatory aspects of this disease process mean that very little or no vasoconstrictive effects occur with conventional local anesthesia. The advantage of tumescent local anesthesia is that the anesthetic solution is injected under pressure, providing vasoconstriction and hemostasis due to compression of the dilated vessels. The rhinophymatous nose is infiltrated with 10 to 15 mL of 1% lidocaine with or without 1:100,000 epinephrine. The diseased tissue is then excised immediately after injection with a Weck blade. Once the tissue volume has been reduced to a level that leaves enough dermal appendages to allow re-epithelialization and is aesthetically acceptable, the ABC is used to achieve absolute hemostasis and to act as a physiologic dressing (Fig. 21–4). The TWA technique combines the advantages of the best techniques with instruments while eliminating the disadvantages of bleeding, scarring, and time. This technique offers results comparable with those

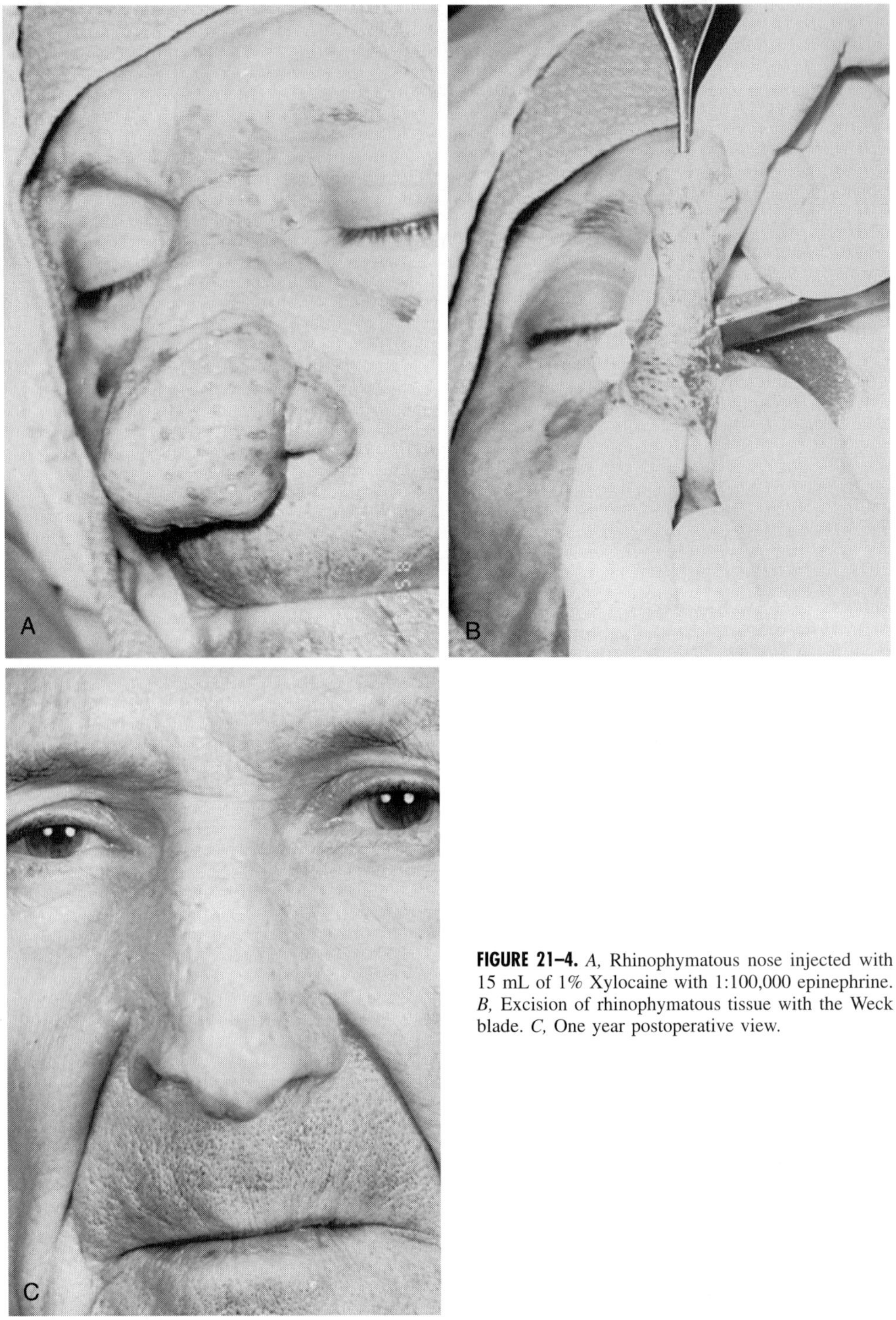

FIGURE 21–4. *A,* Rhinophymatous nose injected with 15 mL of 1% Xylocaine with 1:100,000 epinephrine. *B,* Excision of rhinophymatous tissue with the Weck blade. *C,* One year postoperative view.

obtained with any other technique tried by the senior author. In no case has the total operating time exceeded 10 minutes.

During the past 25 years, the senior author has operated on 134 patients with rhinophyma. In the earlier years the experience with sharp scalpel, dermabrasion, cryosurgery, and electrocautery yielded mixed results and varying complications. When the carbon dioxide laser became available, 34 consecutive patients were managed with this modality. The operating time required for this technique was consistently in excess of 50 minutes. The tumescent local anesthetic allows more careful scalpel excision because the vessels are compressed, which results in much less bleeding. Because of the need to vaporize all anesthetic fluid, this technique is not amenable to the carbon dioxide laser because it would increase an already long operating time. The ABC affords absolute hemostatsis in 15 to 20 seconds.

Our total series of 134 patients included 11 females and 123 males. Five patients had a totally excised basal cell carcinoma. Not all specimens were examined microscopically for skin cancer, and of course this is not possible with some of the techniques.

SUMMARY

Rhinophyma is a functional and cosmetic deformity. Medical therapy has proved to be ineffective. Most surgical therapies that provide decortication with subsequent re-epithelialization of the nose give fair to good results. The carbon dioxide laser was the treatment of choice until 1990. The combination of tissue tamponade with a local anesthetic agent, scalpel excision, and ABC hemostasis is an efficient, simple technique that yields good cosmetic results. One cautionary note should be added, and that is that any surgical excision of tissue must be conservative around the alar rim where the thinner epidermal layer could result in severe alar retraction. There is often a pretreatment contracture in this region, and it is wise to point this out to patients.

REFERENCES

1. Crabtree WC: Rhinophyma. CA West Med 45:485–487, 1936.
2. Odom BL, Odom ER: Rhinophyma. Am J Surg 102:3–16, 1961.
3. Odom BL, Odom ER, Dotz W, Berliner N: Rhinophyma: A master's depiction, a patron's affliction. Am J Dermatopathol 6:231–235, 1984.
4. Plewig G: Rosacea. *In* Fitzgerald TB, Eisen AZ, Wolff K, Freedberg IM, Austin KF (eds): Dermatology in General Medicine, 4th ed. New York, McGraw-Hill, 1993, pp 727–735.
5. Ersek RA, Denton DR: Rhinophyma: Treatment with electrocautery and silver impregnated porcine xenograft. Plast Reconstr Surg 74:269–273, 1984.
6. Freeman BS: Reconstructive rhinoplasty for rhinophyma. Plast Reconstr Surg 46:265–270, 1970.
7. Wiener DR: Rhinophyma. Clin Plast Surg 14:357–365, 1987.
8. Robinson TWE: *Demodex folliculorum* and rosacea: A clinical and histologic study. Arch Dermatol 92:542–544, 1965.
9. Strauss JS, Pochi PE: Intracutaneous injections of sebum and comedones. Arch Dermat 92:443–454, 1965.
10. Clark DP, Hanke CW: Electrosurgical treatment of rhinophyma. J Am Acad Dermatol 22:831–837, 1990.
11. Fisher WJ: Rhinophyma: Its surgical treatment. Plast Reconstr Surg 45:466–470, 1970.
12. Rees TD: Basal cell carcinoma in association with rhinophyma. Plast Reconstr Surg 16:282–287, 1955.
13. Acker DW, Helwig EB: Rhinophyma with carcinoma. Arch Dermatol 95:250–254, 1967.
14. Keefe M, Wakeel RA, McBride DI: Basal cell carcinoma mimicking rhinophyma. Arch Dermatol 124:1077–1079, 1988.
15. Golstein JA, Comite H, Mescon H, Pochi PE: Isotretinoin in the treatment of acne. Arch Dermatol 118:555–558, 1982.
16. Sonnex TS, Dawber RPR: Rhinophyma: Treatment by liquid nitrogen spray cryosurgery. Clin Exp Dermatol 11:284–288, 1986.
17. Roenick RK: CO_2 laser vaporization for treatment of rhinophyma. Mayo Clin Proc 62:676–686, 1987.
18. Shapshay SM, Strong MS, Anastasi GW, Vaughan CW: Removal of rhinophyma with carbon dioxide laser: A preliminary report. Arch Otolaryngol 106:257–259, 1980.
19. Hulsberger Henning JP, Van Gemert MJC: Rhinophyma treated by argon laser. Laser Surg Med 2:211–215, 1983.
20. Eisen RF, Katz AE, Bohigian RK, Grande DJ: Surgical treatment of rhinophyma with the Shaw scalpel. Arch Dermatol 122:307–309, 1986.
21. Staindi O: Surgical management of rhinophyma. Acta Otolaryngol 92:137–140, 1981.
22. Doleyad R, Schultz RC: Early treatment of rhinophyma—a neglected entity? Ann Plast Surg 11:393–396, 1983.
23. Wheeland RG, Bailin PL, Ratz JL: Combined carbon dioxide laser excision and vaporization in the treatment of rhinophyma. J Dermatol Surg Oncol 13:172–177, 1987.
24. Nolan JW: Cryosurgical treatment of rhinophyma. Plast Reconstr Surg 52:437–438, 1973.
25. Gage AA: Cryosurgery for cancer of the ear. J Dermatol Surg Oncol 3:417–421, 1977.
26. Niedelman ML: Rhinophyma: Treatment by electroshaving. Arch Dermatol Syphil 70:91–93, 1954.
27. Tromovitch TA, Glogan RG, Stegman SJ: The Shaw scalpel. J Dermatol Surg Oncol 9:316–319, 1983.
28. Ward PH, Castro DJ, Ward S: A significant new contribution to radical head and neck surgery. Arch Otolaryngol 115:921–923, 1989.
29. Teimourian B, Duda G, Nickodem AM, Jumar A: Application of the argon beam coagulator in plastic surgery. Perspect Plast Surg 5:91–98, 1991.
30. Stucker FJ, Hoasjoe DK, Aarstad RF: Rhinophyma: A new approach to hemostasis. Ann Otol Rhinol Laryngol 102:925–929, 1993.

CHAPTER 22

Facial Soft Tissue Defects and Nasal Deformities in the Pediatric Patient

Fred J. Stucker, M.D.

SOFT TISSUE DEFECTS

Soft tissue reconstruction in the pediatric patient differs from that in the adult patient in a number of ways. Studies show that blunt trauma in adults produces lacerations along relaxed skin tension lines. Due to the inherent elasticity of skin and the lack of skin laxity, traumatic facial injuries in children often result in avulsion defects rather than lacerations. Soft tissue surgical resections require more tension to close than comparable wounds in an older patient. The difficulty of mobilizing local flaps in children renders reconstruction of soft tissue and traumatic defects more challenging. Similar defects in adults are usually amenable to primary closure or local flap reconstruction due to tissue excess and laxity in the adult.

With aging there is marked tissue atrophy in the facial dermal and subdermal adipose tissue. This atrophy is characterized by a loss of elastic fibers and resiliency of the skin. The dermis of the pediatric patient is more contractile and less amenable to stretch. On microscopic examination, the rete ridges are composed of deeper epidermal rete pegs interdigitating with the dermal papillae. This interdigitation helps to secure the overlying epidermis to the underlying dermis. With aging, the dermal-epidermal junction flattens owing to a decrease in the length of the dermal papillae and rete pegs. In the elderly, decreased interdigitation allows dermal-epidermal separation to occur more readily.

In my practice, most challenging cases of soft tissue reconstruction in pediatric patients result from trauma. Benign and malignant facial tumors in children are seen less commonly but provide a significant number of our management dilemmas. The majority of injuries must be handled acutely, but there usually are a variety of options available depending on the experience of the surgeon. I have used the perichondrial cutaneous graft (PCCG) extensively in a variety of applications in the pediatric age group with success. Secondary and multistaged procedures are common in pediatric reconstructive cases.

General Guidelines in Managing Trauma

The following guidelines are advised when the tissue loss is secondary to an injury. A detailed medical history of the patient includes the exact cause of injury, elapsed time since the injury, general medical condition of the patient, tetanus immunization status, and consideration of rabies vaccination in patients with animal bite injuries. The degree and potential for contamination dictate the extent of cleansing needed. The patient's face and scalp are cleansed thoroughly with an antiseptic solution paying careful attention to all matted areas of hair to expose all hidden injuries. The exact extent of the injuries is recorded both on the chart and with photodocumentation. All underlying bony structures are assessed, and radiographs (fine-cut axial and coronal CT [computed tomographic] scans, Panorex x-rays, plain films, and so on) are obtained to detect possible fractures. Treatment of facial fractures is performed prior to soft tissue closure unless there is an overriding reason to delay such repair. Careful examination of facial nerve function is mandatory along with assessment of the parotid duct in all lateral facial injuries. The patient's facial nerve function is evaluated both at rest and during animation.

Management of Soft Tissue Wounds

Lacerations. The typical laceration injury can be closed primarily after thorough cleaning. A minimal number of deeply placed sutures should be used to close any dead space and reduce the tension on the overlying skin. Significantly more tension is required to close pediatric wounds compared to those in adults. There is a direct relationship between the number of deep sutures and the incidence of wound infections.

Meticulous eversion of the skin edges when closing a wound helps to ensure minimal scarring. Eversion can be aided by alternating vertical mattress sutures with simple sutures. Dermabrasion of a scar 3 to 4 weeks after closure can markedly improve the cosmetic results.

Abrasions. Partial-thickness skin loss secondary to traumatic friction to the epidermis is treated with careful wound care. Initial treatment includes adequate debridement of all foreign bodies or embedded materials to prevent traumatic tattooing. Aggressive cleansing and debridement are often required and are performed under local or general anesthesia depending on the patient's tolerance. Occasionally, a wire brush or rotary wheel is required. This experience has indicated to me that dermabrasion, when carefully performed in prudently chosen cases, is a safe procedure in children, including black children (see Fig. 22–4).

Avulsions (Full-Thickness Tissue Loss). Avulsion injuries and their resulting defects present a more complex management problem. These injuries require debridement of all devitalized tissue and foreign bodies. It is essential to examine and explore the depths of the wound for other injuries. Depending on the severity and location of the full-thickness tissue loss, the wound may, under certain circumstances, be allowed to heal by secondary intention. More commonly used options are skin grafting, perichondrial cutaneous grafting, and local, regional, or free flap reconstruction. Rarely and under optimum conditions, and with proper care of the avulsed body part, microvascular reimplantation may be performed.

Surgical Defects

Surgical defects, compared to traumatic injuries, are by their nature cleaner, more precise, and, ideally, more thoughtfully placed. Preoperative planning implies consideration of the various reconstructive options available consistent with the surgical procedure. In managing surgically created soft tissue defects one must consider the histologic diagnosis of the lesion, the potential for recurrence, the possible need for postoperative radiation therapy, the patient's age, size, and maturity, and the impact of future growth on the defect and the method of reconstruction. The reasons for the surgical defect and the likely future implications are of major concern in the young patient. The likelihood of future surgery, the potential for cure, and the psychological impact of the surgery and the reconstruction must enter the management equation. Incisions are placed where they offer the greatest chance for a prudent resection combined with the least cosmetic deformity, such as intraoral placement (Fig. 22–1).

Useful Methods in Managing Soft Tissue Deficits in the Pediatric Patient (Fundamentals)

Perichondrial Cutaneous Grafts (PCCG). Even the thickest full-thickness skin grafts undergo significant contraction. This inherent quality in a growing infant or child can lead to disastrous long-term results (Fig. 22–2). For this reason, I have replaced skin grafts with PCCGs for defects less than 3 to 4 cm in diameter in children. Skin grafts, besides contracting, also are usually too thin and provide a poor color match. Our animal studies as well as a large clinical series indicate that this reliable composite graft actually expands with the growth of the child. Indications for this technique are quite liberal in pediatric patients, in whom primary closure, local flaps, and skin grafts are less likely to be successful than in adults.

In children the most common sites reconstructed with this versatile composite graft are the nose and the eyelids. The tendency to avoid flaps in children and the significant contracture that follows the use of skin grafts has prompted me to use the PCCG in 31 children under the age of 12 over the past 15 years. We have used it in a 9-day-old infant and in 27 other children under the age of 7. I am particularly impressed with its value in children with eyelid injuries, in which it avoids the devastating effects of scarring and contracture (Fig. 22–3). This technique was employed for eyelid reconstruction in 11 children. The graft was harvested from the anterior conchal bowl, where the perichondrium is firmly attached to the skin. The donor site was closed with a posterior auricular island flap rotated through a 1-cm fenestration created in the conchal bowl cartilage. The postauricular defect was closed in a vertical direction, creating a more shallow sulcus. There have been no short- or long-term problems with the donor site reconstruction. Follow-up has extended a minimum of 1 year and as long as 14 years (Fig. 22–4).

Serial Resection. The popularity of tissue expansion has prompted many surgeons to ignore the time-proven technique of serial resection. Serial resection is another method of tissue expansion that may require more procedures but has fewer complications and less of the morbidity that can be so troubling in younger patients. Serial resection is technically easier for the surgeon and in my view generally yields cosmetically superior results. Its one disadvantage is the time required.

My recommendation is not intended to discourage the use of tissue expansion but to highlight the utilitarian value of this technique. Serial resection more easily brings tissue in from desired directions. Tissue expansion is a circumferential three-dimensional phenomenon and as such can produce undesirable deformities as it expands. The complications seen with tissue expansion are well known and have been reported to occur in as many as 40% of cases. Serial resection has essentially the same complication rate as any surgical closure procedure under tension. The technical difficulties encountered and the required expertise are far greater with tissue expansion. At least two or three procedures are required with tissue expansion, but many more may be needed with serial resection. I have experienced no difficulty with scheduling surgery every 6 to 8 weeks in younger patients undergoing serial resection reconstruction. It is wise to consider all aspects of the particular case when deciding which technique to employ. In children, I have found that serial resection is superior to tissue expansion in recruiting extra tissue to the various areas of the face (Fig. 22–5).

Text continued on page 288

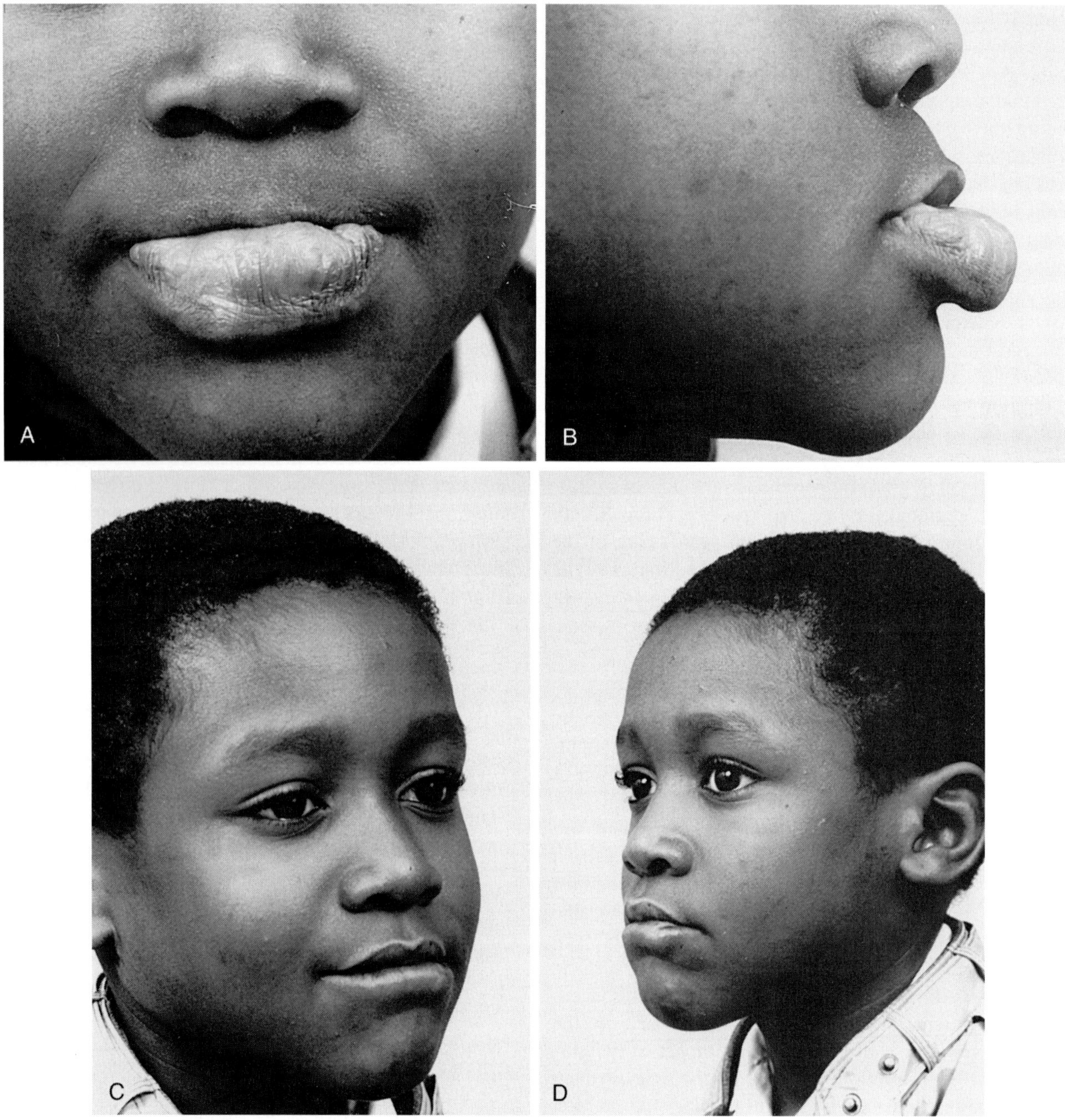

FIGURE 22–1. *A,* Frontal view of lower lip lymphangioma. *B,* Right lateral view. *C,* Two-year follow-up, right oblique view. *D,* Two-year follow-up, left oblique view.

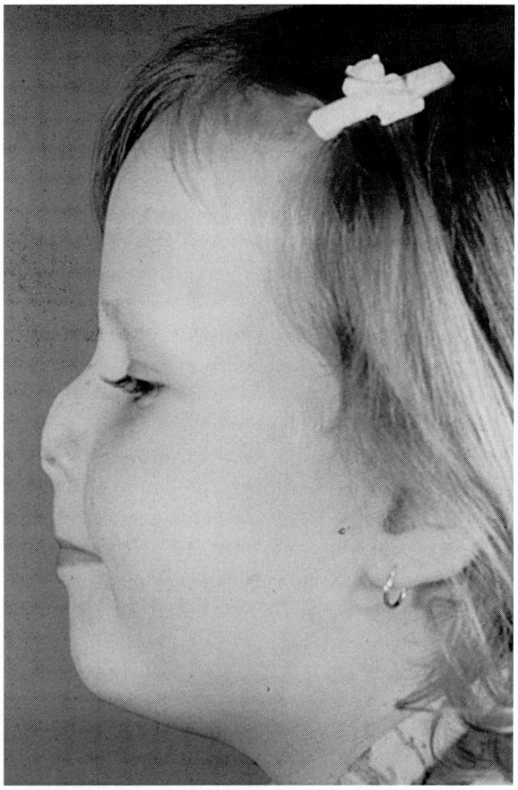

FIGURE 22–2. Seven-year-old who had nasal tip resurfaced with a skin graft at age 6 months.

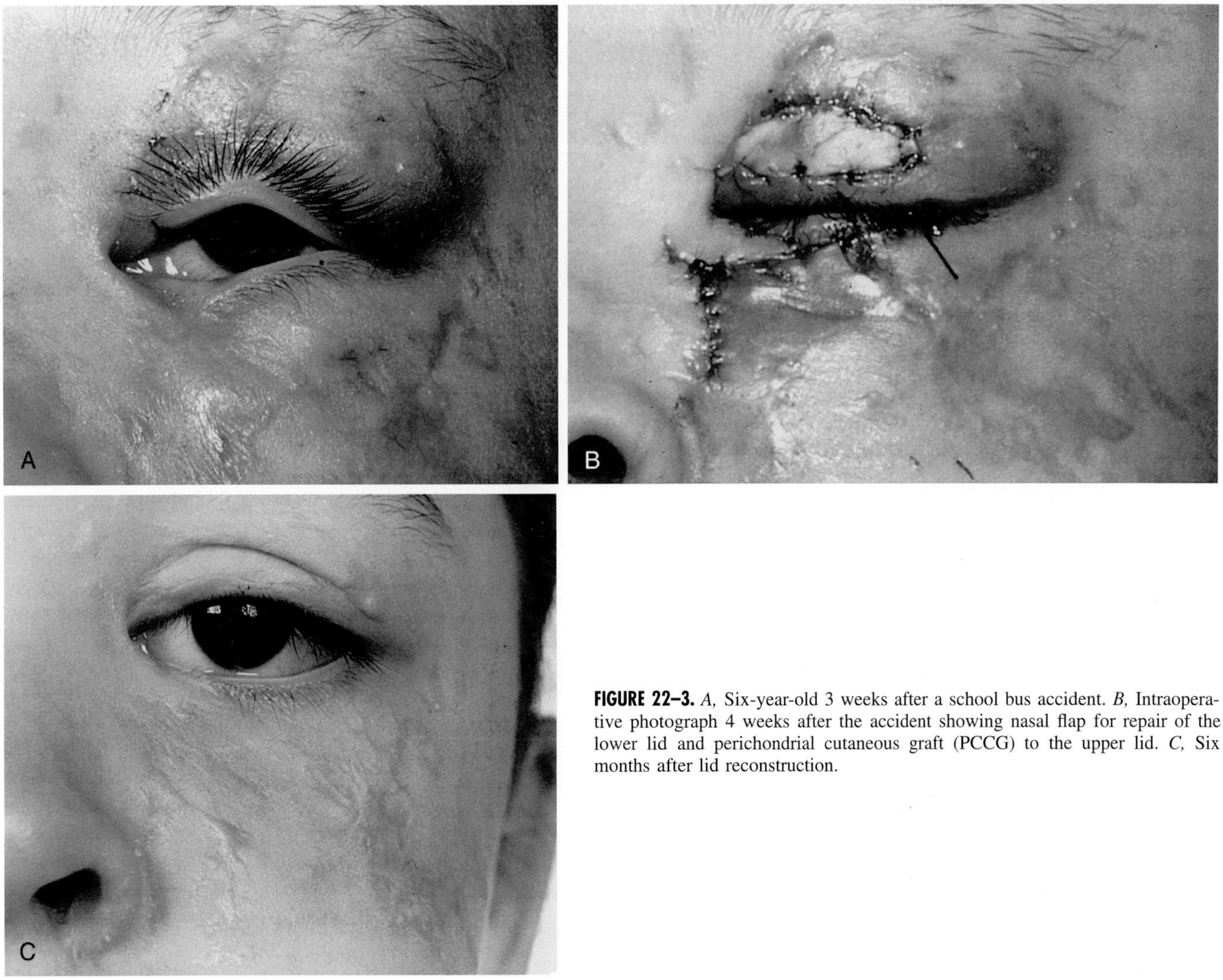

FIGURE 22–3. *A,* Six-year-old 3 weeks after a school bus accident. *B,* Intraoperative photograph 4 weeks after the accident showing nasal flap for repair of the lower lid and perichondrial cutaneous graft (PCCG) to the upper lid. *C,* Six months after lid reconstruction.

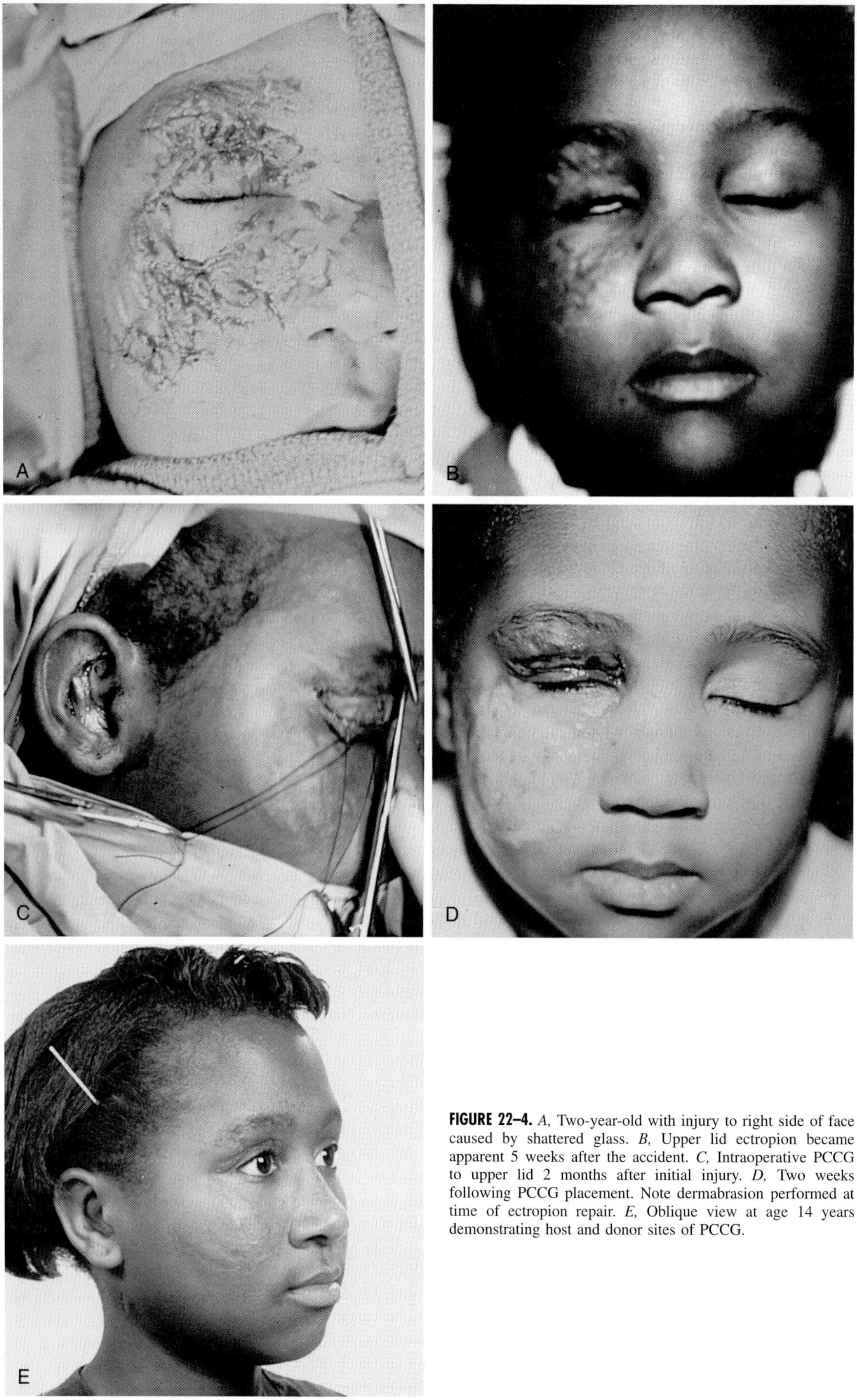

FIGURE 22–4. *A,* Two-year-old with injury to right side of face caused by shattered glass. *B,* Upper lid ectropion became apparent 5 weeks after the accident. *C,* Intraoperative PCCG to upper lid 2 months after initial injury. *D,* Two weeks following PCCG placement. Note dermabrasion performed at time of ectropion repair. *E,* Oblique view at age 14 years demonstrating host and donor sites of PCCG.

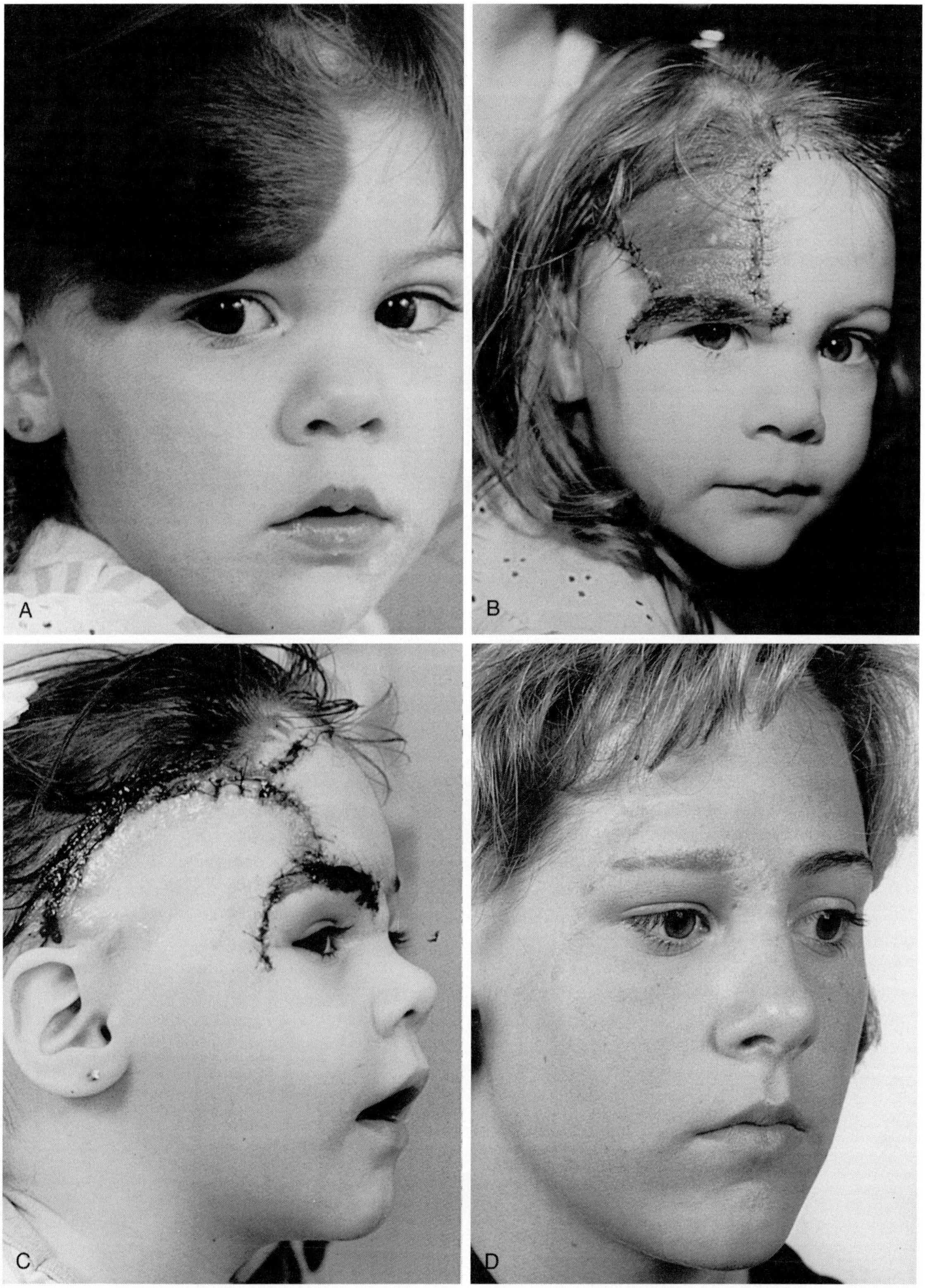

FIGURE 22–5. *A,* Eighteen-month-old child with giant hairy nevus of forehead. *B,* Following second serial resection procedure at 2 years of age. *C,* Postoperative photo following fifth procedure at age 3 years. *D,* Oblique view 14 years after first procedure.

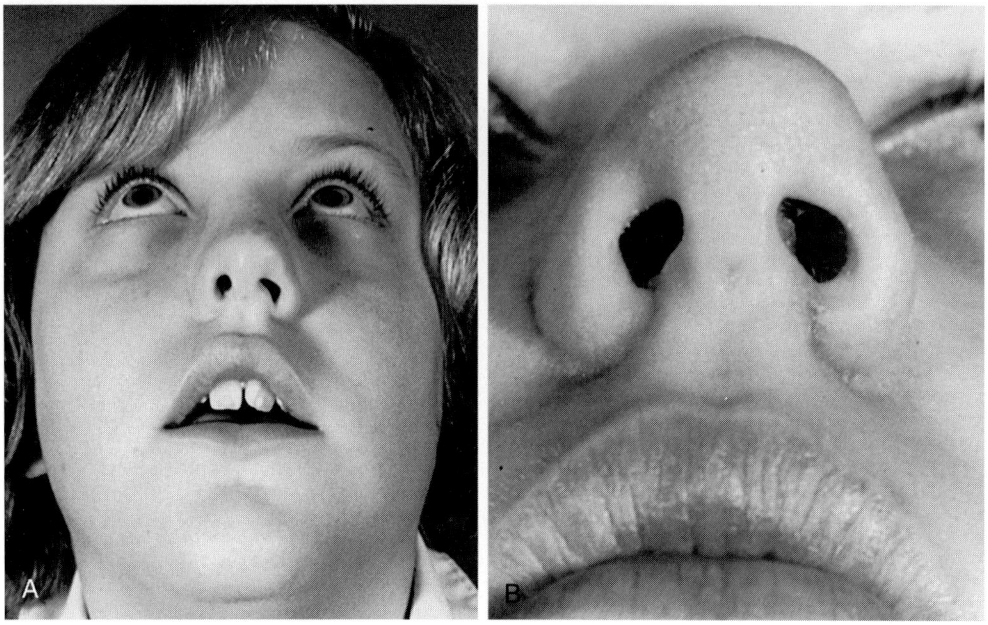

FIGURE 22–6. *A,* Submental view of patient with previous lateral rhinotomy demonstrating asymmetry of nasal ala. *B,* Submental view showing how alar adjustment on normal side creates a more symmetrical appearance.

Creating Symmetry. As with all features on the face, symmetry is one of the most difficult goals to achieve and the most discernible fault when absent. In the pediatric patient the nose and ears are the structures in which a minor deformity is made more obvious because of asymmetry. In some situations it is often prudent to alter the normal side somewhat to achieve a more pleasing symmetrical appearance (Figs. 22–6 and 22–7).

Revision of Scars. Despite meticulous and careful wound closure, some scars heal in a less than satisfactory manner. Waiting 6 months before revising an existing scar to allow for scar remodeling and resolution of erythema is basically a good principle. However, if the scar is causing an obvious deformity such as an ectropion or a gross aesthetic or functional deformity that will not improve with time, an earlier revision is indicated. Techniques using Z-plasty, broken line closures, and skin flaps and grafts are extremely useful in children and must be carefully planned and precisely approximated with sutures (Fig. 22–8). Every attempt must be made to achieve a tension-free skin closure. This can be quite difficult in the pediatric patient. It is useful to support the wound closure with dermal sutures placed some distance from the skin edge and routed deep to the scar bed. These are permanent sutures that can prevent the wound from spreading, a process that can occur up to 2 or 3 months following the revision (Fig. 22–9).

Management of Bites (Animal and Human). Because of their inquisitive nature, children are susceptible to animal bites, particularly dog bites. Most injuries tend to occur on the cheek, forehead, and periorbital areas. Injuries in which there is no loss of tissue should be minimally debrided, thoroughly cleansed, irrigated, and then closed primarily. The wound margins should be loosely approximated to allow egress of any exudate. Human bites tend to occur in adolescents and adults and are notorious for becoming infected. The human oral cavity contains high concentrations of different pathogens, greatly increasing the incidence of infection. Primary closure of human bites must be performed on an individual basis, and secondary management is often indicated. Avulsed tissue, which is the result of an animal bite, has essentially no chance for survival following implantation despite occasional reports to the contrary in the literature (Fig. 22–10).

General Guidelines for Wound Care. During the immediate healing period, wounds should not be allowed to develop blood clots, crusting, or any exudative material. Clots and debris harbor bacteria and encourage bacterial growth, leading to infection and less than optimal healing. An unsightly scar is the ultimate result. The wound, whether closed primarily or allowed to heal by secondary intention, should be cleansed with half-strength hydrogen peroxide several times during the day (or more often as needed) to prevent crusting. While exudative material is still being produced (oozing), iced saline gauze dressings are advocated on wounds closed with nonabsorbable sutures. The saline soak will dissolve absorbable sutures, which will weaken and destroy the closure.

An occlusive ointment, such as vitamin A and D, should then be applied to prevent crusting and to keep the wound margins moist and encourage healing. Antibiotic ointments should be avoided due to the atopic reaction or sensitivity that can develop, especially with bacitracin and neomycin.

Avoidance of sun exposure for 1 year is recommended to prevent unsightly scar formation. A chemical sunscreen of at least 15 sun protection factor (SPF) should be used as well as a physical barrier such as a wide-brimmed hat. Local flaps and grafts can undergo necrosis if not protected from sun exposure.

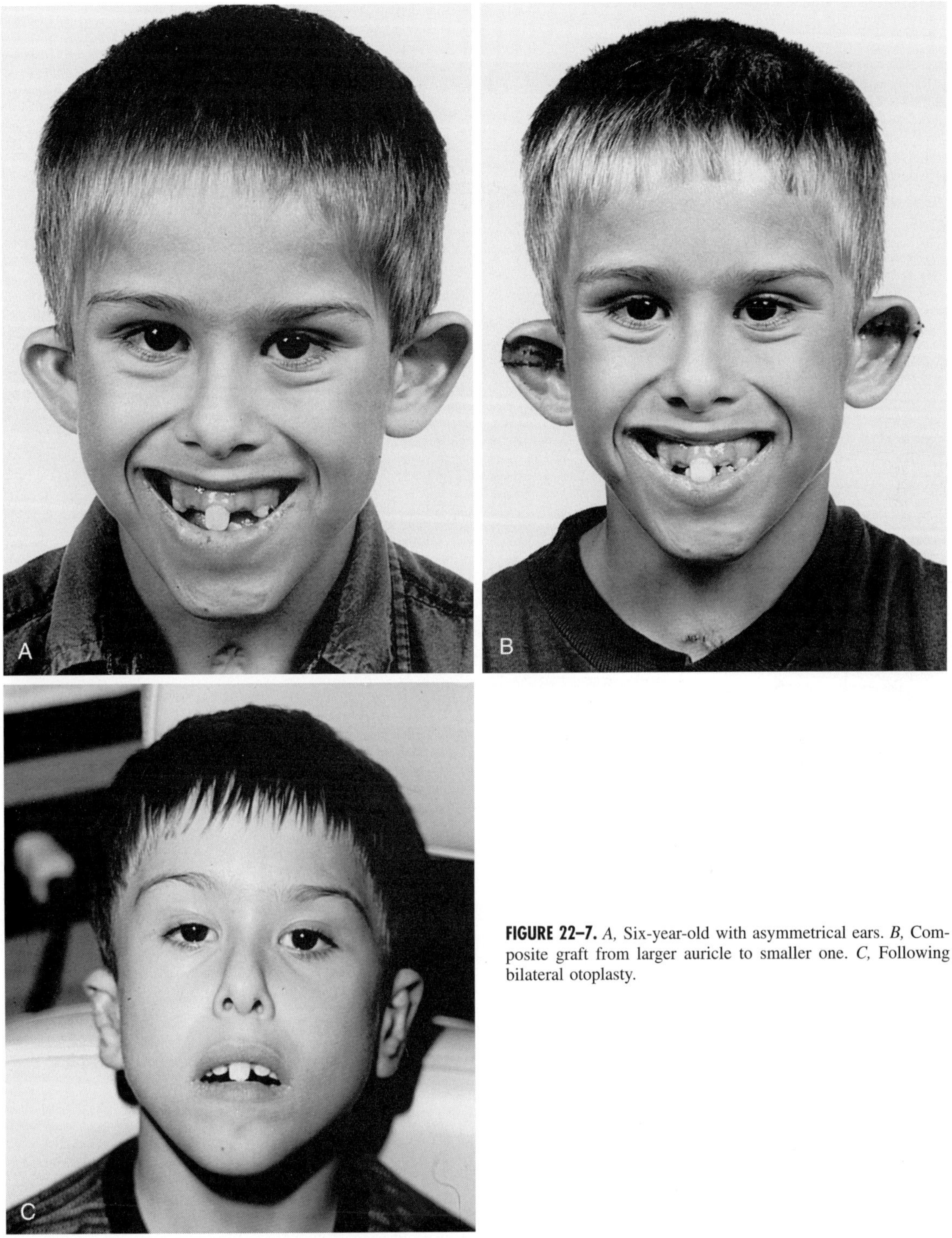

FIGURE 22–7. *A,* Six-year-old with asymmetrical ears. *B,* Composite graft from larger auricle to smaller one. *C,* Following bilateral otoplasty.

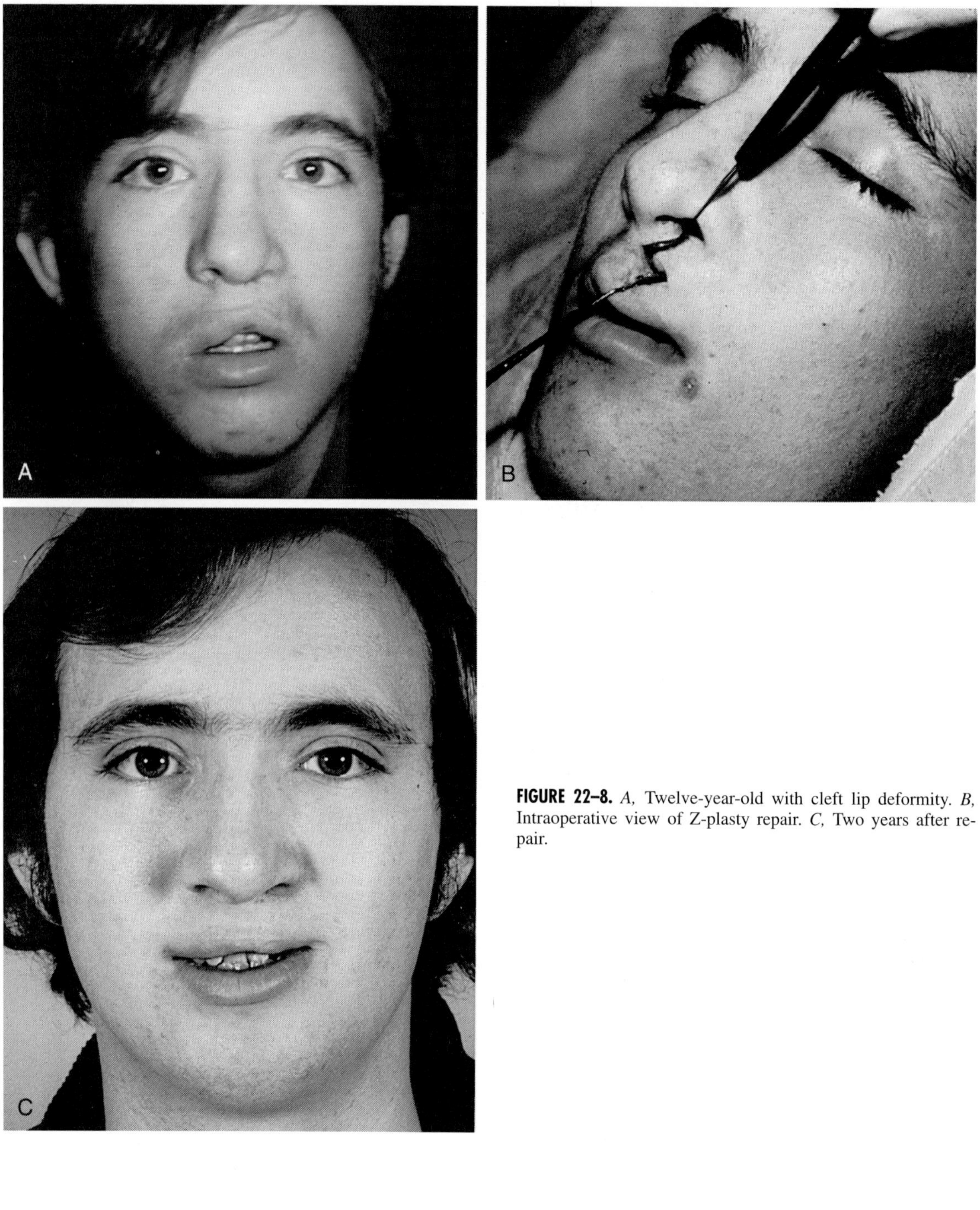

FIGURE 22–8. *A,* Twelve-year-old with cleft lip deformity. *B,* Intraoperative view of Z-plasty repair. *C,* Two years after repair.

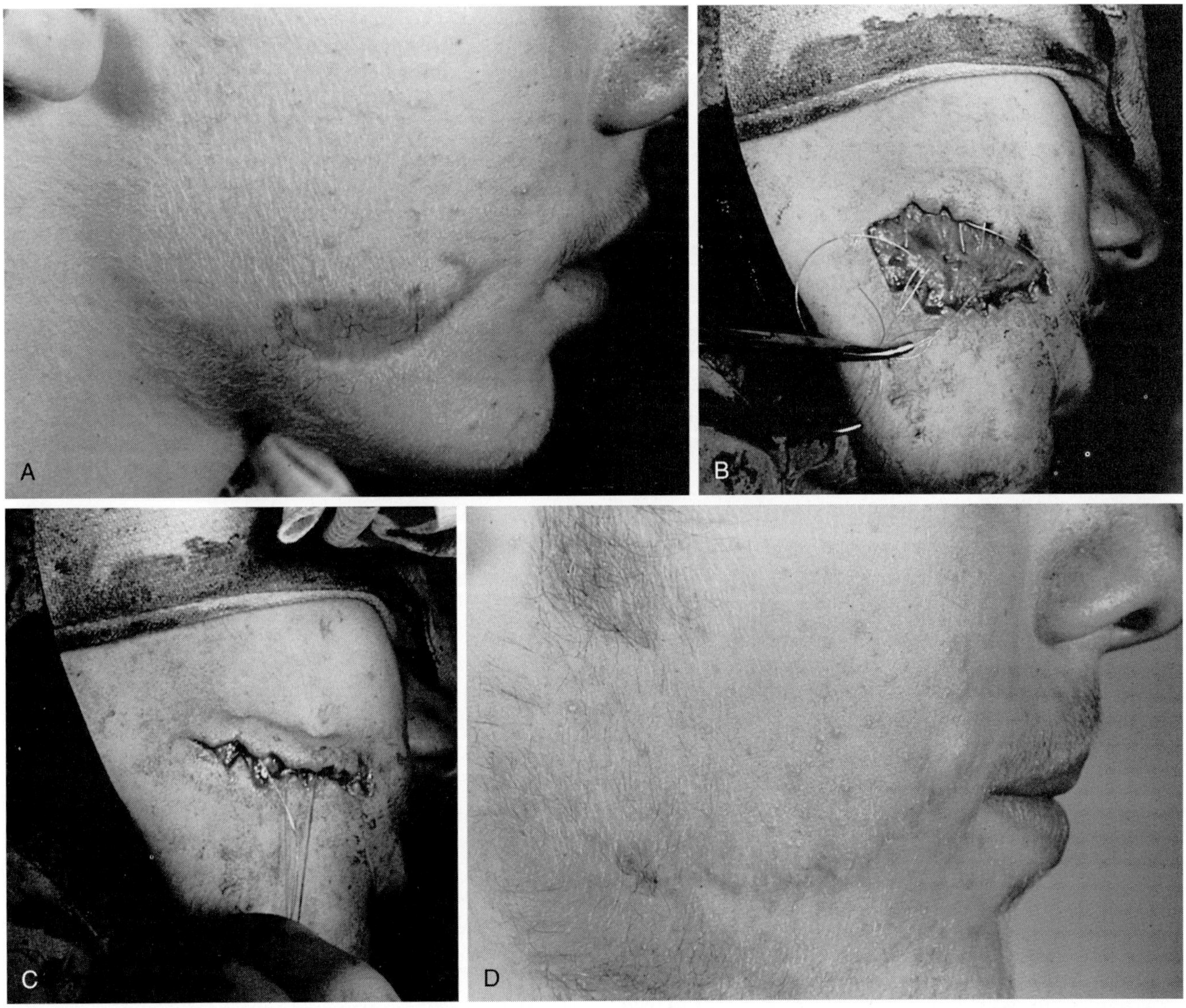

FIGURE 22–9. *A,* Thirteen-year-old with wide atrophic scar over the mandible that spread the mouth following an originally precise closure. *B,* Broken line shows geometric closure with permanent dermal suture passed deep into subcutaneous tissue to reinforce closure. *C,* Traction exhibited by tying the deep suture. *D,* Six-month postoperative view.

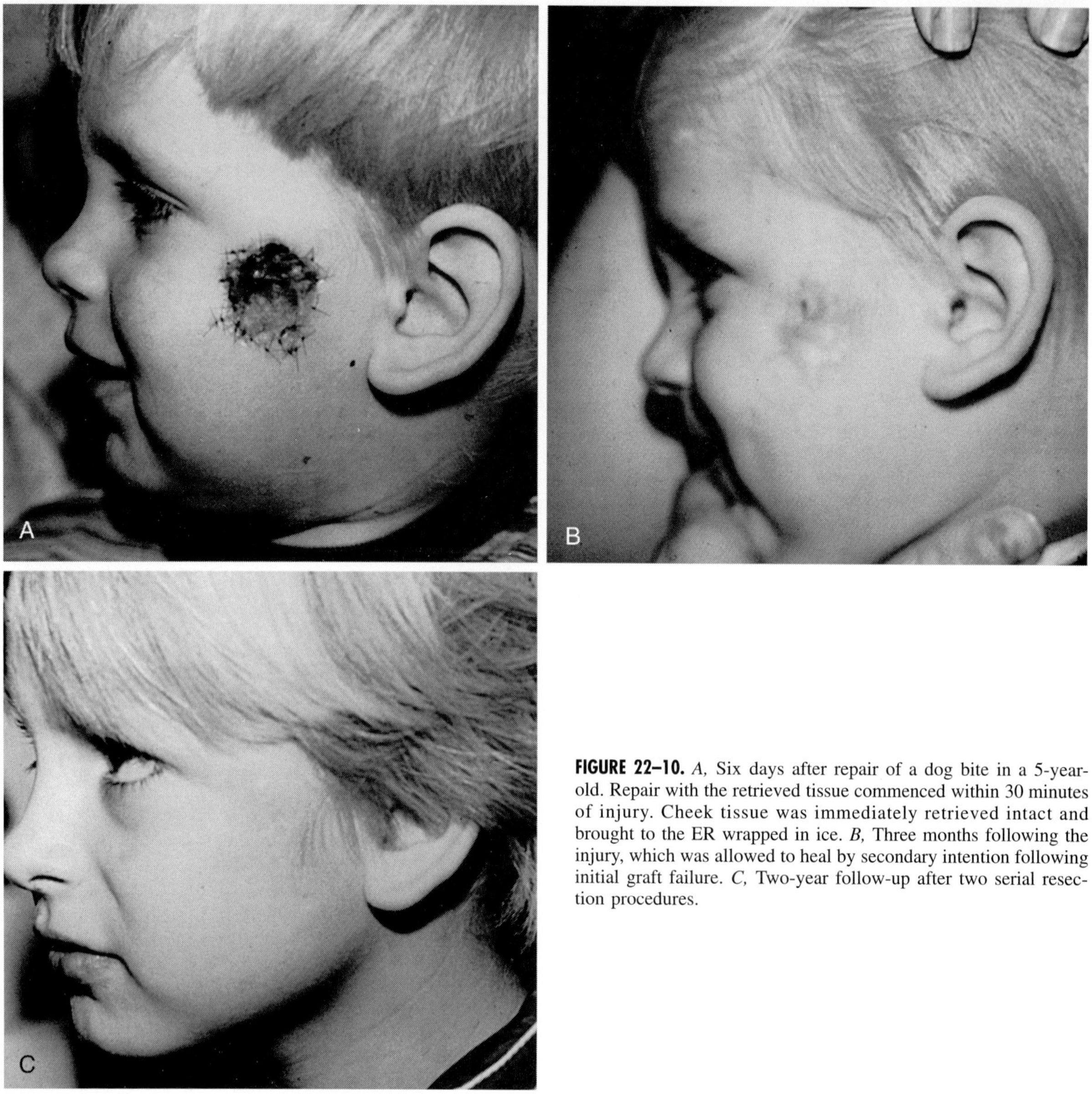

FIGURE 22–10. *A,* Six days after repair of a dog bite in a 5-year-old. Repair with the retrieved tissue commenced within 30 minutes of injury. Cheek tissue was immediately retrieved intact and brought to the ER wrapped in ice. *B,* Three months following the injury, which was allowed to heal by secondary intention following initial graft failure. *C,* Two-year follow-up after two serial resection procedures.

NASAL SURGERY IN THE PEDIATRIC PATIENT

General Principles

My philosophy regarding nasal surgery in children has evolved during the past three decades. Much experience has been gained by managing a large number of trauma patients and noting the subsequent follow-up on them through childhood. Observations of these necessary nasal procedures in children provide guidelines that can be followed in elective surgery. Serial examination of these patients as they pass into adulthood has reinforced my long-held views of therapeutic temperance in regard to pediatric nasal surgery (Fig. 22–11). I have discovered that prudent soft tissue surgery on the nose, including the septal cartilage and the lower lateral cartilages, can usually be carried out safely in children (Table 22–1).

I recommend as conservative an approach as possible consistent with the clinical scenario and the desired goals. In the prepubertal patients I employ the guiding principle of establishing a patent nasal airway. Surgery for nasal neoplasms is expeditiously managed, but again, every consideration for growth is integrated into the planning and performance of extirpative surgery. Cosmetic considerations are secondary at this age except in cases of significant deformity that my experience indicates can be safely corrected.

Technical considerations are much more critical in the pediatric patient. Care is taken to avoid violation and damage to the mucoperichondrium, which is a much more daunting undertaking than it is in the adult owing to the confining space in which one has to work. All dissections are kept to a minimum, and the most conservative resection of septal cartilage is performed. Osteotomies, because of the potential disruption of growth centers associated with them, are avoided in all prepubertal children. A more liberal attitude

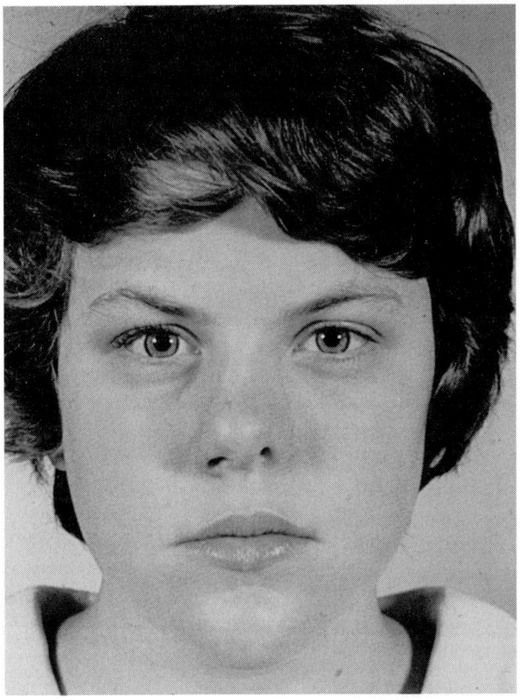

FIGURE 22–11. Eleven-year-old who underwent a lateral rhinotomy at age 6 months for a teratoma. Note arrested growth secondary to osteotomy on left side.

can be taken in the postpubertal adolescent; I continue to recommend conservative principles but do employ osteotomies in selected cases. Restoration of function continues to be the primary indication for nasal surgery in the early adolescent. As the nose approaches adult size, growth disturbances have less significance. When there is no clear need for nasal surgery the general rule of withholding such surgery in boys until age 17 years and in girls until age 15 years is very prudent advice.

Management of Nasal Trauma

Timely operative intervention is indicated for nasal deformities caused by trauma. Most commonly, these are displaced nasal fractures. Most of these deformities can be managed by closed reduction. Diagnosis may be difficult until the edema resolves. Digital compression combined with intranasal elevation of the nasal bones can reduce most fractures if there is no telescoping injury. Elevation with a Sayre elevator or similar instrument is necessary to disimpact the depressed nasal bone. Should closed reduction fail, open reduction is required. Since most children require general anesthesia, I proceed by employing a 2-mm chisel pushed through the mucosa at the piriform aperture and utilize strategic perforations of the bone to allow proper alignment. Development of a unilateral intact mucoperichondrial flap and minimal septal cartilage resection is employed if septoplasty is necessary. Thus, a conservative septorhinoplasty is performed only to obtain adequate alignment and a functional nasal airway. Techniques for further refinement and cosmesis that would require more extensive dissection are delayed.

TABLE 22–1. PRINCIPLES IN MANAGING PEDIATRIC NASAL SURGERY

PEDIATRIC NASAL TRAUMA

1. Examine for septal hematoma
   a. Evacuate, depending drainage
   b. Obliterate with septal whipstitch
2. Reevaluate for fracture after swelling has subsided (day 2 to 4)
3. Be patient with the difficulty in examining children
4. Attempt closed reduction
5. Use 2-mm chisel in open reduction

ELECTIVE NASAL SURGERY

1. Do no harm in elective surgery
2. Avoid elective osteotomies
3. Relieve obstruction
4. Can perform appropriate soft tissue surgery
5. Avoid skin grafts in very young children
6. Think PCCG

CONSERVATION AND PRESERVATION

Most of the problems that necessitate surgical intervention in children are induced by trauma. The majority are secondary to fracture or dislocation of the nasal dorsum and cartilaginous septum. Soft tissue loss, as occurs with lacerations, also requires operative management. The best donor tissue is the skin from the concha of the ear, and this has been described earlier in this chapter under Management of Soft Tissue wounds. Management of a septal hematoma requires first that it be diagnosed. This problem must be anticipated and looked for in all children with nasal trauma. Some of the more severe hematomas can be easily recognized from a basal perspective of the nose, but many are more subtle and can only be diagnosed with vestibular palpation of the septum with a cotton-tipped applicator. Most children require general anesthesia for adequate treatment of a septal hematoma. The consequence of failure to evacuate a septal hematoma properly are manifested by the severe saddle nose deformity seen in adolescents who sustained nasal trauma when they were children.

The recommended treatment includes a generous dependent incision, evacuation of the hematoma, and obliteration of the dead space using a transseptal whipstitch of 4–0 chromic suture. Approximately 10% of septal hematomas are bilateral, and both sides must be addressed. The whipstitch coaptation is the same with unilateral and bilateral involvement. A bilateral hematoma is much more likely to result in septal cartilage dissolution because it interrupts the total nutrient supply from the perichondrium to the cartilage. Progression of a septal hematoma to an abscess also leads to rapid dissolution of the cartilage. All these patients should be given antibiotic coverage.

Elective Nasal Surgery in Children

The patient with a cleft lip-nose requires early intervention to properly align the tissues before the rapid growth phase occurs. Although revisions are often necessary later in life, the results are better when alignment of the cartilage and closure of the cleft occur earlier. The same underlying princi-

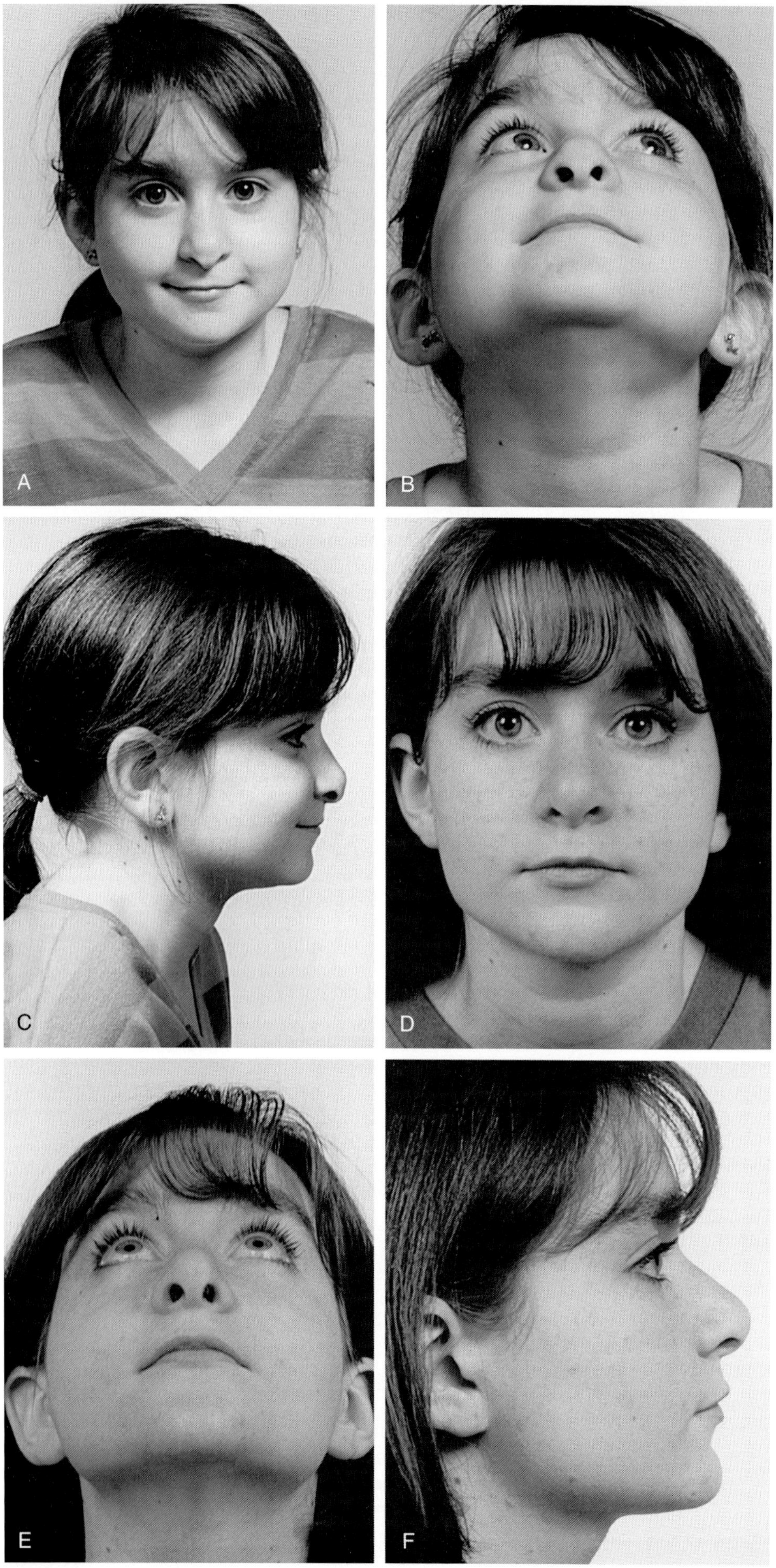

FIGURE 22–12. *A,* Frontal view of 9-year-old with congenital nasal tip deformity. *B,* Submental preoperative view. *C,* Right lateral preoperative view. *D,* Frontal view 5 years postoperatively. *E,* Submental view 5 years postoperatively. *F,* Right lateral view 5 years postoperatively.

ple of surgical management apply—i.e., minimal trauma to the mucoperichondrium at all ages. In the prepubertal patient, soft tissue dissection and mobilization are acceptable along with suspension and mobilization of the lower lateral cartilages as necessary (Fig. 22–12). Extensive dissection of the cartilaginous elements rather than repositioning them in their perichondrial jacket invites damage and a potentially more serious deformity. Growth disturbances of these structures can be the result. Osteotomies usually are not necessary and certainly are to be eschewed as a routine procedure in patients of this age. The postpubertal patient can be handled in the same manner as previously described for the patient of the same age without a cleft.

Airway obstruction as an indication for rhinoplasty in the pediatric patient is related to the severity of the defect. In the prepubertal patient, airway obstruction must be significant to warrant surgical correction. In the postpubertal patient basically the same principle applies, although more minor airway problems may be corrected, especially if they are amenable to minimal dissection.

Problems that should not be corrected in the pediatric patient are racial features and hereditary characteristics. These cosmetic problems are better corrected in the mid and late teens when the decision is more personal and there are fewer adverse consequences to growth. These deformities can require extensive dissection. The question of the desirability of altering these features, especially racial features, is best delayed until the patient reaches adulthood and can make his or her own decisions more rationally.

Regardless of the deformity and its etiology, a plaster splint applied over a base of paper taped to the underlying skin affords excellent stability. It remains remarkably adherent even in the most active child, and its lack of bulk and light weight are other advantages in this age group. It is less conspicuous than the traditional metal and adhesive tape splints, which is a positive feature for the teenage patient, who tends to be more self-conscious.

Bibliography

Barwick WJ, Klein HW: Soft tissue injuries of the face. *In* Serafin D, Georgiade NG (eds): Pediatric Plastic Surgery. St. Louis, C.V. Mosby, 1984, pp. 633–654.

Bennett RG: Anatomy and physiology of the skin. *In* Papel ID, Nachlas NE (eds): Facial Plastic and Reconstructive Surgery. St. Louis, Mosby–Year Book, 1992, pp. 3–13.

Cheney ML: Soft tissue injuries of the face. *In* Cheney ML (ed): Facial Surgery, Plastic and Reconstructive. Baltimore, Williams & Wilkins, 1997, pp. 169–178.

Foster RD, Anthony JP, Singer MI, Kaplan MJ, Pogrel MA, Mathes SJ: Reconstruction of Complex Midfacial Defects. Plast Reconstr Surg 99(6): 1555–1565, 1997.

Funk GF, Laurenzo JF, Valentino J, McCulloch TM, Frodel JL, Hoffman HT: Free-tissue transfer reconstruction of midfacial and cranio-orbito-facial defects. Arch Otolaryngol 121:293–303, 1995.

Key SJ, Thomas DW, Shepherd JP: The management of soft tissue facial wounds. Br J Oral Maxillofac Surg 33:76–85, 1995.

Lee RH, Gamble WB, Mayer MH, Manson PN: Patterns of facial laceration from blunt trauma. Plast Reconstr Surg 99(6):1544–1554, 1997.

Omovie EE, Shepherd JP: Assessment of repair of facial lacerations. Br J Oral Maxillofac Surg 35:237–240, 1997.

Spinelli HM, Forman DL: Current treatment of post-traumatic deformities: Residual orbital, adnexal, and soft-tissue abnormalities. Clin Plast Surg 24(3):519–530, 1997.

Stucker FJ, Bryarly RC, Shockley WW: Management of nasal trauma in children. Arch Otolaryngol 110:190–192, 1984.

Stucker FJ, Shaw GY: The perichondrial cutaneous graft: A 12-year clinical experience. Arch Otolaryngol 118:287–292, 1992.

Stucker FJ, Bryarly RC, Shockley WW: Nasal surgery in the pediatric patient. *In* Plastic and Reconstructive Surgery of the Head and Neck: Proceedings of the Fourth International Symposium. St. Louis, C.V. Mosby, 1984, pp. 62–70.

Stucker FJ, Shaw GY, Boyd S, Shockley WW: Management of animal and human bites in the head and neck. Arch Otolaryngol 116:789–793, 1990.

CHAPTER 23

Treatment of Congenital Craniofacial Anomalies

Jeffrey A. Goldstein, M.D.

Modern craniofacial surgery is a multidisciplinary approach designed to correct major facial skeletal deformities. Its history takes root primarily in the time period after World War II when the main concepts for correcting skeletal deformities were established, primarily in response to the traumatic deformities created in that war. Although there were many contributors to this development, the main innovator of this era was Sir Harold Gillies. In 1950, he reported the early encouraging results of a Lefort III-type midfacial advancement osteotomy to correct a corresponding hypoplasia in a patient with Crouzon's syndrome. Unfortunately, this patient's postoperative course was characterized by a significant relapse.

Building on these earlier contributions, the major pioneer in modern craniofacial surgery was Dr. Paul Tessier. In the late 1960s and early 1970s, Dr. Tessier described a new approach that included a coronal incision for soft tissue retraction, a bifrontal craniotomy for brain retraction and exposure, innovative intracranial and extracranial osteotomies, interposition of bone grafting, and early techniques of internal and external fixation. Dr. Tessier developed radical approaches to the correction of congenital craniofacial deformities that were previously thought to be nonreparable. His underlying philosophy was that these deformities were primarily skeletal in origin and required correction of the underlying skeleton with either osteotomies or autogenous bone grafting. He demonstrated that bones of the cranium and midface could be totally separated from the overlying periosteum and underlying dura, thereby devascularizing them, and could still survive after repositioning. He further demonstrated that the bony orbit could be moved three-dimensionally without affecting vision. In an extensive series of cases, he proved the efficacy, safety, and reliability of a combined intracranial and extracranial approach to cranial orbital reconstruction. Lastly, Dr. Tessier contributed significantly to the next generation of craniofacial surgeons, providing both educational and intellectual stimulus. These colleagues and protégés, along with Dr. Tessier, further applied these techniques to infants with craniofacial anomalies as well to patients of all ages with cranial base tumors.

In the two decades since Dr. Tessier's innovations were published, a number of other craniofacial surgeons have contributed significantly to increase the safety and reliability of this type of surgery. During the past two decades, the advent of rigid fixation and its effect on membranous bone healing have significantly enhanced the stability and long-term results of craniofacial reconstruction. Until recently, fracture repair in the midface and cranial vault was thought to occur by fibrous healing resulting in a fibrous union. In the early 1990s animal and human clinical studies demonstrated that facial bones actually may undergo true osseous union, albeit sometimes with a cartilaginous precursor. The basic function of the facial bones is to protect and support other vital structures as well as to carry a load selectively. Subsequently, the function of the facial bones depends on their characteristics of strength and rigidity. When facial bones are osteotomized, these attributes are diminished, especially when external dynamic forces are applied across the fracture (usually by differential muscular pull), leading to deformation and displacement of the fracture site. As will be demonstrated later in this chapter, correction of major craniofacial deformities often requires extensive osteotomies of the cranium or midface with significant bony advancement. To maintain this advancement, rigid fixation has been shown to be most reliable. Rigid fixation allows for primary rather than secondary bone healing, eliminating the need for a cartilaginous intermediate and diminishing the amount of bony resorption that occurs during the healing process.

The use of plate and screw fixation, originally designed for long bone fracture therapy, was extrapolated for use in the mandible by maxillofacial surgeons. Combining these principles with further technical advances, smaller titanium and vitallium plates and screws were developed for use in the midface and cranium and were pioneered by many, including Champy and Luhr. More recently, resorbable plate and screw systems have been developed to achieve the same goals, primarily in lower weight-bearing bones. To achieve fixation with adequate immobilization, two major fixation systems are used: monocortical miniplate osteosynthesis and compression osteosynthesis. Compression osteosynthesis is primarily employed in the mandible and has been found not to be necessary in the upper two thirds of the face and skull. The use of rigid fixation increased the stability of bony repositioning and bone graft placement because it allowed the bones to withstand the restricting and distracting soft tissue forces, including soft tissue draping, muscular pull, progressive scarring, and postural molding. It also eased the ability to stabilize complex three-dimensional shaping of bone and has decreased the incidence of relapse and infection.

The second major advance in the reliability and stability of craniofacial surgery was the nearly exclusive use of cranial bone grafts. Craniofacial surgery is dependent on bone grafting, in both an inlay and onlay fashion. The majority of the skull is composed of membranous bone, as opposed to endochondral bone, which is primarily present in the long bones of the body. A number of studies beginning in the 1970s and continuing to the present have demonstrated the superiority and enhanced survival of cranial bone over endochondral bone in the head and neck. Compared to endochondral bone (e.g., rib or iliac bone grafts), other advantages of cranial bone grafts include the location of the source of bone within the operative field, significantly diminished donor site morbidity compared to the rib or ileum (e.g., pneumothorax, atelectasis, hematoma), and diminished concerns about patient postoperative pain and scarring. The use of cranial bone grafts combined with rigid fixation have led to the most reliable forms of craniorbital and midfacial reconstruction.

The third major contribution to the advancement of craniofacial surgery has been the major advances made in diagnostic radiography. The introduction of CT scanning, followed by significant refinements in this modality, including three-dimensional reconstruction, has allowed craniofacial teams to better document the underlying abnormalities, plan therapeutic intervention, and, most important, critique the long-term postoperative result. CT scans as well as magnetic resonance imaging (MRI) scanning have further allowed clinicians to diagnose and follow associated intracranial, orbital, and/or sinus abnormalities. Serial CT scans performed in patients with congenital abnormalities have demonstrated the natural growth and progression of the abnormal human skull as well as the effects on it of surgical intervention and osteotomies. Quantitative and biometric measurements can be derived from these scans, further improving planning, observation, and critiques of the postoperative result. Although CT scanning has not replaced cephalometric analysis or anthropometric measurements, it has become the radiographic image most relied on by the craniofacial team.

The last major advance during the past two decades is the importance of the multidisciplinary team approach to the major congenital craniofacial deformities. The team should include a craniofacial surgeon, neurosurgeon, ophthalmologist, neuroradiologist, otolaryngologist, anesthesiologist, speech and language pathologist, geneticist, pediatric dentist, orthodontist, psychologist, photographer, anthropologist, nurse coordinator, social worker, and members of the pediatric intensive care unit. Each member of the team has a role in the decision-making in regard to the actual procedure required, its effect on the surrounding structures, the timing of the procedure, the adequacy of the results, and the further growth and development of the patient's cranium and face. Often one of the most difficult decisions for the team to make is the appropriate timing of surgery. Although some surgeries are not elective, the best timing for the more elective procedures is early enough to diminish the psychosocial aspects of the deformity but not so early that the surgery will interfere with normal growth and development. A number of studies have shown that the skull and periorbital regions reach 90% of adult size by age 5, whereas the mandible does not achieve 90% of its total growth until the age of 14 to 16.

CRANIOSYNOSTOSIS

Craniosynostosis, or premature fusion of the cranial vault sutures, occurs as an isolated event or as part of a larger spectrum of disease. When isolated, it most frequently involves a single suture. In the craniofacial dysostosis syndromes, it involves various forms of cranial vault and cranial base synostosis. These syndromes include Crouzon's syndrome, Apert's syndrome, Pfeiffer's syndrome, and Carpenter's syndrome. Management of craniosynostosis involves a multidisciplinary team approach by the craniofacial team. Single suture craniosynostosis frequently requires only one operative intervention at somewhere between 3 and 12 months of age. Associated intracranial or orbital problems occur less frequently in these patients than in the syndromic cases. Patients with craniofacial dysostosis syndromes usually require cranial orbital reshaping and expansion in infancy, often a repeat reconstruction and advancement in early childhood because of resynostosis or evidence of increasing intracranial pressure, intracranial-extracranial midfacial advancement later in childhood, and maxillofacial surgery at the time of skeletal maturity to balance the jaw relationship and to achieve class I occlusion. The midfacial advancement procedure may be a LeFort III frontal facial advancement or a facial bi-partition if hypertelorism also has to be addressed. The cranial vault anterior cranial base surgery is approached through a coronal skin incision and bifrontal craniotomy. A bifrontal craniotomy allows adequate exposure and retraction of the frontal lobe of the brain, which allows protected osteotomies. Cranial orbital osteotomies are then performed as described later, frequently combined with autogenous cranial bone graft for reconstruction. The following two cases will illustrate the craniofacial approach used for patients with syndromic and nonsyndromic craniosynostosis.

CASE REPORTS

Case 1

Case 1 (Fig. 23–1) is a 5-month-old infant with nonsyndromic metopic craniosynostosis. The skull shape is characterized by trigonocephaly with severe ridging of the anterior medial forehead and bitemporal constriction. There is associated hypotelorism, and the lateral orbital walls are retrusive in nature. There is no associated asymmetry of the nose, midface, or mandible. A CT scan of the craniofacial skeleton demonstrated a metopic suture fusion. There was associated constriction of the anterior cranial fossa but no associated intracranial anomalies. At the time of surgery, a coronal incision was performed followed by a bifrontal craniotomy. Osteotomies were then performed at the zygomaticofrontal suture bilaterally and were extended through the lateral orbital wall and orbital roof to the medial orbital wall and nasal frontal junction bilaterally. A lateral temporal tenon was also removed. This orbital osteotomy unit was then further osteotomized and recontoured to provide a symmetrical appearance, alleviate the hypotelorism with an increase in the intercanthal distance, and redirect the lateral tenons. It was replaced in an anteriorly

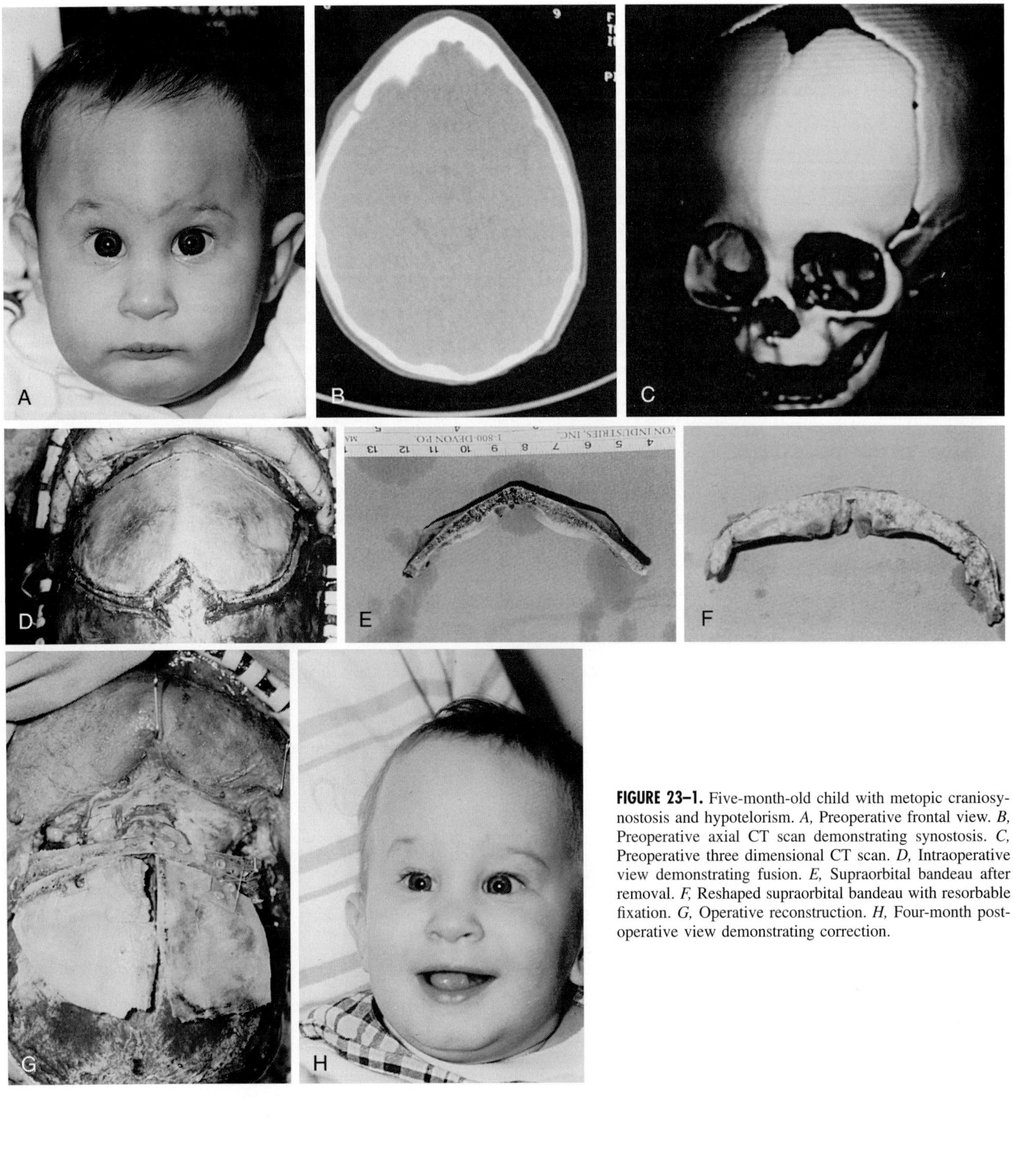

FIGURE 23–1. Five-month-old child with metopic craniosynostosis and hypotelorism. *A,* Preoperative frontal view. *B,* Preoperative axial CT scan demonstrating synostosis. *C,* Preoperative three dimensional CT scan. *D,* Intraoperative view demonstrating fusion. *E,* Supraorbital bandeau after removal. *F,* Reshaped supraorbital bandeau with resorbable fixation. *G,* Operative reconstruction. *H,* Four-month postoperative view demonstrating correction.

advanced position to allow cranial vault and orbital roof expansion. The previously removed anterior cranial vault and forehead was then further osteotomized, and its pieces were repositioned to reconstruct the forehead. Fixation was achieved using a resorbable craniomaxillofacial system. There were no perioperative complications, and the child has continued to do well 1½ years postoperatively.

Case 2—Apert's syndrome

Apert's syndrome is one of the craniofacial dysostoses characterized by brachycephaly, bilateral coronal craniosynostosis, frequent involvement of other sutures, associated hydrocephalus and developmental delay, and bilateral involvement of the upper and/or lower extremities. Hypertelorism and proptosis are common findings. Midfacial hypoplasia is uniformly present presumably associated with anterior cranial base involvement. The 4-month-old infant with Apert's syndrome (Fig. 23–2) shows the usual findings. At the time of surgery, a bicoronal incision was employed for exposure in conjunction with a bifrontal craniotomy. The supraorbital bandeau was again removed using the same type of osteotomies as described in Case 1. Note the shallowness of the orbital roofs. Symmetrical reconstruction of the supraorbital and lateral orbital regions was then achieved on the back table, and the unit was replaced in an advanced expanded position to allow cranial vault expansion and decompression of any early evidence of elevated intracranial pressure. The preoperative CT scan demonstrated evidence of bilateral coronal craniosynostosis, a deficiency of the anterior cranial base as well as hypoplasia of the orbital roof, and no evidence of associated lambdoidal or sagittal craniosynostosis. In fact, the anterior midline sutures were widely patent, most likely as a compensatory measure. After advancement of the supraorbital bandeau, the previously removed anterior cranial vault was again reosteotomized and repositioned to allow appropriate reconstruction and advancement. Fixation was achieved with titanium microplates and screws.

A 6-month postoperative view demonstrated early adequacy of the reconstruction, although the family is aware that resynostosis most likely will occur. The child will also require repeat cranial vault advancement in association with a midfacial advancement somewhere between the ages of 5 and 8. He may in fact require a mono-bloc or facial bipartition to eliminate hypertelorism at

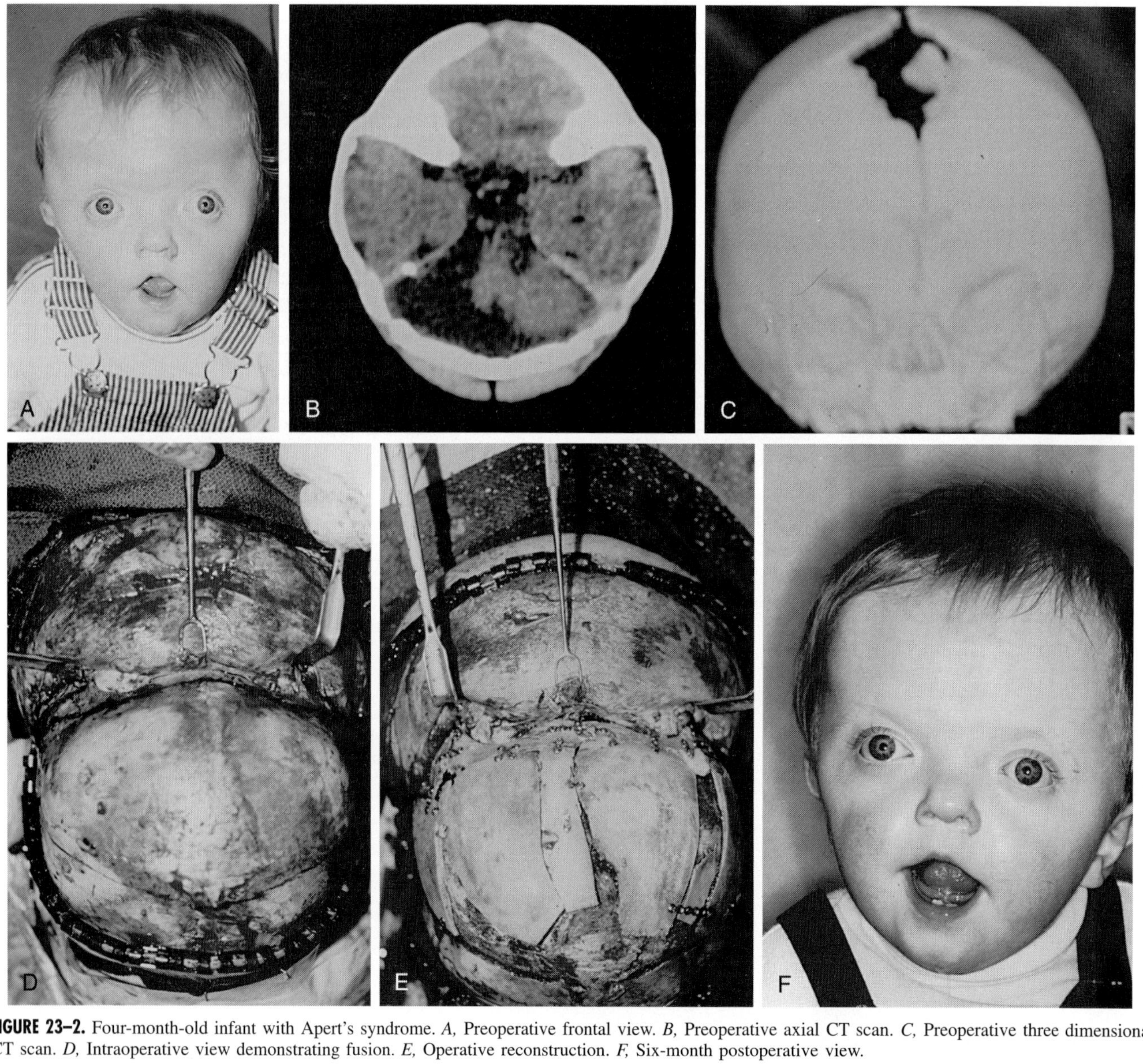

FIGURE 23–2. Four-month-old infant with Apert's syndrome. *A*, Preoperative frontal view. *B*, Preoperative axial CT scan. *C*, Preoperative three dimensional CT scan. *D*, Intraoperative view demonstrating fusion. *E*, Operative reconstruction. *F*, Six-month postoperative view.

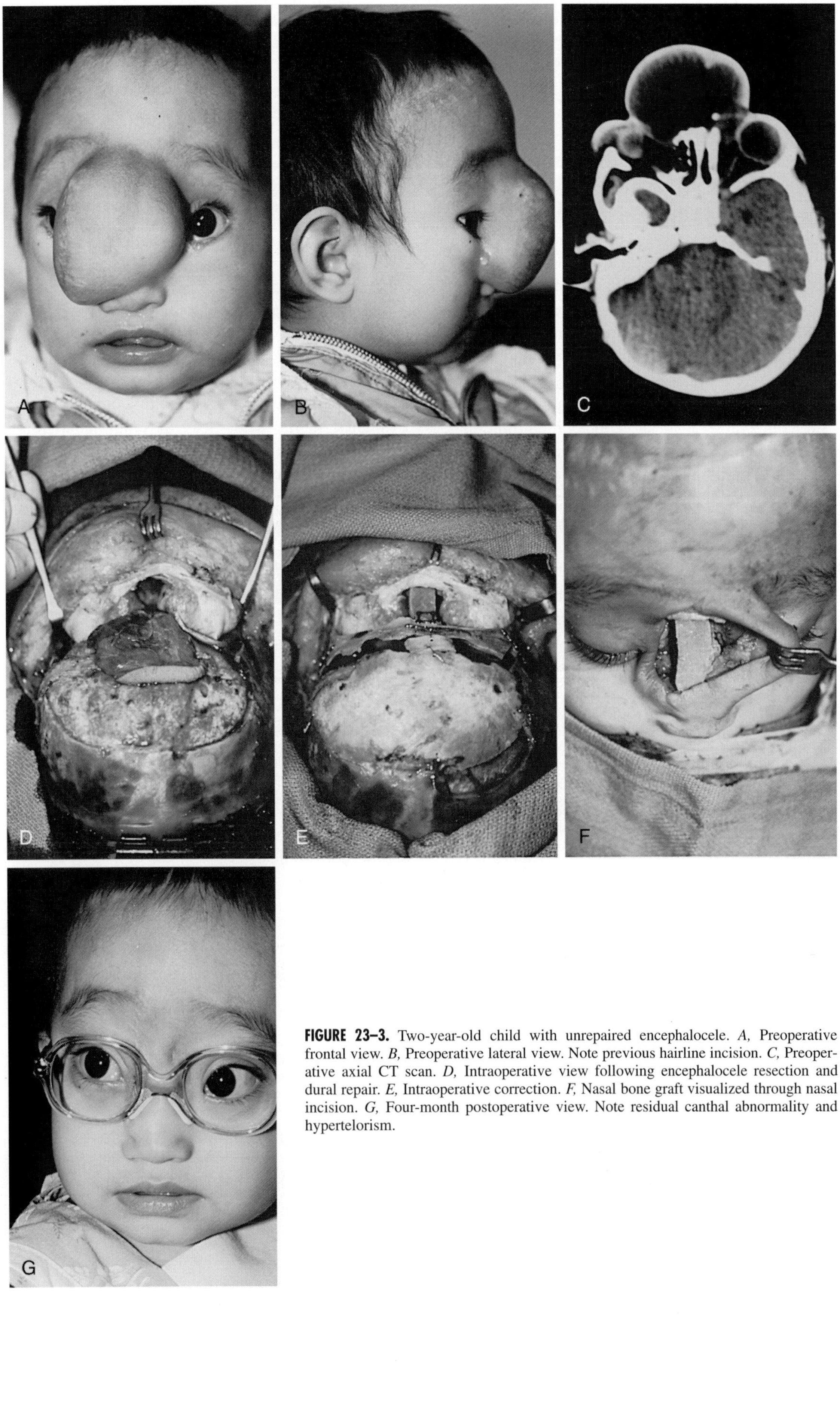

FIGURE 23–3. Two-year-old child with unrepaired encephalocele. *A,* Preoperative frontal view. *B,* Preoperative lateral view. Note previous hairline incision. *C,* Preoperative axial CT scan. *D,* Intraoperative view following encephalocele resection and dural repair. *E,* Intraoperative correction. *F,* Nasal bone graft visualized through nasal incision. *G,* Four-month postoperative view. Note residual canthal abnormality and hypertelorism.

the same time. He will also most likely require orthognathic surgery at skeletal maturity consisting of a LeFort I advancement and most likely bilateral sagittal osteotomies of the mandible to rebalance the jaws and occlusion.

HYPERTELORISM OR ENCEPHALOCELE

Another aspect of craniofacial surgery related to the anterior cranial base is that involving midline craniofacial clefts, hypertelorism, and encephaloceles. Hypertelorism, or increased distance between the bony orbits, can be caused by ethmoidal hyperplasia, tumors such as encephaloceles, or midline craniofacial clefts. These children require multidisciplinary craniofacial evaluation including evaluation by the team neurosurgeon, craniofacial surgeon, ophthalmologists, geneticists, speech and language pathologists, and audiologists. Palatal abnormalities occur frequently including clefting or high arching. The airway is often a concern as well. Figure 23–3 shows a 2½-year-old girl referred from Nicaragua with a congenital frontonasal ethmoidal encephalocele. She had undergone a previous attempt at repair, the details of which were unknown to us except for the anterior hairline incision. Physical examination revealed the presence of a large anterior encephalocele with associated hypertelorism, nasal lacrimal dysfunction, and the above-mentioned scars. CT scans demonstrated the magnitude of the deformity.

At the time of surgery, a coronal incision was again used for exposure in conjunction with a vertical nasal incision. The nasal incision enhanced exposure and allowed for removal of excess tissue. The encephalocele was both excised and plicated. The bifrontal craniotomy with associated orbital osteotomies allowed further exposure and reconstruction. Autogenous cranial bone grafting was required for orbital reconstruction, frontal bone reconstruction, and nasal reconstruction. Titanium microplates and screws were placed for fixation. The patient's perioperative course was uncomplicated, and she returned to Nicaragua where she is reportedly continuing to do well. She will need a second-stage nasal and orbital reconstruction prior to starting school and most likely some further work at the time of skeletal maturity.

CONGENITAL TUMORS

Although congenital tumors in the anterior cranial vault or nasal ethmoidal area are not common they should be evaluated in the same way as craniofacial malformations. Even when benign, they often require early intervention because they may cause progressive deformation and deleterious effects on the surrounding brain, orbits, and nose. There may be intracranial-to-extracranial communication problems such as a congenital midline nasal dermoid or glioma. It should be emphasized that a craniofacial approach is often warranted.

SUMMARY

Modern craniofacial surgery is a multidisciplinary approach used to correct major skeletal deformities. This chapter describes its history and the recent advances that have improved its safety, efficacy, and reliability in treating congenital deformities.

CHAPTER 24

Simultaneous Rhinoplasty and Functional Endoscopic Sinus Surgery

Frank Scaccia, M.D.
David Stepnick, M.D.
Anthony Maniglia, M.D.

Since its introduction in the United States by Kennedy in 1985, functional endoscopic sinus surgery (FESS) has gained widespread acceptance and popularity and has achieved success in treating inflammatory sinus disease.[1] Although complications have been reported, the procedure, when performed properly in trained hands, is usually not only efficacious but also safe.[2–5] Because FESS is an endonasal approach, it avoids external incisions and possible cosmetic problems. Because chronic sinusitis is a very common health problem affecting up to 40 million people each year in the United States, the demands for this surgery will probably continue to grow.

Rhinoplasty is another surgical procedure that has enjoyed increased public interest as members of our society become more conscious of their personal health, their appearance, and the ability to make changes therein. One survey indicated that up to 40% of all adults in the United States are not happy with the external shape of their nose.[2] Like sinus surgery, rhinoplasty is very safe, and its results are satisfying to surgeons and patients alike.

Combining septoplasty or turbinate reduction with rhinoplasty has been done for many years and seems to be a logical outcome of procedures performed on a defined anatomic subsite that can achieve cosmetic enhancement while simultaneously improving the nasal airway. With the advent of endonasal sinus surgery, rhinoplasty candidates who also suffer from chronic nasal and/or sinus ailments such as sinusitis, sinus headache, postnasal drip, and congestion can have these conditions addressed during the same operation. Similarly, patients who are candidates for FESS often desire cosmetic improvement of the external nose and are willing to undergo the cosmetic portion of the procedure during the same operation, whereas they may be reluctant to undergo the surgery for cosmetic reasons alone. The advantages of concurrent surgery are multiple and include the need for only one general anesthetic, less total time needed for recovery (and thereby a shorter absence from work or school), and overall lower medical costs than if the two procedures were performed separately.

This chapter discusses the work-up and preparations needed to perform combined rhinoplasty and sinus surgery procedures, the requirements for a safe surgical approach that will help to ensure a successful outcome, postoperative care recommendations, a review of the current literature, the advantages and disadvantages of performing these procedures at the same surgical setting, and an evaluation of our personal results.

PREOPERATIVE EVALUATION

Virtually all patients who are candidates for simultaneous rhinoplasty and FESS seek the advice and treatment of a physician because of their sinus complaints. As with any presenting problem, the clinician should elicit a thorough medical history with a particular focus on the sinus complaints as well as any functional and nasal deformities. Aspects that should be addressed include the duration of symptoms, associated allergic symptoms, overuse of topical decongestants, prior nasal surgery, failure to respond to medical therapies in the past, and trauma. In addition, if headaches and facial pressure are described, their exact location and possible association with certain allergic factors and visual disturbances should be ascertained. Migraines or neuralgias should be considered in the differential diagnosis.

Patients who are initially seen by the physician for a

cosmetic consultation also need a complete history and physical examination. Occasionally, chronic nasal or sinus problems are diagnosed that require surgery because medical management has failed. These patients may very well welcome the opportunity to have both of their problems handled during the same surgical procedure.

Anterior rhinoscopy is performed both prior to and after decongestion of the nose with 1% Neo-Synephrine to obtain a more accurate assessment of the turbinates' role in nasal obstruction. Following this, a topical anesthetic such as 4% lidocaine is sprayed on pledgets placed in the nasal cavity, so that a small fiberoptic nasal endoscope can be passed painlessly, allowing a more thorough examination of the internal nose. Many surgeons connect the fiberoptic endoscope to a camera or monitor system so that both the patient and possibly the family members can visualize the nasal anatomy during the examination. In addition, preoperative nasal cavity pictures can be taken with this system, allowing documentation in the chart and better communication with the referring physician. Using the fiberoptic scopes, posterior septal spurs and deviations, inferior turbinate pathologies, purulent secretions, polypoid or polyp formation, adenoid hypertrophy, and obstruction of the osteomeatal outflow tract can be identified.

Once the endonasal examination is completed, attention can be directed to the aesthetic assessment of the nose. This is done systematically beginning at the nasofrontal angle and ending at the nasolabial angle. Note is also made of the overall profile, including such elements as the position of the forehead and chin. Spreader grafts for a narrowed nasal valve and/or a strut for a poorly supported tip are at times deemed functionally necessary based on the examination, and their outward effect on the appearance of the nose should be discussed. In addition, the need for an external transcolumellar incision should be discussed with the patient if its need is anticipated. Finally, standard multiple-view photographs of the patient are taken for both medical and legal purposes and enlargement. Some surgeons use computer imaging systems to help explain to their patient how the proposed surgery will affect their appearance. In our experience, however, this often results in unrealistic patient expectations, which may lead to possible dissatisfaction. For enlargements, we use 6 × 9 inch color copies made from our original slides, which can be viewed directly or flipped over and transilluminated on an x-ray viewbox. This allows the surgeon to trace the preoperative patient profile with a pencil and then to draw the anticipated profile on the contralateral view to show the patient in a very basic and understandable way what the likely postoperative result will be.

After a thorough history and physical examination have been completed, there are still a few more important steps that must be taken before a final decision is made about the need for surgery. Sinus surgery, except in emergency situations, should almost never be offered to the patient unless aggressive medical treatment has been attempted in the past and has failed. Such medical therapy may include long-term antibiotics directed at the most likely sinusitis-causing pathogens, oral decongestants, topical steroid preparations, and allergic desensitization therapy, if indicated. If these approaches have failed and rhinoscopic examination demonstrates an obvious anatomic derangement or pathology that could account for the patient's symptoms, a complete coronal CT scan without contrast of the paranasal sinuses is ordered. The completed CT scan is reviewed with the patient, noting any functional deformity or disease that may explain the condition and may be amenable to surgical management.

SURGICAL TECHNIQUE

Once the need for surgery has been established, certain preoperative steps should be followed. Obviously, the possible risks and benefits of both the endoscopic sinus surgery and the rhinoplasty portion of the procedure must be discussed. A detailed explanation of these important issues may be supplemented by other educational materials such as a detailed handout, booklet, or videotape. The patient is informed that the functional (sinus) part of the operation will be performed first and, if for any reason an intraoperative problem occurs that might interfere with further surgery, the cosmetic portion will be abandoned or possibly performed at a later date. He or she is also informed that all aspirin-containing products, nonsteroidal anti-inflammatory agents, and vitamin E must be stopped at least 2 weeks prior to the date of surgery because excessive intraoperative bleeding is often a cause of lack of completion of the sinus procedure as well as potential morbidity. Some physicians routinely use perioperative corticosteroid and antibiotic therapy in all patients unless these are contraindicated. A typical regimen consists of a 6-day course of prednisone and antibiotics begun 1 week preoperatively and extended up to 3 more weeks postoperatively.

At the time of surgery, intravenous antibiotics and steroids may be initiated on call to the operating room. Although deep sedation may be used, general anesthesia is preferred for these combined cases. Hypotensive general anesthesia (systolic 80 to 90 mmHg) may be used to minimize bleeding. A moist throat pack is placed in the oropharynx to collect any bloody runoff and to avoid swallowing of blood during anesthesia, which may cause discomfort and vomiting postoperatively. All CT films and preoperative pictures are displayed in an easily accessible area of the operating room suite. Cocainized 3-inch Cottonoid pledgets are placed in the right and left nasal cavities prior to the skin preparation to maximize internal nasal vasoconstriction. Sinus surgery and septoplasty, if needed, are always addressed first, since bleeding and swelling from the rhinoplasty would make endoscopic visualization difficult. All resected septal cartilage, bone, and turbinate tissue are preserved in saline solution until the completion of the procedure so that grafts may be readily available if they are needed later.

The sinus surgery is performed with both the 4.0-mm, 0-degree and 25-degree wide-angle rigid endoscope utilizing a video monitor to minimize surgeon discomfort resulting from bending over during the procedure. This setup is helpful in a teaching setting. Well-placed injections of 1% lidocaine with 1:100,000 epinephrine at the uncinate process and middle turbinate edge are critical for achieving operative hemostasis. In addition, frequent blotting with topical 1:1000 adrenaline in the ethmoid cavity also minimizes oozing. The basic endoscopic technique utilized by the authors is that described by Messerklinger and others, which has been presented extensively elsewhere.[8] Complete resection of the uncinate process and associated diseased agger nasi cells is imperative to maximize the chances of success and deserves special note.

Often septoplasty must be performed prior to ethmoidectomy in patients with severe deflection so that comfortable access and visualization can be obtained during the surgical procedure. Rarely, partial resection of the septum is necessary in the area of sinus obstruction, and this can be accomplished via an incision made posteriorly using the endoscope and sickle knife. When inferior turbinate reduction is performed, either directly by resection or by tissue ablation with KTP laser, cautery, or cryosurgery, it is always performed after the sinus procedure because bleeding and/or swelling can occur, thereby obscuring the field.

A complete anterior and posterior ethmoidectomy is performed in almost all cases except those in which only limited osteomeatal disease has been identified on CT. Often disease is found in the posterior ethmoid and frontal recess region, even if this is not clearly demonstrated on CT. However, exploration of the sphenoid sinus should be attempted only when disease is clearly demonstrated on preoperative radiographs. There are several advantages to performing a total ethmoidectomy. These include a more thorough exenteration of diseased sinus tissue, easier inspection and assessment of the cavity during the postoperative period, less bleeding intraoperatively and postoperatively when all diseased sinus tissues have been removed, and easier placement of postoperative splints for middle turbinate stabilization. The added operative time and additional risks in performing a total versus partial ethmoidectomy should be minimal in experienced hands.

One of the most discussed and perhaps controversial issues in FESS is the management of the middle turbinate. Postoperative lateralization of a preserved middle turbinate is often cited as the most frequent cause of postoperative failure.[5] The middle turbinate becomes even more of a concern when concurrent rhinoplasty and lateral osteotomies are included as part of the procedure. A floppy middle turbinate in this situation may be even more prone to lateralize and obstruct a newly created osteomeatal outflow tract.

Earlier attempts in our series to prevent this complication by partially resecting the middle turbinate (when combining rhinoplasty and sinus procedures) were successful but appeared to cause a prolonged period of healing of the ethmoid cavity. Edema and granulation tissue were noted to persist up to 3 months postoperatively in some patients. More recently, every effort has been made to preserve the middle turbinate at least partially utilizing the Boomerang middle turbinate glove (Xomed Surgical Products, Jacksonville, FL) to prevent lateralization (Fig. 24–1). Earlier use of an expandable Merocel sponge (Xomed Surgical Products, Jacksonville, FL) for this purpose has been abandoned because it resulted in increased tissue reaction. In our hands, use of the middle turbinate glove appears to be associated with a significant decrease in postoperative edema with almost complete healing of the ethmoid cavity by 3 to 4 weeks. In addition, no middle turbinate lateralization or drift has occurred in these 13 consecutive cases. These splints are now used by us in all cases when both middle turbinates are preserved, even after lateral resections for concha bullosa. When one or both middle turbinates are resected for hypertrophic enlargement, absorbable gelatin film packs are placed lateral to the cut middle turbinate remnants. Both the middle turbinate gloves and absorbable gelatin film, when needed, are placed during the procedure prior to performing rhinoplasty and are left undisturbed for up to 2 weeks postoperatively. Silastic nasal splints, placed bilaterally, minimize the possibility of postoperative scarring.

Rhinoplasty is begun only after endoscopic sinus surgery, septoplasty, and/or turbinate reduction have been completed. The cavities are inspected for persistent bleeding, which must be controlled prior to proceeding with the cosmetic portion of the operation. Surgicel is helpful in packing the nasal cavity temporarily during the steps of rhinoplasty. Additional surgery at this point, especially nasal osteotomies, should not be attempted if complications such as a cerebrospinal fluid (CSF) leak or orbital penetration with fat herniation occurred during the endoscopic sinus procedure. If FESS is uneventful, rhinoplasty can be initiated using the same technique that would be used if it were performed independently. Either an external or an endonasal approach can be used. Nasal osteotomies should not be discouraged, assuming that endoscopic sinus surgery is uncomplicated, if these are needed for nasal pyramid straightening or nar-

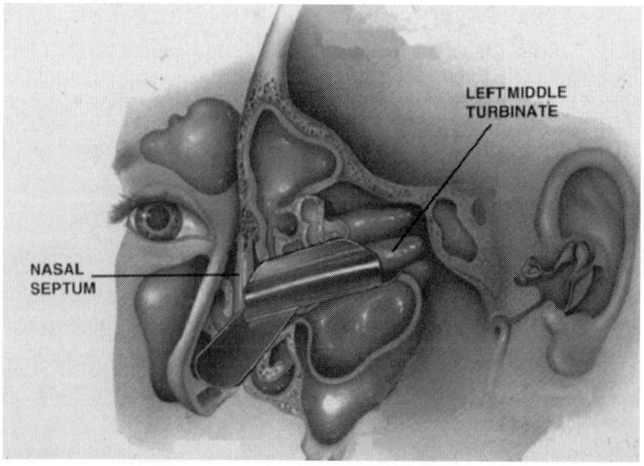

FIGURE 24–1. Middle turbinate glove in place after completion of bilateral ethmoidectomies and (if necessary) septoplasty. Silastic stent extends adjacent to septum and is secured with a mattress suture of 4–0 nylon.

rowing. No significant complications have been encountered in our hands; similar conclusions have been reached by others.[9]

Tip manipulation and grafting are also carried out as necessary. Alloplastic augmentation, however, may be contraindicated if the concurrent sinus procedures were performed on an acutely infected sinus cavity containing purulent material. If infection is suspected preoperatively, antibiotics should be given to eradicate the acute infection. If it is encountered intraoperatively, one should consider abandoning the cosmetic portion of the procedure, especially if cartilage grafts or alloplastic implants are needed.

Alar base narrowing procedures can also be performed, although increased tenderness in this area during the initial postoperative period may restrict some of the postoperative care necessary for ethmoid cavity debridement. This discomfort usually resolves within the first few weeks and is usually not associated with significant problems. At the completion of the procedure, ½-inch Steri-Strips (Medical-Surgical Division/3M, St. Paul, MN) are applied to the nasal skin, an Aquaplast thermoplastic cast is placed externally, and bacitracin-coated Telfa packing (Kendall Healthcare Products, Mansfield, MA) is used for packing. Eight-centimeter-long, 14-F tracheal suction catheters may be placed in each nasal cavity in the packing material to allow some postoperative airflow in an attempt to minimize patient discomfort.

POSTOPERATIVE CARE

Prophylactic antibiotics are prescribed for up to 2 or 3 weeks. In the first postoperative visit the packing is removed, and this is routinely scheduled on the second or third postoperative day. The patient is instructed to begin instilling Ponaris (Jamol Laboratories, Inc, Emerson, NJ) drops into each nasal cavity three times a day for lubrication. One to two weeks later the middle turbinate gloves or, if still present, the absorbable gelatin packs are removed from the nose, and direct endoscopic visualization and debridement of crusts and thickened secretions is instituted on a weekly to biweekly basis until the ethmoid cavities are clean and healed. Daily saline nasal douching utilizing a Water Pik at home is also instituted at this time. Nasal saline spray is also helpful. Occasionally, postoperative injections of 40 mg/mL triamcinolone acetonide into persistent maxillary sinus polyps and oral doses of prednisone are necessary to minimize inflammation and speed healing. Triamcinolone acetonide spray may be used to minimize scarring. Postoperative care involving endoscopic removal of all scarring, granulation tissue, and polypoid mucosa is essential for a successful outcome and to prevent the need for subsequent revision surgery.

Care of the external nose is identical to that recommended if rhinoplasty were performed without concomitant sinus surgery. The Aquaplast thermoplastic splint is generally removed about 1 week postoperatively, and Steri-Strips are replaced as necessary and left in place for up to 3 weeks in all. Triamcinolone acetonide 10 mg/mL is infiltrated beneath the skin–soft tissue envelope if persistent supratip edema appears likely to predispose to a pollybeak deformity.

RESULTS

We reviewed 186 consecutive patients who underwent FESS by one of us (FJS) in conjunction with septoplasty, rhinoplasty, and/or turbinate procedures. Twenty-eight of these patients also underwent cosmetic rhinoplasty. Follow-up ranged from 6 months to 2½ years. Surveys seeking information about perceived postoperative symptomatic results were sent to all 186 patients. Forty-nine patients responded, for an overall response rate of 26 percent. Ninety-six percent of all patients who responded were pleased that they had undergone sinus surgery and felt that it made a positive impact on their general health and well-being. A similar satisfaction rate was seen in that cohort of survey respondents who underwent simultaneous rhinoplasty and sinus surgery. Revision surgery was not required in any of the 28 rhinoplasty patients. No cerebrospinal fluid leak or orbital invasion occurred in patients with planned rhinoplasty procedures, and, as a result, no change was necessary in the procedures done on these patients.

One case of hemorrhage significant enough to require return to the operating room occurred. Bleeding was noted in the region of the sphenopalatine artery, which was probably transected after a very posterior resection of the middle turbinate. This was easily controlled with suction cautery and subsequent packing. We anticipate that this complication will become even less of a problem for us in the future because most middle turbinates are now being preserved. The experience of the other authors (AJM, DWS) in an additional 11 cases revealed no minor or major complications.

Two cases of simultaneous rhinoplasty and sinus surgery are now included to illustrate details of patient management and outcome.

CASE REPORTS

Case 1

A 56-year-old female presented with a history of chronic sinusitis and nasal obstruction. Despite prior aggressive medical treatment with long-term antibiotics, decongestants, and topical nasal steroid therapy, she continued to complain of frontal headaches, postnasal drip, and difficulty in breathing. In addition, she was also unhappy about the appearance of her nose and desired aesthetic improvement. Anterior nasal rhinoscopy demonstrated a deviated nasal septum

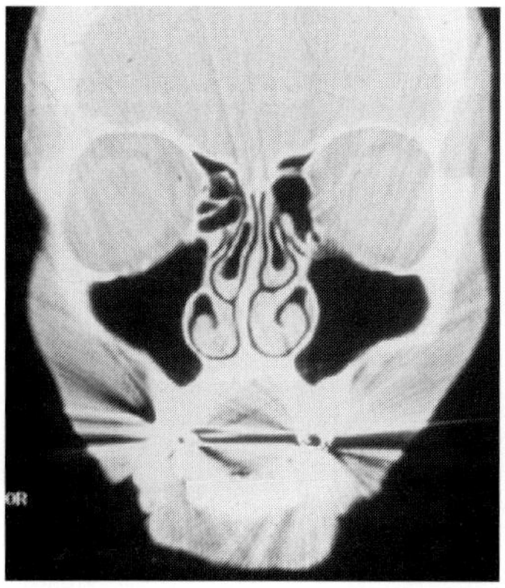

FIGURE 24–2. Case No 1. Preoperative coronal sinus CT scan of patient with minimal anterior ethmoidal disease in the area of the osteomeatal complex along with bilateral concha bullosa, deviated septum, and hypertrophic inferior turbinates.

that partially obstructed the right nasal cavity, enlarged inferior and middle turbinates, and inflammation of the sinus mucosa within the middle meatus bilaterally. External examination of the nose demonstrated a rather marked bony cartilaginous nasal hump and a wide bulbous tip. The patient was also made aware of her moderately recessed chin, which amplified her nasal deformity. A CT scan of the sinuses confirmed the presence of enlarged inferior turbinates and deviated septum. In addition, there was also evidence of mild ethmoiditis and bilateral concha bullosa with narrowing of each of the osteomeatal complexes (Fig. 24–2). Because of these radiographic findings, in conjunction with her history and physical examination and her desire for simultaneous aesthetic improvement, a combined functional endoscopic sinus procedure and aesthetic rhinoplasty was offered and subsequently performed. In addition, an intraoral chin implant was placed to help improve the harmony of the facial profile, KTP laser ablation was performed on the inferior turbinates, and sharp dissection to remove the middle turbinate was used, preserving the medial wall on each side. As depicted in the postoperative pictures, a much more widely patent nasal sinus cavity has been created along with a more pleasing nasal and facial contour

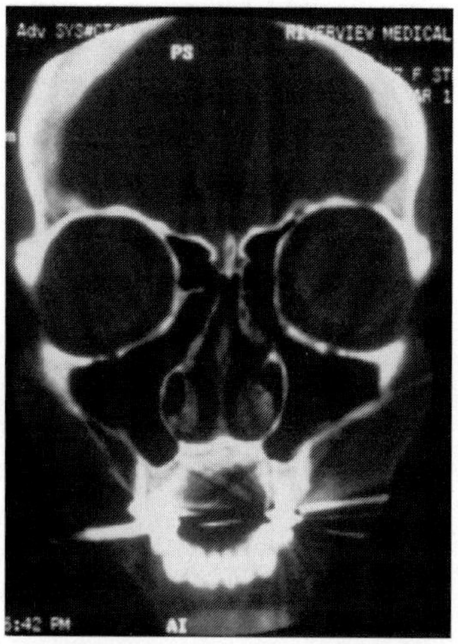

FIGURE 24–3. Case 1. CT scan 1½ years postoperatively of the patient shown in Figure 24–2 after endoscopic sinusotomies, resection of the concha bullosa, and KTP laser ablation of the inferior turbinates and septoplasty.

(Figs. 24–3 to 24–5). At 1½ years follow-up the patient has had total relief from headaches and postnasal drip and reports very significant improvement in nasal function. In addition, she was very satisfied with the appearance of her chin and nose.

Case 2

A 47-year-old female with a history of a prior reconstructive rhinoplasty 20 years earlier presented with chronic sinusitis and nasal obstruction. Maximal medical therapy with multiple antibiotics, decongestants, and steroids were tried over several years but produced little relief from headaches and nasal congestion. The patient was also not satisfied with the cosmetic result of her prior rhinoplasty. Intranasal examination demonstrated a deviated nasal septum to the left, swollen inferior turbinates, and a very inflamed sinus mucosa. External nasal examination demonstrated an irregular nasal dorsum with a mild pollybeak

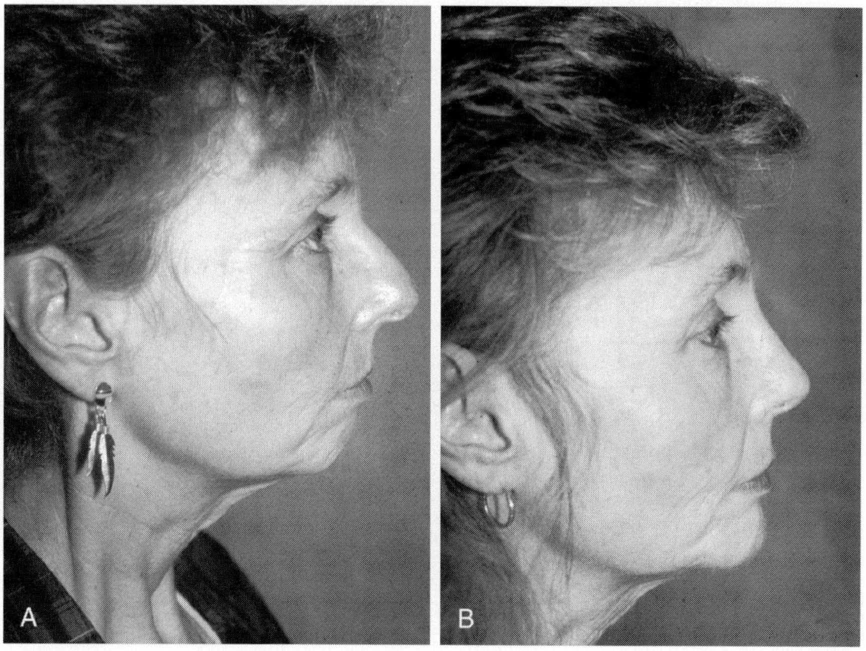

FIGURE 24–4. Case 1. Lateral preoperative *(A)* and postoperative *(B)* photographs of patient who underwent combined rhinoplasty and endoscopic sinus surgery.

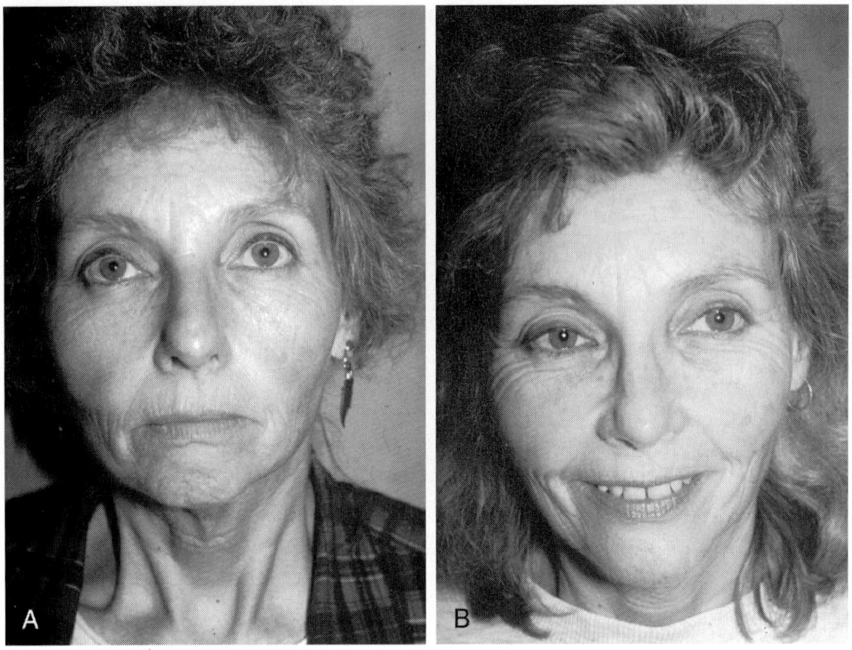

FIGURE 24–5. Case 1. Frontal photographs. Preoperative *(A)* and postoperative *(B)* views.

formation. The tip cartilages were also grossly asymmetrical with a right-sided bossa protuberance and bilateral alar pinching that probably resulted from overzealous cartilage resection in the past. The alar pinching was thought to contribute to the nasal obstruction, especially with deep inspiration. A CT scan demonstrated moderate mucoperiosteal thickening of the ethmoid, maxillary, and frontal sinuses with occlusion of the osteomeatal complexes (Fig. 24–6). Because of the patient's functional complaints and findings and aesthetic desires, a combined endoscopic sinus surgery procedure and open septorhinoplasty was performed. A complete anterior and posterior ethmoidectomy with maxillary antroscopy was done bilaterally. In addition, bilateral middle turbinectomies were performed to prevent postoperative lateralization. An external rhinoplasty approach was used because this was a revision case involving placement of multiple cartilaginous grafts to the tip from both auricles and the remaining septum.

As can be seen in the postoperative CT scan, the nasal and sinus cavities are now widely patent and free of sinus pathology (Fig. 24–7). In addition, the irregularities resulting from the prior rhinoplasty have been corrected (Figs. 24–8 and 24–9). The patient at 1-year follow-up has enjoyed almost total relief from her prior sinus symptoms and is very happy with the more natural appearance of her nose.

DISCUSSION

Although it is uncertain who was first to perform simultaneous rhinoplasty and endoscopic sinus surgery, Sheman and Matarasso[10] are credited with the first published reports of combining these two procedures. Despite an increasing number of patients who are candidates for simultaneous rhinoplasty and endoscopic sinus surgery, a paucity of information

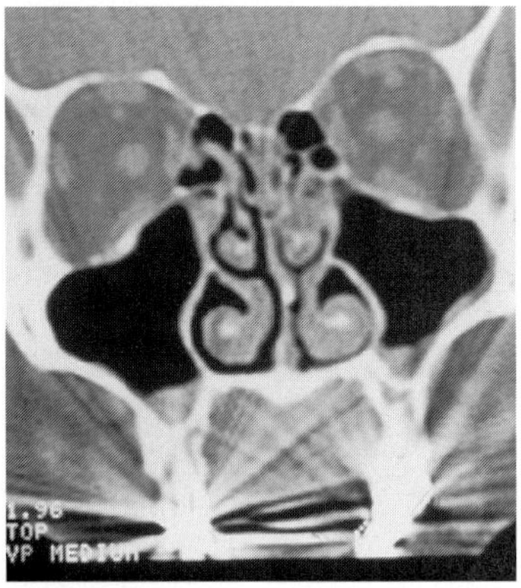

FIGURE 24–6. Case 2. Preoperative coronal sinus CT scan of patient with moderate sinus disease and enlarged turbinates.

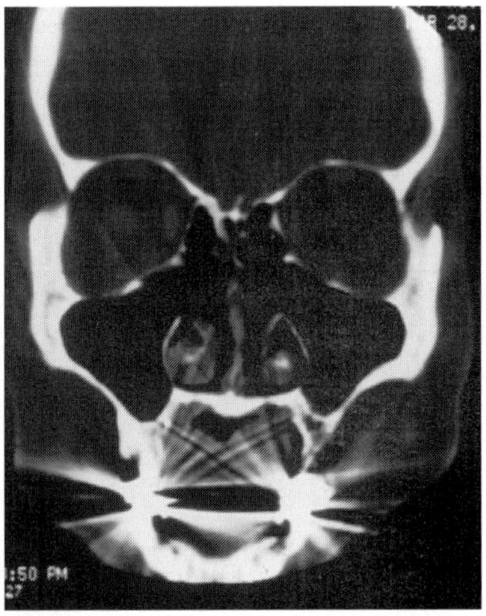

FIGURE 24–7. Case 2. CT scan 1 year postoperatively of same patient shown in Figure 24–6 after endoscopic sinusotomies, middle turbinate resection, and KTP laser ablation of the inferior turbinates.

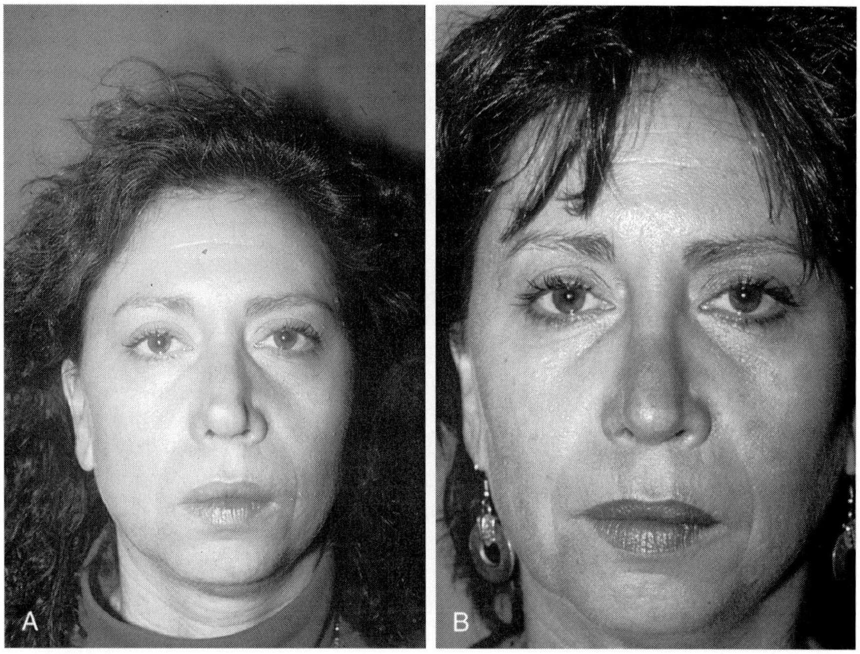

FIGURE 24–8. Case 2. Frontal photographs. Preoperative *(A)* and postoperative *(B)* views of patient undergoing combined rhinoplasty and sinus surgery.

on this topic appears in the literature. In fact, only three subsequent publications have provided information about this concept.[9,11,12]

Toffel, in the first large series reported in the literature, performed simultaneous rhinoplasty and FESS in 122 of 698 cases (19%).[11] He described the technique for each of the two procedures as well as the functional results of the 698 FESS procedures for those patients who were still being followed at 1 and 3 years. Three case reports illustrated the utility of performing these procedures together, but the advantages, disadvantages, and pitfalls of the technique were not addressed.

Glicklich and Lauretano considered the problem of whether it is safe to perform osteotomies, which are often necessary for a rhinoplasty, in the presence of endoscopic ethmoidectomies.[9] In a study using 14 fresh-frozen cadaver heads, extensive ethmoidectomies including marsupialization of the frontal recess and agger nasi areas were followed by medial and lateral osteotomies. There were no major comminutions along the osteotomies, nor did the fractures extend into either the orbit or base of the skull, suggesting that combining the procedures does not jeopardize patient safety. Additionally, the enlarged maxillary ostia created by the sinus surgery was not altered by the osteotomies or by

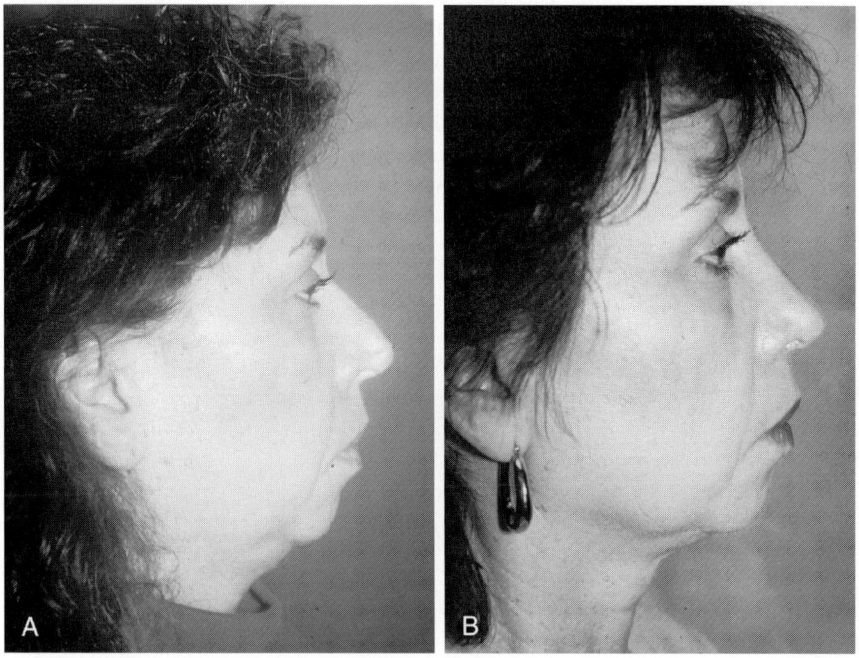

FIGURE 24–9. Case 2. Lateral photographs. Preoperative *(A)* and postoperative *(B)* views of patient who has undergone combined simultaneous rhinoplasty and sinus surgery.

dorsal narrowing. In each case a relatively thick buttress of bone composed of the anterior lacrimal crest and the ascending process of the maxilla separated the ethmoid surgical cavity from the line of osteotomy. The authors advise caution in patients who have undergone previous lacrimal surgery, in those with preexisting pathways into the orbit or skull base, and in those who are to undergo osteotomies by methods that do not preserve the triangular nasal buttress or double osteotomies. Furthermore, they suggest that CT scans should be considered in patients in whom a rhinoplasty is planned who have undergone previous sinus surgery to verify that an iatrogenic skull base or orbital dehiscence has not been created.

Further details about the safety of combining these two procedures are given in the most recent series published. Rizk and colleagues[12] had only one minor complication, postoperative hemorrhage, in a series of 40 patients. They, like us and other authors, recommend completing the endoscopic sinus surgery before beginning the rhinoplasty.

SUMMARY

In summary, the indications for performing these two procedures during the same surgical session are, in essence, the same as for the procedures individually: failure of medical management of sinus disease and the desire of the patient for aesthetic improvement of the nose. Absolute or relative contraindications include a variety of medical conditions (e.g., bleeding disorders, poorly controlled hypertension, diabetes mellitus, or an asthmatic patient with nasal polyposis), gross infection of the sinuses (especially when cartilage grafts or alloplasts are considered necessary for the rhinoplasty), and complications encountered during the endoscopic procedure (excessive bleeding, orbital penetration, or CSF leak). In a patient who may be considered a very poor surgical risk, sinus surgery should be avoided if at all possible. On the other hand, if FESS is absolutely necessary, the procedure can be done with appropriate anesthesia consultation, but the cosmetic portion of the procedure should be avoided. The advantages of performing concurrent surgery are significant and include one anesthetic episode, less total recovery time, and overall lower medical costs than if the two procedures were each performed separately. Disadvantages are minimal and include a potential inability to assess orbital complications from FESS (since osteotomies result in ecchymosis), increased nasal tenderness as a result of the rhinoplasty, possibly compromising the surgeon's ability to perform postoperative cleaning, and more swelling and discomfort than would be likely with either procedure alone. Perioperative and postoperative dexamethasone helps to reduce edema. Our experience and the literature reports support the premise that FESS combined with cosmetic rhinoplasty can be a safe procedure in selected patients and can lead to functional and cosmetic results that are satisfactory to patients and surgeons alike.

REFERENCES

1. Kennedy DW, Zinreich SJ, Rosenbaum AE, et al: Functional endoscopic sinus surgery: Theory and diagnostic evaluation. Arch Otolaryngol 11:576–582, 1985.
2. Maniglia AJ: Fatal and other major complications of endoscopic sinus surgery. Laryngoscope 101:349–354, 1991.
3. Stankiewicz JA: Complications of endoscopic sinus surgery. Otolaryngol Clin North Am 22(4):749–758, 1989.
4. Stankiewicz JA: Blindness and intranasal endoscopic ethmoidectomy prevention and management. Otolaryngol Head Neck Surg 101:320–329, 1989.
5. Neuman TR, Turner WJ, Davidson TM: Complications of endoscopic sinus surgery. Ear Nose Throat 73(8):585–590, 1994.
6. Adams PF, Benson V: Current estimates for the national health interview survey. Vital Health Statistics 10:76, 1990.
7. McCullough G. Personal communication, 1991.
8. Lazar RH, Eunice Y, Ounis RT, Gurucharri MJ: Endoscopic sinus surgery in children. *In* Levine HL, May M. (eds): Endoscopic Sinus Surgery. New York, Thieme, 1993, p 254.
9. Gliklich RE, Lauretano AM: The risks of nasal osteotomies after ethmoid sinus surgery. Arch Otolaryngol Head Neck Surg 121:1315–1318, 1995.
10. Sheman L, Matarasso A: Combined endoscopic sinus surgery and aesthetic rhinoplasty: A pilot study. Am J Rhinol 5:131–135, 1991.
11. Toffel PH: Simultaneous secure endoscopic sinus surgery and rhinoplasty. Ear Nose Throat 73(8):554–573, 1994.
12. Rizk SS, Edelstein DR, Matarasso A: Concurrent functional endoscopic sinus surgery and rhinoplasty. Ann Plast Surg 38(4):323–329, 1997.

CHAPTER 25

Alloplasts in Facial Reconstruction

Cherie-Ann Nathan, M.D.
William Pate, M.D.
Fred Stucker, M.D.

Significant advances have been made in our ability to reconstruct and augment both the soft tissues and the facial skeleton of the head and neck. Fallopius in 1600 was the first one to use a gold implant to repair a calvarial defect.[1] Since then significant technical improvements have been made, and a broad armamentarium of materials has been developed. The ideal implantable material should be inexpensive, easy to shape and use, produce excellent results, be 100% safe, produce no adverse host response, and bond well with the recipient for a lifetime. The biomaterials can be alive or preserved, autogenous or from an exogenous source, or they can be semisynthetic or totally synthetic. The space program and other specialized scientific projects have produced many new technical inventions and materials that have influenced and elevated the standard of medicine.

Patients have high expectations for the outcome of reconstructive surgery and expect little or no morbidity. They desire to be well informed about the procedure, the risks involved, and alternatives to the suggested procedure. They expect implants to last a lifetime and yield excellent functional and cosmetic results. One example of patients' high expectations is the class action suit against the use of silicone that was settled a few years ago. Solid silicone has been used in medicine for approximately three decades, and there is no scientific evidence that it results in systemic complications, but this did not alter or prevent an adverse action in one of the largest medicolegal and product safety lawsuits in history. These and other factors place tremendous pressure on medical personnel to seek ideal materials. It is doubtful that the "ideal" implant will ever be found, but surgeons must have an integrated understanding of the full range of implants that are available. Implant surgeons should understand the biology of these synthetic materials and realize that current law does not protect them from the failure of a device that has been approved by the Food and Drug Administration (FDA). In this chapter we focus on the use of alloplasts in facial reconstruction.

FACTORS AFFECTING THE SUCCESS OF ALLOPLASTS

When planning the reconstruction one should fully evaluate the three components of a successful outcome: the implantable material, the recipient, and the surgeon. All of these are essential and influence the outcome. Tissue injury during the implantation stimulates an inflammatory response. During the inflammatory cascade, the cellular response initiates a drive to debride or remove the material from the wound. The mildness or severity of the response, the retention or rejection of the implant, and whether it forms a granuloma or settles into a state of biologic tolerance determines the biocompatibility of the material.

The Materials of Choice

The facial defect that is to be corrected may require a soft tissue filler, skeletal support, or a combination of both. Many materials have been used in the past, but our clinical experiences support the use of expanded polytetrafluoroethylene, best known as Gore-Tex, as the first choice for a soft tissue polymer implant, and porous polyethylene as the optimum firm polymer for a facial implant. Both of these materials have been shown to cause little tissue reaction, have a low infection rate, are easy to use, stay in position well, and retain their size well. The surgeon must follow the manufacturer's suggestions for handling the implant.

The Recipient (Patient)

Careful consideration must be given to the general health of the recipient, including (but not limited to) nutritional status, medications taken, and immune status. Efforts must be made to correct any nutritional deficiency prior to surgery. Patients who have immune deficiencies, are undergoing chemotherapy, or have received radiation in the area to be reconstructed will be more susceptible to complications and thus to a poor outcome. Infection in the area of the defect must be cleared prior to elective implant surgery. The choice of implant material is determined by the site, size, and type of defect. The thickness of the soft tissue covering the implant markedly influences the body's acceptance of the implant.

The human body has a remarkable ability to repair itself but is conspicuously defensive of all foreign materials. Foreign bodies activate the defense mechanism, which attempts to absorb the foreign material. The surgeon depends on this defense to help secure nonabsorbable implanted material. This process may take a few days or several years. Occasionally the implanted material excites a hypersensitivity reaction that prompts its removal. Hypersensitivity reactions are unpredictable in most cases. They may occur in the early postoperative period or after a long latency period. Hypersensitivity reactions seldom occur with solid polymers.

The Surgeon

The surgeon plays the major role in the final outcome of the procedure. Preoperative evaluation, planning the procedure, knowledge of the implant material, site preparation, and technical skills are all critical factors. The evaluation period reveals the physical and mental status of the patient. Psychological observations should indicate the patient's motive for the reconstruction. It is most important to know the patient's understanding of the procedure and his or her expectations of the outcome. It is not always possible to learn this information, but it is important to try. Evaluation and planning for the procedure may include visual assessment, face masks, plain x-rays, two- and three-dimensional computed tomograms, and computer-controlled milling devices. A knowledge of implantable materials is essential if the surgeon is to select the proper material for the reconstruction. Preparation of the site requires creation of a sterile area for the implant. The surgeon must also have the skills necessary to make any required changes at the time of surgery to ensure a proper outcome.

Once the implantable material is selected and the preoperative evaluation has been completed, the size and shape of the implant are considered. The appropriate personnel should be contacted to ensure that the proper instruments and materials are available in the operating room. Some materials are factory sterile, but some must be sterilized in the operating room. No preoperative evaluation can provide an accurate final plan for the size and shape of the implant. Shaping and sizing in the operating room is required. Most surgeons have developed personal techniques that work for them in most cases.

IDEAL PROPERTIES OF THE IMPLANT

Some materials are less inert than others depending on the chemical composition, physical properties, and surface characteristics of the material. The bulk consistency (i.e., the particulate nature of the material), the presence of impurities, especially at the interface area, the carcinogenic side effects, and the presence of exposed side groups that result in antigenic stimulation are some of the other factors that are responsible for the body's immunogenic response to these materials.

Chemical Composition

The closer the chemical composition or valency of the material to natural elements such as carbon and calcium, the less immunogenic the response because these elements comprise the greatest (nonwater) part of the human body. Silicone, titanium, and hydroxyapatite[2, 3] demonstrate excellent chemical properties for an implant material.

Physical Properties

The two most important physical properties are porosity and particle size, since optimum biocompatibility depends on tissue growth into the pores of the material. Nonporous materials have less chance of being colonized by bacteria because bacteria cannot enter pores of less than 1 μm. On the other hand, macrophages cannot permeate pores less than 50 μm in size, nor can they phagocytize particles larger than 60 μm. Phagocyotsis by macrophages can cause the death of the macrophage, resulting in an intracellular response. Therefore, if an implant with pores of between 1 and 50 μm becomes contaminated with bacteria, phagocytic cells would not be able to clear the bacteria because macrophages are too large to pass through pores smaller than 50 μm. The risk of infection is lowest with pore sizes greater than 50 μm. Particles that resist digestion stimulate monocytes to differentiate into epithelioid cells with focal granuloma formation.[28] Pore sizes between 1 and 50 μm have a greater incidence of bacterial infection.[2] Therefore, pores larger than 50 μm are more likely to allow tissue ingrowth and are less likely to become a source of infection.

The particle size of the biomaterial is equally important, since macrophages cannot ingest particles larger than 60 μm. When larger particles are phagocytized they can cause the death of the macrophages with release of intracellular enzymes and a cascade of cytokines that can stimulate a chronic inflammatory response.[4, 5] Implants that tend to shed particles are at further risk for infection. This problem occurred with the use of Proplast for temporomandibular joint reconstruction, in which particles were produced that caused chronic inflammation.

A biomaterial under investigation known as Bioplastique appears to fit the criteria for particle size. It is composed of silicone particles, all larger than 100 μm, dispersed in a resorbable matrix.[5] It is an injectable viscous liquid, and the large particle size prevents the particles from being ingested by macrophages, thus decreasing the inflammatory response in animal models.

Surface Properties

The surface-tissue interface is the most important relationship in biocompatibility in vivo. The surface, unlike the bulk of the material, determines the host response. For example, with titanium a layer of titanium oxide is formed when titanium is exposed to air, and it is this layer that is important for osseointegration because it acts as a ceramic that promotes excellent biocompatibility.[6]

It is important to handle the biomaterial with care by opening the package just before it is used because surface contamination affects tissue biocompatibility adversely. Preparation of the surface of the implant, in addition to getting rid of contaminants, also increases the surface free energy, exposing ionic groups that then facilitate protein adsorption. This protein layer then stimulates the cellular response, the most important component of which is the fibroblast, which lays down immature collagen that in turn forms a dense capsule around the implant, holding it in place.

Host Factors

As mentioned earlier, the surgical insertion of the implant results in tissue injury. Hence, careful technique and the ability of the host to mount a response that results in biointegration rather than rejection is of equal importance to the composition of the biomaterial.

The host must be well nourished and have a competent immune system and good regional perfusion. Insertion should not be performed in the presence of an acute infection. Systemic conditions such as malnourishment, immunosuppressed conditions, and vascular diseases can all affect the fate of the implant.

In clean contaminated wounds such as the paranasal sinuses and the oral cavity, vascularized implants are preferred to synthetic implants. A few synthetic implants can be used in these wounds, but they must be selected and applied carefully. Implants approved by the FDA are currently used under sterile techniques.[7]

Proper surgical technique involves contouring the implant, selecting an appropriate site and size, and fixing the implant in place without allowing formation of a hematoma. Contouring involves removing all sharp or jagged edges. The pocket created should be sufficient to prevent migration of the implant while at the same time avoiding undue tension on the overlying skin. Excessive tension can cause thinning of the soft tissue overlying the implant, leading to exposure and infection. In addition, fixation of the implant is best done in tissue that has maximal acceptance of that particular implant; for example, titanium osseointegrated implants must be placed in bone that is healthy and of adequate physical strength to bear the load. Implants placed in highly mobile areas are prone to poor wound healing. The implant should be fixed to stable underlying structures.

Adequate soft tissue coverage is important to ensure long-term implantation. It is preferable to bury the implant under subcutaneous fat and muscle as well as skin and dermis. In some areas of the face, such as the nasal dorsum, where very little subcutaneous tissue is present, this is not possible. In such cases, choosing an implant that integrates with the tissue prevents extrusion of the implant. Porous and soft pliable material such as Gore-Tex is an optimum synthetic material for this site.

Systemic diseases or conditions such as diabetes, connective tissue diseases, previous irradiation, and previous surgery can all decrease the blood supply to the implant site. In these circumstances it is better to transfer vascularized tissue to the region before the procedure or at the time of implantation.

Meticulous hemostasis and adequate postoperative wound drainage are important measures to prevent infection of the implant. Fluid accumulation around the implant prevents tissue growth into the pores. It is best to use small closed suction drains for 24 to 48 hours following surgery. Open Penrose drains are best avoided.

ALLOPLASTIC MATERIALS

Polymeric Materials

Polymeric materials can be divided into noninjectable and injectable forms. The noninjectable forms can be either solid, porous, or woven (Table 25–1). In the present medicolegal climate it is important for the reconstructive surgeon to make an informed decision concerning the selection of a synthetic implant based on its chemical composition and application site. We will discuss the synthetic implant materials most commonly used and touch briefly on some of the newer, more promising ones. The composition, tissue response, clinical uses, advantages, and disadvantages of the commonly used alloplasts will be described.

Solid Polymers

Silicone

Silicone has the longest and most widespread use of all polymers.[8] Silicone implants have been used for malar and submalar augmentation, nasal dorsal and chin augmentation, and contouring of the frontal bone and temple area after ablative surgery. In addition, it has been used for soft tissue

TABLE 25–1. ALLOPLASTIC MATERIALS

TYPE OF MATERIAL	EXAMPLE	TRADE NAME
Polymers		
Solid	Silicone Polymethylmethacrylate	
Porous	High-density polyethylene	MedPor
	Polytetrafluoroethylene	Teflon Proplast Gore-Tex
Meshed	Polyester	Mersilene (polyester)
	Polyamide mesh	Supramid (polyamide)
Metals and alloys	Titanium and vitallium Stainless steel Gold	
Ceramics and inorganic implants	Ceramic hydroxyapatite Nonceramic hydroxyapatite	

expansion. Unfortunately, it came under significant scrutiny by the FDA when it was used for mammary augmentation, although there are no statistically significant data to show that the autoimmune problems seen in some of these patients were related to silicone.

Silicone is a polymer made up of covalent repetitive silicon-oxygen bonds with methyl side groups. The most commonly used form is the dimethylsiloxane form. The material's viscosity is determined by the extent of polymerization. With minimal cross-linking, it becomes a liquid (i.e., silicone gel), whereas additional cross-linking changes its physical composition to a more solid form as in Silastic (Dow Corning, Midland, MI). The solid form is used most commonly in facial reconstruction.

With silicone implantation a fibrous capsule forms around the implant. This can cause it to deform in the body. Dacron webbing has been embedded in some implants to prevent such distortion. Silicone gel has been less commonly used because it tends to incite a local inflammatory response, which occurs when the silicone particles are phagocytosed by macrophages.[9] More recently, Bioplastique, an investigational alloplast, seems to have the advantages of the histologic stability and nonreactivity of solid silicone along with the capability of being injected. It is composed of silicone particles greater than 100 μm in size and hence cannot be engulfed by macrophages. These particles are dispersed in a resorbable hydrogel matrix.[5]

Because the surface of most silicone implants is smooth, tissue adherence is decreased, and this may be an important cause of extrusion. Recently, the concept of texturing the implant's surface has been introduced to increase adherence. Occasionally, granulomas can form as a result of the inflammatory response. However, most such cases have been associated with the injection of nonmedical grade liquid silicone. When the implant is placed subperiosteally bone resorption can occur. Hence, it is preferable to place the implant above the periosteum.

Polymethylmethacrylate

Polymethylmethacrylate has not gained wide applicability in the head and neck because it causes an intense inflammatory response and has a potential for thermal injury, both of which result in a high extrusion rate. It is an acrylic polymer cement supplied in a powder form. When mixed with the catalyst it becomes malleable in 5 to 10 minutes and produces a strongly exothermic reaction of over 100°C. A foreign body reaction develops after implantation, and after this abates the implant becomes enveloped in a fibrous capsule. In the head and neck, although it is sometimes used in facial augmentation, it is most commonly used for reconstruction of cranial defects because it can be shaped and contoured intraoperatively.[10] This material works well in this area because of the immobility and relatively low stresses of this environment (Fig. 25–1). Allergic systemic reactions, hypotension, and cardiac arrest have been reported, primarily due to escape of the monomer during curing of this material.

Porous Polymers

High-Density Porous Polyethylene (HDPE [MedPor])

High-density porous polyethylene differs from polytetrafluoroethylene (PTFE) and polyethylene in that it lacks the fluorination of the ethylene monomer.[11] As a result, it is noncompressible and lacks the flexibility of the PTFE group. However, it can be carved with effort. It has regularly spaced pores of between 125 and 250 μm in size and hence allows the ingrowth of soft tissue and to a certain extent bone.[12] It is nonresorbable and causes a minimal foreign body response. It is most useful for chin and malar implants and is preferably inserted in a subperiosteal pocket fixed to the underlying bone.[13] Owing to its stiffness and relatively sharp edges, placement in areas with minimal soft tissue coverage results in a higher extrusion rate. However, specific implants do exist for this purpose. It can also be used for orbital reconstruction following enucleation.

Polytetrafluoroethylenes

Polytetrafluoroethylenes are made up of repeating units of carbon strongly bound to fluorine, which results in chemical and thermal stability. Fluorine is so chemically reactive that once it bonds to carbon atoms, it becomes nondegradable. The body has no enzyme system to break these bonds, and hence the material is biocompatible. The solid forms consist of Proplast and Gore-Tex, and Teflon is available in a paste form.

Teflon was used as a paste for vocal cord augmentation as early as the 1940s.[14] It has a tendency to migrate, especially in the face, where there is no anatomic limit to contain it as is present in the vocal cord. Hence, it has not been approved by the FDA for soft tissue augmentation in the face. Particles ranging in size from 20 to 60 μm are phagocytosed, resulting in macrophage death and chronic inflammation.

Proplast, (Vitek, Houston, TX) is an expanded polytetrafluoroethylene (EPTFE) combined with black vitreous car-

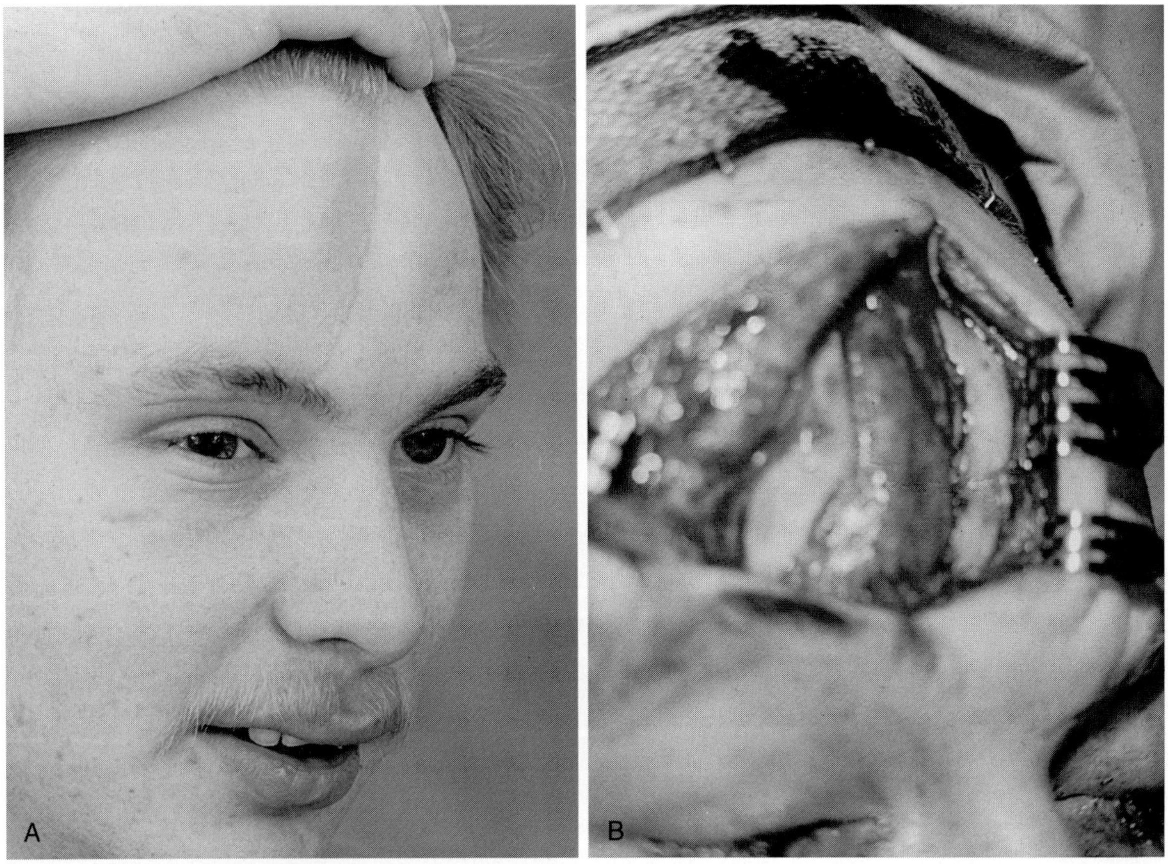

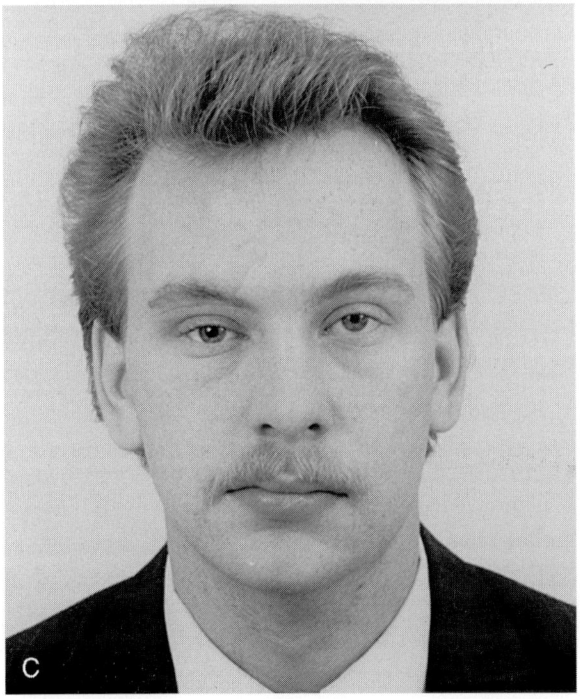

FIGURE 25–1. *A*, Nineteen-year-old patient 1 year after a motorcycle accident showing bony defect of forehead. *B*, Intraoperative view of bony defect showing exposed dura. *C*, Three years after repair of bony defect with methylmethacrylate.

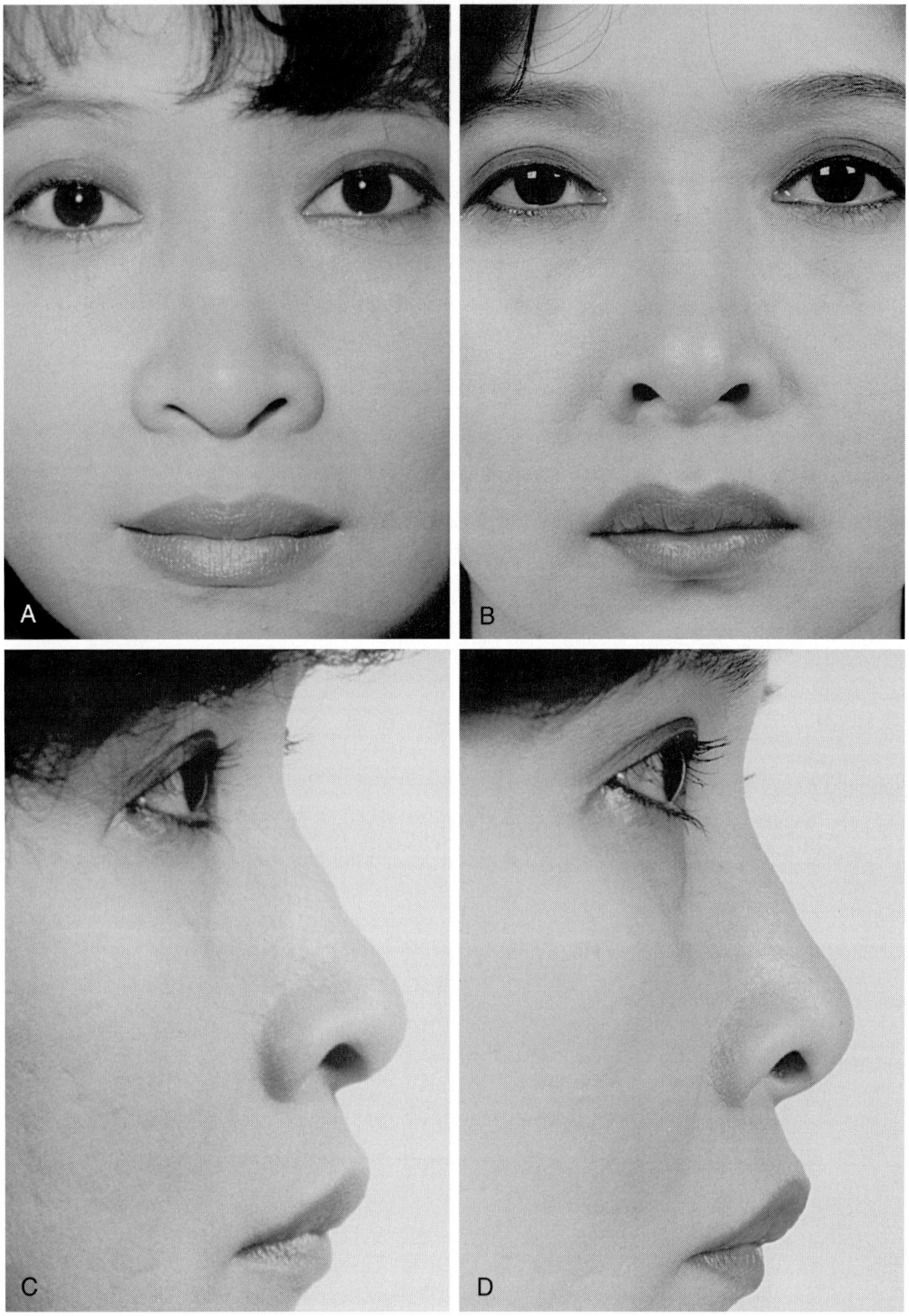

FIGURE 25–2. *A*, Full face view of patient 1 year after augmentation of nasal dorsum with Gore-Tex; note technical error in placement. *B*, One year postoperative view of brief procedure to position the graft. *C*, Right lateral view of patient with malpositoned Gore-Tex graft. *D*, Right lateral view 1 year following graft replacement.

bon fibers (Proplast I) or white aluminum oxide fibers (Proplast II). Proplast I is black and spongy because of its carbon content and hence is aesthetically unpleasing, especially in areas under thin skin. Thus, it has been replaced by Proplast II, which is whiter and harder. Proplast II is combined with hydroxyapatite, which retains the sponge-like consistency of Proplast I while allowing the implant to be fixed to the underlying bone. These implants are compressible sponges with pore sizes varying from 50 to 400 μm. Hence, fibrovascular ingrowth holds the implant in place without fibrous capsule formation.[15]

Proplast is a biologically inert material that causes minimal chronic inflammation. Unfortunately, its use in temporomandibular joint reconstruction resulted in shearing, which caused an intense reaction to the particles. This is a good material for onlay augmentation in nonstress-bearing areas, but because of its inappropriate use and the problems seen in these cases it has been removed from the market by the FDA.

Gore-Tex is the newer fibrillated form of expanded EPTFE that has an average pore size of between 10 and 30 μm.[11] Hence, it allows limited tissue ingrowth, gradually increasing stability without forming a capsule. It has excellent biocompatibility with minimal foreign body reaction, and hence the infection rate is quite low. It is available in 0.4-, 0.6-, 1-, 2-, and 4-mm sheets and in carvable form. It can be resterilized if not used. It is best not to use this material immediately below the dermis, especially in mobile areas such as the lips or nasolabial folds. It should be sutured with nonresorbable monofilament sutures because resorbable ones can result in inadequate anchoring. It can be easily cut and adapted because it is soft and pliable.

The FDA has approved the use of Gore-Tex for "soft tissue deformities." In the face it has been used for filling post-traumatic defects and for augmentation of the chin, malar area, and nasal dorsum. It is easier to work with in secondary procedures (Fig. 25–2). More recently, it has been used instead of fascia lata for reconstruction of static facial paralysis.[16]

Meshed Polymers

Of the meshed polymers, Supramid is composed of polyamide, while Mersilene is composed of polyethylene. Both are supplied in 30 by 30 cm mesh sheets and have similar uses. They stimulate an intense fibrous ingrowth and hence can be extremely difficult to remove should they become infected. They have been seen to resorb several years after implantation and hence are seldom used for facial augmentation.[17] However, the senior author has many patients who have enjoyed excellent long-term results with these polymers. Meshed polymers can be used successfully in nasal tip reconstruction if certain guidelines are followed[18] (Fig. 25–3). However, the mechanical properties of Gore-Tex in comparison to those of the skin and the unreported incidence of resorption with Gore-Tex make it a more optimal synthetic material for nasal tip reconstruction as recommended by Constantino and colleagues.[2]

Supramid

Supramid was the earliest form of polyamide mesh and is now available as Nylamid mesh (S. Jackson, Inc, Minneapolis, MI). It has been widely used in facial augmentation.[19, 20] Owing to the intense fibrous reaction it incites, it is very stable. However, it does tend to contract by approximately 15% to 25% during the first 1 to 2 years.

Mersilene

Mersilene is a nonabsorbable polyester composed of polyethylene terephthalate. It is more commonly used as a permanent suture material. Another name for it is Dacron (Dupont Chemical Corporation, Philadelphia, PA), which has had wide applications in vascular surgery. It has been used commonly for soft tissue augmentation of the chin and nasal tip. The knitted mesh material can be shaped to the desired form and implanted through a cutaneous incision (Fig. 25–4). Mersilene has a slightly higher rate of infection than Supramid but does not exhibit the slow resorption reported with the latter material (see Fig. 25–4)

Metals and Alloys

Metals and alloys are used more commonly for skeletal fixation rather than for soft tissue augmentation and hence are not discussed in detail in this chapter. Percutaneous osseointegrative implants are used to attach restorative facial soft tissue prostheses and are discussed briefly in the next paragraph. In addition, gold implants are used for reanimation of the paralyzed eyelid.[21, 22] The heavy atomic weight and minimal inflammation seen with this element make it ideal for this application.

Percutaneous Osseointegrative Implants

These implants provide a site of attachment for restorative facial prostheses (epitheses). The implant core is embedded in the patient's bone, and the facial prosthesis is then attached to the implant post that protrudes from the core. This method of bone-anchored epithesis has been used in Europe for many years.[23, 24] The bone implants are of two kinds: those that allow osseointegration and those that do not. The osseointegrative implants are the only ones that can be used to anchor the epithesis. The materials that can be used are cobalt-chromium alloys and titanium alloys. Titanium alloys are most commonly used.

Osseointegrative implants stimulate the growth of the underlying bone up to the implant without an intervening layer of fibrous tissue. The bone recognizes the implant as a biologically compatible material with elemental characteristics comparable to those of calcium phosphate.[25] The absence of fibrous tissue prevents loosening over time and decreases the rate of infection because bacteria from the external environment cannot track along the fibrous layer to cause infection. This system has resisted infection even in dental reconstruction, which is a good test of its potential clinical use.

Constantino and colleagues recommend the bone-an-

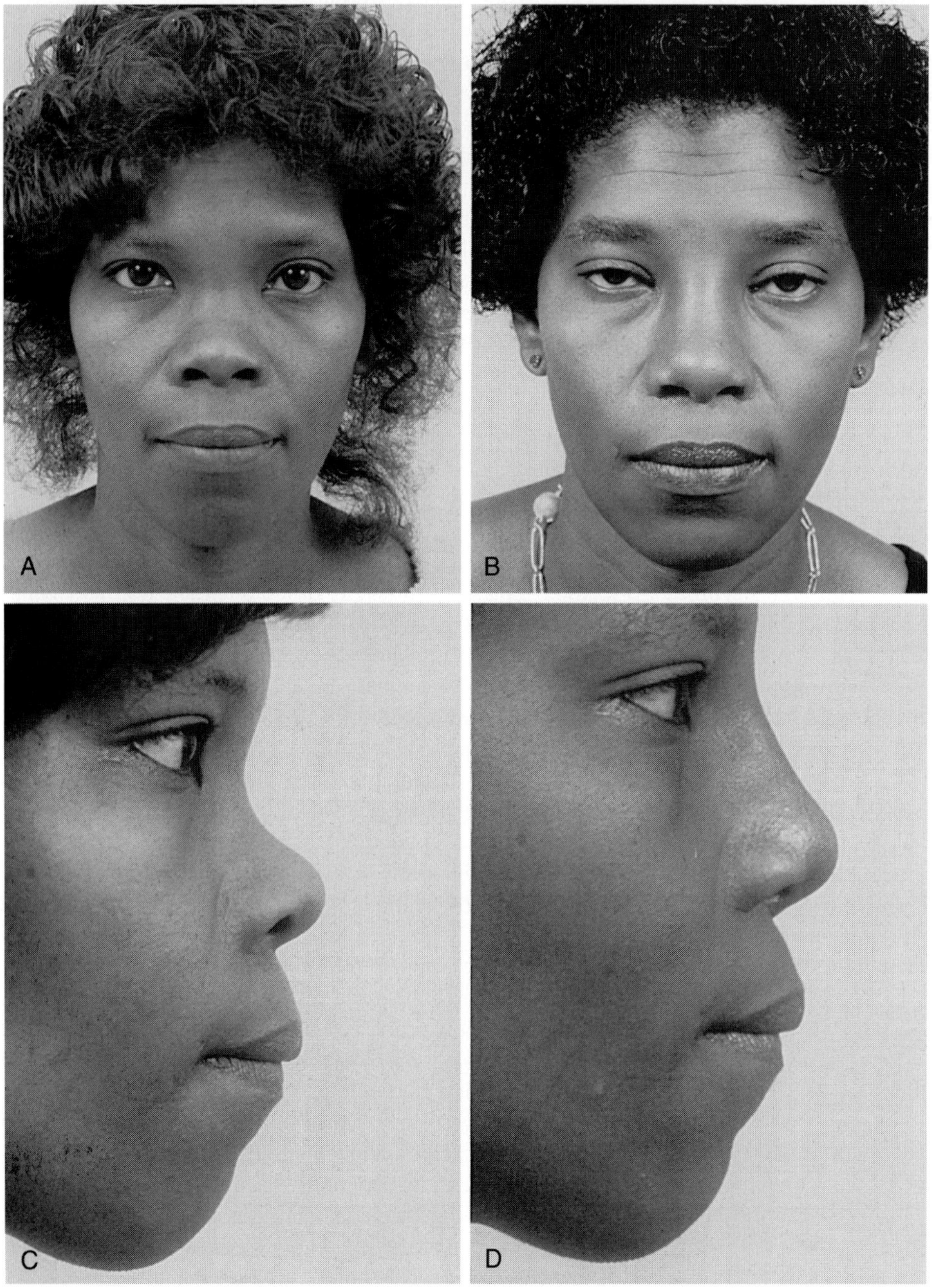

FIGURE 25–3. *A*, Full face preoperative view of 22-year-old patient. *B*, Eight-year postoperative view of augmentation rhinoplasty with polyamide mesh (Supramid). *C*, Right lateral preoperative view. *D*, Right lateral view 8 years after augmentation rhinoplasty.

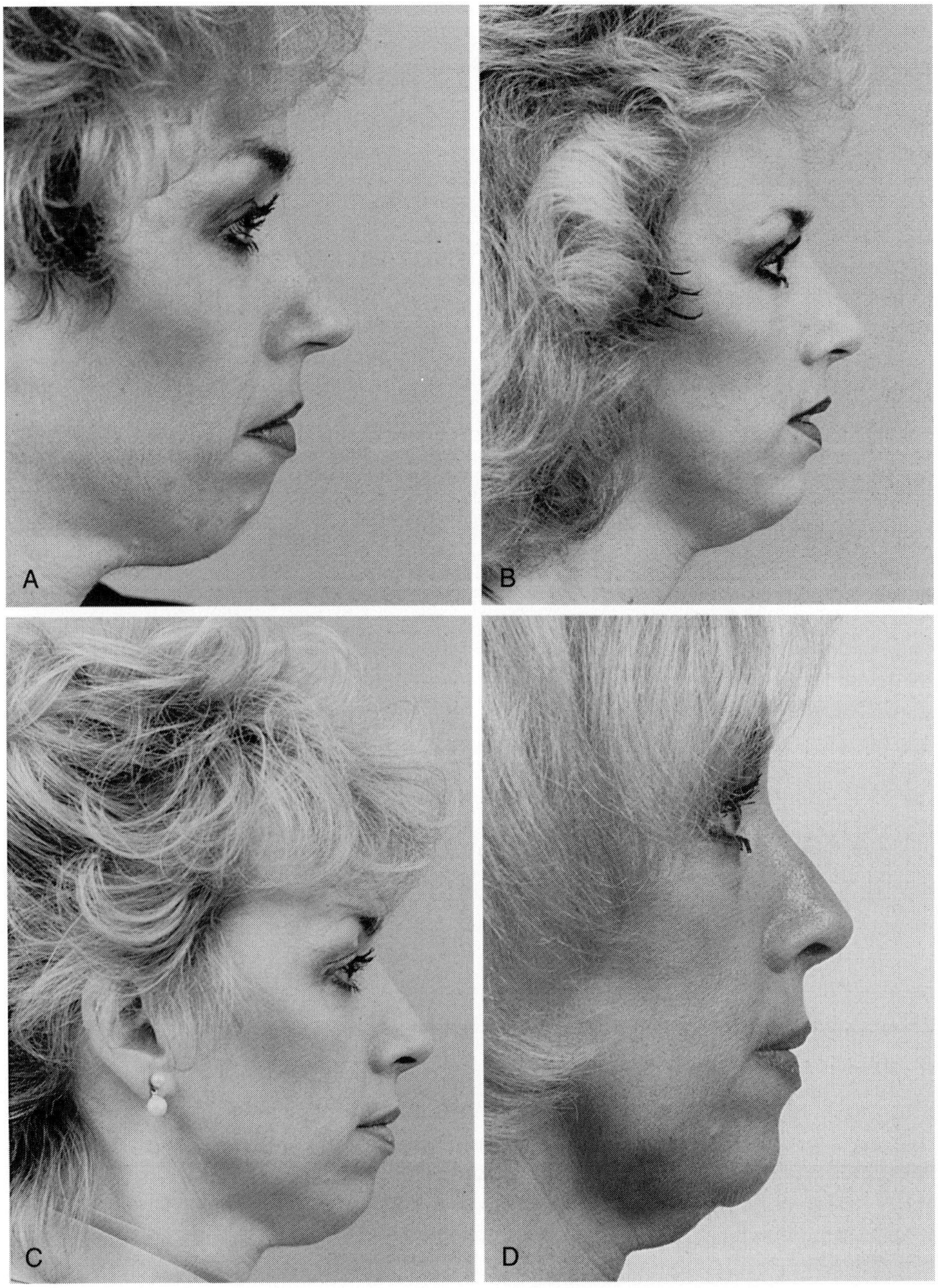

FIGURE 25–4. *A*, Right lateral preoperative view. *B*, Two years after chin augmentation with Supramid. *C*, Eight-year postoperative view; note resorption of implant. *D*, Two years after revision augmentation mentoplasty using Merseline mesh.

chored implant system as the optimal form of reconstruction following oncologic resection.[2] In the presence of postoperative radiation they recommend implant placement 3 to 4 months following radiation treatment.

Ceramics and Inorganic Implants

Ceramic and inorganic implants are also restricted to skeletal augmentation and reconstruction and thus are only briefly discussed here. Calcium phosphate ceramics have a high level of biocompatibility. They bond to viable adjacent bone and, depending on their porosity and structure, can serve as conductors of new bone formation, a process called *osseoconduction*. Its success is based on rigid fixation to the underlying viable bone; otherwise, fibrous encapsulation will result in failure of osseoconduction. The major disadvantage of calcium phosphate ceramics is their brittleness and tendency to fracture. Therefore, in facial reconstruction the material presents technical difficulties with sculpting and initial stabilization, both of which are essential for chemical bonding.[26]

There are two types of hydroxyapatite: ceramic and nonceramic. The primary soft tissue application of the ceramic hydroxyapatite has been in orbital rehabilitation following enucleation. The nonceramic cement form is not sintered to achieve structural stability. This too has been used to augment the soft tissue volume in correction of enophthalmos in patients with orbital floor trauma. It has also been used to correct frontotemporal defects following craniotomy.

GENERAL PRINCIPLES OF PREPARATION AND IMPLANTATION OF ALLOPLASTS

Perioperative intravenous administration of antibiotics is recommended while the patient is hospitalized. If placement is through a clean skin incision, a first-generation cephalosporin is adequate to prevent infection with *Staphyloccocus*. However, if an intraoral or intranasal incision is used, anaerobic coverage in the form of clindamycin is recommended. Postoperatively, 7 days of oral antibiotics are usually adequate. In the presence of an acute infection no implantion attempt should be made.

Soaking the implant in an antibiotic solution containing gentamicin, bacitracin, or clindamycin is appropriate.[27] For porous implants Constantino and colleagues recommend a vacuum-created method of replacing the air in the porous implants with the antibiotic solution, known as "loading" the implant with antibiotic.[2] Whether it actually lowers the rate of infection is not known, but this conclusion is extrapolated from information on polymer catheters used for percutaneous vascular access.

Intraoperatively, the "no touch" technique minimizes the risk of infection. The implant should be removed from the sterile package only after the recipient site has been prepared. Only clean instruments should be used to handle it, not surgical gloves. During insertion of the implant touching the skin can cause contamination by skin flora and should be avoided.

Soft tissue coverage, fixation, and the recipient bed are important factors during implantation and fixation. Soft tissue coverage should be adequate to prevent thinning of the skin overlying the prosthesis and eventual extrusion. This is especially true for stiff, noncompressible implants such as those made of MedPor, for which, in addition to skin and dermis, adipose tissue or muscle coverage should be used. For flexible implants such as Gore-Tex implants, skin and dermis should provide adequate coverage. The biomaterial should be matched to the tissue plane within which it will be implanted.

The implant should be fixed to the most stable underlying structure to decrease mobility and prevent extrusion. The use of implants in highly mobile areas is not recommended.[29] Porous implants require an extended period of immobilization (about 6 weeks) to allow fibrovascular tissue to grow into the pores.[30, 31] In areas of previous surgery with excessive scar tissue the transfer of vascularized tissue prior to implantation is recommended.

The major indications for orbital repair are enophthalmos and/or diplopia secondary to trauma to the orbit. Direct trauma to the globe may produce increased intraorbital pressure. For example, in a direct blow to the orbit the resulting pressure will produce a fracture in the weakest part of the bony orbit, which is most often the floor and less commonly the medial wall. These fractures are usually referred to as "blowout fractures" and may allow the orbital contents to protrude into the maxillary sinus. The rectus (inferior and/or medial) may be trapped in the fracture site, restricting the movement of the globe. A fracture to the medial wall of the orbit seldom requires surgery, but a fracture of the floor frequently requires surgical repair.

EVALUATION AND PREPARATION OF THE DEFECT FOR AUGMENTATION

Orbital Defects

A decision is usually made to repair the defect with an implant. Many materials have been used with good results. Absorbable materials produce a greater inflammatory reaction in the early postoperative period. They are soft and provide little support for the orbital contents. Smooth materials such as silicone may become dislocated and migrate, requiring removal. Metal plates can be secured at the time of surgery with a small metal screw, and the mesh material allows invagination of reparative tissue, which produces natural stabilization. Metal plates have been reported to have a 4.4% infection rate, and biodegradable implants have had an overall infection rate of 8.3%.[32] The overall infection rate is 2.1%. Porous polyethylene, available in sheets of 0.85 and 1.5 mm in thickness, allows rapid soft tissue integration and has a very low infection rate. Because the orbital floor is concave and most implant material is flat, porous polyethylene is sized and placed in some hot water or saline to allow concave contouring. The material is soaked in an antibiotic solution prior to placing it in the orbit. Proper contouring and fitting are essential. If the material is placed too far posterior, the orbital nerve may be damaged. More than one layer of the implant material may be used if necessary to correct enophthalmos. The material may be secured with a metal screw or suture if this is deemed necessary.

Midface Fractures

Delayed reduction of tripod fractures and other midface fractures may result in an asymmetrical appearance of the face. Reconstruction of the original fixation may be considered, but often repair is best attained with an implant. Preoperative assessment depends on the experience of the surgeon and requires a combination of visual assessment, plain x-ray films, and two- and three-dimensional computed tomographic scans. A computer-assisted custom implant usually fits the bony bed well, but it is time-consuming and expensive to make and does not remove the difficulty of determining the necessary thickness of the implant in the presence of the overlying soft tissue and skin. It is best to undercorrect in the presence of enophthalmos because cheek augmentation can accentuate this deformity.

Solid silicone is an excellent implant material but has a high complication rate in most facial sites other than chin implants. Silicone implants are hard and smooth and therefore difficult to stabilize in the cheek area where the skin and soft tissue covering is thin. The force of gravity, motion of the overlying soft tissue, and the likelihood of external trauma make it a poor choice for malar augmentation. Porous polyethylene is easier to shape and mold to the implant site and allows rapid soft tissue integration to stabilize the implant. The material comes in sterile packages from the manufacturer. It becomes more supple when it is heated in hot saline, making it easier to shape and size. This is an ideal implant for cosmetic malar augmentation. The malar eminence is exposed. The desired implant is selected by the surgeon and the material fitted to the defect. If the implant is not preformed, it is sized and shaped on the back table. After the implant has been sized and molded, it is rinsed to remove all debris and then soaked in an antibiotic solution. The implant is then fitted to the bony tissue and is secured with metal screws if necessary. Gore-Tex can be used to augment soft tissue, but it is hydrophobic, and soaking it in an antibiotic solution is of debatable benefit; nevertheless, we routinely soak our Gore-Tex implants and have experienced no difficulties. The wound is then closed.

Nasal Reconstruction

Nasal reconstruction following trauma, ablative surgery, and destructive diseases can be a challenge. The nose is located in the middle of the face and is a focal point of attention in the daily interaction between people. Its major function—to clean and condition inspired air—is overshadowed in the thoughts of most people by its appearance. This mandates reconstruction to produce as near normal an anatomic appearance as possible. Similar defects in other areas would likely go unnoticed. Many manufactured materials have been used in the past to assist in nasal reconstruction but have failed for various reasons. However, some of the newer materials have shown great promise. Expanded polytetrafluoroethylene and porous polyethylene appear to be the most promising. These materials may be used separately or together to repair soft tissue defects and supply skeletal support. Manufacturers have provided numerous sizes and shapes of porous polyethylene that can be molded and trimmed to provide the necessary skeletal support in the operating room, and the expanded polytetrafluoroethylene material can be sized to fill soft tissue defects at the time of use. When these materials are used, they should be well covered by the natural soft tissue and a full-thickness skin layer. This can be done with local flaps if necessary.

Paranasal Sinuses

The paranasal sinuses are exposed to the external atmosphere through the nose, and care must be taken in selecting an implant because these implants are hard to separate from a potential source of contamination and infection. Some potential contamination can be avoided by obliteration of the sinus. Natural materials, metal implants, and other materials are used. Porous polyethylene appears to be an ideal material for these reconstructions but has not been approved by the FDA for this use.

COMPLICATIONS OF FACIAL IMPLANTATION OF ALLOPLASTS

Space age technology has assumed a dominant role in medicine in this century, and patients often develop unrealistic expectations from surgery. The plethora of new technologies and materials has placed tremendous strains on the medical profession to stay current and knowledgeable. Most products are developed for nonmedical reasons and are not subjected to medical conditions. Consumer demand for materials often arises before essential clinical testing periods have been completed. The ideal implant material should be biologically inert, excite no inflammatory reaction, and be permanently accepted by the body; it should also be inexpensive, easily fashioned, produce no adverse effects, and show excellent results. No material meets all these requirements at the present time.

Various materials have been used successfully during this century, and the use of others is increasing almost daily. However, society's demand for immediate and perfect outcomes is inconsistent with its fear of foreign materials. This fear has been highlighted by the class action lawsuit concerning breast implants. Patients with good results and no problems sometimes become frightened by news reports about foreign materials in their bodies and demand that they be removed. These factors have increased the pressure on the development and use of implants.

Universal questions about implantable materials include the following:

- Will it induce cancer?
- Will it produce systemic disease?
- Will a hypersensitivity reaction occur?

Will It Produce Cancer?

An implantable material is expected to remain in the body for the lifetime of the patient. The possibility that an implant may cause cancer is a major concern for the medical community. Many materials have been used during the past three decades. Orthopedic and vascular surgeons are pioneers in implantation. It was estimated that 88,000[33] hips had been replaced by 1975, and it is difficult to estimate the millions of people who have metallic hip implants today. The medical literature reports only 20 cases of cancer associated with metallic implants, with a latency period of 1 to 30 years. One of these cancers was in the head and neck area. It was a squamous cell carcinoma of the gingival and anterior floor of the mouth that was associated with a gold mandible staple plate.[34] The other 19 cases were sarcomas. Clinical reports support the hypothesis that the risk of cancer associated with implanted metallic devices is extremely low. Gillespie and colleagues found a significant increase in the risk of lymphatic and hematopoietic tumors in 1358 patients after total hip replacement. However, the majority of hip replacement patients have arthritis, which may be related to the increased cancer rate.[35]

No cases of cancer have been reported in association with a polymer implant in the face or cranium There are a few case reports of sarcoma associated with Dacron[36–38] vascular prostheses. Two long-term reports, which included more than 14,000 women with breast augmentations with polymer implants, showed no increased risk of cancer.[39, 40]

Will It Produce Systemic Disease?

Metal implants can corrode and in some case dissolve when exposed to air and/or body fluids. Ions are released that leach into the surrounding tissue.[41] These ions accumulate in adjacent areas and in the regional lymph nodes,[42] where they can elicit a local fibroblastic tissue reaction.[43, 44] Postmortem studies on patients with stainless steel and cobalt-chromium long-bone implants reveal elevated levels of the metals in the liver, bone marrow, and distal lymph nodes.[44] Industrial exposure to titanium has shown a necrotizing reaction.[45, 46] No systemic disease has been directly associated with these implants.

Freshly mixed methylmethacrylate releases a free monomer that can produce vasodilatation.[47] Cardiovascular collapse with death has been reported in patients undergoing hip replacement surgery at the time of hip prosthesis insertion. The operating suite must be well ventilated when methylmethacrylate is mixed to prevent the possibility of cardiovascular depression resulting from the release of the free monomer.

Will It Produce a Hypersensitivity Reaction?

Hypersensitivity reactions characterized by pain, nonunion of bone, and local dermatitis have been reported with nickel and stainless steel[48–51] and have been suspected for titanium. Skin tests frequently confirm the sensitivity, and the reaction resolves following removal of the implant. Asthmatic reactions have been reported in operating room personnel exposed to the free monomer of methylmethacrylate.[52] A well-ventilated operating room should eliminate this type of exposure.

Summary of Universal Questions

Clinical experience over several decades of use of implantable materials indicates that there is little chance of cancer, systemic illness, or hypersensitivity reaction to the implants that are in general use in today.

Specific Complications

It is difficult to discern whether individual complications following the use of implants in facial reconstruction are solely the fault of the material, the recipient, or the surgeon. Complications include but are not necessarily limited to the following: infection, fistulas, prominence (i.e., exposure and extrusion), inflammatory reaction, hardware loosening, or patient satisfaction. There is much overlap between the implant material, the recipient, and the skill of the surgeon when discussing complications in implantation surgery.

Infection and Fistulas

Infections are greatly influenced by the site of the defect and the immune response of the recipient. The health of the tissue in the area of the deformity and its blood supply influence the healing of the wound and the acceptance of the implant. Patients who have immune deficiencies, postradiation changes, or are receiving chemotherapy have a much higher incidence of infection. This is especially evident in the oral cavity. It is critical that the reconstruction site be as clean and healthy as practical prior to the procedure. The use of preoperative antibiotics is suggested, especially for implants in high-risk areas. Fistula formation is usually the result of inflammation, usually secondary to an infection.

Often the implanted material must be removed to clear the infection and enable the wound to heal.

Exposure and Extrusion

Exposure and extrusion occur more often in areas with tenuous soft tissue coverage. The mentum, with its abundant soft tissue coverage, is less vulnerable to exposure and extrusion of an implant than are the nose and periorbital area. These implants are easier to palpate because of the scant soft tissue covering them. When the implant is exposed, it is usually prudent to remove it.

Displacement of the Implant

The surface texture and location of the implant and the method of fixation influence the possibility of displacement. Materials that have a smooth surface, like solid silicone, are more likely to be displaced because there is no tissue fixation to help secure them. A site of trauma and tissue mobility places more stress on the fixation of an implant and leads to a greater likelihood of displacement. An example of this is the stability of a silicone implant augmenting the chin compared with an identical implant placed in the periorbital area. The size, molding, and fixation of the implant unquestionably influence its stability. Implants that do not fit well into the recipient site, are too large, are not properly secured, or have a tenuous soft tissue cover have a greater tendency toward displacement.

Implant Fracture

A fractured implant can result from using a material with too little strength to withstand the forces expected to confront it. The mandible encounters far more stress than the forehead, for example, and requires an implant material that is much stronger. The implant material may be improper for the defect, or it may not be properly shaped to fit the defect. The implant may also have been cracked by excessive force used to fixate it during implantation.

Loosening of the Hardware

An implant can be loosened when the tissue to which it is anchored is inadequate. An inadequate implant material or unexpected trauma is sometimes responsible for loosening. The implant may not have been adequately fixed at the time of surgery.

Seroma, Pain, and Inflammatory Reaction

The immune response of the body may produce a seroma secondary to a foreign body reaction. A delayed reaction to the breakdown products of the implant can incite a reaction. A noninfectious inflammatory reaction is more common with absorbable than with nonabsorbable materials. The reaction may occur several years following the time of implant. Pain can be secondary to a cellular mediated reaction, infection, implantation in proximity to a nerve, and occasionally it is a functional response from the patient. The implant may have to be removed in these cases.

Complications of Technique

The following complications and/or poor outcomes are closely related to surgical technique: hematoma, nerve injury, overcorrection, improper sizing of the implant, and improper placement. These complications are usually self-evident. It is very difficult to determine the exact number of successful or unsuccessful outcomes of a specific implant because most physicians do not report or keep records of successes or complications. Even if such records were available it is impossible to determine accurately all the factors involved in the outcome.

SUMMARY

The passage of centuries has added to our knowledge of the art and science of medicine, but the practice of medicine is far from an art or a science. We cannot separate the two. The sophisticated technical world has added invaluable scientific knowledge, but the practitioner must integrate this knowledge with the management of the individual patient. This is what motivates most physicians to accept the long period of training and the lifetime commitment of continuing education. Complications are part of all medical procedures and are a major concern to each and every physician. The international medical community has had several decades of experience with implants, and millions of lives are better as a result. The medical literature supports the safety of many materials for implantation.

REFERENCES

1. Fallopius G: Opera omnia Francofurti. Wecheli A (ed). 1600, p. 1.
2. Constantino PD, Friedman CD, Lane AG: Synthetic biomaterials in facial plastic and reconstructive surgery. Facial Plast Surg 9:1–15, 1993.
3. Morehead JM, Holt GR: Soft-tissue response to synthetic biomaterials. Otolaryngol Clin North Am 27:1:195–201, 1994.
4. Coleman DL, King RN, Andrade JD: The foreign body reaction: A chronic inflammatory response. J Biomed Mater Res 8:199–211, 1974.
5. Ersek RA, Beisang AA: Bioplastique: A new textured copolymer microparticle promises permanence in soft tissue augmentation. Plast Reconstr Surg 87:693–702, 1991.
6. Holt GR: Physical characteristics and biocompatibility of implant materials. *In* Glasgold AI, Silver FH (eds): Applications of Biomaterials in Facial Plastic Surgery. Boca Raton, FL, CRC Press, 1991, pp. 87–97.
7. Merritt K, Shafer JW, Brown SA: Implant site infection rates with porous and dense materials. J Biomed Mater Res 13:101–108, 1979.
8. Brown BL, Neel HB III, Kern EB: Implants of Supramid, Proplast, Plasti-Pore, and Silastic. Arch Otolaryngol Head Neck Surg 105:605–609, 1979.

9. Coleman DL, King RN, Andrade JD: The foreign body reaction: A chronic inflammatory response. J Biomed Mater Res 8:199–211, 1974.
10. Schultz RC: Reconstruction of facial deformities using silicones and acrylics. *In* Glasgol AI, Silver FH (eds) Biomaterials in Reconstructive Surgery. St. Louis, CV Mosby, 1983.
11. Williams D (ed): Concise Encyclopedia of Medical and Dental Materials. Oxford, Pergamon Press, 1990.
12. Maas CS, Merwin GE, Wilson J, et al: Comparison of bimaterials for facial bone augmentation. Arch Otolaryngol Head Neck Surg 116:551, 1990.
13. Rubin LR: Polyethylene as a bone and cartilage substitute: 32-year retrospective. *In* Rubin LR (ed): Biomaterials in Reconstructive Surgery. St. Louis, CV Mosby, 1982, pp. 474–482.
14. LaVern HG, Baberio JR: Tissue reaction to plastics used in surgery with special reference to Teflon. Ann Surg 129:74, 1979.
15. Spector M, Harmon SL, Kreutner A: Characteristics of tissue growth into Proplast and porous polyethylene implants in bone. J Biomed Mater Res 13:677–692, 1979.
16. Konior RJ: Facial paralysis reconstruction with Gore-Tex soft-tissue patch. Arch Otolaryngol Head Neck Surg 118:1188–1194, 1992.
17. Beekhuis GJ: Augmentation mentoplasty with polyamide mesh: Update. Arch Otolaryngol Head Neck Surg 110:364, 1984.
18. Fanous N: Mersilene tip implants in rhinoplasty: A review of 98 cases. Plast Reconstr Surg 87:662–673, 1991.
19. Stucker FJ, Hirokawa RH, Bryarly RC: Technical aspects of facial contouring using polyamide mesh. Otolaryngol Clin North Am 15:123, 1982.
20. Beekhuis GJ: Augmentation mentoplasty using polyamide mesh. Arch Otolaryngol Head Neck Surg 106:642, 1980.
21. Kartush JM, Linstrom CJ, McCann PM, et al: Early gold weight eyelid implantation for facial paralysis. Otolaryngol Head Neck Surg 103:1016, 1990.
22. May M: Gold weight and wire spring implants as alternatives to tarsorrhaphy. Arch Otolaryngol Head Neck Surg, 113:656, 1987.
23. Tjellstrom A, Lindstrom J, Nylen O, et al: The bone-anchored auricular epithesis. Laryngoscope 91:811–815, 1981.
24. Tjellstrom A, Yontachev E, Lindstrom J, Branemark PI: Five years experience with bone-anchored auricular prosthesis. Otolaryngol Head Neck Surg 93:366–374, 1985.
25. Linder L, Albrektsson T, Branemark P, et al: Electron microscopic analysis of the bone-titanium interface. Acta Orthop 54:45–52, 1983.
26. Merwin GE, Rogers LW, Wilson J, et al: Facial bone augmentation using Bioglass in dogs. Arch Otolaryngol Head Neck Surg 112:280, 1986.
27. Fairbanks DNF: Antimicrobial Therapy in Otolaryngology–Head and Neck Surgery, 2nd ed. Alexandria, VA, American Academy of Otolaryngology–Head and Neck Surgery Foundation, 1993.
28. Robbins SL, Cotran RS, Kumar V (eds): Pathologic Basis of Disease, 3rd ed. Philadelphia, WB Saunders, 1984, pp. 64–65.
29. Walen RL: Connective tissue response to movement at the prosthesis/tissue interface. *In* Szycher M (ed): Biocompatible Polymers, Metals, and Composites. Lancaster, PA, Technomick, 1983.
30. Merritt K, Shafer JW, Brown SA: Implant site infection rates with porous and dense materials. J Biomed Mater Res 13:101–108, 1979.
31. Saur BW, Weinstein AM, Klawitter JJ, et al: The role of porous polymeric materials in prosthesis attachment. J Biomed Mater Res Symp 5 (part 1):145–153, 1974.
32. Rubin JP, Yaremchuk MJ: Complications and toxicities of implantable biomaterials used in facial reconstructive and aesthetic surgery: A comprehensive review of the literature. Plast Reconstr Surg 100:1343, 1997.
33. Hori R, Lewis J. Zimmerman J, et al: The number of total joint replacements in the United States. Clin Orthop 132:46, 1978.
34. Freidman KE, Vernon SE: Squamous cell carcinoma developing in conjunction with a mandibular staple bone plate. J Oral Maxillofac Surg 41:265, 1983.
35. Gillespie W, Frampton C, Henderson R, et al: The incidence of cancer following total hip replacement. J Bone Joint Surg [Br] 70:539, 1988.
36. Weiss WM, Riles TS, Gouge TH, et al: Angiosarcoma at the site of a Dacron vascular prosthesis: A case report and literature review. J Vasc Surg 14:87, 1991.
37. Weinberg D, Maini B: Primary sarcoma of the aorta associated with a vascular prosthesis: A case report. Cancer 46:398, 1980.
38. Harrmann J, Kanhouwa S, Kelley R, Burns W: Fibrosarcoma of the thigh associated with a prosthetic vascular graft. N Engl J Med 284:91, 1971.
39. Deapen DM, Pike MC, Casagrande JT, Brody GS: The relationship between breast cancer and augmentation mammoplasty: An epidemiologic study. Plast Reconstr Surg 77:361, 1986.
40. Bryant H, Brasher P: Breast implants and breast cancer—reanalysis of a linkage study. N Engl J Med 332:1535, 1995.
41. Schliephake H, Lehmann H, Kunz U: Ultrastructural findings in soft tissues adjacent to titanium plates used in jaw fracture treatment. Int J Oral Maxillofac Surg 22:185, 1993.
42. Onodera K, Ooya KSD, Harding AF, et al: Titanium lymph node pigmentation in the reconstruction plate system of a mandibular bone defect. Oral Surg Oral Med Oral Pathol 75:495, 1993.
43. Thomas KA, Cook SD, Harding AF, et al: Tissue reaction to implant corrosion in 38 internal fixation devices. Orthopaedics 11:441, 1988.
44. Byrne JE, Lovasko JH, Laskin DM: Corrosion of metal fracture fixation appliances. J Oral Surg 31:639, 1973.
45. Case CP, Langkamer VG, James C, et al: Widespread dissemination of metal debris from implants. J Bone Joint Surg [Br] 76:701, 1994.
46. Moran C, Mullick F, Ishak K, et al: Identification of titanium I human tissues: Probable role in pathologic processes. Hum Pathol 22:450, 1991.
47. Peebles D, Ellis R, Stride S, et al: Cardiovascular effects of methylmethacrylate cement. Br Med J 1:349, 1972.
48. Barranco V, Solomon H: Eczematous dermatitis from nickel. JAMA 220:1244, 1972.
49. Barranco V, Solomon H: Eczematous dermatitis caused by internal exposure to nickel. South Med J 66:447, 1973.
50. Guyuron B, Lasa CI Jr: Reaction to stainless steel wire following orthognathic surgery. Plast Reconstr Surg 89:540, 1992.
51. Halpin DS: An unusual reaction in muscle in association with a vitallium plate: A report of possible metal hypersensitivity. J Bone Joint Surg [Br] 57:451, 1975.
52. Pickering CAC, Bainbridge D, Bithwistle IH, et al: Occupational asthma due to methylmethacrylate in an orthopaedic theatre sister. Br Med J 292:1362, 1986.

INDEX

Note: Page numbers in *italics* refer to illustrations; page numbers followed by t refer to tables.

90038

9 780721 669939